Nursing Research

Methods, Critical Appraisal, and Utilization

Nursing Research
Methods, Critical Appraisal, and Utilization

GERI LoBIONDO-WOOD, Ph.D., R.N.

Associate Professor
University of Texas
Houston Health Science Center
School of Nursing
Houston, Texas

JUDITH HABER, Ph.D., R.N., C.S., F.A.A.N.

Private Practice
Stamford, Connecticut

THIRD EDITION
With **34** *illustrations*

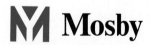 **Mosby**

St. Louis Baltimore Boston Chicago London Madrid Philadelphia Sydney Toronto

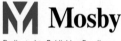

Dedicated to Publishing Excellence

Publisher: Alison Miller
Executive Editor: Darlene Como
Senior Developmental Editor: Laurie Sparks
Project Manager: Patricia Tannian
Senior Production Editor: Betty Hazelwood
Senior Book Designer: Gail Morey Hudson
Manufacturing Supervisor: Karen Lewis

THIRD EDITION
Copyright © 1994 by Mosby–Year Book, Inc.

Previous editions copyrighted 1986, 1990

Printed in the United States of America

Composition by Clarinda Company
Printing/binding by R.R. Donnelley & Sons Company

Mosby–Year Book, Inc.
11830 Westline Industrial Drive
St. Louis, Missouri 63146

Library of Congress Cataloging in Publication Data

Nursing research : methods, critical appraisal, and utililization /
  [edited by] Geri LoBiondo-Wood, Judith Haber. -- 3rd ed.
     p. cm.
   Includes bibliographical references and index.
   ISBN 0-8016-7727-0
   1. Nursing--Research. I. LoBiondo-Wood, Geri. II. Haber,
Judith.
   [DNLM: 1. Nursing Research. WY 20.5 N97445 1994]
  RT81.5.N873 1993
  610.73'072--dc20
  DNLM/DLC
  for Library of Congress   93-32240
                                    CIP

93 94 95 96 97 / 9 8 7 6 5 4 3 2 1

Contributors

Mara M. Baun, D.N.Sc., R.N., F.A.A.N.

Associate Dean for Research
Professor
University of Nebraska Medical Center
College of Nursing
Omaha, Nebraska

Ann Bello, M.A., R.N.

Professor of Nursing
Norwalk Community College
Norwalk, Connecticut

Betty Craft, M.P.N., R.N.

Assistant Professor
University of Nebraska Medical Center
College of Nursing
Omaha, Nebraska

Linda Cronenwett, Ph.D., R.N., F.A.A.N.

Director, Nursing Research and Education
Dartmouth-Hitchcock Medical Center
Lebanon, New Hampshire

Harriet R. Feldman, Ph.D., R.N.

Dean and Professor
Lienhard School of Nursing
Pace University
Pleasantville, New York

Margaret Grey, Dr.Ph., R.N., F.A.A.N.

Independence Foundation Professor of Nursing
Associate Dean for Research and Doctoral Studies
Yale University School of Nursing
New Haven, Connecticut
Formerly, Associate Professor and Director of Primary Care Graduate Program
University of Pennsylvania
School of Nursing
Philadelphia, Pennsylvania

Judith Haber, Ph.D., R.N., C.S., F.A.A.N.

Private Practice
Stamford, Connecticut

Judith A. Heermann, Ph.D., R.N.

Assistant Professor
University of Nebraska Medical Center
College of Nursing
Omaha, Nebraska

Bettie S. Jackson, Ed.D., M.B.A., R.N., F.A.A.N.

Director of Professional Nursing Services
Moses Division
Montefiore Medical Center
Bronx, New York

Patricia R. Liehr, Ph.D., R.N.

Associate Professor
University of Texas Health Science Center-Houston
School of Nursing
Houston, Texas

Geri LoBiondo-Wood, Ph.D., R.N.

Associate Professor
University of Texas Health Science Center-Houston
School of Nursing
Houston, Texas

Marianne Taft Marcus, Ed.D., R.N.

Associate Professor and Chairperson, Nursing Systems and Technology
University of Texas Health Science Center-Houston
School of Nursing
Houston, Texas

Barbara Krainovich Miller, Ed.D., R.N.

Consultant
Garden City, New York

Georgia K. Millor, D.N.S., R.N.

Adjunct Associate Professor
St. John Fisher College
Department of Nursing
Rochester, New York

Carol Ann Mitchell, Ed.D., R.N.

Professor and Chair
Department of Adult Health Nursing
East Tennessee State University
College of Nursing
Johnson City, Tennessee

Cheryl B. Stetler, Ph.D., R.N., F.A.A.N.

Director of Clinical Practice
Project Director
Patient-Centered Redesign Program
Hartford Hospital
Hartford, Connecticut

Helen J. Streubert, Ed.D., R.N.

Associate Professor and Director, Nursing Programs
College Misericordia
Dallas, Pennsylvania

To our families
Pat and Brian and Lenny, Laurie, and Andrew

Foreword

Nurses today are challenged to make quick yet critical and informed decisions about a variety of patient problems occurring within the context of a complex and rapidly changing health care system. Research activity designed to provide new knowledge to inform practice continues to escalate, producing a multitude of conflicting findings that bombard the nurse daily. Thus being a nurse in the 90s requires a far broader repertoire of knowledge, skill, and critical thinking ability than ever before to sort through and apply the best of the research findings to meet the challenges of contemporary health care.

Recognizing these requirements, the authors in this new edition have taken a number of steps to prepare their readers to, as they state in Chapter 1, "make accurate assessments based on research data and protocols in 'tailoring' care for each individual patient" now and into the twenty-first century. To this end, in their typical user-friendly manner, the authors have incorporated into each chapter a wealth of examples focused on the utilization of research in clinical practice, criteria for critiquing the particular aspect of the research process being discussed, and a thorough discussion of issues and future directions.

While retaining the quality content contained in the earlier editions, the authors also have added new content areas, such as research utilization, and expanded others, such as qualitative approaches to research.

Specifically, in the first chapter, the authors do an excellent job of thoroughly and cogently discussing the significance of research to the practice of nursing, emphasizing the importance of nurses as consumers of research. In Chapter 3, the authors present an excellent discussion of research utilization models, strategies, and criteria to determine the applicability of findings in various practice environments and with different patient groups—important content not generally included in a research textbook. Another excellent addition in Chapter 4 is the foundational discussion of strategies for developing critical thinking, reading, and critiquing skills in regard to research, which is then elaborated on in subsequent chapters as each component of the research process is presented in detail. The content on qualitative approaches to research, Chapter 11, has been expanded to provide specific information regarding types of qualitative research, significant issues, especially in regard to ethics, criteria for judging scientific rigor, computer software to assist in data management, and strategies for combining qualitative and quantitative approaches. Then, in Chapter 20, important considerations for evaluating the qualitative research report are specifically discussed and exemplified. Finally, the part opening vignettes by accomplished nurse researchers bring to life the integral nature of nursing practice, education, and research.

Thus once again the authors have combined their unique ability to present difficult yet essential research content in a user-friendly manner with their expert knowledge of research and nursing to prepare a text that will serve their readers well now and into the twenty-first century.

Carolyn F. Waltz, Ph.D., R.N., F.A.A.N.
Professor and Director
Office of Planning and Accountability
School of Nursing
University of Maryland at Baltimore

Preface

The foundation of the third edition of this textbook continues to be the belief that nursing research is integral to all levels of nursing education and practice. At times research still is perceived as a complex process carried out in an ivory tower by expert nurse-scientists and having little or no relevance to the everyday practice of nursing. This dichotomous view of nursing research is changing. Today, more and more nurses are actively involved in doing and using research that shapes nursing care delivery and documents the quality and cost-effectiveness of nursing care. As nurses continue to develop a unique body of nursing knowledge through research, decisions about nursing practice will be increasingly research based.

As editors we believe that all nurses need not only to understand the research process, but to know how to critically read, evaluate, and apply research findings. Though we know that understanding research is a challenge to every student, we believe that the quest for research knowledge can be accomplished in a stimulating, lively, and enlightening manner. However, the kind of knowledge appropriate to different levels of education varies. The research role of the baccalaureate graduate calls for the skills of critical appraisal—that is, the nurse should be a knowledgeable research consumer. Preparing students for this role involves developing their understanding of the research process, their appreciation of the role of the critiquer, and their ability to apply the critical appraisal process to research reports. An undergraduate course in nursing research should teach students how to understand, appraise, and apply research findings. The development of a basic level of competence in this area is essential for full integration of research into clinical practice. This is in contrast to the focus of a graduate level research course in which the emphasis is on carrying out research, as well as understanding it.

The primary audience of this textbook remains undergraduate students who are learning the steps of the research process, learning how to critique published research literature, and learning when and how to apply research findings in clinical practice. This book is also a valuable resource for students at the master's and doctoral levels who want a concise review of the basic steps of the research and critiquing processes. Furthermore, it is a relevant resource for practicing nurses who collaborate with nurse-scientists in the conduct of clinical research or seek to use research findings as the basis for clinical decision making and development of policies, protocols, and procedures rather than tradition, authority, or trial and error. Its use of critiqued published research studies facilitates an understanding of how research can be used in clinical practice.

The third edition of *Nursing Research: Methods, Critical Appraisal, and Utilization* prepares nursing students and practicing nurses to become knowledgeable nursing research consumers by:

- Addressing the role of the nurse as a research consumer with the goal of increasing the value of this role.
- Demystifying research, which is sometimes viewed as a complex process.
- Teaching the fundamentals of the research process and critical appraisal process in a logical, systematic progression that is user-friendly. This approach promotes a lively spirit of inquiry and encourages critical thinking and judgment that will promote enthusiasm on the part of students and nurses about expanding their research knowledge base.
- Elevating the critiquing process to a position of importance comparable to that of producing research. Before becoming research producers, students need to be knowledgeable research consumers. The goal is the stimulation of thoughtful practice that is both creative and innovative through the use of nursing research.
- Developing critical thinking and critical reading skills that facilitate mastery of the critiquing process.
- Emphasizing the role of research utilization as the basis for clinical decision making and theory-based nursing practice that demonstrates quality and cost-effective outcomes of nursing care delivery.
- Showcasing vignettes by renowned nurse researchers whose careers exemplify the link between research, education, and practice.
- Presenting numerous examples from recently published research studies that illustrate and highlight each research concept in a manner that brings abstract ideas to life for students new to the research and critiquing process. The examples are a critical link for reinforcement of the research and critiquing processes.
- Providing pedagogical chapter features including learning objectives, key terms, numerous tables, figures, and boxes, critiquing criteria, and key points at the end of each chapter.

The text is organized into three parts. Part I focuses on roles, approaches, and issues in nursing research. This part of the text provides an overview of the nurse's role as a research consumer. It introduces the sources of human knowledge, characteristics of the scientific approach, and research utilization principles related to the application of research findings in clinical practice.

Part II focuses on the integration of the research and critiquing processes. Chapter 4, which speaks directly to students in the second person, provides an overview of Part II that highlights critical thinking and critical reading concepts and strategies that facilitate student understanding of the research process and its relationship to the critiquing process. The style and content of this chapter is designed to make subsequent chapters more user-friendly for the reader. Chapters 5 through

18 delineate each step of the research process, with clinical research studies used to illustrate each step. The interrelatedness of the steps is examined in relation to the total research process. Both qualitative and quantitative designs are presented. Critical thinking is stimulated by presentation of the potential strengths and weaknesses in each step of the research process. Each chapter includes a section describing the critiquing process related to the focus of that chapter, as well as lists of Critiquing Criteria that are designed to stimulate a systematic and evaluative approach to reading research literature.

Part III focuses on critique and application. In this section the whole process of critical thinking, critical reading, and critiquing is synthesized. Chapters 19 and 20 provide summaries of quantitative and qualitative Critiquing Criteria. These criteria are used to evaluate several recently published quantitative and qualitative research articles, including their applicability to nursing practice.

The accompanying Instructor's Resource Manual and Test Bank, written by Harriet Feldman and Rona Levin, complement the textbook and provide chapter-by-chapter cooperative learning activities and strategies that promote the development of critical thinking and critical reading skills and the competencies necessary for developing informed consumers of nursing research. The study guide, written by Kathy Rose-Grippa and Mary Jo Gorney-Lucero, including a new computer-assisted instruction component for student review and reinforcement, is a new cutting-edge, self-paced teaching/learning strategy designed to enhance student learning outcomes.

The development of a scientific foundation for clinical nursing practice remains an essential priority for future nursing research. The third edition of *Nursing Research: Methods, Critical Appraisal, and Utilization* will help students develop a basic level of competence in understanding the steps of the research process that will enable them to critically analyze research studies, judge their merit, and judiciously apply the findings in clinical practice. To the extent that this goal is accomplished, nursing will have a cadre of clinicians who derive their practice from theory and research specific to nursing.

ACKNOWLEDGMENTS

No major undertaking is accomplished alone. There are those who contribute directly and those who contribute indirectly to the success of a project. We acknowledge with our warmest thanks the help and support of the following people:

- Our students, particularly the nursing students at the University of Texas-Houston Health Science Center School of Nursing, the College of Mount Saint Vincent Department of Nursing, and the University of Nebraska College of Nursing, whose interest and lively curiosity sparked ideas for revisions in the third edition.
- Our chapter contributors, whose expertise, cooperation, and punctuality made them a joy to have as colleagues.
- Our vignette contributors, whose willingness to share evidence of their research wisdom makes a unique contribution to this project.

- Our colleagues, who have taken time out of their busy professional lives to offer feedback and constructive criticism that has assisted us in preparing the third edition.
- Our editors Darlene Como and Laurie Sparks, for their willingness to listen to yet another creative idea about teaching research in a meaningful way and for their help with manuscript production and last minute details.
- Our production editor Betty Hazelwood for her assistance with the editing and last minute details.
- Out typist Betty Vinci, whose painstaking care with our sometimes disorderly manuscripts made the editorial process much smoother.
- Our families, Pat and Brian Wood and Lenny, Laurie, and Andrew Haber, for their unending love, faith, understanding, and support throughout what is inevitably a consuming but exciting experience.

Geri LoBiondo-Wood
Judith Haber

Contents

Glossary, 500

Appendix

PART

I

NURSING RESEARCH
ROLES, APPROACHES, AND ISSUES

Using Research to Improve Patient Care

CHERYL B. STETLER

Once a month for the past few years, I have been meeting with small groups of clinical nurse specialists (CNSs) to explore the process of using research in their practice. This activity has not been a part of my current position; nor has it been a formal expectation of the CNSs. We come together simply and purely because of our interest in and fascination with research utilization. One of the clinical nurse specialists calls it her "monthly facial for the mind." What we do is have the CNSs take turns in presenting research on a topic critical to their daily practice, and then as a group we do the following:

- Systematically review it for its applicability, using the revised Stetler/Marram model
- Help the clinician make a decision whether to use the information; consider use and thus collect more practical information; delay use until there is more scientific information; or reject use
- Review what this discussion has revealed for each of us about the process of research utilization and thus continually improve our own ability to use research effectively

A perinatal clinical nurse specialist decided to present the following study to review with the group. She chose it because it was obviously relevant to her practice, and she soon thereafter was engaged in an excellent example of the value of using research to solve clinical problems:

> Fetal death is obviously a terrible tragedy; but despite existent biophysical tests that can reduce this event, "recent reviews of fetal death indicate that nearly half occur in pregnancies that are not candidates for traditional antepartum testing" (p. 1075). In the past, protocols have thus been developed to use the pregnant woman's perception of fetal movement as a general means of widespread screening; however, they were often reported as problematic for one reason or another, such as low patient compliance. These authors devised a daily movement protocol designed to overcome previously reported problems with such maternal self-screening. They conducted a prospective evaluation, using a control period to collect baseline data; a pilot phase to refine the movement protocol; and a study phase to test the intervention. The results indicated high patient compliance with the procedure and a statistically significant drop in fetal deaths per 1000 births from 8.7 in the control group to 2.1 in the study group. There was also an increase in costly antepartum testing.
>
> Moore, T. & Piacquadio, K. (1989). A prospective evaluation of fetal movement screening to reduce the incidence of antepartum fetal death. *American Journal of Obstetrics & Gynecology, 160*, 1075-1080.

The perinatal clinical nurse specialist had a healthy adolescent who was pregnant with her first child. The CNS had, as usual, instructed the patient to generally watch that the baby moved but found that the young woman was noncompliant (i.e., during her prenatal visits, she indicated no knowledge of her baby's movements). During the "research utilization" session where the study was reviewed, the CNS had decided to consider use of the findings. When she encountered this patient's lack of compliance with *general* movement instructions, the CNS decided to try out and monitor the testing screening protocol. The pregnant teen obviously paid attention to these more specific and yet convenient instructions, because 4 days later she appropriately returned to report a decrease in fetal movement. She was found to have a nonreactive nonstress test (NST) result and a low biophysical score. Labor was therefore induced, and she delivered a healthy baby. The CNS is convinced that without use of this research-based protocol and the patient's corresponding compliance, there would have been another fetal death.

Working with the CNSs on research utilization has been both stimulating and fun. For me it gets at the essence of nursing, which is critical thinking rather than performing a rote set of tasks. More important, however, what application of research does is improve patient care by providing additional alternatives for problem solving, changing ineffective behavior; substantiating the scientific basis of one's current practice, and modifying a way of thinking—one's attitude or appreciation of an issue. By learning about not only the conduct of research, but also ways to *use* the outcomes of research safely and effectively, a nurse can truly engage in professional practice.

CHAPTER

1

The Role of Research in Nursing

GERI LoBIONDO-WOOD
JUDITH HABER

LEARNING OBJECTIVES

After reading this chapter the student should be able to do the following:

- State the significance of research to the practice of nursing.
- Identify the role of the consumer of nursing research.
- Discuss the differences in trends within nursing research before and after 1950.
- Describe how research, education, and practice relate to each other.
- Evaluate the nurse's role in the research process as it relates to the nurse's level of educational preparation.
- Identify the future trends in nursing research.
- Formulate the priorities for nursing research for moving into the twenty-first century.

KEY TERMS

applied research   critique
basic research   research
consumer   research utilization theory

As you begin to read the first chapter of this book you may be wondering, Why on earth is a research course part of my nursing curriculum? You may be asking yourself what research has to do with nursing. You may also wonder how nursing research will help you practice nursing in a better way or how it will help your patients. In answer to such questions, the research course you are taking has everything to do with the practice of professional nursing. As you develop the ability to appraise research studies knowledgeably, your critical thinking skills will become sharper. This, in turn, will help you fine tune your clinical judgment and decision-making skills; the ultimate beneficiary will be your patients! As you may have guessed, many nurses do share the belief that a knowledge of and involvement in nursing research can have a significant effect on the depth and breadth of the professional practice of every nurse. The purpose of this chapter is to help you begin to develop an appreciation of the significance of research in nursing and the research roles of nurses through a historical and futuristic approach.

SIGNIFICANCE OF RESEARCH IN NURSING

The health care environment is changing at an unprecedented pace. Pender (1992) states that "to thrive nursing as a profession must not only keep up with the pace but set the pace for the future of health care" (p. 200). Nurses are challenged to expand their "comfort zone" by offering creative approaches to old and new health problems, designing new and innovative programs that truly make a difference in the health status of our American citizens. This challenge can best be met by integrating rapidly expanding knowledge about behavioral and environmental influences on health into nursing practice. Nursing research provides a specialized scientific knowledge base that empowers the nursing profession to anticipate and meet these constantly shifting challenges and maintain our societal relevancy.

Nationally and internationally the nursing profession has devoted great effort to developing a unique, specialized body of knowledge used in the delivery of health care to patients. Indeed, having a specialized body of knowledge that is scientifically based is one of the hallmarks of a profession and is essential for fostering a sense of commitment and accountability to patients.

The current body of scientific knowledge that is unique to nursing can best be expanded through further research endeavors. But this expansion of knowledge has little meaning for the profession as a whole if it remains located only in research journals or in the minds of researchers. It must be part of a nurse's active repertoire of knowledge and must be put to use by those directly engaged in practice.

You can think of **research utilization** as the actual systematic implementation of a scientifically sound, research-based innovation in a health care setting with an accompanying process to assess the outcome(s) of change (Buckwalter, 1992). Through research utilization efforts, knowledge obtained from research is transformed into clinical practice, culminating in nursing practice that is research based. For example, to help you understand the importance of research utilization, think about the study by Stewart Fahs and Kenney (1991), who sought to determine whether there would be any differences in occurrence or size of bruising when heparin was administered in sites other than the traditional abdominal site and whether administration in other sites would affect the goals of heparin therapy as measured by the activated partial thromboplastin time (aPTT). The findings of their study demonstrated no significant differences in either occurrence or size of bruising or changes in aPTT in relation to differing sites. These findings provided nurses with outcome data that supported scientifically based clinical decision making rather than adherence to tradition. Although the data from this research study have definite potential for utilization in practice, changes in hospital policy will not and should not occur as a result of one study. Replication of this study is necessary to build an adequate knowledge base for implementation in practice, one that has been systematically evaluated over time.

Today more than ever before, nurses *are* required to be accountable for the quality of patient care they deliver. In an era of consumerism that is questioning the quality of health care and skyrocketing health care costs and demanding health care reform, patients are asking health professionals to document the effectiveness of their services. Essentially they are asking, "How do nursing services make a difference?" Reimbursement groups, including insurance companies, managed care organizations, and governmental agencies using prospective payment systems (PPSs) such as Medicare and Medicaid, are also requiring accountability for services provided.

Practice-oriented scientific investigations are but one type of research that can contribute significantly to validating the effectiveness of particular nursing interventions and to improving the quality of patient care. The findings of such studies provide a theory base for decision making about the delivery of nursing care. The nursing profession will be increasingly responsible for preparing *some* of its practitioners to be sophisticated producers of research and *all* of its practitioners to be knowledgeable consumers of scientific literature. Thus the new knowledge being generated can be evaluated and utilized in nursing practice in a meaningful way.

The Commission on Nursing Research of the American Nurses Association (ANA) (1989) has recognized the need for research skills at all levels of professional nursing. The Cabinet proposes that all nurses share a commitment to the advancement of nursing science through the conduct of research and utilization of research findings in practice. Scientific investigation promotes accountability, one of the hallmarks of a profession and a fundamental concept of the ANA Code of Conduct. There is a general consensus that the research role of the baccalaureate graduate calls for the skills of critical appraisal. That is, the nurse must be a knowledgeable **consumer** of research, one who can **critique** research and use existing standards to determine the merit and readiness of research for utilization in clinical practice (ANA, 1989). The remainder of this book is devoted to helping you develop that consumer expertise.

RESEARCH: LINKING THEORY, EDUCATION, AND PRACTICE

Research links theory, education, and practice. Mercer (1984) and Silva (1986) state that research is the process through which the knowledge base for nursing practice grows. *Theory* conceptualizes the abstract nature of the relationship among concepts. *Research*, however, is the systematic inquiry into the possible relationships among particular phenomena. The educational setting provides an environment in which students can learn about the research process. In this setting they can also explore different theories and begin to evaluate them in light of research findings. Theoretical formulations supported by research findings may potentially become the foundations of theory-based practice in nursing. Theoretical knowledge derived from either a qualitative or a quantitative source must have clinical relevance to be useful to professionals in clinical practice and to society in general (Riegal, 1992).

A classic research study by Brooten et al. (1986) illustrates a theory-based investigation that has societal relevance, is clinically oriented, is interdisciplinary, and provides research experience for student research assistants. The study sought to determine the safety, efficacy, and cost savings of early hospital discharge of very-low-birth-weight infants. One group of infants ($n = 40$) was discharged according to routine nursery criteria (weight above 2200 g). Those in the early discharge group ($n = 39$) were discharged before they reached this weight if they met a standard set of conditions. For families of infants in the early discharge group, education, counseling, home visits, and on-call availability of a hospital-based nurse specialist for 18 months were provided. The two groups did not differ in specific outcome criteria, including the number of rehospitalizations and acute care visits and measures of physical and mental growth. The average hospital cost for the early discharge group was 27% less than that for the standard discharge group, and the average physician cost was 22% less. The average cost of the home follow-up care was $576, yielding a net savings of $18,560 for each infant in the early discharge group. Brooten et al. (1986) stated that if only half of the 36,000 very-low-birth-weight infants born in the United States each year were discharged according to the protocol tested, the annual health care savings could be as much as $334 million, with no adverse effect on the infants or their families. These findings have had enormous implications not only for nursing practice but also for related health care disciplines, all of which compose the interdisciplinary health care team involved in the care of very-low-birth-weight infants. Using the team's quality-cost model, Brooten and other researchers have extended their work to three additional patient groups—women with unplanned cesarean births, women with antepartum and postpartum diabetes, and women who have had hysterectomies (Brooten et al., 1988; Brooten et al., 1989; Cohen, Hollingsworth, & Rubin, 1989; Graff, Thomas, Hollingsworth, Cohen, & Rubin, 1992).

Another study examined the experience of living with a wife who is receiving chemotherapy. The descriptive data obtained from interviews with husbands provided the basis for constructing a three-stage explanatory model—identifying the threat, engaging in the fight, and becoming a veteran (Wilson & Morse, 1991). The model illustrates how husbands coped with their experience. The data reveal that husbands engaged in a social process related to role theory called "buffering." In the buffering role, they filtered and reduced the stresses of day-to-day living to protect their wives and they engaged in strategies that preserved self to maintain their own self-control, health, and energy. The findings of this study highlight the need for nurses to assist the healthy spouse, the "primary supporter," in maintaining his critical role within the family while dealing with his wife's response to chemotherapy. Wilson and Morse (1991) also suggested that using the model as an assessment tool would help health care professionals determine appropriate interventions designed to assist the husband's need to engage in buffering behavior.

The preceding examples provide the answer to a question you may have been asking: How will the theory and research content of your course relate to your nursing practice? The data from each study have clearly demonstrated societal and practice implications. The study by Brooten et al. (1986) provided data that illustrated an innovative nursing intervention protocol with very-low-birth-weight infants that was cost-effective *and* maintained high-quality infant outcomes. In an era of skyrocketing health care costs, empirically supported programs that are cost-effective without compromising quality are essential. Given the national concern about women's health issues and the physical, emotional, and financial stress of catastrophic illness in a family, the study by Wilson and Morse (1991) provided important data about a three-stage model for understanding the experience of the husband during his wife's chemotherapy. This model can be used to plan treatment that will support the husband so that he can functionally enact a pivotal role during this stressful process.

At this point you may logically ask how education in nursing research links theory and practice. The answer is twofold. First, it will provide you with an appreciation and an understanding of the research process such that you will become a participant in research activities. Second, it *must* help you become an intelligent consumer of research. A consumer of research uses and applies research in an active manner. To be a knowledgeable consumer, a nurse must have a knowledge base about the relevant subject matter, the ability to discriminate and evaluate information logically, and the ability to apply the knowledge gained. It is not necessary to conduct studies to be able to appreciate and use research findings in practice. Rather, to be intelligent consumers, nurses must understand the research process and develop the critical evaluation skills needed to judge the merit and relevance of findings before applying them in practice.

THE ROLES OF THE NURSE IN THE RESEARCH PROCESS

There are many roles for nurses in research. One of the marks of success in nursing research is the delineation of research activities geared for nurses prepared in different types of educational programs (Fawcett, 1984a; McBride, 1988).

Graduates of associate degree nursing programs should demonstrate an awareness of the value or relevance of research in nursing. They may assist in identifying problem areas in nursing practice within an established structured format, assist in data collection activities, and in conjunction with the professional nurse, appropriately use research findings in clinical practice (ANA, 1989).

Nurses with a baccalaureate education must be intelligent consumers of research; that is, they must understand each step of the research process and its relationship to every other step. Such understanding must be linked with a clear idea about the standards of satisfactory research. This comprehension is necessary when critically reading and understanding research reports, thereby determining the validity and merit of reported studies. Through critical appraisal skills that use specific criteria to judge all aspects of the research, a professional nurse interprets, evaluates, and determines the credibility of research findings. The nurse discriminates between an idea that is interesting but requires further investigation before implementation in practice, and findings that have sufficient support to be considered for utilization (ANA, 1989; Buckwalter, 1992; Massey & Loomis, 1988).

In this context, understanding the research process and acquiring critical appraisal skills open a broad realm of information that can contribute to the professional nurse's body of knowledge and that can be applied judiciously to practice in the interest of providing scientifically based care (Batey, 1982; Duffy, 1987). Thus the role of the baccalaureate graduate in the research process is primarily that of a knowledgeable consumer, a role that promotes the integration of research and clinical practice.

Lest anyone think that this is an unimportant role, let us assure you that it is not. Fawcett (1984b) states that we are all aware of those who assert that research is the bailiwick of "ivory tower" investigators. She goes on to state, however, that it is the staff nurse who is ultimately responsible for utilization of the findings of nursing and other health-related research in clinical practice. To use such research findings appropriately, nurses must understand and critically appraise them. Thus if nursing as a profession is ever to have a genuine theory-based practice, it will be in large part up to nurses in their role as consumers of research to accomplish this task.

Baccalaureate graduates also have a responsibility to identify nursing problems that require investigation and to participate in the implementation of scientific studies (ANA, 1989). It is often clinicians who generate research ideas or questions from hunches, gut-level feelings, intuition, or observations of patients or nursing care. These ideas are often the seeds of further research investigations. For example, a nurse working on a psychiatric unit observed that a certain percentage of discharged patients were readmitted to the unit within 2 months of discharge. She noted that there were differences in the discharge procedure and wanted to find out whether the type of aftercare treatment made a difference in the readmission rate.

Of particular interest was the variation related to whether the patient was connected to the aftercare therapist or facility before discharge and how this influenced the readmission rate. The presence and support of an expert nurse-researcher in the clinical setting can often provide leadership and direction for staff nurses in the systematic investigation of such an idea in an on-site clinical research project. Systematic collection of data about a clinical problem contributes to the refinement and extension of nursing practice.

Baccalaureate graduates may also participate in research projects as members of an interdisciplinary or intradisciplinary research team. The nurse may participate in one or more phases of such a project. For example, a staff nurse may work on a clinical research unit where a particular type of nursing care is part of an established research protocol, let us say, for decubitus ulcers (pressure sores) or urinary incontinence. In such a situation the nurse administers the care according to the format described in the protocol. The nurse may also be involved in the collection and recording of data relevant to the administration of and patient response to the nursing care.

Promotion of ethical principles of research, especially the protection of human subjects, is another essential responsibility of baccalaureate prepared nurses. For example, a nurse caring for a patient who is beginning an antinausea chemotherapy research protocol would make sure that the patient had signed the informed consent and had all his or her questions answered by the research team before beginning the protocol. A nurse who observed the patient having an adverse reaction to the medication protocol would know that his or her responsibility would be not to administer another dose before notifying an appropriate member of the research team (see Chapter 13).

As members of a profession, it is also incumbent on baccalaureate graduates to share research findings with colleagues. This may involve collaborative dissemination of the findings of a study that you have participated in through development of an article or presentation for a research or clinical conference. Or it may involve sharing with colleagues the findings of a research report that you have critiqued and have found to have merit and potential applicability in your practice.

Nurses who are educationally prepared at the master's and doctoral levels must also be sophisticated consumers of research. However, they are also being prepared to conduct research as either a coinvestigator or a primary investigator.

At the master's level, nurses are prepared to be active members of research teams. They are able to assume the role of clinical expert, collaborating with an experienced researcher in proposal development, data collection, data analysis, and interpretation (ANA, 1989). Master's prepared nurses enhance the quality and relevance of nursing research by providing clinical expertise about problems and by providing knowledge about the way that clinical services are delivered. They facilitate the investigation of clinical problems by providing a climate favorable to conducting research. This includes collaborating with others in investigations and enhancing nursing's access to patients and data. At the master's level, nurses conduct research investigations for the purpose of monitoring the quality of the practice of nursing in a clinical setting. They provide leadership by assisting others in applying scientific knowledge in nursing practice (ANA, 1989).

Doctorally prepared nurses have the greatest amount of expertise in appraising, designing, and conducting research. They develop theoretical explanations of phenomena relevant to nursing. They develop methods of scientific inquiry and use analytical and empirical methods to discover ways to modify or extend existing knowledge so that it is relevant to nursing. Two types of research are conducted by doctorally prepared nurses: **basic research** and **applied research**. Table 1-1 provides a definition and an example of each type of research. In addition to their role as

Table 1-1 Types of Nursing Research

Type of research	Definition	Example
Basic research	Theoretical or pure research that generates, tests, and expands theories that describe, explain, or predict the phenomenon of interest to the discipline without regard to its later use (Silva, 1986)	Barrett's (1989, 1990) Power Theory is based on a postulate of Rogers' Science of Unitary Human Beings, i.e., that humans can knowingly participate in change. Barrett proposed that power is the way humans knowingly participate in change, creating their reality by actualizing some potentials for change rather than others. The methodological focus of Barrett's research concerned development of an instrument to measure the theoretical power construct.
Applied research	"Answers questions related to the applicability of basic theories in practical situations" (Donaldson & Crowley, 1978); tests the practical limits of descriptive theories but does not examine the efficacy of actions taken by practitioners	Grey, Cameron, & Thurber's study (1991) of coping and adaptation in children with insulin-dependent diabetes mellitus examined the comparison of preadolescents and adolescents in psychological, physiological, and social adaptational factors by stage of sexual maturation, coping behaviors, and self-care behaviors.

producers of research, doctorally prepared nurses act as role models and mentors who guide, stimulate, and encourage other nurses who are developing their research skills. They also collaborate with and serve as consultants to social, educational, or health care institutions or governmental agencies in their research endeavors. Doctorally prepared nurses are charged with dissemination of their research findings to the scientific community, to clinicians, and, as appropriate, to the lay public. Scientific journals, professional conferences, and the news media are among the mechanisms for dissemination (ANA, 1989; Downs, 1991; Rockwell, 1992).

The most important implication of the delineation of research activities according to educational preparation is the necessity of having a collaborative research relationship within the nursing profession. Not all nurses must or should conduct research. However, all nurses can play some part in the research process. Nurses at all educational levels, whether they are consumers or producers of research or both, need to view the research process as something of *integral value* to the growing professionalism in nursing.

Professionals need to take the time to read research studies and to evaluate them using the standards congruent with scientific research. The critiquing process is used to identify the strengths and weaknesses of each study. Nurses should keep in mind that no study is perfect; whereas the limitations should be recognized, nurses may extrapolate from the study whatever is sound and relevant to be considered for potential use in clinical practice.

HISTORICAL PERSPECTIVE

The history of nursing research comprises many changes and developments. The groundwork for what has blossomed was laid in the late nineteenth century and the first half of the twentieth century. To capture the essence of the development of nursing research and the works of so many excellent researchers, especially in the 1980s and 1990s, is beyond the scope of this chapter. A review of the many nursing journals available provides further support of the efforts of nursing researchers. The box on pp. 12-15 highlights key events that have set the stage for the richness of the current nursing research efforts.

Nineteenth Century—After 1850

In the mid-nineteenth century, nursing as a formal discipline began to take root with the ideas and practices of Florence Nightingale. Her concepts have contributed to and are congruent with the present priorities of nursing research. The promotion of health, prevention of disease, and care of the sick were central ideas of her system. Nightingale believed that the systematic collection and exploration of data were necessary for nursing. Her collection and analysis of data on the health status of British soldiers during the Crimean War led to a variety of reforms in health care (Palmer, 1977). Nightingale also noted the need for measuring outcomes of nursing and medical care (Nightingale, 1863), and she had an expertise in statistics

HISTORICAL PERSPECTIVE

NINETEENTH CENTURY—AFTER 1850

1852   Nightingale wrote *Cassandra*.
1855   Nightingale studied and calculated mortality rates of British in Crimean War and on basis of data developed plans to decrease military overcrowding.
1859   Nightingale's *Notes on Matters Affecting the Health, Efficiency and Hospital Administration of the British Army;* and *Notes on Hospitals* published.
1859   Nightingale's *Notes on Nursing* published.
1860   Nightingale founded St. Thomas's Hospital School of Nursing in England.
1861   Nightingale developed cost accounting system for Army Medical Services.
1872   First nursing schools in the U.S. began: New England Hospital for Women & Children, Boston; Women's Hospital, Philadelphia.
1893   Lillian Wald and Mary Brewster established Henry Street Visiting Nurse Service.
1899   International Council of Nurses organized.

TWENTIETH CENTURY—BEFORE 1950
1900-1909

1902   Lavinia Dock reported school health experiment begun by Lillian Wald for free child health care.
1900   *American Journal of Nursing* publication began.
1909   Nursing programs began at Columbia University Teacher's College and University of Minnesota.
1909   "Visiting Nursing in the United States" conducted by Waters.

1910-1919

1912   American Nurses' Association established.
1914   Metropolitan Life Insurance Company contracted nurses to collect data on health problems and tuberculosis.

1920-1929

1923   Goldmark Report published.
1923   Yale and Case Western Reserve universities' nursing programs began.
1924   First nursing doctoral program began at Teacher's College, Columbia University.
1926   From 1926 to 1934 Committee on Grading of Nursing Schools convened.
1927   Edith S. Bryan became the first nurse to receive a Ph.D. in psychology and counseling from The Johns Hopkins University.

HISTORICAL PERSPECTIVE—cont'd

1930-1939

1934   Nursing doctoral program established at New York University.

1934   Nightingale International Foundation established.

1936   Sigma Theta Tau, National Honor Society for Nursing, began nursing research funding.

1940-1949

1948   *Nurses for the Future—The Brown Report* was published.

1948   United States Public Health Service Division of Nursing conducted nursing surveys and published manuals for the conduct of nursing research.

TWENTIETH CENTURY—AFTER 1950

1950-1959

1950   American Nurses' Association established a Master Plan for Research, 1951-1956.

1952   National League for Nursing was established.

1952   *Nursing Research* publication began.

1953   *Nursing Outlook* publication began.

1953   Institute of Research & Service in Nursing Education was established at Teacher's College, Columbia University.

1955   American Nurses' Foundation was formed.

1956   United States Public Health Service began awarding grants for nursing research.

1956   Predoctoral fellowships for nursing research were first awarded.

1957   Department of Nursing Research was established at Walter Reed Army Hospital.

1957   Western Council on Higher Education in Nursing (WCHEN) sponsored Western Interstate for Higher Education (WICHE) to augment graduate nursing education, especially in nursing research.

1958   Abdellah and Levine study of nursing personnel was published.

1959   National League for Nursing (NLN) Research & Studies Service was established.

1959   First faculty research grants awarded to University of Washington and University of California at Los Angeles.

Continued.

and epidemiology. Nightingale stated, "Statistics are history in repose, history is statistics in motion" (Keith, 1988).

Other than Nightingale's work, there seems to have been little research during the early years of nursing's development, perhaps in part because schools of nursing had just begun to be established in the United States, schools were unequal in ability to educate, and nursing leadership had just begun to develop.

HISTORICAL PERSPECTIVE—cont'd

1960-1969

1962	American Nurses' Association Blueprint for Nursing Research was issued.
1962	Nurse Scientist Graduate Training Grants Program was initiated.
1962	*Nursing Forum* publication began.
1963	*International Journal of Nursing Studies* publication began.
1963	*Surgeon General's Consultant Group on Nursing* report was issued.
1963	Lydia Hall published study of chronically ill at Loeb Center.
1965	American Nurses' Association began sponsoring conferences for nursing research.
1969	Wayne State University College of Nursing established the first nursing research center.

1970-1979

1970	*Abstract for Action—Lysaught Report* was published.
1971	American Nurses' Association Council of Nurse Researchers was organized.
1974	Western Council on Higher Education in Nursing set 5-year goal to triple nursing research.
1974	American Nurses' Association Commission on Nursing Research proposed involvement of various levels of students in research and a clinical thrust for research.
1975	American Nurses' Association testified at President Gerald Ford's Panel on Biomedical Research.
1976	*Research in Nursing: Toward a Science of Health Care.* Published by ANA—Report of nursing research trends.
1976	National League for Nursing set criteria for undergraduate nursing research course in B.S.N. programs.
1978	*Research in Nursing & Health* publication began.
1978	*Advances in Nursing Science* publication began.
1979	*Western Journal of Nursing Research* publication began.
1979	Haller, Reynolds, and Horsley published research utilization criteria.

Twentieth Century—Before 1950

Nursing research in the first half of the twentieth century focused mainly on nursing education, but some patient- and technique-oriented research was evident. The early efforts in nursing education research were made by such leaders as Lavinia Dock (1900), Anne Goodrich (1932), Adelaide Nutting (1912, 1926), Isabel Hampton Robb (1906), and Lillian Wald (1915). Nutting's *The Education and Professional Position of Nurses* (1907) and Nutting and Dock's *A History of Nursing* (1907) were the earliest studies of nursing and nursing education. These pioneering works consist of documentation gathered for the purpose of reforming education in nursing and establishing it as a viable profession.

HISTORICAL PERSPECTIVE—cont'd

1980-1989

1980   Commission on Nursing Research of the American Nurses' Association set research priorities for 1980s.

1983   Institute of Medicine completed report of *Nursing & Nursing Education: Public and Private Action.*

1986   National Center for Nursing Research established at the National Institutes of Health.

1987   *Scholarly Inquiry for Nursing Practice* and *Applied Nursing Research* publication began.

1988   *Nursing Science Quarterly* and *Nursing Scan in Research* publication began.

1988   Conference on Research Priorities in Nursing Science (CORP No. 1) set research priorities known as National Nursing Research Agenda.

1989   National Center for Health Services Research became Agency for Health Care Policy and Research (AHCPR).

1990s

1991   National Pressure Ulcer Advisory Panel gives its first award to Nancy Bergstrom.

1991   *Qualitative Health Research* publication began.

1992   Kathleen McCormick calls for outcome research efforts.

1992   Conference on Research Priorities in Nursing Science (CORP No. 2) met to set updated research priorities.

1992   Clinical Practice Guidelines: *Urinary Incontinence in Adults, Acute Pain Management,* and *Pressure Ulcers in Adults* were published by AHCPR.

1992   *Healthy People 2000* was published by the Public Health Service.

1993   Report was released of a proposed multiyear funding mechanism by National Center for Nursing Research to increase the integration of biological and nursing sciences.

1993   National Center for Nursing Research becomes National Institute of Nursing Research (NINR).

The continued need for reform in nursing education was met by the Nursing and Nursing Education in the United States Landmark Study, known as the Goldmark Report (1923). Sponsored by the Rockefeller Foundation, the Committee on Nursing and Nursing Education was funded to survey on a national level the educational preparation of the faculty and the clinical experiences of the administrators, private duty nurses, public health nurses, and nursing students. The report identified multiple deficiencies and disparate educational backgrounds at all levels of nursing. This study and others in the first half of the century recommended reorganization of nursing education and, most important, its movement into the university setting.

Clinically oriented research emerged in the early half of the century and mainly centered on the morbidity and mortality rates associated with such problems as pneumonia and contaminated milk (Carnegie, 1976). A few of these projects were instrumental in the development of patient care protocols and the employment of nurses in community settings. An experimental project by Wald and Dock conducted in 1902 led to the employment of school nurses in the New York City school system and subsequently in other cities (Roberts, 1954). Although Linda Richards, the first trained American nurse at Bellevue Hospital, did not perform formal research, she was the first nurse to keep written documentation of patient care. This documentation was used by the medical profession for its investigations (Carnegie, 1976).

In 1913 the Committee on Public Health Nursing of the National League of Nursing Education (NLNE) studied such concerns as infant mortality, blindness, and midwifery. The committee called for nursing to distinguish its role in the prevention of disease and the promotion of health through the knowledge and use of the scientific approach.

The 1920s saw the development and teaching of the earliest nursing research course because of the influence of Isabel M. Stewart (Henderson, 1977). The course "Comparative Nursing Practice," first taught by Smith and later by Henderson, introduced students to the scientific method of investigation. Students were encouraged to question all aspects of nursing care and to do laboratory experiments on such topics as measuring the oxygen content in an oxygen tent during a patient's bed bath to assess whether it dropped below a therapeutic level. Also during this period, case studies appeared in the *American Journal of Nursing (AJN)*. These were used as a teaching tool for students and as a record of patient progress (Gortner & Nahm, 1977). Scientific criteria were applied to assess the appropriateness of the methodology used (Gortner & Nahm, 1977).

Other practice-related research focused on improving nursing techniques (Clayton, 1927), handwashing procedures (Broadhurst et al., 1927), and thermometer disinfecting techniques (Ryan & Miller, 1932), among others. Clinical investigations similar to these and subsequent studies of nurses and nursing education were made through the first part of the century.

Social change and World War II affected all aspects of nursing, including research. There was an urgent need for more nurses: increased hospital admissions and military needs created a shortage of personnel. In 1943 the U.S. Cadet Nurses Corps was created after the Nurse Practice Act of 1943 was passed. The Corps provided assistance for nurses and after the war offered information that assisted in planning for nursing education. During the war, investigations focused on hospital environments, nursing status, nursing education, and nursing shortages.

After the war, nursing, like the rest of the world, began to reassess itself and its goals. In 1948 *Nursing for the Future* by Esther Lucille Brown was published. This was the culmination of a 3-year study funded by the Carnegie Foundation. This report reemphasized the inconsistencies in educational preparation and the need to move into the university setting, and it included an updated description of nursing practices. An outgrowth of Brown's report was a number of studies on nursing roles and needs. Also during the immediate postwar period many states carried out studies on nursing needs and resources (Simmons & Henderson, 1964).

Twentieth Century—1950 through 1980

The 1950s saw the blossoming of nursing research. The developments of the 1950s laid the groundwork for nursing's current level of research skill. Nursing schools at the undergraduate and graduate levels were growing in number, and graduate programs were including courses related to research. The worth and benefit of research were appreciated by nursing leadership and were beginning to filter to the various levels of nursing. This period saw the inception of the *Journal of Nursing Research,* which was dedicated to the promotion of research in nursing. In 1955 the American Nurses' Foundation was chartered as a center for research; the audience for its publications consisted of receivers and administrators of research monies. Also at the national level of the ANA a standing Committee on Research and Studies was formed in 1954. This committee was charged with planning, promoting, and guiding research and studies relating to the functions of the Association (See, 1977). A secondary function of the Committee was to collect and unify nursing information that could be used to advise the ANA Board regarding periodic inventories of nurses. Concurrently in 1955 the Commonwealth Fund endowed the National League of Nursing (NLN) with monies for the support of research education and training. Throughout the 1950s these organizations and others, such as the U.S. Public Health Service, put forth funds and personnel to study the characteristics of nursing members and students; the supply, organization, and distribution of nursing services; and job satisfaction.

The first nursing unit for practice-oriented research was set up at the Walter Reed Army Institute of Research. This unit was geared toward chemical research. Although research during this period was focused on nurses and their characteristics, the fields of psychiatric nursing and maternal-child health care received monies from federal grants to develop nursing content and educational programs at the master's and doctoral levels. Grants were also conferred on individuals who studied the social context of psychiatric facilities and its influence on relations between staff and patients (Greenblatt et al., 1955; Stanton & Schwartz, 1954) and the role of the nurse with single mothers (Donnell & Glick, 1954).

In the late 1950s nursing studies began to address clinical problems. In a guest editorial featured in *Nursing Research* (1956), Virginia Henderson commented that studies about nurses outnumber clinical studies 10 to 1. She stated that "the responsibility for designing its methods is often cited as an essential characteristic of a profession" (p. 99).

Thus in the 1960s there began a reordering of research priorities and a targeting of practice-oriented research. These priorities were supported by the American Nurses' Foundation and other major nursing organizations. However, even with this support, research did not flourish. This may be partly attributed to the lack of educational preparation of nurses in research. Where research education did exist, nurses had not yet developed sufficient expertise in research design and methodology to teach their own research courses. Therefore nurses were, until recently, dependent on others from related disciplines such as psychology, education, and sociology who had this expertise to teach these courses. Today this is not usually the case.

Consistent with this need for guidance, many of the studies during the 1950s and 1960s were coinvestigated by individuals from the social sciences and medicine. Another reason for the paucity of research was the small number of nurses with baccalaureate and higher degrees. Although enrollment in these programs had increased by 1960, fewer than 2% of the employed registered nurses held master's degrees and fewer than 7% held baccalaureate degrees (ANA, 1960).

During the 1960s, studies on nurses and nursing continued, but at the same time the pioneers in the development of nursing theories and models, such as Ida Jean Orlando (1961), Hildegarde Peplau (1952), and Ernestine Wiedenbach (1964), called for the development of nursing practice based on theory. Although their theories and those of others have only begun to be tested, the early development of those theories has spurred nurses into a more critical level of thinking regarding nursing practice.

Collaborative efforts in the 1960s on practice-oriented research led to follow-up research by Diers and Leonard (1966) and Dumas and Leonard (1963). These studies done at Yale University explored the effects of nurse-patient teaching and communication on such events as hospitalization, surgery, and the labor experience. Another classic study, the culmination of 8 years of work by Glaser and Strauss (1965), explored various aspects of thanatology among dying patients and their caretakers.

A review of the nursing research studies published during the 1960s reveals that clinical studies were beginning to predominate. These studies investigated a wide gamut of nursing care issues such as infection control, alcoholism, and sensory deprivation. Lydia Hall (1963) published the results of a 5-year study that looked at alternatives to hospitalization for a select group of elderly clients. This study gave rise to a totally nurse-run care facility, the Loeb Center in New York City, which is still in operation and run by nurses today.

The rich history of nursing was also recognized during the 1960s. Nursing archives at Boston University's Mugar Library were established through a federally funded grant with the goal of promoting nursing research. In 1967 the First Nursing Research Conference of the ANA was held. A group of nurses and nursing faculty gathered to report on research and **critique** the findings presented.

The opening of the 1970s saw the publication of the National Commission for the Study of Nursing and Nursing Education Report or the Lysaught Report (1970). This report, conducted with the support of the ANA, NLN, and other private foundations, surveyed nursing practice and education. It offered the conclusions that more practice-oriented and education-oriented research was necessary and that these data must be applied to the improvement of educational organizations and curricula. The call for clinically oriented study was becoming a reality. Carnegie (1976) noted that the majority of research published in the nursing journals was clinically oriented.

The 1970s also saw new growth in the number of master's and doctoral programs for nursing. These programs, along with the ANA, NLN, Sigma Theta Tau, and Western Interstate Council for Higher Education in Nursing, clearly supported nurses learning the research process as well as producing research that could be used to enhance care quality. In the 1970s newer journals such as *Advances in Nursing*

Sciences, Research in Nursing and Health, and *The Western Journal of Nursing Research* that promoted the generation of nursing theory and research were established.

The 1980s

The decade of the 1980s was exciting and productive for research in nursing. The period saw extended growth among upper-level programs in nursing, especially at the doctoral level. By 1989 more than 5000 of the doctorally prepared nurses held their doctorate in nursing. Consistent with the increased numbers of nurses with advanced training, federal funding and support increased not only in universities but also in practice settings for research. Many centers for nursing research exist in educational settings and in hospitals. A number of these centers have programs joining education and practice that provide support and guidance for research efforts.

Mechanisms for communicating research have also increased. A number of journals and reviews now provide additional forums for communicating research. Most nursing organizations also have research sections that serve to foster the conduct and use of research.

Public Law 99-158, which was enacted in 1985, allowed for the establishment of the National Center for Nursing Research (NCNR). Established in 1986, NCNR provided funding programs that focus on studies related to health care outcomes. The NCNR program areas are organized in three broad categories: (1) health promotion and disease prevention, (2) acute and chronic illness, and (3) nursing systems and special programs (Hinshaw, 1988). The National Advisory Council of the NCNR in 1988 identified the following nursing research priorities:

1. Low birth weight—care of mothers and infants
2. Patients, partners, and families with human immunodeficiency virus
3. Long-term care
4. Symptom management
5. Information systems
6. Health promotion
7. Technology dependency across the life span

The efforts of the 1980s were aimed at the refinement and development of research and the utilization of research findings in clinical practice. The developments and strides in the area of research made in the 1980s suggested that nursing was ready to rise to the societal and professional demands that now confront the discipline in the 1990s.

FUTURE DIRECTIONS—THE 1990S: TOWARD A HEALTHY 2000

During the 1990s, nursing research continues to grow and flourish. There are 54 nursing doctoral programs in the United States and 25 nursing doctoral programs outside the United States, and additional programs are under development

(1992). At the conduct level the efforts of nurse researchers are primarily geared toward the development of clinically based outcome studies. The mechanisms for the utilization of the research produced are being refined and identified as a priority (see Chapter 3). Nurse researchers and nurse leaders are visibly involved at the national level, participating in policy making, representing nursing on expert panels, and lobbying for needed funding dollars. A review of the twentieth century reveals that nursing has truly risen to the challenges of the development of nursing science with the ultimate goal of improving health care.

Nursing's research efforts now have further recognition. In June 1993, the National Institutes of Health (NIH) reauthorization bill gave the National Center for Nursing Research institute status. NCNR is now the National Institute of Nursing Research (NINR). Hereafter in the text, NCNR will be referred to as NINR.

Promoting Depth in Nursing Research

In a complex, health-oriented society such as ours that is increasingly responsive to consumer concerns related to the cost, quality, availability, and accessibility of health care, it is of paramount importance to define the future direction of nursing research and establish research priorities (Hinshaw, 1988, 1990).

Nursing leaders unanimously agree that the essential priority for nursing research in the future will be promotion of excellence in nursing science (Hinshaw & Heinrich, 1990; Jennings, 1991; Phillips, 1988; Riegel et al., 1992). This priority is linked to the efforts of the discipline's scholars to develop a knowledge base that can accurately guide nursing practice (Hinshaw, 1990).

Research-based practice reflects the characteristics of the research from which it is derived. The quality of research by which nursing science is generated and information is provided to guide practice will be one of the major keys to producing predictable patient outcomes and improving patient care for our own discipline (Hinshaw, 1990). Essential to the achievement of this goal will be the continuing development of a national and international research environment (Hinshaw & Heinrich, 1990; Shaver, 1992). Within this environment an increasing number of nurses who have significant expertise in appraising, designing, and conducting research will continue to emerge within the profession. They will provide a "critical mass" of investigators who will be at the forefront of the ongoing development and refinement of our scientific knowledge base for nursing practice.

To maximize utilization of available resources and prevent wasteful duplication, researchers must develop intradisciplinary and interdisciplinary networks in similar areas of basic and applied study across disciplines (Hinshaw & Heinrich, 1990). Clinical consortia will help delineate the common and unique aspects of patient care for the various health professions. Cluster studies, multiple-site investigations, and programs of research will facilitate the accumulation of evidence supporting or negating an existing theory and thereby contribute to defining the base of nursing practice.

Depth in nursing science will be evident when replicated, consistent findings exist in a substantive area of inquiry. Programs of research that include a series of studies in a similar area of study, each of which builds on the prior investigation, both replicating and adding to the research question being studied, will promote depth in nursing science (Hinshaw, 1990). An example of a program of research is provided by the work of Nancy Bergstrom, the principal investigator funded by a 3-year grant from the NINR for the multisite study of the Nursing Assessment of Pressure Sore Risk. Approximately 1200 patients in a variety of health care settings were studied. The study further validated the use of the Braden scale developed by Barbara Braden for evaluating pressure sore risk. The outcome of this study leads to improved patient care and ultimately to cost savings in terms of equipment use and reduction of hospital stays caused by complications of pressure sores. Consistent and replicable findings across sites will yield a body of practice-relevant, in-depth knowledge of pressure sore prevention.

The preceding example illustrates the value of replication studies that are built into programs of research. Hinshaw (1990) proposes that the adoption of research findings in practice, with their potential risks and benefits, including the cost of implementation, should be based on a series of replicated studies. As such, replication studies will have much more credibility in the future and will play a crucial role in developing depth in nursing science.

Nursing research is increasingly addressing physiological as well as psychological responses to actual and potential health problems (Cowan, Heinrich, Lucas, Sigmon, & Hinshaw, 1993). Investigations that reflect state-of-the-art science will examine the interface of the biological sciences with the evolving knowledge base of nursing. Nurse researchers will also have increased opportunity to participate in clinical trials. This will provide direction to improve aspects of care such as symptom assessment, management, and interventions to prevent and reduce physical distress such as pain (Hinshaw, 1991).

Nurse researchers will continue to have increased methodological expertise. They are increasingly sophisticated about the development and application of computer technology to the research process. A greater emphasis will be placed on measurement issues such as the development of tools that accurately measure clinical phenomena.

The increasing focus on the need to use multiple measures to assess clinical phenomena accurately is also apparent. Related to the need to measure clinical phenomena accurately will be the development of noninvasive methods to measure physiological parameters of interest in high-technology settings. These methods may well be another aspect of using multiple measures to assess particular clinical phenomena. The development of qualitative measures and new qualitative computer analysis packages is also expanding as the qualitative mode of inquiry is more frequently used in research.

Nurse researchers will employ new, more diverse, and advanced methods for the design of research studies and analysis of findings. For example, qualitative research methods have become increasingly respected as a mode of scientific inquiry, contributing to theory development and providing essential descriptive data that provide direction for clinical practice and future research studies. Consider the importance of the findings of Beck's qualitative studies (1992, 1993) of the Lived Experience of Postpartum Depression, which revealed that the fundamental structure of postpartum depression, as described by the study subjects, differed significantly from that assessed by the questions contained in the most frequently used depression assessment tools. Beck (1992) suggests that quantitative assessment tools should include the gamut of possible behavioral manifestations from which a mother can rate her depressive symptoms. Beck proposes that the fundamental structure of postpartum depression developed from this study can be a starting point for future methodological research focused on developing a quantitative instrument to measure postpartum depression specifically. Researchers using quantitative research methods will expand the frontiers of empirically derived knowledge through the use of advanced analytical programs related to causation.

Outcome Research Studies

Another trend is the proliferation of outcomes research that is both patient- and delivery system–focused (Jennings, 1991). Stimulated by the need for cost-effective care that makes a difference without compromising quality, outcome studies will provide an unprecedented opportunity for nurses to pursue research that will contribute to the scientific basis of nursing practice. By verifying the relationship between nursing interventions and patient outcomes, nurse researchers will be adding to the body of nursing interventions that are scientifically sound *and* document the impact of nursing care. The outcome study of Brooten et al. (1986) described earlier in this chapter, which tested an innovative client care delivery model for very-low-birth-weight infants, is a classic example of an outcome study that documents the impact of nursing care.

Through examination of outcomes related to organizational systems outcomes, the most cost-effective models for the delivery of high-quality collaborative care are being identified. For example, the pioneering work of Ethridge and Lamb (1989) in nursing case management illustrates a research program designed to describe the process of case management and evaluate its impact on quality and costs of care for high-risk patients. Lamb (1992) reports that a series of research studies, which have incorporated both qualitative and quantitative research designs, have convincingly demonstrated that the previously cited community-based nursing care delivery model has a positive impact on quality outcomes such as greater confidence in self-care, symptom management, and patient satisfaction and on cost-effectiveness outcomes such as hospital length of stay, hospital admissions, and emergency department visits. It is clear that nurses must capitalize on the opportunity to lead other health care providers in ensuring that outcomes are measured fully.

Programs of Research

Research training for the scientific role will increasingly become an essential component of a research career plan. Nurse researchers will be committed to developing programs of research that are supported by public and private funding sources. They will also subscribe to a life-style of periodic education and retraining that will be funded by awards, grants, and fellowships. For example, the NINR awards funding for predoctoral, postdoctoral, midcareer, and senior scientist programs of study. These programs facilitate growth in the depth and breadth of research expertise and recognize the need of some researchers to be retrained as they develop or shift the emphasis of their research, seek to broaden their scientific background, acquire new research capabilities, and enlarge their command of an allied research field.

Nurses who are prepared to direct the conduct of research will head an expanding number of nursing research departments in clinical settings. Currently there are more than 100 clinical research centers in as many as 32 states. Nurse researchers who head these centers will involve the nursing staff in generating and conducting research projects and critically evaluating existing research data before using it to guide changes in clinical practice. An expanded number of centers for nursing research will be established in university settings as faculty members become qualified to direct them.

An International Perspective

With the discipline's emphasis on cultural aspects of nursing care and the influence of such factors on practice, increasing international research is a natural futuristic trend. Access to multiple populations as a function of globalization allows the generation and testing of nursing science from many different perspectives. Interaction with colleagues from other countries provides a rich context for the generation and dissemination of research issues (Hinshaw & Heinrich, 1990).

Alliances with international organizations committed to the goal of health for all will create natural research partnerships. For example, the World Health Organization (WHO), through the Pan-American Health Organization, has designated that four WHO Collaborating Centers for Research and Clinical Training in Nursing be located in American schools and colleges of nursing. These centers will provide research and clinical training in nursing to colleagues worldwide. The International Council of Nurses (ICN) and the ANA Council of Nurse Researchers International conferences are examples of international nursing research forums designed to inform nurses of the global breadth of health problems. Such forums for dissemination of research will continue to increase, challenging nurse researchers in various regions of the world to form collaborative research relationships in which they share research expertise, educational opportunities, and the ability to conduct research projects of mutual interest and, perhaps, ultimately create an international research agenda (Shaver, 1991; University of California, San Francisco, 1992).

Future Research Priorities

In 1992 the Department of Health and Human Services published the summary report, "Healthy People 2000." This document, a product of 22 expert working groups and nearly 300 national organizations, including nursing bodies, contains 22 objectives geared to the improvement of the health of the nation. The National Research Agenda identifies priorities that are consistent with the goals of the national health agenda. By the year 2000 and into the twenty-first century, a cost-effective, community-based health care delivery system that emphasizes primary care and promotes prevention in partnership with members of a culturally diverse society will actualize a high-quality health care vision. One of the objectives, for example, is "to reduce physical abuse directed at women by male partners to no more than 27 instances per 1000 couples" (Department of Health and Human Services, 1990). Several nurse researchers, such as Campbell (1989a; 1989b; 1991); Campbell, Poland, Waller, and Ager (1992); McFarlane (1989, 1991); McFarlane, Anderson, and Helton (1987); McFarlane (1992); and Sampselle (1992), have been conducting research, developing theoretical perspectives, and conducting synthesis conferences in the area of abuse of women. In at least one case a study conducted by Campbell and Alford (1989) was used to assist in legislative change.

By the year 2000 the population will include a higher proportion of children and elderly adults who are chronically ill or disabled. The health problems of mothers and infants will continue to spur concern for dealing effectively with the rising maternal-infant mortality rate. Individuals who have sustained life-threatening illnesses will live by means of new life-sustaining technology that will create new demands for self-care and family support. Cancer, heart disease, arthritis, chronic pulmonary disease, diabetes, and Alzheimer's disease are prevalent during middle and later life and will command large proportions of the available health care resources. Mental health problems will result from rapid technological and social change. Alcohol and drug abuse will continue to be responsible for significant health care expense. The impact of human immunodeficiency virus (HIV) on individuals, families, and communities dealing with the crisis of acquired immunodeficiency syndrome (AIDS) will have a major effect on the health care delivery system. Increasingly, the settings where care is provided will be homes, schools, workplaces, and primary care centers. Over the next 10 years many hard questions of cost containment and access to care will be addressed through an interdisciplinary approach.

The emphasis of research studies will be related to clinical and systems issues and problems. The preeminent goal of scientific inquiry by nurses will be the ongoing development of knowledge for use in the practice of nursing. Consequently, priority will be given to nursing research that generates knowledge to guide practice in the areas listed in the box on p. 25.

In light of the priority given to clinical research issues, the funding of investigations will increasingly emphasize clinical research projects in relation to populations of interest. For example, the historical exclusion of women from clinical research is now well documented. Men have been the subjects in the major contemporary research studies related to adult health. The findings of such studies have been generalized from men to all adults, despite the lack of female representation (Brink, 1991). The Baltimore Longitudinal Study on Aging began in 1958 but did not include women as subjects until 1978. Although women now make up about 60% of those in the United States who are 65 or older, the study's well respected 1984 report, "Normal Human Aging," contained no data specific to women.

PRIORITY AREAS FOR NURSING RESEARCH

Promoting health, well-being, and competency for personal health in all age
  groups
Minimizing or preventing health problems that compromise the quality of life and
  reduce productivity
Ensuring that the special care needs of vulnerable populations are met through
  appropriate strategies
Designing and developing health care systems that demonstrate high-quality
  outcomes and cost-effectiveness in meeting the health care needs of the
  population
Classifying nursing practice phenomena
Developing instruments to measure nursing outcomes
Developing integrative methodologies for the holistic study of human beings as
  they relate to their families and life-styles
Ensuring that ethical principles guide research
Evaluating the effectiveness of alternative approaches to nursing education
Identifying and analyzing historical and contemporary factors that influence the
  shaping of nursing professionals' involvement in national health policy
  development

From The National Nursing Research Agenda: CNR invites your input. (1991.) *Communicating Nursing Research, 18*(3), 3.

Women of color have been even more likely to be excluded from research studies; as a result, research data on women of color are extremely scarce. Funding for research related to women's health issues and problems such as infertility, menopause, breast and ovarian cancer, and osteoporosis has been less than equitable. Given the indisputable nature of this research bias, the Office of Research on Women's Health has been established at the National Institutes of Health (NIH) to redress historical inequities in research design and allocation of federal resources. Research on women's health is likely to be a major funding focus in the future.

The most recent conference on research priorities in nursing practice conducted by the NINR (formerly NCNR) (NCNR, 1993) established the following future research priorities:

To develop and test community-based nursing models designed to promote access to, utilization of, and quality of health services by rural and other underserved populations

To assess the effectiveness of biobehavioral nursing interventions to foster health-promoting behaviors of individuals at risk for HIV and AIDS and the effectiveness of biobehavioral interventions to ameliorate the effects of illness in individuals who are already infected. The focus is on persons of different cultural backgrounds—especially women. The need to incorporate biobehavioral markers is noted

To develop and test biobehavioral and environmental approaches to remediating cognitive impairment

To test interventions to strengthen individuals' personal resources in dealing with chronic illness

To identify biobehavioral factors and test interventions to promote immunocompetence

Other types of research investigations such as those using historical, feminist, or case study methods embody the rich diversity of extant nursing research methods. Brink (1990) states that the enormous, exponential growth in nursing research since the early 1950s seems attributable to the diversity of methodological approaches that have been used to answer the profession's research questions. The nursing profession must continue to value and promote creativity and diversity in research endeavors at all educational levels as a way of empowering nursing practice for the future. As opportunities are recognized and gaps in science are observed, nurses will engage in the conduct, critique, and utilization of nursing research in ways that give voice to how nursing care makes a difference.

Nurse researchers will have an increasingly strong voice in shaping public policy. Hinshaw (1992) states that disciplines such as nursing, which focus on treatment of chronic illness, health promotion, independence in health, and the care of the acutely ill, are going to be central to shaping health care policy, since these are heavily emphasized values for the future. Research data providing evidence that supports or refutes the merit of health care needs and programs focusing on these issues will be timely and relevant. Thus nursing and its science base will be strategically placed to shape health policy decisions (DeBack, 1991).

Since we will continue to live in the "information age," dissemination of nursing research will become increasingly important in professional and public arenas. Research findings will continue to be disseminated in professional arenas such as international, national, regional, and local publications and conferences, as well as in consultations and staff development programs. However, dissemination of research findings in the public sector is an exciting future trend that has already begun. Nurse researchers are increasingly asked to present testimony at governmental hearings and to serve on commissions and task forces related to health care. Traditionally nurses have rarely been quoted in the media when health care topics are addressed, but this is changing. Today nurses and nurse researchers are participating in teleconferences, starring in videos, and appearing in interviews on television and radio and in printed media such as newspapers and lay magazines. Nurses have their own radio shows and are beginning to have their own television shows. Dissemination of research through the public media provides excellent exposure to thousands of potential viewers, listeners, and readers (Rockwell, 1992).

It is apparent from the previous discussion that nursing has a research heritage to be proud of and a challenging and exciting future direction. Both consumers and producers of research will engage in a united effort to give voice to research findings that make a difference in the care that is provided and the lives that are touched by our commitment to research-based nursing practice.

KEY POINTS

- Nursing research provides the basis for expanding the unique body of scientific knowledge that forms the foundation of nursing practice. Research links education, theory, and practice.
- Nurses become knowledgeable consumers of research through educational processes and practical experience. As consumers of research, nurses must have a basic understanding of the research process and critical appraisal skills that provide a standard for evaluating the strengths and weaknesses of research studies before applying them in clinical practice.
- In the first half of the twentieth century, nursing research focused mainly on studies related to nursing education, although some clinical studies related to nursing care were evident.
- Nursing research blossomed in the second half of the twentieth century; graduate programs in nursing expanded, research journals began to emerge, the ANA formed a research committee, and funding for graduate education and nursing research increased dramatically.
- Nurses at all levels of educational preparation have a responsibility to participate in the research process. The role of the baccalaureate graduate is to be a knowledgeable consumer of research. Nurses prepared at the master's and doctoral levels must be sophisticated consumers as well as producers of research studies.
- A collaborative research relationship within the nursing profession will extend and refine the scientific body of knowledge that provides the grounding for theory-based practice.
- The future of nursing research will continue to be the extension of the scientific knowledge base for nursing expertise in appraising, designing, and conducting research and will provide leadership in both academic and clinical settings. Collaborative research relationships between education and service will multiply. Cluster research studies and replication of studies will have increased value.
- Research studies will emphasize clinical issues, problems, and outcomes. Priority will be given to research studies that focus on promoting health, diminishing the negative impact of health problems, ensuring care for the health needs of vulnerable groups, and developing cost-effective health care systems.
- Both consumers and producers of research will engage in a collaborative effort to further the growth of nursing research and accomplish the research objectives of the profession.

REFERENCES

Acute Pain Management Guideline Panel. (1992). *Acute pain management: Operative or medical procedures and trauma. Clinical practice guideline* (AHCPR Publication No. 92-0032). Rockville, MD: U.S. Public Health Service, Agency for Health Care Policy and Research.

American Nurses' Association. (1960). *Facts about nursing* (pp. 109-116). New York: Author.

American Nurses' Association. (1981). *Guidelines for the investigative function of nurses* (pp. 2-3). Kansas City, MO: Author.

American Nurses' Association. (1989). Commission on Nursing Research: Education for preparation in nursing research, Kansas City, MO: Author.

Barrett, E.A.M. (1989). A nursing theory of power for nursing practice: Derivation from Rogers' paradigm. In J. Riehl (Ed.), *Conceptual models for nursing practice,* 3rd ed. Norwalk, CT: Appleton & Lange.

Barrett, E.A.M. (1990). Rogers' science-based nursing practice. In E.A.M. Barrett (Ed.), *Visions of Rogers' science-based nursing.* New York: National League for Nursing.

Batey, M.V. (1982). Research: A component of undergraduate education. In *Evaluating research preparation in baccalaureate nursing education: National conference for nurse educators.* Published proceedings. Ames: University of Iowa College of Nursing.

Beck, C.T. (1992). The lived experience of postpartum depression: A phenomenological study. *Nursing Research, 41*(3), 166-170.

Beck, C.T. (1993). Teetering on the edge: A substantive theory of postpartum depression. *Nursing Research, 42*(1), 42-48.

Brink, P.J. (1990). The discipline is the method. *Western Journal of Nursing Research, 22*(3), 432.

Brink, P.J. (1991). Feminist research. *Western Journal of Nursing Research, 13*(3), 304-305.

Broadhurst, J., and others. (1927). Hand brush suggestions for visiting nurses. *Public Health Nursing, 19,* 487-489.

Brooten, D., Brown, L., Munro, B., York, R., Cohen, S., Roncoli, M., & Hollingsworth, A. (1988). Quality-cost model of early hospital discharge and nurse specialist transitional follow-up care. *Image, 20*(2), 64-68.

Brooten, D., Kumar, S., Brown, L., Butts, P., Finkler, S., Bakewell-Sachs, S., Gibbons, A., & Delivoria-Papadopoulos, M. (1986). A randomized clinical trial of early hospital discharge and home follow-up of very-low-birth-weight infants. *New England Journal of Medicine, 315*(8), 934-939.

Brooten, D., Munro, B., Roncoli, M., Arnold, A., Brown, L., York, R., Hollingsworth, A., Cohen, S., & Rubin, M. (1989). Development of a program grant using the quality-cost model of early discharge and nurse specialist transitional follow-up care. *Nursing and Health Care, 10*(6), 315-318.

Brown, E.L. (1948). *Nursing for the future.* New York: Russell Sage Foundation.

Buckwalter, K.C. (1992). Research utilization awards, utilization versus dissemination? *Reflections, 18*(3), 8.

Campbell, J.C. (1989a). A test of two explanatory models of women's responses to battering. *Nursing Research, 38,* 18-24.

Campbell, J.C. (1989b). Women's response to sexual abuse in intimate relationship. *Health Care for Women International, 8,* 335-347.

Campbell, J.C. (1991). Health care system response to family violence. In D. Knudson & J. Miller (Eds.), *Abused and Battered.* New York: Aldine de Gruyter.

Campbell, J.C., & Alford, P. (1989). The effects of marital rape on women's health. *American Journal of Nursing, 89,* 946-949.

Campbell, J.C., Poland, M.L., Waller, J.B., & Ager, J.A. (1992). Correlates of battering during pregnancy. *Research in Nursing & Health, 15*(3), 219-226.

Carnegie, E. (1976). *Historical perspectives of nursing research,* Boston: Boston University, Nursing Archive, Special Collections.

Clayton, S.L. (1927). Standardizing nursing techniques: Its advantages and disadvantages. *American Journal of Nursing, 27,* 939-943.

Cohen, S., Hollingsworth, A., & Rubin, M. (1989). Another look at psychologic complications of hysterectomy. *Image, 21*(1), 51-54.

Committee on Nursing and Nursing Education in the United States, Josephine Goldmark, sec. (1923). New York: Macmillan.

Cowan, M.J., Heinrich, J., Lucas, M., Sigmon, H., & Hinshaw, A.S. (1993). Integration of biological and nursing sciences: A 10-year plan to enhance research and training. *Research in Nursing & Health, 16*(1), 3-9.

DeBack, V. (1991). Nursing needs health policy leaders. *Journal of Professional Nursing, 6*(2), 69-74.

Diers, D., & Leonard, R.C. (1966). Interaction analysis in nursing research. *Nursing Research, 15,* 225-228.

Dock, L.L. (1900). What we may expect from the law. *American Journal of Nursing, 1,* 8-12.

Donaldson, S.K., & Crowley, D.M. (1978). The discipline of nursing. *Nursing Outlook, 26,* 113-120.

Donnell, H., & Glick, S.J. (1954). The nurse and the unwed mother. *Nursing Outlook, 2,* 249-251.

Downs, F. (1991). Informing the media. *Nursing Research, 40*(4), 195.

Duffy, M.E. (1987). The research process in baccalaureate nursing education: A ten-year review. *Image, 19,* 87-91.

Dumas, R.G., & Leonard, R.C. (1963). The effect of nursing on the incidence of postoperative vomiting. *Nursing Research, 12,* 12-15.

Ethridge, P., & Lamb, G. (1989). Professional nursing case management improves quality, access and cost. *Nursing Management, 20*(1), 30-37.

Fawcett, J. (1984a). Another look at utilization of nursing research. *Image, 16,* 59-61.

Fawcett, J. (1984b). Hallmarks of success in nursing research. *Advances in Nursing Science, 1,* 1-11.

Glaser, B.G., & Strauss, A.L. (1965). *Awareness of dying* [Observations series]. Chicago: Aldine.

Goodrich, A. (1932). *The social and ethical significance of nursing: A series of addresses.* New York: Macmillan.

Gortner, S.R., & Nahm, H. (1977). An overview of nursing research in the United States. *Nursing Research, 26,* 10-33.

Graff, B., Thomas, J., Hollingsworth, A., Cohen, S., & Rubin, M. (1992). Development of a postoperative self-assessment form. *Clinical Nurse Specialist, 6*(1), 47-50.

Greenblatt, M., and others. (1955). *From custodial to therapeutic patient care in mental hospitals.* New York: Russell Sage Foundation.

Grey, M., Cameron, M.E., & Thurber, F.W. (1991). Coping and adaption in children with diabetes. *Nursing Research, 40*(3), 145-149.

Hall, L.E. (1963). A center for nursing. *Nursing Outlook, 11,* 805-806.

Haller, K., Reynolds, M., & Horsley, J. (1979). Developing research-based innovative protocols: Process, criteria and issues. *Research in Nursing & Health, 2,* 45.

Healthy People 2000: Summary Report (1992). Department of Health and Human Services. Boston: Jones & Bartlett.

Henderson, V. (1956). Research in nursing practice: When [editorial]. *Nursing Research, 4,* 99.

Henderson, V. (1977). We've "come a long way," but what of the direction? [guest editorial]. *Nursing Research, 26,* 163-164.

Hinshaw, A.S. (1988). The new National Center for Nursing Research: Patient care research program. *Applied Nursing Research, 1,* 2-4.

Hinshaw, A.S. (1990). National center for nursing research: A commitment to excellence in science. In J.C. McCloskey & H.K. Grace (Eds.), *Current Issues in Nursing* (pp. 357-362). St. Louis: Mosby.

Hinshaw, A.S. (1991). Interfacing nursing and biologic science. *Journal of Professional Nursing, 7*(5), 264.

Hinshaw, A.S. (1992). The impact of nursing science on health policy. Silver threads: 25 Years of nursing excellence. *Communicating Nursing Research, 25,* 15-26.

Hinshaw, A.S., & Heinrich, J. (1990). New initiatives in nursing research: A national perspective. In R. Bergman (Ed.), *Nursing research for nursing practice: An international perspective* (pp. 20-37). London: Chapman.

Jennings, B.M. (1991). Patient outcomes research: Seizing the opportunity. *Advances in Nursing Science, 14*(2), 59-72.

Johnson, T.L. (1992). Health research that excludes women is bad science. *Chronicle of Higher Education,* October 14, 1992, B1-2.

Keith, J.M. (1988). Florence Nightingale: Statistician and consultant epidemiologist. *International Nursing Review, 35*(5), 147-149.

Lamb, G.S. (1992). Conceptual and methodological issues in nurse case management research. *Advances in Nursing Science, 15*(2), 16-24.

Larson, E. (1981). Nursing research outside academia: A panel presentation. *Image, 13,* 75-77.

Lindemann, C. (1984). Dissemination of nursing research. *Image, 16,* 57-58.

Massey, J., & Loomis, M. (1988). When should nurses use research findings? *Applied Nursing Research, 1,* 32-40.

McBride, A.B. (1988). Making research an activity for all nurses. *Reflections, 14,* 2.

McCormick, K. (1992). Areas of outcome research for nursing. *Journal of Professional Nursing, 8,* 71.

McFarlane, J. (1989). Battering during pregnancy: Tip of an iceberg revealed. *Women and Health, 15,* 69-83.

McFarlane, J. (1991). Violence during teen pregnancy: Health consequences for mother and child. In. B. Levy (Ed.), *Dating violence: Young women in danger.* Seattle: Seal Press.

McFarlane, J. (1992). Battering in pregnancy. In C.M. Sampselle (Ed.), *Violence against women* (pp. 205-218). New York: Hemisphere.

McFarlane, J., Anderson, E., & Helton, A. (1987). Response to battering during pregnancy: An educational program. *Response, 10,* 23-25.

Mercer, R.T. (1984). Nursing research: The bridge to excellence in practice. *Image, 16,* 47-50.

National Commission for the Study of Nursing and Nursing Education. (1970). *An abstract for action.* New York: McGraw-Hill.

National Nursing Research Agenda: CNR invites your input. (1991). *Communicating Nursing Research, 18*(3), 3.

NCNR (1993, March). Priorities resulting from Second Conference on Research Priorities in Nursing Practice. NCNR.

Nightingale, F. (1863). *Notes on hospitals.* London: Longman Group.

Nursing doctoral programs in the United States. (1992). *Reflections, 18,* 14-15.

Nursing research on an international level. (1992). *The Science of Caring.* San Francisco: School of Nursing, University of California at San Francisco, *3*(2), 2-6.

Nutting, M.A. (1912). *Educational status of nursing* (Bulletin No. 7). Washington, DC: U.S. Bureau of Education.

Nutting, M.A. (1926). *A second economic basis for schools of nursing and other addresses.* New York: G.P. Putnam's Sons.

Nutting, M.A., & Dock, L.L. (1907-1912). *A history of nursing* (4 vols.). New York: G.P. Putnam's Sons.

Orlando, I.J. (1961). *The dynamic nurse-patient relationship.* New York: G.P. Putnam's Sons.

Palmer, I. (1977). Florence Nightingale: Reformer, reactionary, researcher. *Nursing Research, 26,* 84-89.

Panel for the Prediction and Prevention of Pressure Ulcers In Adults. (1992). *Pressure ulcers in adults: Prediction and prevention. Clinical practice guideline* (AHCPR Publication No. 92-0047). Rockville, MD: Public Health Service, Agency for Health Care Policy and Research.

Pender, N.J. (1992). Environmental compatibility: Accepting the challenge. *Nursing Outlook, 40*(5), 200-201.

Peplau, H.E. (1952). *Interpersonal relations in nursing: A conceptual frame of reference for psychodynamic nursing.* New York: G.P. Putnam's Sons.

Phillips, J.R. (1988). The reality of nursing research. *Nursing Science Quarterly, 1,* 48-49.

Pollock, S. (1986). Top-ranked schools of nursing: Network of scholars. *Image, 18,* 58-60.

Riegel, B., Omery, A., Calvillo, E., Elsayed, N.G., Shuler, P., & Siegal, B.E. (1992). Moving beyond: A generative philosophy of science. *Image, 24*(2), 115-120.

Robb, I.H. (1906). *Nursing: Its principles and practice for hospitals and private use* (3rd ed.). Cleveland: E.C. Koeckert.

Roberts, M.M. (1954). *American nursing: History and interpretation.* New York: Macmillan.

Rockwell, T. (1992). Emerging role for nurses in health communication. *Reflections, 18*(4), 4-5.

Rogers, M. (1992). Nursing science and the space age. *Nursing Science Quarterly, 5:*1, 27-34.

Ryan, V., & Miller, V.B. (1932). Disinfection of clinical thermometers: Bacteriological study and estimated costs. *American Journal of Nursing, 32,* 197-206.

Sampselle, C.M. (1992). *Violence against women.* New York: Hemisphere.

See, E.M. (1977). The ANA and research in nursing. *Nursing Research, 26,* 165-176.

Shaver, J. (1991). Global perspectives: The ANA and CNR international nursing research conference. *Council of Nurse Researchers Newsletter, 18*(3), 1-6.

Shugars, D.A., O'Neil, E.H., & Bader, J.D. (Eds.). (1991). *Healthy America: Practitioners for 2005: An agenda for action for U.S. health professional schools.* Durham, NC: The Pew Health Professions Commission.

Silva, M.C. (1986). Research testing nursing theory: State of the art. *Advances in Nursing Science, 9,* 1-11.

Simmons, L.W., & Henderson, V. (1964). *Nursing research: A survey and assessment.* New York: Appleton-Century-Crofts.

Stanton, A.H., & Schwartz, M.A. (1954). *The mental hospital: A study of institutional participation in psychiatric illness and treatment.* New York: Basic Books.

Stetler, C.B., & Marram, G. (1976). Evaluating research findings for applicability in practice. *Nursing Outlook, 24,* 559-563.

Stewart Fahs, P., & Kinney, M. (1991). The abdomen, thigh, and arm as sites for subcutaneous sodium heparin injections. *Nursing Research, 40*(4), 204-207.

Taylor, N., Hutchison, E., Milliken, W., & Larson, E. (1989). Comparison of normal versus heparinized saline for flushing infusion devices. *Journal of Nursing Quality Assurance, 3*(4), 49-55.

U.S. Department of Health and Human Services. (1992). *Healthy People 2000: Summary report* (Publication No. PH591-50213). Boston: Jones & Bartlett.

Urinary Incontinence Guideline Panel. (1992). *Urinary incontinence in adults: Clinical practice guideline* (AHCPR Publication No. 92-0038). Rockville, MD: Public Health Service, Agency for Health Care Policy and Research.

Wald, L.D. (1915). *House on Henry Street,* New York: Henry Holt & Co.

Wiedenbach, E. (1964). *Clinical nursing: A helping art.* New York: Springer.

2

The Scientific Approach to the Research Process

HARRIET R. FELDMAN
GEORGIA K. MILLOR

LEARNING OBJECTIVES

After reading this chapter the student should be able to do the following:

- Describe the relationship between philosophy and science.
- Identify the major sources of human knowledge.
- Contrast the strengths and weaknesses of the major sources of human knowledge.
- Compare the inductive and deductive modes of logical reasoning.
- Identify the characteristics of the scientific approach.
- Define theory.
- Examine the relationship between theory and research methods.

KEY TERMS

assumption	inductive reasoning
deductive reasoning	metaphysical
determinism	proposition
empirical	research
generalize	scientific approach
hypothesis	theory

As stated in Chapter 1, the importance of research to nursing is in the development of a scientific base for nursing practice. Nursing knowledge comes from many sources, such as intuition, tradition, trial and error, logical reasoning, and scientific inquiry, and is developed within the context of a particular philosophical stance. Philosophy, representing the belief system of nursing, also guides research approaches of the discipline.

This chapter examines the sources or origins of human knowledge and the components of the scientific approach that guide the process of inquiry. In addition, the approaches to developing theory and the relationship between theory and method are discussed.

THE PHILOSOPHY OF SCIENCE

Philosophers and scientists pursue a common goal of developing and expanding knowledge. However, their approaches to understanding reality are different. A philosopher uses intuition, reasoning, contemplation, and introspection to examine "the purpose of human life, the nature of being and reality, and the theory and the limits of knowledge" (Silva, 1977, p. 60). On the other hand, the scientist observes, verifies, constructs definitions, makes and verifies predictions, and conducts experiments to derive scientific laws and interpret reality. Another contrast is in the kinds of questions philosophers and scientists ask. Philosophy deals with abstract (**metaphysical**) questions about the nature of being or reality, for example, "What is knowledge?" or "Are people inherently good or bad?" Science deals with questions that are **empirical,** that is, they come from experience and observation, such as "How are X and Y related?" and "Does the application of ice result in reduced muscle swelling?"

The development of knowledge about the discipline of nursing depends on both philosophy and science. Gortner (1990) says that "philosophy represents the belief system of the profession and . . . provides perspectives for practice, for scholarship, and for research" (p. 101). Beliefs influence our thinking about nursing,

nursing science, and the metaphysical or empirical knowledge needed to support or further the discipline's development. These beliefs are reshaped as the discipline of nursing changes over time. "At least four major schools of thought have influenced (covertly or overtly) nursing's philosophy of science: logical positivism, and the paradigmatic, evolutionary, and feminist schools" (Riegel et al., 1992, p. 116). A generative philosophy was proposed by Riegel et al. (1992) because of a "poor fit between existing philosophies of science and practice disciplines" and in an effort to represent "nursing in its complexity and richness" (p. 116).

Many views have influenced the development of nursing's philosophy of science, such as the following:

1. Science as wholly objective and tested by traditional, experimental methods (Silva & Rothbart, 1984)
2. Science as an orderly process, accepted and directed by the discipline and changed by revolution within the discipline (Kuhn, 1970)
3. ". . . science as an economical, problem-solving process that advances in an orderly, progressive fashion" (Riegel et al., 1992, p. 116)
4. Science that takes into account the "influences of gender, culture, society, and shared history" (Riegel et al., 1992, p. 116), as typified by feminism and critical theory perspectives

Thus a nurse scientist-researcher's philosophy of human behavior, health, and patient care guides the intent and direction of a research project. If a researcher thinks that health behaviors can be shaped (reflecting the nature of human beings) and are influenced by the amount of information patients have, investigations of that researcher may focus on the effects of different teaching strategies on specific patient outcomes, for example, an outcome related to specific blood sugar levels in a patient with diabetes who has received a teaching program. Furthermore, the researcher-scientist uses logic and reasoning to organize, formulate, and verify ideas and relationships, a process known as the scientific approach. In this way the investigator's philosophical stance shapes the framework for studying problems.

According to Millor et al. (1992), investigators develop their philosophical stance on the basis of education and experience. In selecting a research approach, the following conditions are considered:

(a) The investigator's perceptions and understanding of life, including a preference for one mode of reasoning as opposed to another;
(b) The level of pre-existing, research-based knowledge about the phenomenon [to be studied];
(c) The specific purpose of the research, that is, to discover, to expand, or to verify information about a phenomenon; and
(d) The ability to obtain information in a manner that will be acceptable as valid, reliable, and meaningful evidence of the phenomenon. (pp. 6-7)

As a research consumer, you can critically appraise the content, methods, and usefulness of research projects in light of the philosophy of science that guides the research. For example, you might ask the following questions:

How does the philosophical perspective of the researcher support the usefulness or benefit of studying the relationship between knowledge (through teaching) and behavior (study outcome) in patients with diabetes?

Does the research reflect a philosophical view of reality as a cause-and-effect relationship or as an interactional relationship?

Does it reflect a philosophical view of human beings that is consistent with the methods used to collect and evaluate data?

On what basis was the type of patient to be studied determined?

Why were identified study outcomes selected?

In the research example cited earlier, would persons with brittle diabetes be appropriate or would a more stable sample provide a better basis for evaluating the teaching strategy in relation to the outcome of blood sugar level?

What content area(s) would be emphasized in the teaching? In other words, what knowledge is essential to impart to a person with diabetes that, if learned and applied, can ultimately produce the desired effect of lowered blood sugar level?

Science can be viewed from two perspectives: as a body of theoretical knowledge (Andreoli & Thompson, 1977; Johnson, 1974) or as a method or process of inquiry (Beckwith & Miller, 1976; Newman, 1979). As a body of knowledge, science is specifically concerned with interrelated principles, laws, and theories, not with random or unrelated data. Viewed as the method or process of inquiry, science becomes the medium for systematically collecting, analyzing, and evaluating data. When defining science, it is useful to include both of these perspectives.

SOURCES OF HUMAN KNOWLEDGE

Ideas are generated in many ways. Some sources of knowledge are highly structured and are generally bound by defined rules of process or method. Examples include scientific inquiry, critical thinking, and logical reasoning. Other sources are less structured and have few defined rules; they include empathy, intuition, trial-and-error experience, and meditation. These approaches are summarized in the box below. Because it is important to nurses as research consumers to know how information is approached in a research or scientific context, several of these sources of knowledge are discussed in this chapter.

APPROACHES TO GENERATING KNOWLEDGE

UNSTRUCTURED	STRUCTURED
Intuition	Induction
Trial and error	Deduction
Tradition	Nursing process
Authority	Research

Unstructured Sources of Knowledge
Intuition

Webster's New Universal Unabridged Dictionary (1983) defines intuition as "the power of knowing, or knowledge obtained, without recourse to inference or reasoning; innate . . . knowledge." Intuition is a frequently used method of problem solving. It can operate in one of two ways: as a form of inference in which intuition closely resembles sensory perception or as an extrasensory experience independent of sensory input. Intuition helps people gain a "deeper understanding of reality than can be obtained from analyzing data" (Noddings & Shore, 1984, p. 21). In describing Aristotle's view of intuition, Noddings and Shore (1984) call it "a leap of understanding, a grasping of a larger concept unreachable by other intellectual means, yet still fundamentally an intellectual process" (p. 8).

Intuition depends on some familiarity with a subject area; ". . . people do not produce 'intuitions' in subject areas where they are ignorant . . . generally, the people most knowledgeable in an area are those who have the most frequent and most reliable intuitions" (Noddings & Shore, 1984, p. 64). Intuitive leaps in science and the arts, made by such people as Albert Einstein and Ludwig van Beethoven, have led to great contributions to humanity. The following situation illustrates an intuitive leap, or an "ah ha," experienced by students enrolled in a course on change theory. Each time the course in change theories and strategies was taught, the instructor listed the stages of the change process. A few years ago a student enthusiastically blurted out, "That's the same as the nursing process," and another student said, "It's also like the research process." Both students expressed an insight; consequently that insight helped them have a clearer understanding of the change process. How many times have you unsuccessfully sought a solution to a problem, only to awaken in the middle of the night with a creative answer? Some people even keep writing materials or a tape recorder near their beds to catch the insights while they are fresh. According to Gortner (1990), "intuition and practical reasoning may well underlie all forms of reasoning including scientific reasoning and the production of scientific knowledge" (p. 103).

In the case of research pursuits, intuition also plays a role. Although intuition is not a sufficient means to approach information in a research context, it can serve as a guiding and creative adjunct. Often, it is an initial "hunch" or inference that leads investigators to the examination of anticipated relationships or a later hunch that opens new avenues for understanding analyzed data. Furthermore, structured processes of inquiry are often complemented by intuitive insights that bring depth and breadth to the total research experience. For example, a nurse senses a pervasive attitude of anxiety among parents of patients who are treated in a particular well-baby clinic. Curious to know whether this situation is typical or atypical, the nurse visits a second well-baby clinic in a nearby town. Although the physical attributes and clientele of the two clinics are similar, intuitively the nurse senses a difference in these settings. This intuition prompts an investigation of what makes these two seemingly similar clinics different.

When you are reviewing research reports, the use of intuition throughout the research process may or may not be apparent. Sometimes the introductory section of a research report identifies how the investigators first became aware of the problem they studied, and this may reflect the use of intuition. Authors do not always include this information in the introduction, nor do they necessarily document insights that arose along the way.

Trial-and-Error Experience

One approach to solving problems of interest to the discipline of nursing is the process of elimination. When a problem is identified, a solution is attempted. Depending on whether the solution works, the practitioner either adopts the trial solution or tries another one. When the second trial solution fails, the practitioner keeps trying, eliminating one possible solution after another until the problem is actually solved. For example, a nurse may try five or six approaches to promoting the healing of a decubitus ulcer before finding the one that works for a particular patient. For another patient with a similar problem the solution found for the first patient may not work, so other trials are implemented until a successful method for groups of similar patients is discovered. This method of problem solving can be inefficient in terms of both time and energy, because it may take a long time to find a successful solution. In addition, that solution may have already been determined by someone else. A more structured approach to evaluating solutions that work would certainly save time, money, and inconvenience to patients. The nurse may wonder whether a solution has already been found and how the trial-and-error method can be shortened. Ways to find out whether alternative solutions exist include reading the literature pertinent to that problem to see what solutions have been determined through research and asking a consultant about possible solutions.

Tradition and Authority

Often people are tricked into believing that something is right or acceptable because it is backed by tradition and authority. When trial-and-error experiences lead to problem resolution, a ready source of known solutions becomes available. That resource pool forms the basis for tradition or precedent. As individuals become more invested in those traditional solutions, the solutions take on an air of authority. In nursing the temperature-taking ritual is an example of this problem-solving evolution from trial and error to authority. In many instances nurses have come to accept that individuals require temperature readings every 4 hours, simply because they are admitted to an acute care facility. The initial rationale for this procedure has been long forgotten, and more current investigations have refuted this practice. In fact some hospitals have discontinued this temperature-taking routine on the basis of their own research. Another example is the procedure used for charting information about patients. Tradition has often dictated the charting procedure(s) used in each health care institution, and although newer methods of charting may have been shown to do a better job of communicating critical information among health care professionals, the institution continues to follow what it sees as "tried and true."

Although it is important to look at what has existed for a long time and listen to what those in authority are saying, both of these sources of knowledge must be critically evaluated in light of other available data, for example, related literature and experts in the field. As research consumers, nurses have a responsibility to examine the validity and applicability of knowledge derived from these sources. They do this by questioning, identifying, and synthesizing all available data sources and noting the ones that clearly and logically support valid solutions. The more research consumers challenge the kind of practice that evolved solely by precedent, the sooner nursing will advance in its development of a scientific basis for practice.

The study by Stewart Fahs and Kinney (1991) exemplifies a challenge to the traditional practice of using the abdomen as the injection site for sodium heparin injections "although the basis for this recommendation is unclear" (p. 204). In this study, low-dose heparin therapy was administered via three different subcutaneous sites, the abdomen, thigh, and arm. The investigators evaluated the effectiveness of these injections in terms of the activated partial thromboplastin time (aPTT), the occurrence of bruising at the injection sites, and the size of bruises at the injection sites. They found that there were no differences in aPTT or bruising at 60 and 72 hours postinjection among the three injection sites. Therefore the traditional practice of abdominal injection of sodium heparin was not supported by research.

Structured Sources of Knowledge

The **scientific approach** or research approach involves the mental processes of logical reasoning concerning the existence and properties of phenomena about which more information, new knowledge, is sought through a systematically planned investigation. Logical reasoning about abstract concepts and empirical observations permit the researcher to consider creatively how best to formulate the scientific inquiry to obtain the desired information.

Logical Reasoning

The two major modes of logical reasoning are inductive and deductive, as reflected in their respective approaches to inquiry, the qualitative and quantitative approaches. As nurses tackle daily problems, they often use these logical approaches or mental operations without realizing it. **Inductive reasoning** involves the observation of a particular set of instances that belong to and can be identified as part of a larger set. This reasoning moves from the particular to the general and underlies qualitative approaches to inquiry (see Chapter 11). On the other hand, **deductive reasoning** uses two or more variables or related statements that, when combined, form the basis for a concluding assertion of a relationship between the variables, called *relational statements*. This reasoning moves from the general to the particular and is typically applied through quantitative inquiry approaches (see Chapters 8 to 10). The two approaches are compared in the box on p. 40.

Inductive reasoning. As stated, inductive reasoning moves from the particular to the general. Conclusions are developed from specific observations. For example, Sigmund Freud gathered much information by listening to his patients report their dreams before drawing conclusions about the symbolism he identified. Two clinical nursing applications of inductive reasoning illustrate how conclusions are derived by this scientific approach to answering questions. In the first applica-

---

DIFFERENCES IN THE RESEARCH PROCESS WHEN USING INDUCTIVE AND DEDUCTIVE REASONING

INDUCTIVE	DEDUCTIVE
State problem	State problem
Review literature	Review literature
Select method	Identify theoretical framework
Collect data	State hypothesis
Analyze data	Select method
Interpret results	Collect data
Develop concepts	Analyze data
Draw conclusions	Accept/reject hypothesis
Examine universality	Interpret results
Create hypotheses	Examine generalizability
Communicate results	Communicate results

---

tion, a nurse may observe that many hospitalized children needing nursing care behave in a particular way and may conclude that the unfamiliar setting of the hospital is stressful to those children. The nurse may arrive at this conclusion by inductively organizing similar bits of information (empirical data) into a more cohesive statement about what those behaviors represent based on existing general knowledge about the behavior of children under stressful conditions. However, one individual with a limited number of patients to observe cannot generalize that the hospital setting is stressful for *all* children. Additional studies of the phenomena in other hospitals will be necessary to confirm that unfamiliarity with hospitalization, rather than illness or uncomfortable treatments, is contributing to the children's behaviors. When study findings are repeatedly observed among other children and in other unfamiliar situations, the practitioners-researchers can make a generalization that hospitalization is stressful for children.

In the second application of inductive reasoning, a nurse may notice that more and more newborns in the nursery are developing rashes on their backs. The nurse may inductively reason that a problem exists with the method of laundering the sheets on which the newborns lie. However, it is not reasonable to conclude that the laundromat is using harsh detergents on all the sheets. The problem may just as well be caused by inadequate rinse water. The nurse can attribute the problem to the method of laundering but has insufficient information to conclude that the detergent is the culprit and is causing skin rashes in the nursery.

Inductive reasoning is exemplified in the qualitative study (see Chapter 11) conducted by Hutchison and Bahr (1991), which focused on caring behaviors demonstrated by elderly nursing home residents. The behavior of elders has been characterized both as socially unproductive and as involved and reaching out to others. Research in gerontology has mainly focused on the former behavior, not the latter. Hutchison and Bahr were interested in identifying the types of caring behaviors engaged in by elders and the personal meaning of these behaviors. Through observation and in-depth interviews of nursing home residents, the researchers were able to identify four types of caring behaviors. They labeled the concepts they discovered as follows:

1. Protecting (for example, verbalizing concern or directing others to a particular place)
2. Supporting (for example, helping someone cope or comforting someone)
3. Confirming (for example, confirming to others that they were respected and cared about)
4. Transcending (for example, praying for the benefit of others)

Hutchison and Bahr (1991) reasoned that these kinds of behaviors were important in maintaining elders' self-esteem, self-identity, and continuation of personhood. They concluded that although their model of caring requires further verification and expansion, it shows how elders in a nursing home setting can engage in meaningful acts of caring and be socially productive. The authors stated:

> This study offers a beginning explanation of the meaning of the concept of care as related to a specific client group that engages in caring behaviors. . . . The current findings as well as others . . . can be used as a base upon which to develop further studies of defining the concepts of care/caring. (p. 88)

The inductive approach, then, begins with an observation or some other way of obtaining information and leads to a conclusion. When conclusions are arrived at using very specific or limited data, results may be narrowly focused and erroneous. "Research using inductive reasoning based on naturalistic observations and field notes has a respected place in modern science, going back at least as far as the nineteenth-century biologists. . . . [This is] a uniquely human form of data" (Schumacher & Gortner, 1992, p. 5).

Deductive reasoning. Deductive reasoning moves from the general to the particular. A specific **hypothesis** (prediction) can be deduced from a theory or an organizing statement about abstract concepts that serves as a more general statement or network of interrelated concepts (see Chapter 7). As a result of deduction, observations can be made and predictions tested. Rather than generating or discovering sources of new information, deductive reasoning can serve as an approach to unveiling and confirming existing relationships. For example, if it is known that theory R has been substantiated, the nurse researcher could anticipate what outcomes and behaviors are logically expected. The following are examples of how a nurse can use deductive reasoning.

1. It is known that certain physiological changes take place in bedridden clients as a result of continuous or uneven pressure to bony prominences. A nurse could deduce that pressure-relieving methods will decrease the incidence and intensity of decubitus ulcer development. In research-based practice the nurse would apply this knowledge of specific relationships to the prevention of decubiti by relieving pressure on a client's bony prominences.
2. The gate control theory of pain identifies the interaction of motivational,

affective, and sensory processing that modulates the perception of and response to pain. According to that theory, such variables as anxiety, attention, age, culture, meaning of the present pain experience, and pathophysiological findings are associated with the pain experience. Since anxiety and the pain sensation tend to reinforce each other, thereby increasing the intensity of the pain experience, the nurse could deduce that anxiety-reducing measures such as empathic interaction, a back rub, an explanation to the patient, and prompt administration of pain medication would result in decreased pain. If the nurse wanted to know which of these methods worked best to relieve distress in patients with certain painful conditions, a research study could be designed to test which of the hypothesized or predicted relationships between pain relief method and relief would be confirmed.

3. Social support can be viewed as "a characteristic of the social situation that buffers the effect of stress on the health of the individual" (Northouse, 1988). In other words, social support helps an individual to see an event as less stressful, so the person can cope with it more effectively. One stressful situation that affects the health of an individual is breast cancer. On the basis of what is known about social support and its effects on stress and health, a researcher studying the adjustment of women to mastectomy might deduce that breast cancer patients who receive social support after mastectomy would have fewer adjustment problems than those who do not receive social support.

Becker, Grunwald, Moorman, and Stuhr (1991) conducted a quasiexperimental clinical study (see Chapter 9) that evolved through deductive reasoning. The following statements show how logical deduction was used by these investigators to develop their study of very-low-birth-weight infants:

1. The relatively high incidence of deficits in information processing and attention-related disorders at preschool and school ages [in children who were premature infants] . . . may represent injury to the developing brain resulting from the stressful nature of the intensive care environment;

2. There is accumulating evidence that the NICU [neonatal intensive care unit] environment is more apt to involve sensory overload than deprivation, exposing the infant to experiences that are not only stressful but also inappropriate;

3. It has been shown that even very fragile infants can communicate both positive and negative reactions through motor behavior, postural tone, facial expression, and alterations in behavioral state, as well as through autonomic and visceral responses, and that this behavioral repertoire can be reliably assessed;

4. It is postulated that individualizing care based on the infant's cues has the potential not only to avoid behavioral and physiological disorganization but also to enhance the normal development of the infant's physiological, motor, state, and interactive systems. (pp. 150-151)

On the basis of their observations and documented research findings, the researchers deduced that a program of nursing staff education (with ongoing support from and consultation with a neonatal clinician and occupational therapist) for the purpose of implementing an individualized developmental care plan could significantly improve such outcomes as respiratory status, feeding status, weight gain, length of hospital stay, behavioral organization, and degree of morbidity.

As with inductive reasoning, there may be inherent problems in using the deductive approach. First, not all deductions can be verified, particularly when the measurement methods are poor or undeveloped. Second, a deduction that is based on a tentative premise may result in a conclusion that is logically valid, yet unsound. Third, an unsound conclusion may be assumed sound, especially if it seems reasonable. If a systematic, scientific approach is used to test a prediction deduced from a theory, the conclusion is more likely to be sound and to be useful to the discipline.

Scientific Approach

The scientific approach is a system of logical and orderly elements that direct a formal, structured inquiry process in the effort to obtain knowledge. By combining several elements, such as logical reasoning, order and control, empiricism, and generalization, sophisticated systems of inquiry have been developed. **Research** is accepted as a scientific approach to knowledge generation when the processes that are used adhere to principles of logic, standards for data collection and analysis, absence of investigator bias, and rules governing generalizability or universality of findings. This is obviously a complex system of interrelated components.

Scholars of each discipline determine which scientific approach will yield reasonable and useful information to expand the empirical knowledge upon which a discipline builds its scientific base. In nursing, no single approach has gained acceptance as the primary one to be used to generate knowledge. The nursing discipline is embedded in both practice and science, and these shape the philosophical stance and research approaches that are accepted by the discipline as ways of generating scientific information (Riegel et al., 1992).

In evaluating reported studies for the investigators' adherence to the scientific approach, research consumers ask such questions as the following: What controls were in effect for this study? What research method was used? How was the sample selected, and was it representative of the defined population? Was the approach carried out in logical, orderly, objective fashion?

Scientific approach and nursing process. The research and nursing processes are both used to solve problems. They require specific steps of inquiry, obtaining and making sense of information, making decisions about the meaning and usefulness of the results of the research study or intervention, and ultimately communicating the new information to colleagues. Wide dissemination of new knowledge enables other practitioners or scientists to test hypotheses further or evaluate the intervention with similar or diverse samples (replication of studies), which will then confirm or refute the generalizability of this knowledge. The information derived from the research process contributes to building the discipline's scientific base, and the nursing process contributes to advancing nursing practice in a specific context.

The scientific approach to knowledge generation through research and the nursing process of problem solving are similar in that they both involve the following:

1. Observation and the recording of empirical information concerning the phenomenon or problem being described or measured
2. Analysis and classification of information (data)
3. Conclusions derived from the data about the phenomenon or the problem and its solution
4. Further testing of hypotheses or evaluation of interventions

The effectiveness of the research or the nursing process is contingent upon the user's logical organization of each process, that is, the congruency between existing knowledge or theory and the approach selected to answer the research question or to develop an intervention. When planning a study, for example, the researcher does a thorough review and critique of the relevant nursing and nonnursing scientific literature to identify what is already known and what specific gaps in knowledge exist regarding the problem to be studied (see Chapter 5). The nurse, because of constraints of time or of access to the literature, relies on widely known scientific information and prior experience to apply the nursing process to an individual or a group of patients. The absence of a complete literature review limits the nurse's or the researcher's ability to relate the data to prior knowledge, which could guide the design of an intervention or a research study.

The primary differences between these two processes are strict application of scientific versus clinical methods and control over the phenomenon. In the scientific process the investigator is expected to adhere strictly to the rules and steps of a specific research approach and attempt to control any circumstances that might contribute to any change in the phenomenon, regardless of the intervention. That is, the researcher wants to be certain that the intervention, not some other extraneous factor(s), is responsible for the outcome or change in study participants, so he or she adheres to standards for administering the data collection and analytical procedures. The nurse, unlike the scientist, is unable to exert the same degree of control over the situation or patients for which interventions are provided. However, the nurse can provide clinical interventions in a consistent manner from patient to patient with the same nursing diagnoses when evaluating planned changes in nursing care for a group of patients, and the nurse can draw conclusions about the usefulness of the intervention for other, similar patients. In this manner the nurse applies principles of the scientific approach to advancing nursing practice.

The scientific approach has limitations; among them are moral and ethical constraints, difficulty ensuring precise measurement and control, and problems associated with performing research on human subjects (see Chapters 12 and 13). However, the scientific approach has been found to be more useful and predictive than other sources of human knowledge, such as intuition, trial and error, or tradition and authority.

CRITICAL ELEMENTS IN RESEARCH INQUIRY

For research to yield results that are minimally biased by investigative processes, the researcher pursues a logical inquiry process and applies research methods that increase the likelihood that the data collected are truly representative of the phenomenon. There are standard procedures and research methods of data collection and analysis. These are selected by the researcher to optimize the outcomes; that is, research methods are chosen that will best answer the question or test the hypotheses. Research designs and methods are described in later chapters. For now, it is important to discuss critical elements of any research investigation that influence credibility.

Order and Control

As a systematic method of problem solving, the scientific approach requires the use of clearly delineated, ordered steps. For example, when a researcher begins the deductive inquiry process, a thorough search of the literature is always made (see Chapter 5). Not only does this search inform the researcher about prior research on a particular phenomenon, but also it shapes the decision about which research design and methods are appropriate to the research problem or question (see Chapters 8 to 11). Similarly, an investigator cannot draw conclusions before collected data are analyzed (see Chapters 16 and 17). This predetermined system of orderly steps guides a research study so that consumers have greater confidence in the investigator's predictions and outcomes. When reviewing a research report, the research consumer should look for the investigator's problem statement, research methods, results, and conclusions to see whether they adhere to the expected order in conceptualizing and carrying out the study. The specific rationale and design criteria for studies using varied approaches are discussed in Chapters 8 to 11.

Although total control is almost impossible to achieve, control is an important facet of research, particularly research in which a deductive approach is used, such as experimental studies. To isolate and study specific variables that represent abstract concepts, it is necessary to control as completely as possible the influences, events, and conditions that can alter the theorized relationships. For example, it is known that pain perception is influenced by age, sex, culture, and other factors. In examining the relationship between self-esteem and pain perception, the investigator must specify which age-group, sex, and culture will be included and excluded (delimited). An alternate approach would be to select a large sample reflecting a variety of ages, sexes, and cultures (a heterogeneous sample) (see Chapter 12). Then the data could be analyzed for both the total sample and each of the influencing factors (variables). These analyses would yield information about the strength of each factor in terms of study outcomes. Research consumers need to determine the nature and extent of control in sampling and procedures used to collect data. For example, was the sample representative of the defined population or was there bias in the selection process? Were the data collection procedures administered under identical conditions for all research subjects?

Empiricism

Empiricism refers to information that is described or observed and can be verified. It is also the component of the scientific approach that is objective or real.

In research approached through deductive reasoning, reality is usually defined as what can be measured directly or indirectly by instruments that are free from bias that may be introduced by either the investigator or the subject(s) regarding the variables being examined in the study. In studies approached through inductive reasoning, reality is defined by the perceptions of the participants (subjects) as these are verbalized to the investigator. In both approaches, findings are grounded in the reality of the phenomenon and observations are made and verified on the basis of actual information, not on the basis of personal beliefs or biases of the researcher. The research consumer evaluates how well the investigator captured the reality of the information collected (see Chapters 12, 14, and 15 for discussions of sampling and measurement).

Generalization

One goal of science is to understand relationships among phenomena in order to be able to **generalize**, that is, to predict future outcomes and relationships (see Chapters 8 and 18). Focusing on isolated events does not make it possible to "explain a wide variety of phenomena in a manner that consistently holds and therefore is not tentative" (Chinn & Kramer, 1991, p. 61). The following example clarifies the intent of generalization.

When nurse researchers wanted to learn whether implementing an individualized, developmental approach to nursing care of low-birth-weight babies in a neonatal intensive care unit (NICU) would enhance the infants' development, they designed a clinical study that specified the nursing intervention behaviors in five areas: two aimed at reducing the stress in the environmental context of the infants' care, and three aimed at caring behaviors designed to promote sleep-wake organization, gross motor development, and development of feeding behaviors in the infants (Becker, Grunwald, Moorman, & Stuhr, 1991). Outcome data indicate that light and noise levels decreased as indicators of developmentally facilitative nursing behaviors and infant outcomes, such as morbidity, length of hospitalization, and age at first oral feeding, were lower in the group of infants who received the individualized, developmental approach to care compared with the infants who did not receive this care. The differences between the two groups supported the conclusion that "a developmental approach to nursing care of very-low-birth-weight infants can have a positive impact on their progress during hospitalization" (Becker et al., 1991, p. 153). The results suggest that the benefits of an individualized nursing care strategy provided to a group of NICU infants can be generalized to other hospitalized low-birth-weight infants. The generalization can be validated through similar studies in other NICUs. Although knowledge that an individualized care plan for a specific infant can facilitate development is important clinically, research-based information about the positive outcomes of a strategic, organized approach to caring for a group of infants has a wider application for nursing practice.

Questions that elicit information about generalization include the following: When and to whom do the conclusions apply? What are the limits and scope of the findings? Did the investigator generalize beyond the sample on which the study was based? Did the sample include the appropriate referent subjects? The following questions may clarify the latter: If a laboratory sample was studied, was the generalization inappropriately extended to include a clinical population? If the study involved subjects from a predominantly Caucasian population, was the generalization extended to all ethnic groups? If only young adults were sampled, were conclusions generalized to older adults (see Chapter 12)?

Theory

A **theory** can be defined as an organizing statement about abstract concepts that gives them meaning in relation to the real world. Theories describe, explain, or predict relationships among abstract concepts. Abstract concepts are mental images of reality; they may be highly abstract and nonobservable, such as intelligence, or relatively concrete and directly measurable, such as caring behaviors. Theories are linked to the real world through definitions that specify how concepts will be known, experienced, observed, and measured. Theories guide decision making by providing the "supporting conceptualizations for the study, such as, 'significance of the problem,' 'background,' and 'problem definitions or statement of the problem' " (Phillips, 1986, p. 111).

As current research findings are linked to knowledge of the concepts as reported in the literature, a body of scientific knowledge about a phenomenon accumulates. Theories are always evolving as new information is discovered or verified about particular concepts through both inductive and deductive research. In research conducted through the discovery or inductive approach, theories are derived from conceptual clustering of the actual data. The conceptual reasoning about the observations is usually linked to a broad, highly developed theoretical base, for example, role theory or caring. What is discovered must be verified, what is verified must be tested to establish the validity and reliability of the information, and so the process of theory development continues. New knowledge becomes accepted by members of a discipline who decide that the information contributes to their particular science or matrix, the "structure and tradition that lends a unique identity to the discipline" (Riegel et al., 1992, p. 117).

A theory that comprises abstract concepts provides a framework for the deductive approach to research by guiding the selection of research variables. Variable selection in the study of the coping behaviors of children with diabetes (Grey, Cameron, & Thurber, 1991), for example, was directed by existing theories of coping and adaptation, and particular attention was paid to substantiating empirically that developmental maturation influences coping processes. Developmental maturation was measured by using the children's chronological ages, and a standardized method was used to assign levels of pubertal growth.

Theory also guides decision making with regard to subsequent interpretation of results. In the Hutchison and Bahr (1991) caring study, their review of the literature provided descriptions of the concept of caring as developed and researched by others. Although this information did not direct variable selection, the researchers found that their inductive clustering of the data resulted in a conceptual model of caring similar to what had been reported in the literature. They interpreted this similarity as evidence of the universality of the structure and meaning of their theory of caring.

A number of nursing theories further exemplify how theories provide a framework for the research process. Nursing theories and theoretical models are congruent with the discipline's beliefs that human phenomena result from the interaction of the holistic person with social and environmental circumstances and that these interactions can promote or discourage health (Meleis, 1985). The various nursing theorists define these concepts clearly and describe the conceptual linkages in their respective theories.

King's Theory of Goal Attainment

King's theory of goal attainment (1986) was derived from the interpersonal system component of her Interacting Systems Conceptual Framework. The theory proposes that:

> . . . nurse and client interactions are characterized by verbal and nonverbal communication, in which information is exchanged and interpreted; by transactions, in which values, needs, and wants of each member of the dyad are shared; by perceptions of nurse and client and the situation; by self in role of client and self in role of nurse; and by stressors influencing each person and the situation in time and space. (King, 1981, p. 144).

Hypotheses derived from the propositions of this theory include the following (King, 1986):

> Goal attainment will be greater in patients who participate in mutual goal setting than in patients who do not participate.
>
> Mutual goal setting will increase the morale of elderly patients.
>
> Goal attainment decreases stress and anxiety.
>
> Goal attainment increases patients' learning and coping abilities in nursing situations. (p. 206)

Theories Developed From Orem's Self-Care Conceptual Framework

Three theories developed from Orem's Self-Care Conceptual Framework are the theory of self-care deficit, the theory of self-care, and the theory of nursing systems (Orem, 1991). The theory of self-care proposes that "self-care and care of dependent family members are learned behaviors that purposely regulate human structural integrity, functioning, and human development" (Orem, 1991, p. 69). From the theory of self-care, Orem (1991) proposed that "the individual's abilities to engage in self-care or dependent care are conditioned by age, developmental state, life experience, sociocultural orientation, health, and available resources" (p. 71). Hypothesis testing of this **proposition,** or linking of concepts, of Orem's framework is in the early stages of development. The characteristics of self-care behaviors among older adults are described in a study derived from Orem's concept of self-care requisites (Conn, 1991).

Roy Adaptation Model

Individual theories of the four adaptive modes of the Roy Adaptation Model, that is, physiological, self-concept, role function, and interdependence, have been developed. A proposition taken from the theory of interdependence states that "adequacy of seeking nurturance and nurturing positively influences interdependence" (Roy & Roberts, 1981, p. 277). A hypothesis developed from the theory of independence is the following: "If the nurse provides time and space for private family visits, the patient will demonstrate more appropriate attention-seeking behavior" (Roy & Roberts, 1981, p. 280).

A more detailed discussion of the theoretical framework is provided in Chapter 6. As a research consumer, you might ask the following questions: Is the theoretical rationale explicitly stated? Are the hypotheses explicitly substantiated, that is, are they grounded in the theory? Are the concepts defined and measured in a manner consistent with the theory?

Assumptions about Reality and Causality (Determinism)

An **assumption** is a basic principle about existence that is accepted as true, with no need for scientific proof. The abstract concepts embedded in assumptions are independent of an individual's perceptions. That people will have pain during their lives, that people are mortal, that self-actualization motivates behavior (Maslow, 1970), and that prenatal role sufficiency influences the transition to maternal role (Gaffney, 1992) are all assumptions. The first two assumptions are broad and apply to humans in general; the last two are part of the foundations of specific theories. An underlying assumption of Rogers (1991) espouses a particular view of human beings as more than and different from the sum of their parts. This underlying assumption is one of several that form the basis for testing relationships using Rogers' conceptual model of unitary human beings. Hypotheses based on this model are concerned with the nature of the self and personal growth, which evolve through mutual process between person and environment.

Determinism is an assumption related to causality of events and situations. In the traditional scientific explanation of causality the world is conceptualized as real, that is, observable and in some manner measurable, orderly, and predictable. This conceptualization assumes that an intervention determines an outcome and that the causal relationship can be known. For example, cancer may be the result of several phenomena such as smoking and exposure to certain chemicals and pollutants, and the inflammatory response occurs as a result of the presence of certain conditions. This example of linear reasoning is associated with the traditional, deductive approach to science. Not all persons who have contact with these precausal conditions, however, develop cancer. Can other explanations of carcinogenesis exist? Can conditions of the person or of interactional processes influence health outcomes? The traditional assumption about causal relationships has been challenged in favor of assumptions about mutual process among phenomena from which new phenomena emerge. Beliefs about humans and the universe of experiences that are elements of both Rogers' (1992) theory of unitary human beings and Watson's (1985) theory of human caring permit the nurse-scientist to consider nondeterministic approaches to explaining the existence of human situations.

Assumptions are not always stated in an obvious way. They may be implicit rather than explicit, and the research consumer asks whether the assumptions are implicit or explicit when examining the underlying values and beliefs about the problem being investigated. The research consumer should also identify what the value orientation is and whether there are logical consistencies between the assumptions. These questions are essential to examining the conceptual operations that shape the investigator's approach to a study and to judging whether the conclusions are reasonable.

THE RELATIONSHIP BETWEEN THEORY AND METHOD

Consistency and congruence between the conceptual reasoning and the overall study design, its conduct, and its interpretation of the results are critical elements in the research process. As stated earlier, relationships are examined by testing hypotheses that are based on propositions, which are linkages of concepts (see Chapter 6) derived from a theoretical framework. Such examination takes place under the aegis of order and control, empiricism, assumptions, theory, and generalization.

When little is known about a phenomenon, research is usually conducted for the purpose of discovery and exploration of descriptions of the phenomenon as it occurs in the natural world. At this level of inquiry the researcher may use either inductive or deductive logic to organize the study. As research-based information becomes available, quantitative research methods are used to test the hypothetical relationships among concepts by means of deductive methods of data collection and analysis. A variety of methods can be used to address the problem under study; however, there must be consistency between the hypothesis and the type of method used. To verify hypotheses, an overall method for gathering and processing information must be implemented. That method must also operate in a systematic, controlled way to ensure that "the reality indicators for the conceptual relationship specified by the theory are valid" (Chinn & Kramer, 1991, p. 94). Fig. 2-1 illustrates the components or "links" of the research process that connect theory with method. There must also be logical, conceptual consistency from each one of these important links to the next.

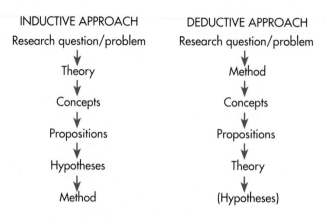

INDUCTIVE APPROACH	DEDUCTIVE APPROACH
Research question/problem	Research question/problem
Theory	Method
Concepts	Concepts
Propositions	Propositions
Hypotheses	Theory
Method	(Hypotheses)

Fig. 2-1   Links between theory and method.

A study in which a deductive approach is used is described here to further clarify the link between theory and method. In the earlier section on theories, the relationships among abstract concepts, hypotheses, and variable selection were discussed. Now, the focus is on linking those elements in the research process with data collection and analysis and interpreting the results. When the results are not consistent with what the theory had led the investigator to believe was true about the phenomenon, the investigator critically reexamines the original conceptualization of the study and methodological procedures to see whether limitations in either concepts or methods may have influenced results.

In a study of children's coping with diabetes (Grey et al., 1991) the investigators defined the concepts of coping and adaptation on the basis of a review of the literature. They "proposed that adaptation would be influenced by age, coping behaviors, and self-care behaviors" (p. 144). They selected a questionnaire to measure coping behaviors, which included items consistent with the concepts identified in the theoretical framework, and used behavioral items that were age-appropriate for the children in the study. Similarly, questionnaires were used to measure the children's social adaptation. In the discussion of the results the investigators explained the ways in which their findings were consistent and inconsistent with the theoretical framework. They noted that, as expected, there were age differences in coping and adaptation. The investigators could not conclude, however, that differences in adaptation could be attributed to development rather than to the illness process, because the study lacked a comparison group. They provided specific suggestions for future research studies to create additional explanatory information about children's coping with stress and illness. Their discussion of the results revealed the continuity of theoretically derived concepts and logical reasoning throughout the study.

When an investigation is undertaken from the inductive perspective, the relationship between theory and methods proceeds from empirical data collection and content analysis to the discovery of abstract concepts that best capture both the objective and subjective aspects of the phenomenon. As in deductive studies, specific methodological procedures for data collection and analysis are followed, and from them new concepts emerge. The investigator compares these concepts with what has been reported in the literature in order to demonstrate the congruence between the new conceptualizations and what is already known about the phenomenon. When the findings are discrepant with what is already known, the investigator reviews the original design and methods for limitations, such as misclassification of the data or other limitations related to the occurrence of the phenomenon. It is critical to the acceptance of this new theoretical knowledge that the investigator's inductive reasoning be logical, that the concepts be specific to the findings, and that the conclusions make sense.

An example of how the conceptual and research processes of an inductive study reveal the fit between theory and method is demonstrated in the study "Quality of life of hospitalized persons with AIDS" (Ragsdale, Kotarba, & Morrow, 1992). The researchers' conceptualizations of the problem of living with acquired immunodeficiency syndrome (AIDS) and quality of life were consistent with a nursing philosophy related to holistic human life and provided the philosophical organization for their study. Their discussion of what was already known justified their asking the question "What is the quality of life from the perspective of the hospitalized person with AIDS?" The central theme, labeled "management style," emerged from the clustering of interview and observational data. The theme was conceptualized and defined as "efforts to generate and maintain a semblance of control" over the meanings of the participants' lives and what they were experiencing (Ragsdale et al., 1992, p. 261). Although the six identified management styles seemed independent of treatment regimes, the researchers noted that the voluntary nature of the sample precluded accepting the universality of the central theme or theory. The study concepts seem logically derived from the data. The researchers' discussion of the implications of their concepts for nursing practice suggests hypotheses about the interactions between nurses and AIDS patients with each management style. This study of persons with AIDS illustrates how the cycle of knowledge development proceeds from holistic exploratory inductive inquiry to description and testing of specific interactional hypotheses about nurse-patient relationships arising from that theory.

When links between theory and methods are made explicit in a research report, it is easier for the research consumer to examine the study for definitional consistency and congruency of the concepts in the theoretical framework with their application or derivation through data collection, analysis, and interpretation of the results. Some questions to ask include the following: Are the analytic methods appropriate to answer the research questions or test the hypotheses? Is the interpretation of the results congruent with the conclusions? Was the research carried out in a logical, orderly process so that the findings are believable? The greater the conceptual integrity, the more likely that the conclusions will be accepted as true, representative, and useful by members of the discipline.

KEY POINTS

- It has been demonstrated that knowledge generated through structured approaches is more likely to be valid and generalizable than that which is arrived at through intuition, authority, or trial and error.
- The relationship between the philosophy of nursing, which values humans as holistic, interacting persons, and science as both process and product underlies nursing's efforts to create a unique body of knowledge. The scientific approaches used to generate nursing knowledge reflect both inductive and deductive conceptualizations of phenomena and utilize varied research methods developed within other disciplines but applied from the unique nursing perspective of the discipline's researchers.
- Theories help to organize the discipline, both in practice and in research endeavors, by providing explanations and making predictive statements about concepts.
- Concept formulation and concept testing are purposes of nursing research. These theoretical conceptualizations permit nursing to propose assumptions from which the evolving science will grow.
- Consistency and congruency in the development and use of nursing concepts and

their validation through credible research will contribute to the quality of nursing's scientific base and to the acceptance of new knowledge within the discipline and by other scientists.

REFERENCES

Andreoli, K., & Thompson, C. (1977). The nature of science in nursing. *Image, 9,* 32-37.

Becker, P.T., Grunwald, P.C., Moorman, J., & Stuhr, S. (1991). Outcomes of developmentally supportive nursing care for very-low-birth-weight infants. *Nursing Research, 40*(3), 150-155.

Beckwith, J., & Miller, L. (1976). Behind the mask of objective science. *The Sciences, 16,* 16-19.

Chinn, P., & Kramer, M. (1991). *Theory and nursing: A systematic approach* 3rd ed. St. Louis: Mosby.

Conn, V. (1991). Self-care actions taken by older adults for influenza and colds. *Nursing Research, 40*(3), 176-181.

Gaffney, K. (1992). Nursing practice model for maternal role sufficiency. *Advances in Nursing Science, 15*(2), 76-84.

Gortner, S.R. (1990). Nursing values and science: Toward a science philosophy. *Image, 22*(2), 101-105.

Grey, M. Cameron, M.E., & Thurber, F.W. (1991). Coping and adaptation in children with diabetes. *Nursing Research, 40*(3), 144-149.

Hutchison, C., & Bahr, R.T. (1991). Types and meanings of caring behaviors among elderly nursing home residents. *Image, 23*(2), 85-88.

Johnson, D. (1974). Development of theory: A requisite for nursing as a primary health profession. *Nursing Research, 23,* 372-377.

King, T. (1981). *A theory for nursing: Systems, concepts, process.* New York: John Wiley & Sons.

King, T. (1986). King's theory of goal attainment. In P. Winstead-Fry (Ed.), *Case studies in nursing theory* (pp. 197-312). New York: National League for Nursing.

Kuhn, T. (1970). *The structure of scientific revolutions.* Chicago: University of Chicago Press.

Maslow, A. (1970). *Motivation and personality.* New York: Harper & Row.

Meleis, A.I. (1985). *Theoretical nursing: Development and progress.* Philadelphia: J.B. Lippincott.

Millor, G.K., Haber, J.E., Carter, E., Feldman, H.R., Hott, J.R., & Jacobson, L. (1992). What is nursing research: Evolving approaches to methods and content. *Journal of the New York State Nurses Association, 23*(3), 4-9.

Newman, M. (1979). *Theory development in nursing.* Philadelphia: F.A. Davis.

Noddings, N., & Shore, P.J. (1984). *Awakening the inner eye.* New York: Teachers College Press.

Northouse, L. (1988). Social support in patients' and husbands' adjustment to breast cancer. *Nursing Research, (1991). 37,* 91-95.

Orem, D. *Nursing: Concepts of practice* (4th ed.). St. Louis: Mosby.

Phillips, L.R. (1986). *A clinician's guide to the critique and utilization of nursing research.* Norwalk, CT: Appleton & Lange.

Ragsdale, D., Kotarba, J., & Morrow, J. (1992). Quality of life in hospitalized persons with AIDS. *Image, 24*(4), 259-265.

Riegel, B., Omery, A., Calvillo, E., Elsayed, N.G., Lee, P., Shuler, P., & Siegal, B.E. (1992). Moving beyond: A generative philosophy of science. *Image, 24*(2), 115-120.

Rogers, M.E. (1992). Nursing science and the space age. *Nursing Science Quarterly, 5:*1, 27-34.

Roy, C., & Roberts, S. (1981). *Theory construction in nursing: An adaptation model.* Englewood Cliffs, NJ: Prentice-Hall.

Schumacher, K.L., & Gortner, S.R. (1992). (Mis)conceptions and reconceptions about traditional science. *Advances in Nursing Science, 14*(4), 1-11.

Silva, M. (1977). Philosophy, science, theory: Interrelationships and implications for nursing research. *Image, 9,* 59-63.

Silva, M.C., & Rothbart, D. (1984). An analysis of changing trends in philosophies of science on nursing theory development and testing. *Advances in Nursing Science, 6*(2), 1-13.

Stewart Fahs, P.S., & Kinney, M.R. (1991). The abdomen, thigh, and arm as sites for subcutaneous sodium heparin injections. *Nursing Research, 40*(4), 204-207.

Watson, J. (1985). *Nursing: Human science and human care.* Norwalk, CT: Appleton-Century-Crofts.

Webster's new universal unabridged dictionary (deluxe 2nd ed.). (1983). Ohio, Dorset & Baber.

ADDITIONAL READINGS

Agor, W.H. (1986). *The logic of intutitive decision making.* New York: Quorum Books.

Broome, M.E., Lillis, P.P., & Smith, M.C. (1989). Pain interventions with children: A meta-analysis of research. *Nursing Research, 38,* 154-158.

Cohen, L.J. (1989). *An introduction to the philosophy of induction and probability.* Oxford: Clarendon Press.

Fawcett, J. (1989). *Analysis and evaluation of conceptual models of nursing* (2nd ed.). Philadelphia: F.A. Davis.

Hinds, P.S. (1989). Method triangulation to index change in clinical phenomena. *The Western Journal of Nursing Research, 11,* 440-447.

Howson, C., & Urbach, P. (1989). *Scientific reasoning: The bayesian approach.* La Salle, IL: Open Court.

Hyman, R.B., Feldman, H.R., Harris, R.B., Levin, R.F., & Mallory, G.B. (1989). The effects of relaxation training on clinical symptoms: A meta-analysis. *Nursing Research, 38,* 216-220.

Kidd, P., & Morrison, E.F. (1988). The progression of knowledge in nursing: A search for meaning. *Image, 20*(4), 222-224.

Schultz, P.R., & Meleis, A.I. (1988). Nursing epistemology: Traditions, insights, questions. *Image, 20*(4), 217-221.

Strauss, A., & Corbin, J. (1990). *Basics of qualitative research: Grounded theory, procedures, and techniques.* Newbury Park, CA: Sage Publications.

3

The Evolution of Research: From Science to Practice

CAROL ANN MITCHELL

LEARNING OBJECTIVES

After reading this chapter the student should be able to do the following:

- Value research participation and use of research findings to improve nursing practice and patient outcomes.
- Cite examples of research findings that have contributed to improvements in nursing practice, patient outcomes, and health policy.
- Use research utilization criteria to determine the applicability of findings in various practice environments and with different patient groups.
- Evaluate clinical environments that facilitate or hinder the use of research findings in nursing practice.
- Select strategies and resources to promote research utilization.
- Use research findings to improve nursing practice and influence health policies.

KEY TERMS

basic research   research utilization
downlink   uplink
replication

The knowledgeable consumer of research becomes part of an extraordinary professional cycle by contributing to the development and refinement of nursing theory, practice, and research. Why? Because, according to Dickoff and James (1968), theory is born in practice, is refined in research, and returns to improve practice. If research is not returned to practice, it is only draining off energy from the main business of nursing; theory then becomes nothing more than idle speculation or personal opinion. Bock (1990) predicts that better patient care will result when research findings are translated into daily nursing practice, suggesting that nursing research should be conducted primarily to bring about improvement in delivery of nursing care. This chapter gives evidence that this prediction is accurate.

The succeeding chapters provide background for understanding the central purpose of research utilization in nursing and its importance in improving outcomes of care, including quality and cost-effectiveness, and influencing health policy. This background is essential for understanding the research process and developing evaluation skills needed to judge the merit and relevance of research findings before attempting to apply them in clinical practice.

This chapter emphasizes critical thinking and the importance of research utilization and provides decision-making models for choosing studies to be considered for use in clinical practice. Numerous examples are given of how nurses who conduct research and clinicians who use research findings make a difference in developing nursing science, professional credibility, and influence on policies that affect nursing care and patient outcomes.

THE WHAT AND WHY OF RESEARCH UTILIZATION

In Chapter 1, **research utilization** is defined as a systematic method of implementing sound, research-based innovations in clinical practice, evaluating the outcomes, and sharing the knowledge through the process of research dissemination. Communicating findings regarding the success or failure in implementing research innovations is essential so that nursing interventions can be modified, improved, or, as necessary, abandoned. In 1974, Gortner proposed that the quality of nursing care would not improve until scientific accountability was as valued as humanitarianism in nursing.

Much momentum has been gained in using research findings in nursing practice. Nurses must remember that as professionals they are accountable to the public who are the consumers of health care and for the scientific basis of nursing practice. This in no way means that all nurses must *conduct* research. Rather, it means that all nurses must *use* research as the foundation for clinical practice. Through utilization of research findings the quality of care provided by nurses improves because care is based on empirical findings—findings that demonstrate which interventions are effective and which are not.

When decisions about nursing care delivery and choice of nursing interventions are based on research data, the profession is positioned to have a greater impact on health care by demonstrating how nursing care can make a difference. In an era of spiraling health care costs, when containing costs while maintaining or improving quality is a crucial issue, it is essential that the nursing profession provide evidence that it *does* make a difference. Using research findings that document cost-effective quality outcomes as the basis of nursing practice is one way to accomplish this goal (Feldman, Penney, Haber, Hott, & Jacobson, 1993). The following examples illustrate this idea.

Consider the study by Stewart Fahs and Kinney (1991) (see Appendix A), which sought to determine whether there would be any differences in occurrence or size of bruising when heparin was administered in sites other than the traditional abdominal site, and whether administration in other sites would affect the goals of therapy as measured by the activated partial thromboplastin time (aPTT). The findings of their study demonstrated no significant differences in either occurrence or size of bruising or changes in aPTT in relation to differing sites. These findings provide nurses with outcome data that support scientifically based clinical decision making rather than adherence to tradition. Although the data from this research study have definite potential for use in practice, changes in hospital policy will not and should not occur as a result of one study. Replication of this study is necessary to build an adequate knowledge base for implementation in practice, one that has been systematically evaluated over time.

In another study Kruszewski, Lang, and Johnson (1979) examined the effect of positioning on discomfort caused by intramuscular injections in the dorsogluteal site. Findings demonstrated that internal rotation of the femur during injection into the dorsogluteal site, with the client in either the prone or the side-lying position, reduced discomfort from the injection. This is an example of a research-based nursing intervention that is simple for an individual nurse to implement at no harm or cost to the patient. Failure to use this innovation has potential effects on patient discomfort and may well contribute to a patient's dissatisfaction with care (Brett, 1987).

A third study, a large-scale, randomized clinical trial prompted by concerns about the risks of heparin-induced thrombocytopenia (HITP), evaluated the effects of heparinized and non-heparinized flush solutions on the patency of arterial pressure monitoring lines in 5139 subjects from 198 participating sites (American Association of Critical-Care Nurses, 1993).

The findings of this study, known as the Thunder Project, indicate that arterial pressure monitoring lines maintained with heparinized flush solutions have a significantly greater probability of remaining patent over time than lines maintained with non-heparinized flush solutions. In addition to heparin, four other variables significantly influenced the probability of lines remaining patent: receiving other anticoagulants, having a catheter longer than 2 inches, a femoral insertion site, and male gender. The results of this study are different from those reported in studies examining the effect of heparinized versus non-heparinized flush solutions on intravenous peripheral access devices (IVPAD) (Goode et al., 1991), which report no significant difference in patency between heparinized and non-heparinized flush solutions (see Chapter 1).

The authors conclude that clinicians will need to make decisions about the risks of HITP compared with the risks of nonpatency of the arterial line. When long-term patency is critical, decisions may be different from those made when short-term use is contemplated. Clinicians will now have research data on which to base those decisions.

Rather than basing nursing care on the sacred cows of tradition, authority, and trial-and-error experience, nurses can use the findings of these and other research studies to validate the merit of current practice and provide the basis for decision making about making changes in practice (see Chapter 2). Such changes should be reflected in the development and revision of organizational policies and protocols that spell out the best research-based method for implementing a nursing intervention and include the supporting documentation.

Research utilization also plays a powerful role in professional image enhancement. When nurses use data from research as the basis for their practice, they have a sound rationale for *why* they are taking a particular action. They are able to articulate this rationale to others, be they patients, families, administrators, or legislators.

The data from the classic study by Brooten et al. (1986) illustrate how research findings can be used to enhance nursing image and credibility and shape health policy. This study examined the effectiveness of an innovative nursing care delivery system for very-low-birth-weight (VLBW) infants. It focused on early discharge and home follow-up care by a clinical nurse specialist. Those in the treatment group went home 11 days earlier than those in the control group, which resulted in an average savings of $18,500 per treatment group infant with no increase in acute care visits or rehospitalization and no difference in developmental outcomes. If only half of the 36,000 VLBW infants born in this country each year could be cared for by using this patient care delivery system, the annual savings would be approximately $334 million (Brooten et al., 1986). Similar cost savings have been demonstrated with adult hospitalized patients who received a comprehensive discharge and follow-up care program. These are powerful data that demonstrate the effectiveness and credibility of the innovative nursing care VLBW program, one that maintains quality of care while demonstrating cost-effectiveness. The findings of this study (Brooten et al., 1986) have been used by numerous policy officials and legislators to shape health policy regarding this high-risk population.

RESEARCH UTILIZATION MODELS

Consumers of research have the skills to appraise studies critically for potential application to practice. These skills are used to identify sound clinical studies and determine scientific merit. Integrating research findings or replicating a study can be simple or complex, requiring little time and few resources or a great deal of both. Findings of studies can be implemented or the studies themselves replicated on a small to a grand scale.

There are several sets of criteria and models that can be used for deciding whether to incorporate the findings of a study into practice. One may be easier to use than another. Remember, consultation from and collaboration with expert colleagues in research utilization may be needed.

One of the first research utilization efforts of the 1970s was a regional model funded by the U.S. Department of Health, Education and Welfare and instituted by the Western Interstate Commission for Higher Education (WICHE). The major goal was to increase nursing research activities in order to develop a body of validated nursing knowledge so that client outcomes could be improved (Krueger, Nelson, & Wolanin, 1978).

Another goal was to promote interaction of researchers and practitioners, thereby making the vital, necessary link in identifying problems that needed a research-based answer and developing clinician research utilization skills. These skills included the ability to critique research, function as change agents in implementing research-based interventions, and prepare reports, analyses, and evaluations of the utilization projects. The implications of the 6-year program led to the recommendations listed in the box below, which laid the groundwork for future research utilization efforts.

The next major research utilization effort was the Conduct and Use of Research in Nursing (CURN), a 5-year project sponsored by the Michigan State Nurses' Association. The aims of the project were to promote clinical research activities and to assist nurses in integrating research findings into their practice. Examples of clinical problems studied were pain, prevention of pressure ulcers, reduction of diarrhea in tube-fed patients, and provision of structured preoperative teaching.

WICHE REGIONAL NURSING RESEARCH DEVELOPMENT, COLLABORATION, AND UTILIZATION PROJECT RECOMMENDATIONS

1. Nurse-researchers need to include implications for nursing practice in reports.
2. Reports must be prepared so that they can be easily read and used by practicing nurses.
3. Researchers need to conduct more clinical studies.
4. Researchers must collaborate with skilled clinicians in identifying important clinical research problems.

Horsley, the principal investigator, and other colleagues (Horsley, Crane, Crabtree, & Wood, 1983) developed criteria for judging the applicability of research findings and the strategies to extend the innovation or intervention to other clinical arenas. Hinshaw (1988) asserts that these criteria are one of the better developed sets for making decisions related to shaping practice and policy.

Criteria used to identify studies of sufficient quality to implement in nursing practice included the following:

Scientific merit
Replicability
Relevance to practice
Importance as a patient problem
Feasibility of implementation
Risk-benefit ratio

Participants in the project used research findings to develop protocols for implementation and evaluation of effectiveness in practice. Each protocol was constructed to include the format and content listed in the box below. After implementation and evaluation, a decision was made to accept, modify, or abandon the intervention.

This model is used today in a number of educational programs to teach research utilization. Students and faculty may consider the following example in a growing field of research, that of validating the origins of nursing diagnoses so that nurses can make more accurate diagnoses and thus plan more focused and effective interventions. A feasible, modified small-scale utilization or replication project is the study of McKieghen, Mehmert, and Dickel (1990) across age-groups of the characteristics and related factors and diagnostic related groups (DRGs) in acute care settings. This descriptive, retrospective study was conducted to validate the nursing diagnosis of bathing-hygiene self-care deficit. Data were obtained from a computerized patient care–planning data base. Analysis revealed that the major characteristic, "inability to wash body or body parts," and the major related factor, "decreased activity tolerance," were supported in 80 DRGs and across all age-groups, from 9 to 92 years of age. Using the CURN format, these findings might be developed into a protocol for use in clinical practice. For the fifth CURN content area, description of the intervention implementation, modifications might include selecting only two

---

CURN PROTOCOL FORMAT AND CONTENT

1. Description of a practice problem
2. Research-based summary
3. Nursing intervention or innovation design
4. Identification of the research-based principle to direct the intervention
5. Description of how the intervention is to be implemented
6. Evaluation of the outcomes of the intervention
7. Summary and references

age-groups and only DRGs related to surgical interventions in developing the protocol.

The third major research utilization project was the Nursing Child Assessment Satellite Training (NCAST) project. Its primary objectives were to determine whether satellite communication technology is an effective method for disseminating nursing research and whether an interactive communication facility would promote effective application of new health assessment techniques. The findings of the study supported the use of satellite communication as an effective research dissemination strategy (King, Barnard, & Hoehn, 1981). A research utilization model with four components was proposed as a vehicle for educating individual nurses about research utilization:

> *Recruitment.* Using specific nurse learners for whom the results would be applicable (i.e., educators and practicing nurses)
>
> *Translation.* Expressing research findings into language practicing nurses can understand
>
> *Dissemination.* Research findings are shared in an effective and efficient manner
>
> *Evaluation.* The program's overall cost benefit and the effectiveness of each of its components are evaluated

Today advances in technology make the preceeding utilization model highly effective for involving nurses in research utilization and replication. A grand-scale utilization project implementing these components of recruitment, translation, dissemination, and evaluation might be applied to findings of the study by Brooten et al. (1986), which were discussed earlier and are summarized in the box below.

If satellite communication, such as that used in the NCAST project, were readily available, research findings, like those in the Brooten et al. study, could be shared rapidly with nurses in the United States and around the world as well.

EARLY DISCHARGE PROGRAM
FOR VERY-LOW-BIRTH-WEIGHT INFANTS

Brooten et al. (1986) conducted a randomized clinical trial of early hospital discharge and home follow-up care by a clinical nurse specialist of very-low-birth-weight (VLBW) infants to determine safety, usefulness, and cost-effectiveness. Infants in the experimental group were sent home, on average, 11 days earlier, 2 weeks younger and weighing 200 g less than infants in the control group. At infant age of 18 months the findings indicated no differences in hospital readmissions, acute care visits, and physical and mental growth indicators of the two groups of babies. In terms of cost-effectiveness the clinical nurse specialist model of care resulted in a cost savings of $18,560 for each infant in the experimental group.

Brooten, D., Kumar, S., Brown, L., Butts, P., Finkler, S., Bakewell-Sachs, S., Gibbons, A., & Delivora-Papadopoulos, M. (1986). *New England Journal of Medicine, 315,* 934-939.

A utilization model originally developed by Stetler and Marram (1976) and refined and expanded over the years is the Stetler Model (in press), which can be used in daily clinical practice. The model, illustrated in Fig. 3-1 and outlined in Table 3-1, involves the following phases for evaluating the applicability of research findings to practice: (1) preparation, (2) validation, (3) comparative evaluation, (4) decision making, (5) translation/application, and (6) evaluation. This model is similar to processes nurses use informally, as described by Gennaro and Vessey (1991).

The Stetler Model (in press) is an interactive practitioner-oriented model whose assumptions and actions are grounded in research on knowledge utilization and the nature of research. The user's interactive frames of reference, other internal factors, and the external environment all have an influence on knowledge and research utilization. In this model (Stetler, in press), the individual nurse may or may not need to involve the organization in the utilization process. For example, if in the decision-making phase a cognitive type of use is considered, no organizational involvement is required of the nurse who uses qualitative research data about the experience of living with a wife who is receiving chemotherapy (Wilson & Morse, 1991) to deepen understanding of how husbands cope with this experience. On the other hand, if instrumental use is appropriate because the nurse, after appraising the literature on non-nutritive sucking in low-birth-weight infants (McCain, 1992), wants to implement a policy change, administrative involvement is needed. Specifically, the findings of a study in low-birth-weight infants summarized in the box below might be used to change protocols for oral feedings, which are then evaluated to determine such outcomes as better sucking and weight gain.

It should be evident now that research dissemination and utilization are major responsibilities of every nurse. Research utilization models such as the ones presented provide frameworks for continually refining knowledge and improving practice. Decisions made by nurses that are derived from research findings provide the foundation of science-based nursing practice, which becomes the basis for develop-

---

NONNUTRITIVE SUCKING IN LOW-BIRTH-WEIGHT INFANTS AND MOTHERS

Author: McCain, G. (1992)

Title and publication: Modulation of preterm infant behavioral state and heart rate prior to oral feeding. *Proceedings of the Robert Wood Johnson Foundation First Annual Meeting of Clinical Nurse Scholars Alumni*, Nashville, TN.

Purpose: Examine the effects of 10 minutes of nonnutritive sucking (NNS), NNS and rocking, and stroking on preterm infant behavioral state and heart rate prior to oral feeding.

Findings: The NNS treatments were significantly effective in changing infant behavior from sleep and restless states to the optimal state of quiet and awake prior to oral feeding.

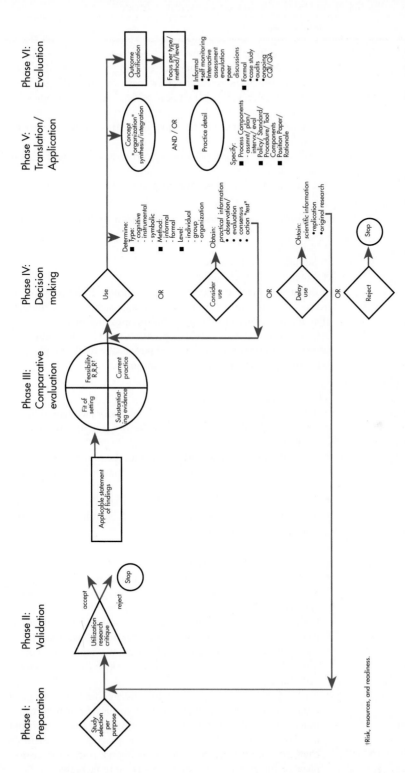

Fig. 3-1 The Stetler model for research utilization. (*Note:* From Refinement of the Stetler/Marram model for application of research findings to practice by C.B. Stetler, *Nursing Outlook* (in press).

†Risk, resources, and readiness.

Table 3-1   Phases of the Stetler Research Utilization Model

Phase	Description
Phase I Preparation	Potential users of a particular study or studies are required to specify the purpose of the research review including the following: • Need to solve a difficult clinical, educational, or managerial problem • Interest in maintaining the most up-to-date knowledge base in a specialty area • Validation or revision of a policy/procedure/standard teaching document • Preparation of an in-service program
Phase II Validation	A utilization research critique is conducted to determine the following regarding the study: • Scientific merit • Significance for practice • Potential for applicability A decision is made to accept or reject a study. If the decision is to accept, the user moves on to an applicable statement of findings that should reflect (1) the probabilistic meaning of study statistics relative to the related patient population and (2) the studied relationships in terms that could be pragmatically used in daily activities, such as assessments or interventions.
Phase III Comparative evaluation	The following are assessed: • Fit of setting, including factors that inhibit or facilitate utilization • Feasibility: R, R, R, including Risk factors, potential need for Resources, and Readiness • Substantiating evidence that recognizes the potential value of both research, and, within recognized limitations, nonresearch-based information • Current practice to determine whether theory does or can provide a relevant basis for practice and understanding the level of effectiveness of *current* practice
Phase IV Decision making	Four kinds of decisions are possible: • To Use—data provide scientific substantiation for current practice or for formally or informally instituting change in practice (instrumentally), thinking (cognitively), or influencing (symbolically) others to support change on an individual, group, or organizational level without waiting for additional data. • To Consider Use—available findings appear applicable, but additional pragmatic, short-term information is desirable before actual use. • To Delay Use—although there may be a clinical need or great interest in the findings, there may be too little research, too much conflict in current studies, or too much risk or the political climate is not conducive to change; practice will remain unchanged until needed replication or original research is complete or the political climate becomes more favorable.

Table 3-1   Phases of the Stetler Research Utilization Model—cont'd

Phase	Description
Phase IV—cont'd Decision making—cont'd	• To Reject or Not Use—no further consideration is given to the available data because of (1) the lack of consistent or strong findings, (2) the cost of implementation, or (3) the strength of current practice.
Phase V Translation/Application	The potential user does the following: • Integrates or synthesizes interrelated findings into a generalization • Identifies the exact nature of the practice implications • Specifies the extent to which implementation in practice represents adaptation versus adoption of research findings
Phase VI Evaluation	Evaluation includes the following: • Clarification of expected outcomes relative to the originally defined purpose • Differentiation of formal and informal application • Determination of feasibility

ment and revision of protocols and policies. An example of a protocol derived from research findings is provided in Fig. 3-2 (pp. 66-69). Science-based practice is essential to the development of professional credibility.

CURRENT BARRIERS TO RESEARCH UTILIZATION

Research findings tend to be implemented readily by nurses who are knowledge seekers and innovators. Those struggling with clinical problems and dissatisfied with traditional procedures that do not substantively affect outcomes are also likely to use research findings to make decisions about clinical practice. Yet, barriers that inhibit research utilization do exist. To overcome barriers, strategies are necessary because clinicians may be limited in their attempts to close the gap between knowledge produced by research and its clinical use. A study by Funk, Champagne, Wiese, and Tornquist (1991) identified 28 barriers to the use of research results. The greatest barriers were related to settings in which nurses believe that they have neither the authority nor the time to implement innovations in nursing care that affect patient outcomes.

Personal and Professional Barriers

Often the word *research* elicits a reaction among nurses similar to that produced by words such as *mathematics* and *physics*. Initially they may not understand

TITLE	Epidural Catheter Analgesia Protocol
PURPOSE	To outline the nursing responsibilities associated with the care of a patient with an epidural catheter.
LEVEL	Interdependent.
SUPPORTIVE DATA	An epidural catheter is placed in the lumbar or thoracic epidural space by Anesthesia for the purpose of local anesthesia and/or analgesia. The agents administered may be local anesthetics or synthetic narcotics alone or in combination. Temporary epidural catheters are used in obstetrical, pediatric, and adult patients. Permanent epidural catheters are useful for chronic pain management.

Patients receiving epidural catheter analgesia with a synthetic narcotic solution (fentanyl or sufentanil) alone or in combination with Bupivacaine in a 0.125% concentration or lower may be cared for on the clinical floor units. Patients receiving solutions containing greater than 0.125% Bupivacaine require monitoring in the SCU or ICU for the first 24 hours or as patient's condition warrants.

The Anesthesia Department manages the analgesic regimen in pain control for all patients receiving epidural catheter therapy. *Notify Anesthesia initially for any problems related to the epidural catheter and/or the patient's pain management.*

CONTENT

Nursing Assessment

After arrival from post anesthesia recovery room (PARR)

1. Assess VS q 1 hr × 4 hr. If stable, q 4 hr × 24 hr, then q shift until cessation of the epidural infusion.
2. a. For epidural infusions with ≤0.125% Bupivacaine, assess sensory and motor function q 4 hr × 24 hr, then q shift per Flowsheet guidelines until cessation of the infusion.
   b. For epidural infusions with >0.125% Bupivacaine, assess sensory and motor function q 2 hr × 4, and then q 4 hr per Flowsheet guidelines until cessation of the infusion.
   c. For epidural infusions without Bupivacaine, no sensory and motor assessment is necessary.
3. Assess pain relief q 4 hr per Flowsheet guidelines.
4. Assess sedation level q 4 hr × 24 hr, then q shift per Flowsheet guidelines for patients receiving a synthetic narcotic.
5. Assess skin integrity per Immobility Protocol.
6. Assess bladder function q 8 hr per Urinary Catheter Protocol.

(Source: Diann Miner, RN, MS, CS, Neuroscience Clinical Specialist, Department of Nursing Education and Research, Mary Imogene Bassett Hospital, Cooperstown, New York.)

Fig. 3-2 Example of a research-based protocol.

	7. Instruct patient to report S/S of CNS toxicity: tinnitus, metallic taste, headache, paralysis, circumoral numbness, and dizziness.
	8. Inspect catheter insertion site q 4 hr × 24 hr, then q shift for intact dressing and/or leakage, redness, swelling, local pain, and drainage.
Interventions	9. Administer the correct epidural solution and rate per Anesthesia order to provide adequate pain relief per patient report.
	10. Sit, stand and/or ambulate patients only with a Physician Order and with the assist of two initially and PRN. Do not attempt to stand or ambulate patients with motor weakness without checking with a physician.
	11. Elevate HOB 30 degrees.
	12. Monitor I&O for first 24 hours and as indicated by patient's condition.
	13. Maintain a patent IV site for first 72 hours or 4 to 8 hours after removal of the epidural catheter.
Reportable conditions	14. REPORT TO ANESTHESIA any of the following:
	a. Changes in the VS outside the parameters established by Surgery. Report to Surgery also.
	b. Increasing level in the loss of sensation on chest or abdomen in patients receiving local anesthetics.
	c. Loss of motor control in patients receiving local anesthetics.
	d. Respiratory rate <6 bpm.
	e. Development of S/S CNS toxicity.
	f. Breakage or displacement of catheter.
	g. S/S of infection or leakage at insertion site.
	h. Score of 3 on Sedation Scale.
	i. Poor pain control post increasing infusion to maximum ordered rate.
Safety	15. Label all epidural catheters with the appropriate label as shown:

EPIDURAL CATHETER

16. TAPE OVER ALL INJECTION SITES on epidural infusion sets with adhesive tape and label as "Epidural Catheter."
17. Secure all connection sites on infusion tubing.
18. Secure Millipore filter on catheter if present.
19. Administer no PRN narcotic analgesics while an epidural narcotic infusion is running without consulting with Anesthesia.

Continued.

Fig. 3-2—cont'd

20. Maintain resuscitation equipment and naloxone 0.04 mg (in STAT Box) on units.
21. Administer all epidural infusion by infusion pump.
22. All epidural admixtures will be prepared by Pharmacy.
23. All bolus medications through the epidural catheter will be administered only by Anesthesia.
24. Epidural admixtures are ordered by Anesthesia.
25. Do not clamp epidural catheter.
26. DO NOT INFUSE ANY OTHER SOLUTION OR MED THROUGH EPIDURAL CATHETER.

Complications and Management

Respiratory depression <6 bpm

27. Initiate the following interventions for respiratory depression:
    a. Stop infusion.
    b. Notify Anesthesia.
    c. Stimulate the patient.
    *d. Bolus with Naloxone 0.1 mg IVP q 2-3 min until respiratory rate is >6 breaths per minute (mix Naloxone 0.4 mg in 3 ml NS [1 ml = 0.1 mg]). CAUTION: This will reverse analgesia.

Sympathetic blockade
  BP < parameters

  P < parameters

28. Initiate the following for hypotension and/or bradycardia:
    a. Notify Anesthesia and Surgery.
    b. Place patient flat.
    c. Remain with patient.
    d. Monitor BP q 5-10 min until condition stable.

Nausea and vomiting

29. Initiate the following for nausea and vomiting:
    a. Notify Surgery.
    b. Check patient's VS.
    c. Institute interventions outlined for hypotension/Sympathetic Blockade if appropriate.
    d. PREVENT ASPIRATION.
    e. DO NOT INSTITUTE NAUSEA AND VOMITING PROTOCOL.

Ascending level in loss of sensation or motor control

30. Initiate the following if the patient reports an increasing level of diminished sensation per the sensory/motor assessment:
    a. Notify Anesthesia.
    b. Ensure that the HOB is elevated 30°.

Skin impairment

31. Initiate Skin Care Protocol

Urinary retention

32. Initiate the Urinary Catheter Protocol. (Patients with diminished sensation will be unable to report subjective symptoms of urinary retention.)

*Indicates a standing physician order; therefore the nurse may administer this medication without prior notification of the physician.

Fig. 3-2—cont'd

Catheter separation or breakage	33. Initiate the following if catheter separates or breaks:
	    a. Notify Anesthesia.
	    b. Stop infusion.
	    c. Cover catheter with sterile 3×3.
	    d. Tape remaining catheter in place.

Dressing Change	34. Change dressing per procedure q 72 hours or PRN.
Removal	35. All epidural catheters will be removed by Anesthesia.
Documentation	36. Document all assessment findings on the Epidural Flow-sheet according to guidelines.
	37. Document all epidural medications solutions, dosages, rate, amount infused on the IVAR.
	38. Document the Epidural Protocol on the Nursing Account-abilities and Protocol Flowsheet.
	39. Document all patient responses, effectiveness of therapy, any untoward effect, or special interventions in progress notes or on unit-specific Flowsheets.

REFERENCES

1. Baggerly, J. (1986). Epidural catheters for pain management: The nurse's role. *Journal of Neuroscience Nursing. 18*(5), pp. 290-293.
2. Grunde, J., Grine, R., & Gellatly, T. (1984). Pain management by epidural analgesia: The challenge for nursing. *Heart and Lung. 14*(2), pp. 164-173.
3. (1989). Care of the patient receiving epidural analgesia for pain management. *University of Washington Hospital Division for Nursing Procedure Manual,* pp. 1-15.
4. Simpson, T., Wahl, G., DeTraglia, M., Speck, E., & Taylor, D. (1992). The effects of epidural versus parenteral analgesia on postoperative pain and pulmonary function in adults who have undergone thoracic and abdominal surgery: A critique of research. *Heart and Lung. 21*(2), pp. 125-137.

Fig. 3-2—cont'd

just how integral to nursing practice mathematics related to dosage calculation, the physics of body movement, and nursing research are. This barrier can be overcome with knowledge and attitude change. Especially for the novice nurse who is beginning clinical practice, insufficient time to read research and think about how it might be used in a clinical setting is a problem. Resistance to reading research studies and lack of confidence in skills needed to use research findings seem to be attitudes left over from an era of dependence on tradition and authority. Research is now being valued starting much sooner in educational programs, and strides are being made in adopting research attitudes and behaviors in clinical practice rather than doing something because it has *always* been done that way (see Chapter 2). Illustrating this idea is the study by Stewart Fahs and Kinney (1991). Discussed earlier, this study examined the effect of administering heparin in sites other than the abdomen. As you may recall, the findings demonstrated no significant differences in number or size of bruise or changes in aPTT in relation to use of differing injection sites. These data provide a *scientific* reason for considering a change from the *traditional* abdominal site to other sites such as the arm and thigh. Indeed, for nursing practice to be scientific, it *must* be research-based rather than tradition-based.

Educational and Communication Barriers

Educational barriers include nursing programs that emphasize theory- and research-based knowledge only in a research course, not in every course. When faculty have limited experience in research or research utilization in clinical practice, they may not be effective role models in demonstrating research utilization behaviors. As a result, graduating nurses may be inadequately prepared in the research process and utilization.

Communication barriers are (1) time lag between conducting a research study and its publication, (2) findings communicated primarily between researchers rather than to practitioners, (3) too few readable studies published in practice journals, and (4) research published without clear-cut practice implications. Another communication barrier may be the perceived inequalities among researchers, educators, and practicing nurses. Nurses may feel that researchers and educators are telling them what to do rather than asking them what might work best in their practice, thus setting up resistance. Funk et al. gives this notion credence (1991) in noting that "rarely have the potential adopters themselves, the clinicians, been asked what they perceive to be barriers to using research in practice" (p. 39).

Practice Setting and Public or Societal Barriers

A lack of cooperation from other health care providers, lack of administrative support, and lack of resources to implement and evaluate new ideas are often cited as inhibiting factors. According to Hinshaw (1988), members of society and public agencies who may not be enamored with nursing research and do not understand the importance of the type of research conducted by nurses may serve as formidable barriers because they are then unlikely to commit resources needed for research utilization projects.

Nursing's unique perspective on the client and health care, commitment to professional accountability, and concern for cost-effective care is leading to increasing professional credibility. That perspective is what Davis (1988) describes as nursing's ever-present concern "with human responses to health-related problems in all types of situations—prevention, maintenance, cure, and restoration" (p. 292). Decisions about the delivery of nursing care based on science are giving the profession credibility, control, and influence in shaping health care policy, which in turn lessens societal and political barriers.

STRATEGIES AND RESOURCES FOR ENHANCING RESEARCH UTILIZATION

External driving forces such as the National League for Nursing's accreditation criteria and the American Nurses Association's Guidelines for the Investigative Functions of Nurses (ANA, 1981) contribute to strengthening research and research utilization. More important, internal driving forces probably have been most instrumental in maintaining the momentum of research utilization. These include the excitement and pride in realizing the influence research has on changing practice and policy, the growing energy of researchers in developing programs of research that build knowledge systematically, and the increasing momentum of a strong, integrated research utilization movement involving practicing nurses, researchers, educators, and leaders at local, state, regional, and national levels (see Chapter 1).

Consumer Strategies and Resources

As consumers of research, nursing students, faculty, and practicing nurses must hold themselves responsible and accountable for research utilization, but responsible and accountable for what? Research competence, varying only in degree, is required in every educational program today. All nurses need to know not only the investigative functions of their own level of preparation but also those of nurses prepared at other levels (see Chapter 1). This knowledge helps promote more complete and effective collaboration in integrating research findings into practice and building the science base of the profession. Students (and faculty) should ask themselves the questions listed in the boxes below.

THOUGHT QUESTIONS
FOR THE EDUCATIONAL ENVIRONMENT

1. Do the faculty share research findings during class or at the clinical agency?
2. How often do oral and written assignments require that I use research findings to support a position, a plan, or an intervention I recommend?
3. Do students participate in some way in a faculty's program of research?
4. Besides a research course, do faculty integrate research findings in every course in the program?

THOUGHT QUESTIONS
FOR THE PRACTICE ENVIRONMENT

1. Does the clinical agency have a clinical nursing research department, researcher, or nursing research committee?
2. Do staff nurses mention research findings during report or in discussions about patients?
3. Is there a library? Are nursing references adequate? Is the library used by nurses?
4. Is there a journal club for nurses? Are the meeting times posted?
5. Is there a sharing of research among faculty, staff nurses, and students?
6. When clinical nurse educators offer courses to staff and students, is the content based on research findings?

Acquiring the professional behavior of systematically collecting, analyzing, and sharing results of nursing interventions needs to begin among faculty and students and extend beyond the educational environment to include nurses and other health colleagues in the practice arena. Specific strategies and resources for the research consumer require only that you initiate the following simple but important activities.

Read articles on your own, start a journal club or a research committee. Bock (1990) asserts, "All nurses need to read research! Challenge yourself . . . challenge your colleague . . . share your information" (p. 51). As a student, aspire to being elected a member of the National Nursing Honor Society, Sigma Theta Tau, joining others who value scholarship, service, and research. As a member, you receive the journals *Image* and *Reflections.* The first carries scholarly and research articles; the second is primarily informational but includes a "Research News" column that highlights research briefs. For example, in the winter issue in 1992 Heyne, the column editor, highlighted three important research projects, two of which are described here.

One of these, "Healthy Kids Project," investigates comprehensive preventive health services for children enrolled in Medicaid from birth to 21 years of age. When this federally funded nursing research project is used, health care cost improves. Because it is underused, especially in rural areas with health care problems of access and equity, federal legislation (policy) has mandated increased state use up to 80% by 1995. Another study reviewed in the previously mentioned column was "Wound Care in the Elderly," in which Mitraflex, a new polyurethane dressing, was used. The findings indicated that when this inexpensive, versatile wound care product was used, a wide range of wounds healed with no risk of infection (especially important in elders, who often have a suppressed immune system) and little nursing time (e.g., no wound cleaning) and few supplies were required. The dressing was comfortable and promoted healing. Often such research briefs or reviews stimulate enough interest for the nurse or student to contact the researcher or to read the full research report to learn how to evaluate its use in practice or to replicate the study. If you should contact a researcher to ask questions about evaluating findings or replicating a study in your practice, you will probably get an enthusiastic response and a lot of assistance.

Another strategy is to question practice. Ask the following questions: "Why are we doing this?" "What is the scientific basis for this?" "What change is necessary to create a scientific basis for this practice?" There are many ways to bring about change, but first, commitment to change is necessary. Kirchhoff (1991) advocates welcoming change, supporting it, communicating with researchers, and interacting with those collecting data. Use technology such as a researchers' electronic bulletin board to learn more about research, share research findings, and learn to incorporate research findings into your practice. For example, Nursing Care Research (NUCARE) is an on-line conference presented by Lister Hill National Center for Biomedical Communications, a part of the National Library of Medicine. It is a national computer system that allows nurses to share nursing care information and use technology to facilitate more nursing research. This system can be accessed on the Educational Technology Network and on Sprintnet or Internet at no charge. The Health and Psychosocial Instruments (HAPI) data base at the Sigma Theta Tau International Virginia Henderson Library is another electronic computer research information resource. This data base includes more than 12,000 information records about research instruments and is updated every 3 months.

Take advantage of the media and technology. More practice journals and professional organizational newspapers are now carrying "research briefs" columns or reports (see Chapter 5). Read them. They are short and concise and can keep your knowledge current in research related to your practice interests. Review research computer-assisted instruction (CAI) or interactive video disc (IVD) programs. Find out whether your agency has a **downlink** (a receiver for programs beamed from other agencies) that allows you to participate in telecommunications conferences. You may find that your agency has an **uplink,** which broadcasts conferences so that you can attend from a distance.

Barriers related to not having enough time to read about research can be overcome by using the reading skill of scanning and by selecting research columns in practice journals or research reviews or briefs in research journals (see Chapter 4). For example, in *The American Nurse,* the official newspaper of the American Nurses Association, a recent column, "Focus on Patient Care," highlighted Cassetta's discussion (Cassetta, 1993) about the appropriateness of restraints in nursing homes. Citing the nursing research findings of Evans and Strumpf (1990), Cassetta noted that the benefits of not using restraints included improved quality of care, decreased length of recovery, and improved quality of life for patients. For nurses specializing in care of elders, this discussion not only provides the names and topics that a research consumer may need in conducting a more in-depth search of the literature for studies and scholarly discussions about the topic, but also presents the implications for health care policy.

In 1990, *Image* published the discussion of Evans and Strumpf "Myths about Elder Restraint." A further search of the literature would reveal a program of research that these investigators are pursuing, which is related to restraint myths (for example, that elders do not mind restraints) and the legal liability associated with not using restraints. These investigators are demonstrating through research that the myths supporting the continued use of restraints as "customary care" are no longer acceptable. They note also that to provide additional data supporting the reduction of this harmful practice, further research is essential. Evans and Strumpf propose that application of their findings to clinical practice, as well as further replication studies, would make a significant contribution to the development of research-based versus myth-based standards for practice.

As illustrated by the study of Evans and Strumpf, which reveals that restraints contribute to falls, agitation, pressure sores, incontinence, and general decline in functional status, the findings of nursing research can have considerable impact not only on practice but also on public policy. For example, on the basis of the body of nursing research pertaining to restraint use, the Health Care Financing Administration (HCFA) issued a proposal for policy change calling for stricter nursing home regulations for monitoring and prohibiting the inappropriate use of physical and chemical restraints. Again, research can lead to and direct policy changes to improve patient outcomes.

Another consumer strategy is to attend conferences or request the proceedings from conferences to keep yourself up-to-date on current research related to your interest areas. Technology again makes this strategy fairly efficient. Most conferences now provide audiotapes on important topics presented, and some provide videotapes.

Researcher Strategies and Resources

Researchers and practicing nurses must interact more with each other to maintain the momentum that is building in research utilization. Kirchhoff (1991), a clinically based nurse-researcher, provides a number of insights about how researchers can more effectively reach their audience, the consumers of research. She suggests that nurse researchers develop the ability to talk in a language understood by nurses who work directly with patients so that interpreters are not necessary. She believes that researchers who are not in regular contact with nursing staff will find that their ideas may become out-of-date or irrelevant. She proposes that staff nurses can be the source for pressing, relevant research ideas. Kirchhoff highly recommends that students who conduct research studies report their results to the nursing staff so that they will be enthusiastic about participating in future studies. Furthermore, nurses may be motivated to use the completed research results. Faculty and students who participate in research utilization projects need to invite their clinically based colleagues to participate with them.

Researchers need to be close to clinical practice to be current, identify priorities, study clinically important problems, and forge relationships with practitioners. This proximity can be accomplished, for example, by faculty practice, joint positions between education and practice, and presentations at practice conferences as well as research conferences. Part of a nurse's responsibility is to be persistent with researchers in helping them to make research understandable and establish the connections between their research and ways to improve practice.

Administrative Strategies and Resources

Administrative support and encouragement have been identified most often as factors that facilitate research utilization (Funk et al., 1991). Administrative incentives that promote research involvement include budgeting time and resources to establish a nursing research committee, conduct a literature search, attend a conference, or offer in-service education programs that focus on research. Many hospitals have established Research and Development Centers (RDCs) or Nursing Research Committees (NRCs) that are instrumental in fostering a research climate, supporting clinically relevant research, and encouraging research involvement of nurses (Vessey & Campos, 1992). Institution-based nurse researchers can provide consultation, conduct seminars and workshops on research utilization, and serve on institutional review committees.

Nursing research departments and committees can assist in setting up unit-level nursing research committees. At the unit level committee members can review research findings specific to their special interests, propose clinical evaluation trials, standardize care based on research for policy and procedure manuals, and share relevant findings and knowledge gained from these activities with other staff members. Campbell (1993) recently described an effective, efficient method for accomplishing unit-based research and research utilization. Having implemented unit-based research, she found focus groups to be an excellent way of identifying research priorities, establishing time lines, and selecting the right topic to investigate. The project could involve design of an original study, a **replication,** or systematic implementation of findings from completed studies. Campbell's ideas, as shown in the box below, lend themselves to the Stetler utilization model (Table 3-1) for groups of nurses, not just individuals.

FOCUS GROUPS: A MECHANISM FOR IDENTIFYING RESEARCH UTILIZATION PRIORITIES

RESEARCH PRIORITIES
1. Select high-volume patient diagnosis.
2. Identify common patient problems.
3. Consider frequent nursing interventions and new technology.

TIME LINES
1. All work is done by focus group members in a dedicated 1-hour period each week during scheduled work time.
2. Allow 1 to 2 years for the research or research utilization. Allot time in the following percentages:
   To identify the question or the problem—25%
   To develop the proposal or protocol—50%
   To collect and analyze the data—25%
3. Allow 1 year for writing up and presenting the research or for evaluation of outcomes of an innovation.

THE RIGHT RESEARCH TOPIC
   The findings to be implemented or study to be replicated should:
1. Be clinically relevant to the population of patients on the unit.
2. Be easy to implement in the context of available human and environmental resources.
3. Be realistic in scope.
4. Have a potential financial impact or improve nursing practice.
5. Allow for data collection during normal patient care.

ADMINISTRATIVE STRATEGIES TO PROMOTE RESEARCH UTILIZATION

1. Include research utilization in mission, philosophy, and outcomes statements.
2. Specify research utilization and dissemination responsibilities in job descriptions.
3. Increase, incrementally, research responsibilities in clinical ladder programs.
4. Support joint or reciprocal positions for faculty and nursing staff to foster collaborative research activities.
5. Maintain a research library with nursing practice and research journals, computer terminals for literature searches, and convenient hours for access.
6. Develop collaborative or consortium agreements with other health care agencies to test application of findings, and share them locally or regionally.
7. Negotiate library privileges for nurses at nearby health science libraries.
8. Provide budgetary assistance to units for subscriptions to research briefs and newsletters.
9. Provide incentives for conducting research grand rounds.
10. Promote interdisciplinary research activities.
11. Host a Research Day and provide budgetary support for research poster presentations.

Staff can work collaboratively with administrators to build a research climate, provide incentives, and reward the translation of science into practice (see the box above). Campbell (1993) notes that outcomes of unit-based research (and by logical extension, research utilization) include staff nurses functioning as investigators and innovators, validating clinical practice. Additionally the unit-based managerial outcomes include a decreased staff turnover rate, increased institutional visibility, recruitment without costs, and educational advancement for nursing staff. She stresses that unit-based research and research utilization effectively bring about changes in policy and procedures, attitudes, knowledge, and use of research to improve practice.

STATE, REGIONAL, AND NATIONAL STRATEGIES AND RESOURCES

Soaring health costs, geographic differences in health care, and demands for changing the health care system have brought into being unexpected strategies and resources for nursing. Major private foundations, such as Pew, the charitable trust, Kellogg Foundation, and Robert Wood Johnson Foundation, are funding collaborative studies emphasizing disease prevention, health promotion, elder independent functioning, primary and home care, and other topics. Federal research and project initiatives are similar in focus.

Private and federal funding for nurses who are conducting clinical research and studies of health care delivery systems is increasing. For example, the findings of a recent study, highlighted in the box below, concern the primary health care system and the effectiveness of two major groups of primary care providers, physicians and nurse practitioners and nurse midwives; these findings will be helpful to federal commissions as they develop plans for cost-effective primary health care and create policies for access to care and equity.

This study builds on similar studies deriving similar findings and conclusions. Such studies, when replicated, substantiate scientific merit and thus can be used with confidence in making policy decisions.

Nurses are also being sought for membership in prestigious organizations such as the Institute of Medicine (IOM) and the National Institutes of Health (NIH) task forces. The work of prominent nurse researchers has been recognized at the national level, as is evident in the Agency for Health Care Policy and Research (AHCPR) (see Chapter 2). The Medical Treatment Effectiveness Program (MEDTEP), an agency coordinated by AHCPR, addresses the following elements:

Medical treatment effectiveness research
Development of data bases for such research
Development of clinical guidelines
Dissemination of research findings and clinical guidelines

Three expert panels focusing on pain, pressure sores, and incontinence have been either chaired or cochaired by nurse-researchers. The AHCPR sought input from a panel of expert nurses to provide nursing's perspective on clinical guideline development. The nursing panel, chaired by Norma Lang, recommended that

---

A METAANALYSIS OF PROCESS OF CARE, CLINICAL OUTCOMES, AND COST-EFFECTIVENESS OF NURSES IN PRIMARY CARE ROLES: NURSE PRACTITIONERS AND NURSE MIDWIVES

Brown and Grimes (1993) conducted a metaanalysis for the American Nurses Association comparing nurses in advanced practice and physicians as providers of primary care. Major health care delivery concerns are the severe shortage of physicians and the millions of people in need of health care services. The findings were as follows:

Nurses provided more health promotion activities such as patient education.
Although nurses ordered slightly more tests, the cost was somewhat lower.
Nurses scored higher on quality of care measures such as diagnostic accuracy and completeness of the care process.
Nurses and physicians prescribed medications equally.

Other findings related to clinical outcomes revealed equivalent or greater patient satisfaction with the health care provider and compliance with health care recommendations.

From Brown, S., & Grimes, D. (1993, February). *The American Nurse*, p. 3.

guidelines be used as a mechanism for translating science-based knowledge into clinical actions easily accessible to clinicians (Hernandez & Hastings, 1991). Further, the panel recommended expanding the narrow term *medical diagnosis* to *clinical condition,* which encompasses most conditions that nurses deal with daily, such as pain, incontinence, impaired functional status, and pressure sores, for which guidelines have been developed. As Hernandez and Hastings conclude, "Our health care system is deteriorating and needs to be nurtured back to health. Who is more qualified to do this than the nurturing profession?" (p. 199).

The influence of nursing research and nursing leaders in shaping policy is evident in the key positions they occupy in AHCPR and on the guidelines committees. Many of the research studies cited in the guidelines were drawn from programs of research by nurse-researchers. A synopsis of the work of these panels is given in the box below and the two boxes on p. 79.

The guidelines provided by AHCPR are in essence protocols for interventions derived from **basic research.** Clinicians are urged to use these protocols, evaluate the outcomes, and share the information with the agency and other practitioners. Using the Stetler (1993) research utilization model for validation, comparative evaluation, and decision making, a protocol could be selected for implementation. Campbell's idea of focus groups in a variety of clinical specialties would be an efficient way to implement research findings. Satellite technology similar to that used in

---

ACUTE PAIN MANAGEMENT GUIDELINE PANEL
(FEBRUARY 1992)

Cochair: Ada Jacox, PhD, FAAN.

Panel: Five of the 18 members and 18 of the 51 interdisciplinary peer reviewers are nurses.

Task: Review research, review scholarly literature, and use expert opinion to develop guidelines.

Control: Clinical surveys reveal that pain managed by routine orders for intramuscular injections of opioids as needed fail to relieve pain in about half of postoperative patients. There is widespread inadequacy in pain management. Guidelines are corrective action that might become policy.

Review of the research literature: The literature was heavily nurse dominated. Note the following examples:

Beyer, J.E., McGrath, P., & Berde, C. (1990). Discordance between self-report and behavioral pain measures in children age 3 to 7 years after surgery. *Journal of Pain and Symptom Management, 5,* 350-356.

Johnson, J., Rice, S., Fuller, S., & Endress, P. (1978). Sensory information, instruction, in a coping strategy and recovery from surgery. *Research in Nursing and Health, 1,* 4-17.

Tesler, M., Savedra, M., Holzemer, W., Wilkie, A., Ward, J., & Paul, S. (1991). The word-graphic rating scale as a measure of children's and adolescents' pain intensity. *Research in Nursing and Health, 14,* 361-371.

PANEL FOR THE PREDICTION AND PREVENTION OF PRESSURE ULCERS IN ADULTS (MAY 1992)

Chair: Nancy Bergstrom, PhD, RN, FAAN.

Panel: Seven of 13 panel members and 14 of 27 interdisciplinary reviewers are nurses.

Task: Review research, review scholarly literature, and use expert opinion to develop guidelines.

Executive summary: Twenty-three percent of ulcers occur in skilled care and nursing home facilities. The incidence in acute care facilities is 9.2%. Elderly persons with fractures have a 66% incidence.

Review of the literature: Forty of more than 100 articles were by nurses. An example is the following:

Bergstrom, N., & Braden, B. (in press). A prospective study of pressure sore risk among institutionalized elderly. *Journal of the American Geriatrics Society.*

URINARY INCONTINENCE GUIDELINE PANEL (MARCH 1992)

Cochair: Kathleen McCormick, PhD, FAAN.

Panel: Four of 15 panel members and 6 of 26 interdisciplinary reviewers are nurses.

Task: Review research, review scholarly literature, and use expert opinion to develop guidelines.

Executive summary: Urinary incontinence affects 15% to 30% of noninstitutionalized persons over 60, or 10 million Americans, mostly elderly, at an estimated annual cost of $10 billion. It is prevalent, widely undiagnosed, and underreported.

Review of the literature: For example, the following research of a well-known geriatric nurse researcher is cited:

Wells, T., Rink, C., Diokno, A. et al. (1991). Pelvic muscle exercise for stress urinary incontinence in elderly women. *Journal of the American Geriatrics Society. 38,* 296-299.

---

the NCAST project could rapidly disseminate findings to AHCPR and agencies across the country.

THE IMPACT OF RESEARCH: FROM SCIENCE TO PRACTICE IN THE PRESENT AND FUTURE

One of the most important achievements in nursing research was the creation in 1986 of the National Center for Nursing Research (NCNR). In 1993 the NCNR was converted to a National Institute of Nursing Research (NINR) equal in status to the other National Health Institutes. The priorities of the NINR have been updated for 1995 to 2000; these include chronic illness, self-care and community care, and the elderly. Research utilization is now one of the main priorities of NINR. To promote research utilization, NINR has held regional and national conferences and made funding available. The following priority areas have already been studied: human immunodeficiency virus (HIV) infection, long-term care for older adults, symptom management, nursing informatics, health promotion among children and adolescents, and technology dependency across the life span.

Four research utilization models have been presented in this chapter. Use one of these models to consider how the implementation of findings of an innovation, intervention, or health service related to the NINR priorities described in the box on p. 81 could take place in a practice setting.

Nurse researchers and clinicians also are addressing national priority problems such as obesity, smoking, lack of immunizations, and access to and equity in care. One study related to equity in care that could be considered for research utilization is Barsevic's investigation of changes in reimbursement for health care of elders with hip fractures, described in the box on p. 82.

Studies of other clinical therapies being conducted also related to maintaining functioning in elders, reducing disabilities, preventing pressure ulcers, and promoting wound healing. For the most part, other research activities fit well with the emphasis on self-care and responsibility advocated in "Healthy People 2000."

"Healthy People 2000: National Health Promotion and Disease Prevention" (DHHS, 1990) is a statement from the federal government based on input from more than 300 professional organizations. The document acknowledges that responsible behavior of every individual is the key to good health (Department of Health and Human Services, 1990). In addition to care of the sick in hospitals, the focus on education, self-responsibility, care of the disadvantaged, and health problems of communities has always been a nursing emphasis.

The national health promotion and disease prevention objectives are deliberately comprehensive and allow states and communities to address their highest-priority needs by choosing from the various recommendations. The objectives address not only health promotion and disease prevention but also health protection, need for surveillance and data systems, age-related needs, and needs of special populations. Nurse-researchers are conducting studies in almost every one of these areas. Programs of research and the research base established in certain areas are too numerous to list in this chapter. However, several studies that are related to various "Healthy People 2000" objectives and contribute to research utilization are summarized in the box on pp. 83-84. Again, select a model and decide whether you would attempt research utilization and how you would proceed.

Each of the research examples cited can be substantiated by similar studies or replications. Ideally you have made a decision for cognitive application, or what Stetler (1985, p. 42) describes as using the research base to affect your "way of thinking, approaching and/or observing situations."

To utilize nursing research actively, practice, using the strategies discussed

EXAMPLES OF RESEARCH RELATED TO NINR PRIORITIES

HIV INFECTION

Author: Kiethley, J., Zeller, J., Szeluga, D., & Urbanski, P. (1992).

Title and publication: Nutritional alterations in persons with HIV infection. *Image: Journal of Nursing Scholarship, 24,* 183-189.

Purpose: Describe nutritional status of HIV-infected persons at various points on the HIV continuum and examine the potential interrelationships of nutritional changes with immune function and quality of life.

Findings: Asymptomatic patients, as well as those with AIDS-related complex (ARC) or stable AIDS, are able to maintain body weight and composition. As a function of disease, percentages of T-helper cells were significantly lower but absolute T-helper cell numbers were not. Quality of life was difficult to measure because the homosexual population has a different type of available family support; thus the instrument was inaccurate for this group.

SYMPTOM MANAGEMENT

Author: Oberle, K., Wry, J., Paul, P., & Grace, M. (1990).

Title and publication: Environment, anxiety, and postoperative pain. *Western Journal of Nursing Research, 12,* 745-757.

Purpose: Compare pain and anxiety levels in surgical patients in two environments: an old and a new hospital.

Findings: Postoperative patients in the old building were significantly more anxious, and there was a trend of decreasing anxiety in patients in the new building. Pain scores and usage of analgesics were relatively the same between both groups, and a significant relationship between pain and anxiety was found in both groups, although the new hospital group scores were lower.

TECHNOLOGY DEPENDENCY ACROSS THE LIFE SPAN.

Author: Wilson, D.M. (1992).

Title and publication: Ethical concerns in a long-term tube-feeding study. *Image: Journal of Nursing Scholarship, 24,* 195-199.

Purpose: Conduct a secondary analysis to examine ethical concerns related to long-term tube-feeding practices.

Findings: Tube-feeding practices are not standardized and patients did not appear to benefit functionally from tube feeding, since none regained any ability to perform activities of daily living. Tube feeding was found to be capable of sustaining life for a long time. Deciding to initiate and continue tube feeding did not appear to be adequately based on a weighing of burdens and benefits. This study demonstrated that respect for the patient's autonomy does not guide tube-feeding decisions.

ACCESS AND EQUITY OF CARE

Author: Barsevic, A. (1991, April).

Title and publication: The impact of Medicare payment systems on outcomes of the elderly with hip fractures. *Proceedings of the Robert Wood Johnson Annual Meeting of Clinical Nurse Scholars Alumni,* Scottsdale, AZ.

Purpose: Compare the impact of changes in Medicare to prospective payment plan based on diagnostic related groups (DRGs) on outcomes of care for the elderly with hip fractures.

Findings: With the new system, the following occurred:

The proportion of elders who died within the year after hip fracture increased significantly, by 20%.

Length of stay decreased from 23 to 20 days.

The proportion of elders staying in nursing homes after a fracture decreased from 55% to 39%.

---

earlier in the chapter, is needed. Success in research utilization can be enhanced by involving all nurses concerned about improving practice and client outcomes—clinicians, students, faculty, and researchers. Nonetheless, each nurse is responsible for reading current research, refining clinical problem-solving skills, and modifying practice based on research. Research utilization must be an integral part of each nurse's practice, a habit of knowledge seeking and application.

KEY POINTS

- Research utilization is a systematic method of implementing a sound, research-based innovation in clinical practice, evaluating the outcome, and sharing the knowledge through the process of research dissemination.
- Utilization of research findings improves quality and cost-effectiveness of patient care and provides the foundation of science-based professional practice.
- The findings of research studies validate the merit of current practice and provide the basis for decision making about initiating changes in practice.
- Research utilization contributes to professional image enhancement.
- Research utilization models include the WICHE, CURN, NCAST, and the Stetler models. They can be used for deciding whether to incorporate the findings of a study in practice.
- Barriers to research utilization include personal and professional barriers, educational and communication barriers, and practice setting and societal barriers.
- Strategies and resources for enhancing research utilization include external and internal forces. External forces include National League for Nursing accreditation criteria and standards promulgated by professional organizations like the ANA. Internal forces include motivation and pride in utilizing research to validate and change practice and shape health policy.

NATIONAL HEALTH PROMOTION AND DISEASE PREVENTION AREAS, HEALTH STATUS OBJECTIVES, AND RESEARCH EXAMPLES*

AREA: HEALTH PROTECTION

9. Unintentional Injuries
10. Occupational Safety and Health*
11. Environmental Health
12. Food and Drug Safety
13. Oral Health

Health status objective 10.9: Increase hepatitis B immunization levels to 90% among occupational exposed workers.

Research example

Author: Pennie, R., O'Connor, A., Garvock, M., & Drake, E. (1991).

Title and publication: Factors influencing the acceptance of hepatitis B vaccine by students in health disciplines in Ottawa. *Canadian Journal of Public Health, 82,* 12-15.

Purpose: Determine immunization prevalence and factors influencing intentions of students to accept hepatitis B vaccine.

Findings: Only 14% were immunized. There was significant variability among students regarding the risk of hepatitis, beliefs about the efficacy of the vaccine, and willingness to pay for it.

Implications: Different educational interventions are needed for nurses and doctors; doctors can be told to be immunized, and nurses need to be convinced of the efficacy. Low-cost hepatitis B vaccination programs need to be developed to encourage immunization.

AREA: PREVENTIVE SERVICES

14. Maternal and Infant Health
15. Heart Disease and Stroke*
16. Cancer
17. Diabetes and Chronic Disabling Conditions
18. HIV Infection*
19. Sexually Transmitted Diseases
20. Immunization and Infectious Diseases
21. Clinical Preventive Services

Health status objective 15.1: Reduce coronary heart disease deaths . . .

Research example

Author: Redeker, N.S. (1992).

Title and publication: The relationship between uncertainty and coping after coronary bypass surgery. *Western Journal of Nursing Research, 14*(1), 48-68.

Purpose: Explore the nature and dynamics of coping following coronary artery bypass surgery.

Findings: The most frequently used coping strategy in the first week following surgery was to seek social support, followed by problem-focused coping and emotion-focused coping such as self-blame and avoidance. There was an overall decrease in coping, suggesting a general decline in stress of recovery.

Implications: Nurses need to individualize interventions based on assessment of whether the particular strategy, e.g., blaming self, is protective or destructive.

*Indicates the objective that is illustrated by the examples below.   *Continued.*

NATIONAL HEALTH PROMOTION AND DISEASE PREVENTION AREAS, HEALTH STATUS OBJECTIVES, AND RESEARCH EXAMPLES—cont'd

Health status objective 18.14: Extend to all facilities where workers are at risk for the occupational transmission of HIV regulations to protect workers . . .

Research example

Author: McNabb, K., & Keller, M. (1991).

Title and publication: Nurses' risk taking regarding HIV transmission in the workplace. *Western Journal of Nursing Research, 13,* 732-745.

Purpose: To explore nurses' representation regarding transmission of HIV in the workplace, to determine whether risk-taking behavior is influenced by representation, and to explore situations that are associated with risk-taking behavior.

Findings: Nurses have accurate knowledge about HIV transmission in the workplace; that knowledge is not the most important determinant. Rather, situational demands take precedence, resulting in exposures. The most frequent situations resulting in exposure were starting intravenous infusions, being in a rush but not in an emergency situation, difficulty with "clumsy" gloves, and carelessness.

Implication: Education needs to focus more on risk behaviors than on general prevention.

AREA: AGE-RELATED OBJECTIVES

5. Children
6. Adolescents and Young Adults*
7. Adults
8. Older Adults

Health status objective 6.3: Reduce to less than 10% the prevalence of mental disorders among children and adolescents . . .

Research example

Author: Kettner, B., Kettner, D., & Farren, E. (1990).

Title and publication: Family routines and conduct disorders in adolescent girls. *Western Journal of Nursing Research, 12*(2), 161-174.

Purpose: Identify which family characteristics were related to adolescent female social behavior and to what extent family characteristics were predictive of conduct disorders among female adolescents.

Findings: Girls with conduct disorders were from homes that claimed less religious affiliation; fewer parents had college educations, and families of these girls had lower incomes and few family routines.

Implications: Routine assessment of families may be a potentially useful screening and predictive measure for adolescent behavior disorders.

- Strategies that enhance research utilization include reading research articles, starting or joining journal clubs, questioning practice traditions, using electronic bulletin boards and satellite teleconferences, and attending conferences.
- Researchers must communicate research findings in understandable language and involve practicing nurses in identifying research problems.
- Administrative support facilitates research utilization by providing financial resources, time, and sanction for research activities. Nursing research departments, committees, and staff development programs are ways of demonstrating administrative and organizational support for research utilization.
- Nursing research is being utilized to shape health policy on state, regional, and national levels.

REFERENCES

Acute Pain Management Guideline Panel. (1992). *Acute pain management: Operative or medical procedures and trauma.* Clinical Practice Guideline. (AHCPR Pub. 92-0032.) Rockville, MD: Agency for Health Care Policy and Research, Public Health Service, U.S. Department of Health and Human Services.

American Association of Critical-Care Nurses. (1993). Evaluation of the effects of heparinized and nonheparinized flush solutions on the patency of arterial pressure monitoring lines: The AACN Thunder project. *American Journal of Critical Care 2,* (1):3-14.

American Nurses' Association. (1981). *Guidelines for the investigative function of nurses.* Kansas City, MO: Author.

Barsevic, A. (1991, April). The impact of medicare payment systems on outcomes of the elderly with hip fractures. *Proceedings of the Robert Wood Johnson Foundation Annual Meeting Clinical Nurse Scholars Program,* Scottsdale, AZ.

Bergstrom, N. & Braden, B. (1992). A prospective study of pressure sore risk among institutionalized elderly. *Journal of the American Geriatrics Society, 40* (8), 747-758.

Beyer, J.E., McGrath, P. & Berde, C. (1990). Discordance between self-report and behavioral pain measures in children age 3-7 years after surgery. *Journal of Pain and Symptom Management, 5,* 350-356.

Bock, L.R. (1990). From research to utilization: bridging the gap. *Nursing Management, 21*(3), 50-51.

Brett, J.L.L. (1987). Use of nursing practice research findings. *Nursing Research, 36:*6, 344-349.

Brooten, D., Kumar, S., Brown, L., Butts, P., Finkler, S., Bakewell-Sachs, S., Gibbons, A., & Delivoria-Papadopoulos, M. (1986). A randomized clinical trial of early hospital discharge and home follow-up of very low birth weight infants. *New England Journal of Medicine, 315,* 934-939.

Brown, S. & Grimes, D. (1993, February). A meta-analysis of process of care, clinical outcomes, and cost-effectiveness of nurses in primary care roles: Nurses practitioners and nurse midwives. *The American Nurse,* p. 3.

Campbell, G. (1993, February). Staff nurse involvement in clinical research: Achieving the impossible. Keynote address, Annual Research Day, Sigma Theta Tau, Epsilon Sigma Chapter, Johnson City, TN.

Cassetta, R. (1993, February). Nurses grapple with restraint issue. *The American Nurse,* p. 11.

Davis, G.C. (1988, November/December). Nursing values and health care policy. *Nursing Outlook,* 289-292.

Department of Health and Human Services. (1990). *Healthy people 2000: national health promotion and disease prevention objectives.* Full Report. (DHHS Pub. 91-50212). Washington, DC: U.S. Government Printing Office, Public Health Service, U.S. Department of Health and Human Services.

Dickoff, J., & James, P. (1968). Theory in a practice profession. Part I. Practice oriented research. *Nursing Research, 17,* 425-435.

Evans, L.K. & Strumpf, N.E. (1990). Myths about elder restraint. *Image: Journal of Nursing Scholarship, 22*(2), 124-128.

Feldman, H.R., Penney, N., Haber, J., Hott, J., & Jacobson, L. (1993). Bridging the nursing research practice gap through research utilization. *The Journal of the New York State Nurses Association, 24*(3), 4-9.

Funk, S.G., Champagne, M.T., Wiese, R.A., & Tornquist, E.M. (1991). BARRIERS: The barriers research utilization scale. *Applied Nursing Research, 4*(1), 39-45.

Gennaro, S., & Vessey, J. (1991). Making practice perfect. *Nursing Research, 40*(5), 259.

Goode, C.J., Titler, M., Rakel, B., Ones, D.S., Klieber, C., Small, S., & Triolo, P.K. (1991). A meta-analysis of effects of heparin flush and saline flush: Quality and cost implications. *Nursing Research, 40,* 324-330.

Gortner, S. (1974). Scientific accountability in nursing. *Nursing Outlook, 22*(12), 764-768.

Hernandez, G.A., & Hastings, K.E. (1991). The effectiveness initiative: Implications for nursing practice and research. *News Outlook, 39*(5), 198-199.

Heyne, C. (Ed). (1992, Winter). Research news: Sigma Theta Tau, reporting on Healthy Kids project by investigators, Selby, M., Riportella-Muller, R., Sorensson, J., Quade, D., Stearns, S., Farel, A., and DeClerque, J. and wound care in the elderly research by Resinck, B. *Reflections* p. 3.

Hinshaw, A.S. (1988, January/February). Using research to shape health policy. *Nursing Outlook,* pp. 21-24.

Horsley, J.A., Crane, J., Crabtree, M.T., & Wood, D.J. (1983). *Using research to improve nursing practice: A guide, CURN Project.* New York: Grune and Stratton.

Johnson, J., Rice, S., Fuller, S., & Endress, P. (1978). Sensory information, instruction, in a coping strategy and recovery from surgery. *Research in Nursing and Health, 1,* 4-17.

Kettner, B., Kettner, D., & Farren, E. (1990). Family routines and conduct disorders in adolescent girls. *Western Journal of Nursing Research, 12* (2), 161-174.

Kiethley, J., Zeller, J., Szeluga, D., & Urbanski, P. (1992). Nutritional alterations in persons with HIV infection.

King, D., Barnard, K.E., & Hoehn, R. (1983). Disseminating the results of nursing research. *Nursing Outlook, 29*(3), 164-169.

Kirchhoff, K.T. (1991) Who is responsible for research utilization? *Heart & Lung, 20*(3), 308-309.

Krueger, J., Nelson, A., & Wolanin, J. (1978). *Nursing research: development, collaboration and utilization.* Germantown, MD: Aspen Systems.

Kruszewski, A., Lang, S., & Johnson, J. (1979). Effect of positioning on discomfort from intramuscular injections in the dorsogluteal site. *Nursing Research, 28,* 103-105.

McCain, G. (1992, March). Modulation of preterm infant behavioral state and heart rate prior to oral feeding. *Proceedings of the Robert Wood Johnson Foundation First Annual Meeting Clinical Nurse Scholars Alumni.* Nashville, TN.

McKeighen, R., Mehmert, P., & Dickel, C. (1990). Bathing/hygiene self care deficit: Characteristics and related factors across age groups and diagnosis related groups in an acute care setting. *Nursing Diagnosis, 1*(4), 155-161.

McNabb, K., & Keller, M. (1991). Nurses' risk taking regarding HIV transmission in the workplace. *Western Journal of Nursing Research, 13,* 732-745.

National League for Nursing. (1993). NCNR charged to investigate women's health and long-term care. Washington Focus Column. *Nursing and Health Care, 14*(1), 6-7.

Oberle, K., Wry, J., Paul, P., & Grace, M. (1990). Environment, anxiety and postoperative pain. *Western Journal of Nursing Research, 12*(6), 745-757.

Panel for the prediction and Prevention of Pressure Ulcers in Adults. (1992, May). *Pressure ulcers in adults: prediction and prevention.* Clinical Practice Guideline, Number 3. (AHCPR Pub. 92-0047). Rockville, MD: Agency for Health Care Policy and Research, Public Health Service, U.S. Department of Health and Human Services.

Pennie, R., O'Connor, A., Garvock, M., & Drake, E. (1991). Factors influencing the acceptance of hepatitis B vaccine by students in health disciplines in Ottawa. *Canadian Journal of Public Health, 82,* 12-15.

Redeker, N.S. (1992). The relationship between uncertainty and coping after coronary artery bypass surgery. *Western Journal of Nursing Research, 14*(1), 48-68.

Stetler, C.B. (1985). Research utilization: Defining the concept. *Image, 17:*2, 40-44.

Stetler, C.B. (in press). Refinement of the Stetler/Marram Model for application of research findings to practice. *Nursing Outlook.*

Stetler, C.B., & Marram, G. (1976). Evaluating research findings for applicability in practice. *Nursing Outlook, 24*(9), 559-563.

Stewart Fahs, P.S., & Kinney, M.R. (1991). The abdomen, thigh, and arm as sites for subcutaneous sodium heparin injections. *Nursing Research, 40,* 204-207.

Tesler, M., Savedra, M., Holzemer, W., Wilkie, A., Ward, J., & Paul, S. (1991). The word graphic rating scale as a measure of children's and adolescent's pain intensity. *Research in Nursing and Health, 14,* 361-371.

Urinary Incontinence Guideline Panel. (1992, March). *Urinary incontinence in adults.* Clinical Practice Guideline. (AHCPR Pub. 92-0038). Rockville, MD: Agency for Health Care Policy and Research, Public Health Service, U.S. Department of Health and Human Services.

Vessey, J., & Campos, R. (1992). The role of nursing research committees. *Nursing Research, 41*(4), 247-249.

Wells, T., Rink, C., Diokno, A. et al. (1991). Pelvic muscle exercise for stress urinary incontinence in elderly women. *Journal of the American Geriatrics Society, 38,* 296-299.

Wilson, D.M. (1992). Ethical concerns in a long-term tube feeding study. *Image: Journal of Nursing Scholarship, 24*(3), 195-199.

Wilson, S. & Morse, J.M. (1991). Living with a wife undergoing chemotherapy. *Image: Journal of Nursing Scholarship, 23,* 78-84.

PART
II

THE RESEARCH PROCESS

Using Research in the Care of Patients

LINDA CRONENWETT

In my early years at Dartmouth-Hitchcock Medical Center, I disseminated summaries of current research in a publication that we called *Nursing Research Review*. I will never forget the story that came back to me after the appearance of the following entry:

> Reduced appetite following parenteral nutrition (TPN) may be due to physiological causes rather than lack of patient cooperation or disease pathology. In early studies, investigators found that patients reported feeling hungry while on TPN, but when oral food was reintroduced, 75% reported rapid satiety and were able to consume only a few mouthfuls per meal. Martyn and her colleagues monitored the effects of TPN on oral intake, body weight, and gastric motility in four healthy rhesus monkeys. Once the TPN was discontinued, they looked at how long it took before the monkeys returned to baseline oral intake. It took two days of TPN before the monkeys' oral food intake declined to match their decreased need for calories. When terminating TPN after 7 days of infusion, food intake was significantly less than baseline for 6 to 8 days. Body weight decreased 5-7% in response to the continued appetite suppression. If human physiological responses parallel monkey responses, patients could be prepared for the lack of appetite-suppression when TPN is initiated. Likewise, nurses and patients could expect a transition period post-TPN during which patients are unable to consume enough food to maintain body weight.
>
> Martyn, PA, Hansen, BC, Jen, KC: The effects of parenteral nutrition on food intake and gastric motility. *Nursing Research* 1984; 33:336-342.

A week after dissemination, the clinical nurse specialist (CNS) from our neurological/neurosurgical unit visited me with the introduction "You'll never believe what I was just told by one of our patients." Apparently, an elderly man had been receiving TPN for some time. The parenteral feedings were discontinued a few days earlier, and his wife was visiting during almost every meal to urge him to eat. Their interchanges were difficult, leading occasionally to accusations by the wife that he must not want to get better or he would eat more. The CNS was following this couple and stopped in to make a nutritional assessment. On this particular day, husband and wife were feeling more positive about his recovery. The man said that he and his wife had been arguing lately about his lack of ability to eat enough food; however, this morning his nurse had told him that she had read about some research that seemed to indicate that the lack of ability to eat after TPN might be a normal physiological response that would pass in a few days. Both husband and wife were looking at his food intake problem in a new way. They were sure he would be able to increase his intake soon.

The staff nurse in this story did not *use* research employing the formal methods or processes that you will read about in this book. She had not reviewed the literature to see whether multiple studies corroborated the cited study's findings. In fact, she did not know whether the findings of an animal model applied to humans. But this nurse read about scientific findings that had relevance for her practice and thought about her practice in a new way. She offered a distressed couple a new, and potentially valid, way to interpret their experiences. She used research to make a difference in the quality of their lives as they coped with a new challenge to recovery from illness.

Research can be used in many ways, from formal to informal, from dramatic changes in protocols to minor alterations in the processes and interactions of care. The important point is that new knowledge, the product of research, is or should always be a stimulus to professional thought and behavior. By using research, nurses commit themselves to the process of continuously evaluating and improving the quality of patient care.

CHAPTER
4

Overview of the Research Process

GERI LoBIONDO-WOOD
JUDITH HABER
BARBARA KRAINOVICH MILLER

LEARNING OBJECTIVES

After reading this chapter the student should be able to do the following:

* Identify the importance of critical thinking and critical reading for the reading of research articles.
* Identify the steps of critical reading.
* Use the steps of critical reading for reviewing research articles.
* Use identified strategies for critically reading research articles.
* Identify the format and style of research articles.

KEY TERMS

abstract   critique
critical reading   critiquing criteria
critical thinking

As you venture through this text you will see the steps of the research process unfold. The steps are systematic and orderly and relate to both nursing theory and nursing practice. Understanding the step-by-step process that researchers use will assist in judging the soundness of research studies. Through the chapters, research terminology pertinent to each step is identified and illustrated with many examples from the research literature. Three completed research studies are found in the appendixes and are used as examples to illustrate significant points in each chapter. The steps of the process generally proceed in the order outlined in Table 4-1 (pp. 100-101) but may vary, depending on the nature of the research problem. It is important to remember that a researcher may vary the steps slightly, but the steps must still be addressed systematically. This chapter provides an overview of critical thinking, critical reading, and critiquing skills; introduces the overall format of a research article; and provides an overview of the subsequent chapters in the book. These topics are designed to help you read research articles more effectively and with greater understanding, thereby making this book more "user-friendly" for students learning about the research process.

CRITICAL THINKING AND CRITICAL READING SKILLS

As you read a research article for the first time you may be struck by the difference in style or format between a research article and a theoretical article. The terms are new, and the focus of the content is different. You may be wondering, "How will I possibly learn to evaluate all the steps of a research study as well as all the terminology? I'm only on Chapter 4; this is not so easy." The answer, which may seem trivial, is that it occurs with time and help. First reading research articles is frustrating and difficult. However, the best way to become an intelligent consumer of research is to use critical thinking and reading skills to read research articles. Students are not expected to understand a research article or critique it perfectly the first time. Nor are they expected to develop this skill on their own. An essential objective of this book is to help you acquire these critical thinking and reading skills so you can reach this goal. Remember that critical thinking and reading, like learning the steps of the research process, are learning processes that take time.

Critical thinking is the rational examination of ideas, inferences, assumptions, principles, arguments, conclusions, issues, statements, beliefs, and actions

(Bandman & Bandman, 1988, p. 5). This means that you are engaging in the following:

1. The art of thinking about your thinking so as to make it more clear, precise, accurate, relevant, consistent, and fair
2. The art of constructive skepticism
3. The art of identifying and removing bias, prejudice, and one-sidedness of thought (Paul, 1990, p. 32)
4. The art of clarifying what you do understand and what you don't know

In other words, you are consciously thinking about your own thoughts and what you say, write, read, or do, as well as what others say, write, or do. While thinking about all of this, you are questioning the appropriateness of the content, applying standards or criteria, and seeing how things measure up, or thinking about alternative ways of handling the same situation. Although this is considered a highly rational process, it is a highly emotional and at times anxiety producing one (Brookfield, 1991).

Developing the ability to evaluate research critically requires not only critical thinking skills, but critical reading skills. Paul (1990), a noted theorist on critical thinking, defines **critical reading** as

> an active, intellectually engaging process in which the reader participates in an inner dialogue with the writer. . . . [It] means entering into a point of view other than our own, the point of view of the writer. A critical reader actively looks for assumptions, key concepts and ideas, reasons and justifications, supporting examples, parallel experiences, and any other structural features of the written text, to interpret and assess it accurately and fairly. (p. 544)

This means that the reader actively looks for assumptions—those supposedly true or accepted statements that are actually unsupported. It is perhaps easier to understand how you do this by thinking about one of the early assumptions of nursing education and practice. In the late 1950s and early 1960s the nursing process was presented as "the" framework for practice. The formulation of a nursing diagnosis was viewed as an essential step of this process. Initially there was no scientific evidence to support this assumption. Yet schools of nursing began to teach these concepts and nurses began to use them in their practice. Eventually, nursing process became a part of the American Nurses Association (ANA) (1980) social policy statement's definition of the practice of nursing.

At the same time these assumptions were introduced, nurse researchers questioned them and devised studies to examine the concepts in relation to nursing process. The results of these studies provided data to support or refute the assumptions. Numerous studies conducted over the years offer evidence that these concepts are more than assumptions.

Currently students are formally introduced to critical thinking skills through the nursing process (Lewis & Eakes, 1992). Critical thinking and critical reading skills are further developed through learning the research process. You will find that beginning critical thinking and reading skills used in activating the nursing process can easily be transferred to understanding the research process and reading research articles. Gradually you will be able to read an entire article and reflect on it by identifying and challenging assumptions, identifying key concepts, questioning rationales, and determining whether supporting evidence exists and finally be able to re-read it to "accurately and fairly assess it" (Paul, 1990, p. 544).

THE PROCESS OF CRITICAL READING

To accomplish the purpose of critically reading a research study, the reader must have skilled reading, writing and reasoning abilities. It is quite common for a research study to require several readings. A minimum of three or four readings and even as many as six readings, with your research textbook at your side, facilitate and are necessary to do the following:
- Identify concepts
- Clarify unfamiliar concepts or terms
- Question assumptions and rationale
- Determine supporting evidence

Critical reading can be viewed as a process that involves various levels or stages of understanding:
- Preliminary understanding
- Comprehensive understanding
- Analysis understanding
- Synthesis understanding

Preliminary Understanding: Familiarity

Preliminary understanding is gained by quickly or lightly reading an article to familiarize yourself with its content or to get a general sense of the material. During the preliminary reading the title and **abstract** are read closely but the content is skimmed. The abstract, a brief overview of a study, keys the reader to the main components of the study. The title keys the reader to the main variables of the study. "Skimming" includes reading the introduction, major headings, one or two sentences under a heading and the summary or conclusion of the study. The preliminary reading includes use of the following strategies:
- Highlighting or underlining the main steps of the research process
- Making notes on the photocopied article
- Writing key variables at the top of the photocopied article
- Highlighting or underlining on the photocopy new and unfamiliar terms and significant sentences
- Looking up the definitions of new terms and writing them in the margins of the photocopy
- Reviewing old and new terms before the next reading
- Writing comments, questions, and notes on the photocopy
- Keeping a research text and a dictionary by your side

Using these strategies enables the reader to identify the main theme or idea of the article and bring this knowledge to the second comprehensive reading.

Comprehensive Understanding: Content in Relation to Context

Gagne (1985) refers to this level as *skilled reading*. The purpose of comprehensive understanding is to understand the article—to see the terms in relation to the context or the parts of the study in relation to the whole article. For example, when reading Hutchison and Bahr's (1991) study (see Appendix C) for comprehension, it is essential to understand that their framework for caring is based on the results of their grounded theory study, that is, the context of caring. To simply recall that the major variable of the study was caring behaviors among the elderly would be inadequate. At comprehension level reading, you would be able to discuss the four major properties of caring: protecting, supporting, confirming, and transcending.

When reading for comprehension keep your research text and dictionary nearby. Although during the preliminary reading some terms may have seemed clear, on the second reading they may be unclear. Do not hesitate to write cues or key relationships words on the photocopy. If after this reading the article still does not make sense, ask for assistance before reading it again. One suggestion is to make another copy and ask your professor to read it. Indicate on the copy the unclear areas and write out your specific questions. Often what is or is not highlighted or the comments on the copy help the faculty person to understand your difficulty. The problem may be that further reading on the topic is necessary to comprehend the article. For example, if a student is unfamiliar with Rogers' Science of Unitary Human Beings (1990), reading a study testing a proposition of this model may be difficult unless Rogers' model is read.

Comprehensive understanding is facilitated by the following strategies:
* Reviewing all unfamiliar terms before reading for the second time
* Clarifying any additional unclear terms
* Reading additional sources as necessary
* Writing cues, relationships of concepts, and questions on the photocopy
* Making another copy of your annotated article and requesting that your faculty member read it
* Stating the main idea or theme of the article, in your own words, in one or two sentences on an index card or on the photocopy

Comprehensive understanding is necessary to analyze and synthesize the material. Understanding the author's perspective for the study reflects critical thinking (Paul, 1990) and facilitates the analysis of the study according to established criteria. The next reading or two allows for analysis and synthesis of the study.

Analysis Understanding: Breaking into Parts

The purpose of reading for analysis is to break the content into parts to understand each aspect of the study. Some of the questions that you can ask yourself as you begin to analyze the research article are as follows:
* Did I capture the main idea or theme of this article in one or two sentences?
* How are the major parts of this article organized in relation to the research process?

- What is the purpose of this article?
- How was this study carried out? Can I explain it step by step?
- What are the author's(s') main conclusions?
- Can I say that I understand the parts of this article and summarize each section in my own words?

In a sense you are determining how the steps of the research process are presented or organized in the article and what the content related to each step is all about. This is also the time that you begin to answer the questions in the critiquing sections of each chapter. You are beginning the critiquing process that will help determine the study's merit.

The **critique** is the process of objectively and critically evaluating a research report's content for scientific merit and application to practice, theory, and education. It requires some knowledge of the subject matter and knowledge of how to critically read and how to use critiquing criteria. An in-depth exploration of the criteria for analysis required for quantitative research critiques is given in Chapters 5 through 10 and 12 through 18 and summarized in Chapter 19; the criteria for qualitative research critiques are covered in Chapter 11 and summarized in Chapter 20.

Critiquing criteria are the measures, standards, evaluation guides, or questions used to judge (critique) a product or behavior. The reader, in analyzing the research report, must evaluate each step of the research process. The reader must ask questions about whether each explanation of a step of the process meets or does not meet these criteria. For instance, Chapter 5 states that one of the objectives of a literature review is to determine gaps and consistencies and inconsistencies in the literature about a subject, concept, or problem. One critiquing guide question in Table 19-1 (see Chapter 19, p. 443) is "What gaps in knowledge about the problem are identified, and how does this study intend to fill those gaps?" In this example the purpose of the objective of the literature review is the evaluation question or criterion for critiquing the review of the literature.

The review of the literature section of a study by Haber and Austin (1992) entitled "Marital Decision Making" illustrates how that criterion is addressed. In this section the authors reviews many studies; in the summary of the literature review, which appears before the hypotheses, they highlight the impact of each study on the hypotheses. They conclude the following:

> Therefore, none of the prior studies included a method for examining the behavior of married couples when they were involved in an actual episode of decision making. . . . Thus this study provides a more objective test of selected aspects of the model. (p. 324)

This example implies that reading for analysis took place. Understanding gained by reading for analysis is facilitated by the following critiquing strategies:
- Being familiar with critiquing criteria
- Reaching the comprehensive reading stage before applying critiquing criteria; rereading if necessary
- Applying the critiquing criteria to each step of the research process in the article
- Asking whether the content meets the criteria for each step of the research process

- Asking fellow students to analyze the same study with the same criteria and comparing results
- Writing notes on the copy about how each step of the research process measures up against the established criteria

Synthesis Understanding: Putting Together

Synthesis is the "combination or putting together; combining of parts into a whole" (New Webster's Dictionary and Thesaurus, 1991, p. 384). The purpose of reading for synthesis is to pull all the information together to form a new whole (Kerlinger, 1986); to make sense of it; to explain relationships. Although the process of synthesizing the material may be taking place as the reader is analyzing the article, a fourth reading is recommended. It is during the synthesis reading that the understanding and critique of the whole study are put together. During this final step you decide how well the study meets the critiquing criteria (Chapters 19 and 20) and how useful it is to practice (Chapter 3). It is the point at which the reader decides how well each step of the research process relates to the previous step. Synthesis can be thought of as looking at a jigsaw puzzle once it is completed. Does it form a comprehensive picture, or is there a piece out of place? In the case of reviewing or reading for synthesis of several studies, the interrelationship of the studies is assessed. Reading for high-level synthesis is essential to critiquing research studies. The previous example of Haber and Austin's (1992) summary statement of their review of the literature also reflects synthesis reading.

Reading for synthesis is facilitated by the following strategies:

1. Reviewing your notes on the article on how each step of the research process measured up against the established criteria
2. Briefly summarizing the study in your own words, including in your summary:
   a. The components of the study
   b. The study's overall strengths and weaknesses
3. Following the suggested format of:
   a. Limiting the summary to one page, computer-typed or handwritten on a 5 × 8 index card
   b. Including the citation at the top of the page in the specified reference style
   c. Stapling the summary to the top of the photocopied article

This type of summary is viewed as the first draft of a final written critique. It teaches brevity, facilitates easy retrieval of data to support your critiquing evaluation, and increases your ability to write a scholarly report. In addition, the ability to synthesize one study prepares you for the task of critiquing several studies on a similar topic and comparing and contrasting their findings (see Chapter 5).

PERCEIVED DIFFICULTIES AND STRATEGIES FOR CRITIQUING RESEARCH

Critiquing research articles is difficult for the beginning consumer of research and is somewhat frustrating at first. However, the best way to become an intelligent consumer of research is to use critical thinking and reading skills to read articles. The box below presents some highlighted strategies for reading and evaluating a research report. As mentioned, a helpful strategy when reading research articles for the first few times is to keep your text nearby so that unfamiliar or unclear terms can be looked up and if necessary each step of the research process can be reviewed as you read. No matter how difficult it may seem, read the entire article and reflect on it. Critically read for the levels of understanding described in this chapter. Most important, draw on previous knowledge, common sense, and the critical thinking skills you already possess.

Another important overall strategy is to ask questions; remember that questioning is essential to developing critical thinking. Asking faculty questions and sharing your concerns about what you are reading or their own published work is an

---

HIGHLIGHTS OF CRITICAL THINKING AND READING STRATEGIES

- Read primary source data-based articles from refereed journals (see Chapter 5, Table 5-6)
- Read secondary source data-based critique/response/commentary articles from referred journals (see Chapter 5, Table 5-9)
- Photocopy primary and secondary source articles; make notations directly on the copy
- While reading data-based articles:
  - Keep a research text and a dictionary by your side
  - Review the chapters in a research text on various steps of the research process, critiquing criteria, unfamiliar terms, and so on
  - List key variables at the top of photocopy
  - Highlight or underline on photocopy new terms, unfamiliar vocabulary, and significant sentences
  - Look up the definitions of new terms and write them on the photocopy
  - Review old and new terms before subsequent readings
  - Highlight or underline identified steps of the research process
  - Identify the main idea or theme of the article; state it in your own words in one or two sentences
  - Continue to clarify terms that may be unclear on subsequent readings
  - Make sure you understand the main points of each reported step of the research process you identified before critiquing the article
- Determine how well the study meets the critiquing criteria
  - Ask fellow students to analyze the same study using the same criteria and compare results
  - Consult faculty members about your evaluation of the study
- Type a one-page summary and critque of each reviewed study
  - Cite references at the top according to APA or another reference style
  - Briefly summarize each reported research step in your own words
  - Briefly describe strengths and weaknesses in your own words

effective way of developing your reading skills. Do not hesitate to write to or call a researcher if you have a question about his or her work. You will be pleasantly surprised by how willing researchers are to discuss your questions.

RESEARCH ARTICLES: FORMAT AND STYLE

Before one considers the reading of research articles, it is important to have a sense of their organization and format. Many journals publish research, either as the sole type of article in the journal or in addition to clinical or theoretical articles. Although many journals have some common features, they also have unique characteristics. All journals have guides for manuscript preparation and submission, which generally are published in each journal. A review of these guides will give you an idea of the format of articles that appear in specific journals. It is important to remember that even though each step of the research process is discussed at length in this text, you may find only a short paragraph or a sentence in the research article giving the details of the step in a specific study. Because of the journal's space limitations or other publishing guidelines, the published study that one reads in a journal is a shortened version of the total work done by the researcher(s). Readers will find also that some researchers devote more space in an article to the results, whereas others present a longer discussion of the methods and procedures. In recent years most authors give more emphasis to the method, results, and discussion of implications than to details of assumptions, hypotheses, or definitions of terms. Decisions about the amount to present on each step of the research process within an article are bound by the following:
- A journal's space limitations
- A journal's author guidelines
- The type or nature of the study
- An individual researcher's evaluation of what is the most important component to report.

The following discussion provides a brief overview of each step of the research process and how it might appear in an article. Table 4-1 indicates where the step usually can be located in a journal article and where it is discussed in this textbook. It also is important to remember that a published article about a quantitative study will differ from one about a qualitative study. The primary difference is that a qualitative study does not test a hypothesis but may generate hypotheses based on the results. Another difference is the manner in which literature reviews are conducted and used in the study (see Chapters 2, 11, and 20).

Abstract

An abstract is a short comprehensive synopsis of a study at the beginning of an article. An abstract quickly focuses the reader on the main points of a study. A well-presented abstract is accurate, self-contained, concise, nonevaluative, coherent, and readable (American Psychological Association, 1983). Abstracts vary in length from 50 to 250 words. A number of journals that publish research provide abstracts;

Table 4-1   Steps of the Research Process and Journal Format

Research process steps and/or format issue	Usual location in a journal heading or subheading	Text chapter
Research problem	Abstract and/or in the Introduction (not labeled) or in a separate labeled heading: Problem	7
Purpose	Abstract and/or in the Introduction or at the end of the literature review, theoretical framework section, or labeled as a separate heading: Purpose	7
Literature review	At the end of the heading Introduction but not labeled as such, or labeled as a separate heading: Literature Review, Review of the Literature, or Related Literature; or not labeled but the variables reviewed appear as headings or subheadings	5
Theoretical framework (TF) and/or Conceptual framework (CF)	Combined with Literature review or found in a separate heading as TF or CF; or each concept or definition used in the TF or CF may appear as a separate heading or subheading	6
Hypothesis/research questions	Stated or implied near the end of the introductory section, which may or may not be labeled or found in a separate heading: Hypothesis or Research Questions; or reported for the first time in the Results section	7
Research design	Stated or implied in the Abstract or in the Introduction or under the heading: Methods	8, 9, 10, 11
Sample: type and size	"Size" may be stated in the abstract, in the Methods section, or as a separate subheading under Methods section as sample, sample/subjects or subjects, or participants "Type" may be implied or stated in any of previous headings described under size	12, 11
Legal-ethical issues	Stated or implied in labeled headings: Methods, Procedures, Sample or Subjects	13
Instruments (meaurement tools)	Found in Headings labeled Methods, Instruments, or Measures	14, 15

Table 4-1   Steps of the Research Process and Journal Format—cont'd

Research process steps and\or format issue	Usual location in a journal heading or subheading	Text chapter
Validity and reliability	Specifically stated or implied in headings labeled Methods, Instruments, Measures, or Procedures	15
Data collection procedure	Stated in Methods section under subheading Procedure or Data Collection, or as a separate heading: Procedure	14
Data analysis	Stated in Methods section under subheading Procedure or Data Analysis	16, 17
Results	Stated in separate heading: Results	18
Discussion of findings and new findings	Combined with Results or as separate heading: Discussion	18
Implications, limitations, and recommendations	Combined in Discussion or presented as separate or combined major headings	18
References	At the end of the article	4, 5
Communicating research results	Research articles, poster and paper presentations	1, 2, 3, 4, 18, 19, 20

however, several do not. *Western Journal of Nursing Research,* for example, does not have an abstract at the beginning of its articles.

An example of a succinct abstract can be found at the beginning of the study by Rice, Mullin, and Jarosz (1992). It reads as follows:

> Fifty adult coronary artery by-pass (CABG) patients were randomly assigned to preadmission self-instruction or posthospital admission instruction of therapeutic exercises (e.g., coughing). Self-instructed subjects reported higher positive mood scores, performed correctly significantly more exercise behaviors and required less teaching time following admission. (p. 253)

Within the first sentence of this example, the authors provide a view of the following information: sample composition (CABG patients), sample size (50), type of sampling method (probability), design (experimental), and type of procedure (two-group comparison of intervention effectiveness). The second sentence gives a synopsis of the variables measured and the results. The three studies in Appendixes A, B, and C all have abstracts.

Identification of a Research Problem

Early in a research article, in a section that may or may not be labeled Introduction, the researcher presents a picture of the area researched. This is the presentation of the *research problem* (see Chapter 7). Reading the study by Grey, Cameron, and Thurber (1991) (Appendix B), the reader can find the research problem in the opening paragraph of the article:

> It is important to determine the factors associated with adaptation to chronic illness in preadolescents and adolescents, because current approaches to the care of these children assume that the factors predicting adaptation are similar. (p. 144)

Definition of the Purpose

The purpose of the study is defined either at the end of the researcher's initial introduction or at the end of the literature review or conceptual framework section. These components of the research process may or may not be labeled as such (see Chapters 5, 6, and 7). Following along in the study by Grey et al. (1991) (Appendix B), in the paragraph before the "Review of the Literature," the purpose is clearly stated:

> The purpose of this study was to determine the adaptation of preadolescent and adolescents with insulin dependent diabetes mellitus (IDDM). (p. 144)

In the study by Stewart Fahs and Kinney (1991) (Appendix A), the reader will find the purpose stated clearly, though positioned differently than in the previous example, in the last sentence of the first paragraph before the section labeled "Literature Review":

> Therefore, this study was undertaken to determine whether alternate sites were effective in accomplishing the goals of low-dose heparin therapy and to identify any differences in bruising at the injection site. (p. 204)

Literature Review and Theoretical Framework

Authors of studies and journal articles present the literature review and theoretical framework in different ways. Many research articles merge the literature review and theoretical framework. The section heading may include the main concepts investigated; may be called "review of the literature," "literature review," "theoretical framework," or conceptual framework"; or may not be labeled at all (see Chapters 5 and 6). By reviewing Appendixes A and B, the reader will find the headings "Literature Review" (Stewart Fahs & Kinney, 1991) and "Review of the Literature" (Grey et al., 1991). These sections contain both the literature review and the theoretical frameworks of the studies. An example of a study where these sections are discussed separately can be found in the study by Gass, Gaustad, Oberst, and Huges (1992). One style is not better than another; all three studies identified contain all the critical elements but present them differently.

Hypothesis/Research Question

A study's research question and hypotheses can also be presented in different ways (see Chapter 7). They may be labeled as "Hypotheses," as in Stewart Fahs and Kinney's (1991) study (Appendix A):

I. There is no difference in effectiveness of low-dose heparin therapy, as measured by activated partial thromboplastin time (aPTT), when administered in three different subcutaneous sites. (p. 204)

Or they may be implied, as in a study by Grey et al. (1991) at the end of the introduction:

It was proposed that adaptation would be influenced by age, coping behaviors, and self-care behaviors. (p. 144)

Research Design

The type of research design can be found in the abstract, within the purpose statement, in the introduction to the procedures or methods section, or not stated at all (see Chapters 8, 9, 10, and 11). For example, of the three studies in the appendixes, only one identified the type of study design used: Hutchison and Bahr (1991) (Appendix C) identified their study as one using the grounded theory method.

One of the first things to determine is whether the study is qualitative or quantitative (see Chapters 8 and 11). This is important because the critiquing criteria differ for qualitative and quantitative studies. In quantitative studies in particular, the way the steps of the research process are used provides clues to determine a study's design.

Do not get discouraged if you cannot easily determine the design. Unfortunately, as stated, more times than not the specific quantitative design is not stated or if an advanced design is used, the details are not spelled out. One of the best strategies is to review the chapters in this text that address quantitative designs (Chapters 8, 9, and 10) and to ask your professors for assistance after you have read the chapters! Determining designs is not an easy process. The following are a few tips to help you determine whether the study you are reading uses a *quantitative design:*
• Hypotheses are stated or implied (See Chapter 7)
• The terms *control* and *treatment group* appear (See Chapter 9)
• The term *survey, correlational,* or *ex post facto* is used (see Chapter 10)
• The term *random* or *convenience* is mentioned in relation to the sample (see Chapter 12)
• Variables are measured by instruments or tools (see Chapter 14)
• Reliability and validity of instruments are discussed (see Chapter 15)
• Statistical analyses are used (see Chapters 16 and 17)

In contrast, generally *qualitative studies* do not deal with "numbers." However, some qualitative studies use standard quantitative terms, such as *subjects,* rather than the qualitative term for a phenomenological study, *informants;* they may or may not mention the number of informants used in the study (see Chapter 20). It can be confusing, so one of the best strategies is to review this text's chapter on qualitative design (Chapter 11), as well as critiquing qualitative studies (Chapter 20). Do not hesitate to ask faculty members for assistance after you have read the chapters.

Sampling

The population from which the sample was drawn is discussed in the methods section entitled "Methods" or "Methodology" under the subheadings of Subjects or Sample (see Chapter 12). For example, Stewart Fahs and Kinney's (1991; Appendix A) study discusses the sample of their quantitative study under the heading "Method" and with the subheading "Subjects." These researchers discuss the subjects used in great detail in two paragraphs. They state the following at the end of the first paragraph:

> The final sample included 101 subjects classified as general medical/surgical patients. Final group sizes were Abdomen (A) = 33, Thigh (B) = 33, and Arm (c) = 35. (p. 205)

Although the type of sampling was not indicated, it can be inferred that it was a nonprobability sampling method (see Chapter 12).

In contrast, the qualitative grounded theory study by Hutchison and Bahr (1991; Appendix C) drew its sample from a group of nursing home residents who met the following criteria:
- Age of 62 years or older
- Cognitively intact
- Expectation of living in the nursing home indefinitely
- Length of stay of at least 2 months

The researchers also noted that they were guided by a theoretical sampling strategy.

Instruments: Reliability and Validity

The discussion related to method used to measure the variables of a study is usually included in a Methods section under the subheading of Instruments or Measures (Chapter 14). The researcher usually describes the particular measure (instrument or tool) used by discussing its reliability and validity (Chapter 15). Grey et al. (1991; Appendix B) discuss the measures they used in their Method section under the subheading Instruments. Multiple instruments (questionnaires) were used. The researchers reported the reliability of all and indicated the validity of some. However, the validity and reliability of instruments are not always reported. In some cases researchers do not use space in the article to report on commonly used valid and reliable instrument(s) such as Spielberger's State-Trait Anxiety Inventory (STAI) (1983). Seek assistance from your instructor if you are in doubt about the validity or reliability of a study's instruments.

Another example is the discussion by Stewart Fahs and Kinney (1991; Appendix A). In their Method section under the subheading Measures they state in the first paragraph that blood was measured for calculation of aPTT and bruising, as measured by two methods.

Procedures and Data Collection Methods

The procedures used to collect data or the step-by-step way that the researcher(s) used the measures (instruments or tools) is generally headed Procedures (see Chapter 14). In the study by Stewart Fahs and Kinney (1991; Appendix A), the researchers not only define what a bruise is, but describe how they assessed for bruising and the details of the two methods used for measuring the bruises.

Data Analysis

The *data analysis procedures,* that is, the statistical tests used in quantitative studies and the results of descriptive and/or inferential tests applied, are presented in the section labeled Results or Findings (Chapters 16 and 17). Although qualitative studies do not use statistical tests, the procedures for analyzing the themes, concepts, and/or observational or print data are usually described in the Method or Data Collection section and reported in a section labeled Results or Findings (Chapters 11 and 20).

When researchers do not indicate in a separate section what statistical test they used, it is presented in the Results section. For example, in the studies by Stewart Fahs and Kinney (1991; Appendix A) and Grey et al. (1991; Appendix B), the inferential statistical tests used were reported with the results under the heading Results (see Chapter 17). Hutchison and Bahr (1991; Appendix C) report the results of their qualitative grounded study, which used the analysis method of constant comparison (Method section), in the section headed Findings.

Results/Discussion

The last section of a research study is the Results or Discussion section. As you will find when you read Chapter 18, the researcher in this section ties together all the pieces of the study and gives a picture of the study as a whole. Often researchers report the results in one section and the discussion in a separate section. Again, one is no better than the other. Both quantitative studies in Appendixes A and B report each separately.

New findings or unexpected findings are usually described in the Discussion section. In the case of Grey et al. (1991; Appendix B), the researchers stated the following:

> It was not expected that investing in close friends as a coping strategy would be associated with poorer metabolic control. (p. 148)

The researchers were not expecting this finding and discuss the possible reason for it.

Recommendations and Implications

In some cases the researcher reports the implications, based on the findings, for practice and education and recommend future studies in a separate section; in other cases they appear at the end of the Discussion section (see quantitative studies in Appendixes A and B). In contrast, the qualitative study found in Appendix C includes the recommendations based on the findings under the heading Discussion and Recommendations and includes a separate heading labeled Further Research (Chapter 18). Again, one is no better than the other—only different.

References

Included at the end of a research article or any scholarly article, are all references cited in the article. The main purpose of the reference list is to support the material presented by identifying the sources in a manner that allows easy retrieval by the reader (APA, 1983).

Communicating Results

Communicating the results of a study can take the form of a research article, a poster, or a paper presentation (Chapter 3). All are valid ways of providing nursing with the data and the ability to provide high-quality patient care based on research findings. Research-based nursing care plans and patient protocols are outcome measures that indicate effectively communicated research.

As you develop critical thinking and reading skills by using the strategies presented in this chapter, you will become more familiar with the research and critiquing processes. Gradually your ability to read and critique research articles will improve. You will be well on your way to becoming a knowledgeable consumer of research from nursing and other scientific disciplines.

KEY POINTS

- The best way to become an intelligent consumer of research is to use critical thinking and reading skills to read research articles.
- Critical thinking is the rational examination of ideas, inferences, principles, and conclusions.
- Critical thinking enables you to question the appropriateness of the content of a research article, apply standards or criteria to assess the study's scientific merit, or consider alternative ways of handling the same topic.
- Critical reading involves active interpretation and objective assessment of an article, looking for key concepts, ideas, and justifications.
- Critical reading requires four stages of understanding: preliminary, comprehensive, analysis, and synthesis. Each stage includes strategies to increase your critical reading skills.
- Preliminary understanding is gained by quickly and lightly reading an article to familiarize yourself with its content or to get a general sense of the material.

- Comprehensive understanding is skilled reading designed to increase understanding of the terms in relation to the context or the parts of the study in relation to the whole article.
- Analysis understanding is designed to break the content into parts so that each part of the study is understood; the critiquing process begins at this stage.
- The goal of synthesis understanding is to combine the parts of a research study into a whole. During this final stage the reader determines how each step relates to all the steps of the research, how well the study meets the critiquing criteria, and the usefulness of the study for practice.
- Critiquing is the process of objectively and critically evaluating a research article for scientific merit and application to practice, theory, or education.
- Critiquing criteria are the measures, standards, evaluation guides, or questions used to judge the worth of a research study.
- Research articles have different formats and styles depending on journal manuscript requirements and whether they are quantitative or qualitative studies.
- Basic steps of the research process are presented in journal articles in various ways. Detailed examples of such variations can be found in chapters throughout this book.

REFERENCES

American Nurses Association. (ANA). (1980). *A social policy statement.* Kansas City, MO: Author.

American Psychological Association. (APA). (1983). *Publication manual of the American psychological association.* (3rd ed.). Washington, DC: Author.

Bandman, E.L., & Bandman, B. (1988). *Critical thinking in nursing.* Norwalk, CT: Appleton & Lange.

Brookfield, S.D. (1991). *Developing critical thinkers.* San Francisco: Jossey-Bass.

Gagne, E.D. (1985). *The cognitive psychology of school learning.* Boston: Little, Brown.

Gass, K.A., Gaustad, G., Oberst, M.T., & Hughes, S. (1992). Relocating appraisal, functional independence, morale, and health of nursing home residents. *Issues in Mental Health Nursing, 13,* 239-253.

Grey, M., Cameron, M.E., & Thurber, F.W. (1991). Coping and adaptation in children with diabetes. *Nursing Research, 40*(3), 144-149.

Haber, L.C., & Austin, J.K. (1992). How married couples make decisions. *Western Journal of Nursing Research, 14*(3), 322-342.

Hutchison, C.P., & Bahr, R.T. (1991). Types and meanings of caring behaviors among elderly nursing home residents. *Image, 23*(2), 85-88.

Kerlinger, F.N. (1986). *Foundations of behavioral research.* (3rd ed.). New York: Holt, Rinehart & Winston.

Lewis, J.B., & Eakes, G.G. (1992). The AIDS care dilemma: An exercise in critical thinking. *Journal of Nursing Education, 31*(3), 136-137.

New Webster's Dictionary and Thesaurus. (1991). New York: Book Essentials.

Paul, R.W. (1990). *Critical thinking: What every person needs to survive in a rapidly changing world.* Rohnert Park, CA: Center for Critical Thinking & Moral Critique.

Rice, V.H., Mullin, M.H., & Jarosz, P. (1992). Preadmission self-instruction effects on postadmission and postoperative indicators in CABG patients: Partial replication and extension. *Research In Nursing & Health, 15,* 253-259.

Rogers, M.E. (1990). Nursing: Science of unitary, irreducible, human beings: Update 1990. In E.A.N. Barrett (Ed.), *Visions of Rogers' science-based nursing* (pp. 5-11). New York: National League for Nursing.

Spielberger, C.D., Gorsuch, R.L., Lushene, R., Vagg, P.R., & Jacobs, G.A. (1983). *Manual for the state-trait anxiety inventory.* Palo Alto, CA: Consulting Psychologists Press.

Stewart Fahs, S., & Kinney, M.R. (1991). The abdomen, thigh, and arm as sites for subcutaneous sodium heparin injections. *Nursing Research, 40*(4), 204-207.

ADDITIONAL READINGS

Allen, D.G., Bowers, B., & Dickelmann, N. (1989). Writing to learn: A reconceptualization of thinking and writing in the nursing curriculum. *Journal of Nursing Education, 28*(1), 6-11.

Brooks, K.L., & Shepherd J.M. (1990). The relationship between clinical decision-making skills in nursing and general critical thinking abilities of senior nursing students in four types of nursing programs. *Journal of Nursing Education, 29*(9), 391-399.

Carnevali, D.L., Mitchell, P.H., Woods, N.F., & Tanner, C.A. (1984). Diagnostic reasoning in nursing. Philadelphia: J.B. Lippincott.

Cross, K.P. (1987). *Adults as learners.* San Francisco: Jossey-Bass.

Miller, M.A., & Malcolm, N.S. (1990). Critical thinking in the nursing curriculum. *Nursing & Health Care, 11*(2), 67-73.

Radwin, L.E. (1990). Research on diagnostic reasoning in nursing. *Nursing Diagnosis, 1*(2), 70-77.

Watson, G., & Glaser, E.M. (1980). *Watson-Glaser critical thinking appraisal manual.* San Antonio: The Psychological Corporation.

CHAPTER
5

The Literature Review

BARBARA KRAINOVICH MILLER

LEARNING OBJECTIVES

After reading this chapter the student should be able to do the following:

- Discuss the relationship of the review of the literature to nursing theory, research, education, and practice.
- Discuss the purposes of the literature review for research and nonresearch activities.
- Discuss the use of the review of the literature for quantitative designs and qualitative approaches.
- Discuss the major objectives for the consumer of research in relation to the review of the literature.
- Differentiate between conceptual and data-based literature.
- Differentiate between primary and secondary sources.
- Compare the advantages and disadvantages of the most commonly used computer and print data-base sources for conducting a relevant review of the literature.
- Identify the characteristics of a relevant literature review.
- Critically read (summarize and critique), at a beginning consumer of research level, conceptual and data-based resources.
- Apply critiquing criteria to the evaluation of literature reviews in selected research studies.

KEY TERMS

CINAHL on-line or CD-ROM   print data bases
computer data bases   refereed journal
conceptual literature   review of the literature
data-based literature   scholarly literature
empirical literature   scientific literature
MEDLINE on-line or CD-ROM   secondary source
primary source   theoretical literature

The reader may wonder why an entire chapter is devoted to the review of the literature. It is because the literature review is a key step in the research process. A more personal question you might ask yourself is "Will knowing more about the literature review really help me in my student role or later in my research consumer role as a practicing professional nurse?" The answer is that most certainly it will. The ability to review the literature is a skill essential to your role as a student and your future role as a research consumer.

The **review of the literature** is traditionally considered a systematic and critical review of the most important published **scholarly literature** on a particular topic. The term *scholarly literature* can refer to published and unpublished **data-based literature** and **conceptual literature** materials found in print and nonprint forms. Data-based resources are reports of completed research. Conceptual literature can be reports of theories, some of which underlie reported research, as well as other nonresearch material. For example, an article that discusses a particular theory or reviews the literature related to a concept such as anxiety is considered conceptual rather than data-based literature.

This chapter introduces the review of the literature as a concept essential to the growth of nursing theory, research, education, and practice, as illustrated in Fig. 5-1. In turn, knowledge, generated from theorists, researchers, educators, and practitioners, builds the literature through scholarly publications and presentations. In relation to these four concepts, a critical review of the literature does the following:

- Uncovers new knowledge that can lead to the development, validation, or refinement of *theories.*
- Reveals appropriate *research* questions for the discipline.
- Provides the latest knowledge for *education.*
- Supplies *practice* with new knowledge, especially as research-based nursing interventions.

The purpose of this chapter is to introduce you to the use of the review of

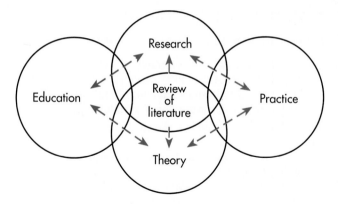

Fig. 5-1   Relationship of the review of the literature to theory, research, education, and practice.

the literature in quantitative research* and other scholarly nonresearch activities. The primary focus of the discussion is the perspective of the consumer of research rather than the "conductor of research." The use of the literature review in qualitative approaches is discussed in depth in Chapter 11.

REVIEW OF THE LITERATURE: PURPOSES
Overall Purpose: Knowledge

The overall purpose of a review of the literature, as illustrated in the box, p. 112, is to discover knowledge (Philips, 1992). The goal is to develop a strong knowledge base to carry out research and other nonresearch scholarly activities in the educational and clinical practice settings (Glass, 1991; Kirchhoff, 1991). The 10 objectives listed in the box relate to research and nonresearch purposes. The knowledge uncovered from a critical review of the literature contributes to the development, implementation, and results of both quantitative and qualitative studies. Such knowledge enhances the writing of scholarly papers by students and faculty. In the clinical practice arena, the knowledge from a critical literature review contributes to the implementation of research-based practice interventions, protocols, and evaluation programs that improve the quality of patient care (see Chapter 3).

Research Purpose of the Literature Review

The first eight objectives in the box best reflect the literature review as it pertains to the research process. Critically reading the literature is essential to meeting

---

*Parts of this chapter are from Grey, M. (1990). The literature review. In G. LoBiondo-Wood & J. Haber (Eds.). *Nursing research: Methods, critical appraisal, and utilization.* (pp. 78-88). St. Louis, MO: Mosby.

OVERALL PURPOSES OF A REVIEW OF LITERATURE

MAJOR GOAL: TO DEVELOP A STRONG KNOWLEDGE BASE TO
CARRY OUT RESEARCH AND OTHER SCHOLARLY EDUCATIONAL
AND CLINICAL PRACTICE SETTING ACTIVITIES

Objectives: A review of the literature does the following:

1. Determines what is known and not known about a subject, concept, or problem
2. Determines gaps, consistencies, and inconsistencies in the literature about a subject, concept, or problem
3. Discovers unanswered questions about a subject, concept, or problem
4. Describes the strengths and weaknesses of designs/methods of inquiry and instruments used in earlier works
5. Discovers conceptual traditions used to examine problems
6. Generates useful research questions or projects/activities for the discipline
7. Determines an appropriate research design/method (instruments, data collection and analysis methods) for answering the research question
8. Determines the need for replication of a well-designed study or refinement of a study
9. Promotes development of protocols and policies related to nursing practice
10. Uncovers a new practice intervention, or gains support for changing a practice intervention

---

these objectives. The main goal is to develop a sound study that will contribute to further knowledge development for theory, research, education, and practice. A research proposal must meet all the criteria of each step of the research process. Subsequent chapters present the criteria for each remaining step of the research process. Table 5-1 summarizes the main focus of the literature review for qualitative approaches and its use in the steps of the research process for quantitative designs. Its use in the steps of the research process is discussed later.

Nonresearch Purposes of the Literature Review

The major nonresearch focus of the literature review is on uncovering knowledge for use in educational and clinical practice settings. Objectives 1 through 6, 9, and 10 in the box above address nonresearch purposes. Critically reading the literature generates useful projects for education and clinical practice. Table 5-2 (p. 114) illustrates a few examples of the use of the literature review in nonresearch scholarly activities.

From a student perspective a critical review of the literature is essential to acquiring knowledge for the development of scholarly papers, presentations, and debates. Nursing students' patient care plans usually require the use of data-based literature resources for the written or documented rationale for each nursing intervention used.

Table 5-1   Examples of the Uses of Review of Literature for Research Process: Qualitative and Quantitative

Qualitative process	Quantitative designs and steps

The use of the literature review depends on the selected designs/types and phases; usually an extensive data base is not available, conceptual data are somewhat limited, and for this reason a qualitative design is being used.
 	
The following examples highlight the predominant use of the literature review for the particular qualitative approach:
Phenomenological—compare *findings* with information from the review of the literature (Oiler, 1986)
Grounded theory—constantly compare literature with *data being generated* (Hutchison, 1986).
Ethnographic—more conceptual than data based, *provides framework* for study (Germain, 1986)
Historical—review of literature is *source of data* (Matejski, 1986)
	The review of the literature is used for all designs/levels:
	Experimental and quasiexperimental
	Nonexperimental
	
	The review of the literature is usually defined as a step of the research process. When a research study is written as a proposal or is published, the literature review often is written as a separate aspect of the study. However, the actual review of the literature (i.e., the results of the review) is used in developing all steps of the process.
	
	The review of the literature is essential to the following steps of the research process:
	Problem
	Need/significance
	Question/hypothesis(es)
	Theoretical/conceptual framework
	Design/methodology
	   Specific instruments (validity and reliability)
	   Data collection method
	   Type of analysis
	Findings (interpretation)
	Implications of the findings
	Recommendations based on the findings

Differences of Research and Nonresearch Purposes

How does the literature review differ when it is used for research versus non-research purposes? Traditionally for research, the literature review is used in the development of a sound research proposal ready for implementation. It includes a critical evaluation of both conceptual and data-based literature related to the proposed study; the weaknesses, strengths, conflicts, and gaps in the literature are discussed. It is *not* a rehash or simple paraphrasing of what each article stated. Essential to the review is relating the proposed study to the reviewed research. However, it can be argued that a literature review, whether for research or nonresearch purposes, should be critical, framed in the context of previous data-based and conceptual literature, and pertinent to the objectives presented in the box on p. 112.

Table 5-2   Examples of the Uses of the Literature for Nonresearch Purposes: Educational and Practice Settings

Educational setting	Clinical/professional setting
The literature review is used *by students:* To develop academic scholarly papers (i.e., researching a topic, problem, or issue) To prepare oral presentations or debates of a topic, problem, or issue The literature review is used *by faculty:* To develop and revise curricula To develop theoretical papers for presentations and/or publication	The literature review is used **by nurses** in the clinical setting: To implement research-based nursing interventions To develop hospital-specific nursing protocols or policies related to patient care To develop and substantiate hospital specific QA, CQI, or TQM* projects or protocols The literature review is used *by professional nursing organizations/governmental agencies* To develop ANA's major documents (e.g., Social Policy Statement (1980, in revision), Standards of Clinical Practice (1991) To develop ACHPR's practice guidelines (e.g., Acute Pain Management . . . . (1992)

*QA, Quality assurance; *CQI,* continuous quality improvement; *TQM,* total quality management.

A critical review of the literature is essential to meeting ANA's (1991) Practice Standard VII related to nonresearch implementation activities of the baccalaureate prepared nurse. Table 5-2 lists a number of nonresearch projects conducted in the educational and clinical/professional settings. A critical literature review is central to developing and implementing these nonresearch activities. It would be unconscionable to think that new practice protocols or nursing interventions would be implemented in various health care settings solely on the basis of nurses' "noncritical" literature reviews, or the reading of only one study's results without evaluating it in the context of prior research. For example, in 1992 the Acute Pain Management Guideline Panel (APMGP) of the Agency for Health Care Policy and Research (AHCPR) published practice pain management guidelines that were based on an extensive critical review of the literature (review Chapter 3). Their extensive literature review was conducted for the development of these practice guidelines rather than as a step in a research project. The literature review was most certainly placed in the context of previous research and met all the other objectives related to critically reading the literature as represented on p. 112. Therefore, whether a nurse is developing a research study, a curriculum, or a patient protocol, he or she should base that project on a critical review of the literature. In essence the difference lies in the type of outcome produced. The research purpose produces a sound study proposal that can be implemented. Nonresearch purposes typically produce sound curricula or patient protocols for implementation or scholarly papers for publication or presentation.

REVIEW OF THE LITERATURE: CONDUCTOR OF RESEARCH PERSPECTIVE

The literature review is considered essential to all steps of the research process. From this perspective the review is a broad but not exhaustive, systematic, and critical collection and evaluation of the important published scholarly literature (conceptual and data-based), as well as unpublished scholarly print materials (e.g., doctoral dissertations and master's theses), audiovisual materials (e.g., audiotapes and videotapes), and personal communications (e.g., presentations and one-to-one interviews).

Objectives 1 through 8 represent different ways of thinking about the literature. From the perspective of a producer of research, these objectives direct the questions the researcher asks while reading the literature to determine a useful research question(s) and an appropriate design and method and/or the need for replication or refinement of a particular study.

The following is a brief overview of the use of the literature review in relation to the steps of the quantitative research process. (For an in-depth presentation in relation to qualitative research, see Chapter 11.) A critical reading of relevant literature is done in the following quantitative steps of the research process.

- *Theoretical framework:* The literature review reveals conceptual traditions and/or theories from nursing and other related fields that can be used to examine problems. The literature defines concepts and terms in relation to the study. The study's theoretical framework is based on the review and is considered useful in nursing research because the findings of the study (when appropriate) can be used for theory development and/or clarification.
- *Problem statement and hypothesis:* The literature review helps to determine what is known and not known; to uncover gaps, consistencies, or inconsistencies; and/or to reveal unanswered questions in the literature about a subject, concept, or problem. The review allows for refinement of research problems and questions and/or hypotheses. How far back a search must extend often depends on the newness of the topic or problem. The literature review is critical to developing useful research questions for the discipline.
- *Design and method:* The literature review reveals the strengths and weaknesses of designs and methods of previous research studies. The review is crucial to choosing an appropriate design, data collection method, and sample size; valid and reliable instruments; and effective data analysis method, as well as assisting in the development of an appropriate consent form that addresses ethical concerns. The literature review is necessary for answering a useful research question for the discipline. The appropriateness

of a design can determine whether a previous study should be replicated and/or refined. It also can uncover instruments that lack validity and reliability, as well as the need for instrument refinement, testing, or development.

* *Outcome of the analysis (findings, implications, and recommendations):* The literature review is used to discuss the results or findings of a study. The discussion relates the study's findings to what was or was not found in the review of the literature. As noted, this is important to the development and refinement of nursing theory, as well as nursing practice, education, and research. Implications for practice based on the findings in relation to the literature are presented. Recommendations for further study are based on the study's results and their relationship to the findings of the literature review. For example, the review of the literature may have revealed additional methodologies that the researcher may wish to recommend on the basis of the experience of conducting the current study.

It is apparent that the review of the literature is essential to all aspects of conducting and/or writing the results of quantitative studies. It is integral with a useful scholarly discussion of the findings, the implications for practice, and recommendations for further study. The schema illustrated in Fig. 5-2 relates the literature review to all aspects of the research process.

REVIEW OF THE LITERATURE: CONSUMER OF RESEARCH PERSPECTIVE

As discussed, consumers of research are not expected to write a complete scholarly review of the literature on their own but are expected to know how to conduct a literature review. In addition, as a consumer of research, it is essential for the student to understand the purpose(s) of a review of the literature for research and nonresearch purposes (see box, p. 112). Embedded in the purposes is the ability to do the following:

* Efficiently retrieve an adequate amount of scholarly literature using computer and print resources
* Critically evaluate data-based and conceptual material based on accepted reviewing criteria for the respective literature
* Critically evaluate a review of the literature (i.e., the entire compilation of conceptual and data-based literature) based on accepted reviewing criteria

The preceding objectives reflect both academic and professional expectations for a beginning consumer of research (see Chapter 1). Fig. 5-3 presents an overview of the steps for conducting a literature search. This process is the same whether the purpose is critiquing or writing a literature review. The schema reflects the cognitive processes and manual techniques of retrieving and critically reviewing sources from the literature. The remainder of this chapter presents the essential material for accomplishing these goals.

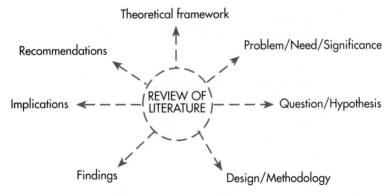

Fig. 5-2   Relationship of the review of the literature to the steps of the quantitative research process.

Table 5-3   Literature Review Synonyms

Conceptual literature	Data-based literature
Theoretical literature	Empirical literature
Scholarly nonresearch literature	Scientific literature
Scholarly work	Research literature
Soft- versus hard-science literature	Scholarly research literature
Review of the literature article	Research study
Concept analysis article	Study

SCHOLARLY LITERATURE: WHAT DO I KNOW ABOUT LITERATURE REVIEWS?
Conceptual and Data-Based Literature Synonyms and Sources

Students read many reviews of the literature in conceptual and data-based articles, as well as theory and data-based texts and books. Synonyms for conceptual and data-based scholarly literature are presented in Table 5-3. Often these terms are used interchangeably. Most frequently the term **theoretical literature** is interchanged with *conceptual literature;* the terms **empirical literature** and **scientific literature** are interchanged with *data-based literature.* Definitions and general examples of conceptual and data-based literature are presented in Table 5-4 (p. 119).

A large body of scholarly nursing literature does not consist of reported theories or the testing of relationships for linking the concepts of a theory. Some conceptual articles are an extensive review of the conceptual and data-based literature on a particular concept. Conceptual literature, like data-based literature, contributes to

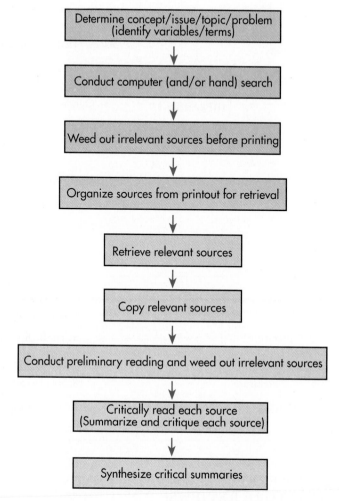

Fig. 5-3   Steps for searching the literature.

nurse's knowledge base for use in education and practice. An example of a conceptual article is Bridges' (1990) "Literature Review on the Images of the Nurse and Nursing in the Media." The author reviewed both conceptual and data-based material. Hawks (1991) developed a paper using a concept analysis strategy to refine the concept of power. The reference list at the end of the article indicates both conceptual and data-based resources. LeMone (1991) analyzed the human phenomenon of self-concept. Ouellet and Rush (1992) synthesized selected literature on the concept of mobility. The purpose was to consolidate the literature on mobility for possible use in nursing practice. Owens and Ehrenreich (1991) titled their conceptual article "Literature Review of Nonpharmacologic Methods for the Treatment of Chronic Pain." Whitley's concept analysis on anxiety (1992a) and fear (1992b) serves to

Table 5-4   Types of Information Sources for a Review of Literature

Conceptual literature	Data-based literature
Published articles, documents, or books of theories, conceptual frameworks, and/or models of a concept(s), constructs, theorems, concept analyses, literature reviews that directly underlie or are related to the intended research or nonresearch problem/issue/topic	Published studies in journals or books directly related or indirectly related to the problem of interest
	Unpublished studies: master's theses and doctoral dissertations dealing directly or indirectly with the intended research problem or topic
Proceedings and audiotapes and videotapes from scholarly conferences containing abstracts of a conceptual paper or the entire conceptual presentation	Unpublished proceedings from research conferences that contain abstracts of research studies

clarify nursing diagnosis categories for their use in nursing practice, as well as their contribution to theory development (Avant, 1990).

The common sources of both conceptual and data-based literature are books, chapters of books, journal articles, abstracts, critique reviews, abstracts published in conference proceedings, professional and governmental reports, and unpublished doctoral dissertations.

Abstracts, as defined in Chapter 4, are concisely written summaries of the main aspects of a study or conceptual paper. They may or may not be written by the person who conducted the study or wrote the original conceptual article. Research proceedings often contain abstracts of studies. These usually include the purpose, designs/methods, findings, and implications. Some published data-based and conceptual articles have a very brief summary or abstract on the first page, set off from the beginning of the article. Some entries of a computer search, such as **CINAHL** (Cumulative Index in Nursing and Allied Health Literature), provide a brief abstract of the source.

Other sources of abstracts are specific abstract publications. For example, *Nursing Scan in Research: Application for Clinical Practice* publishes abstracts of studies called *synopses,* as well as written critiques and clinical applications of the study. These abstracts or summaries are written by someone other than the person who carried out the study. This type of source will be discussed later in the consideration of primary and secondary sources. The term *abstract* also is used in relation to print sources for searching the literature (see print sources, Table 5-5). The reference librarian is an excellent source for discussing the various sources of scholarly literature and available abstracts.

Less common and less used sources of scholarly material are audiotapes, videotapes, personal communications (letters or telephone or in-person interviews), and unpublished master's theses and papers. However, qualitative studies, by their nature, depend on this type of material (see Chapter 11).

Table 5-5   Primary and Secondary Sources

Primary: essential	Secondary: useful
Data-based or conceptual articles or books written by the person who conducted the study or developed the theory (model) or concept.	Data-based or conceptual articles or books written by someone other than the person who conducted the original study(ies) or developed the theory (i.e., an author who presents, summarizes, or critiques (analysis and synthesis) someone else's work.
HINT: Critical evaluation of *mainly* primary sources is essential to a thorough and relevant review of the literature.	*HINT:* Use secondary sources sparingly; *however,* secondary sources, especially of studies that include a critique by a seasoned researcher, are a valuable learning tool for a beginning consumer of research.
Example: A researcher's report of his or her research study (e.g., question, design, method, findings, results) is a primary source whether published or unpublished.	*Examples:* Response/commentary/critique articles; review of literature articles published in a refereed scholarly journal; summary and critique published in an abstract review scan; doctoral dissertation review of the literature.

Differentiating Data-Based and Conceptual Material

An article's abstract usually indicates whether it is a data-based (study) or conceptual report. Examples of data-based studies (research literature) are found in Appendixes A, B, and C. Stewart Fahs and Kinney's (1991; Appendix A) quantitative study's abstract begins, "The purpose of this *study* was to evaluate . . . ." (p. 204). Appendix B's abstract of Grey, Cameron, and Thurber's (1991) study begins, "The purpose of this study was to investigate . . . ." (p. 144). Appendix C represents a qualitative data-based article. Hutchison and Bahr's (1991) abstract states, "This grounded theory *study* explored and described . . . ." (p. 85). Most databased articles indicate that they are research-based by stating that a study was conducted.

Conceptually based articles also indicate their type in the abstract or introductory section. They commonly state the following: "This literature review considers research . . . ." (Shade, 1992, p. 408); "This article presents strategies . . ." (Stepnick, McDaniel, & Bach, 1991, p. 61); "The purpose of this paper is to compare and contrast . . . ." (Lefort, 1993, p. 57); or "The purpose of this article is to present a consolidated review of the literature . . . ." (Ouellet & Rush, 1992, p. 72).

EXAMPLES OF NURSING JOURNALS FOR LITERATURE REVIEWS

Advances in Nursing Science
AORN Journal
Applied Nursing Research
Archives of Psychiatric Nursing
Clinical Nursing Research
Computers in Nursing
Heart & Lung
Holistic Nursing Practice
Image
Journal of Professional Nursing
Journal of Obstetric, Gynecologic
   and Neonatal Nursing

Journal of Qualitative Research
Journal of Nursing Scholarship
NACOG
Nurse Educator
Nursing Diagnosis
Nursing & Health Care
Nursing Research
Nursing Science Quarterly
Research in Nursing & Health
Scholarly Inquiry for Nursing Practice
Western Journal of Nursing Research

Main focus: **Primary sources** of research studies and conceptual articles; sources of some **secondary sources,** such as an extensive review of literature on a particular concept, issues and responses or critiques of data-based and conceptual articles; most are refereed journals; all can be searched through CINAHL print and computer data bases.

The following section on primary and secondary sources highlights examples of data-based and conceptual articles and books. The student can find specific additional examples of data-based and conceptual literature in this chapter's critiquing section on synthesis examples.

Refereed Journals

A major portion of most literature reviews consists of journal articles. Journals are a ready source of the latest information on almost any conceivable subject. Books usually take longer to publish; therefore journals are the preferred mode for communicating the latest theory or results of a research study. As a beginning consumer of research you must use **refereed journals** or (peer-reviewed journals) as sources of scholarly literature. A refereed journal uses a panel of external and internal reviewers or editors who review submitted manuscripts for possible publication. The external reviewers are drawn from a pool of nurse scholars who are experts in various fields. In most cases these reviews are "blind": that is, the reviewers do not know who the author of the article is. The review panels use the same set of scholarly criteria to judge whether the manuscripts are worthy of publication. The box above lists several nursing journals that contain scholarly literature.

PRIMARY AND SECONDARY SOURCES

Reading scholarly journals, especially refereed ones, will facilitate the role of the research consumer. A credible literature review reflects the use of *mainly* primary sources. Table 5-5 gives the general definition and examples of these sources.

A **primary source** is written by a person(s) who developed the theory or conducted the research. Most primary sources are found in published literature. A **secondary source** is written by a person(s) *other than* the individual who developed the theory or conducted the research. Often a secondary source represents a response to, or a summary and critique of, a theorist's or researcher's work.

The box on p. 121 illustrates journal sources that contain both primary and secondary articles. Table 5-6 presents conceptual and data-based examples of primary and secondary sources. The first column of Table 5-6 represents primary sources. For example, Rogers developed and published the Science of Unitary Human Beings. Rogers' (1970) book is a primary source because the author is also the theorist (i.e., firsthand information). The second column of Table 5-6 represents

Table 5-6   Conceptual and Data-Based Examples of Primary and Secondary Journal Articles, Books, Chapters in Books, or Documents

Primary	Secondary
Journal Article: Stewart Fahs, P., & Kinney, M. (1991). The abdomen, thigh, and arm as sites for subcutaneous sodium heparin injections. *Nursing Research. 40*(4), 204-207.	*Journal Article:* Quellet, L. L., Rush, K. L. (1992). A synthesis of selected literature on mobility: A basis for studying impaired mobility. *Nursing Diagnosis, 3*(2), 72-80.
Book: Rogers, M. E.(1970). *An introduction to the theoretical basis of nursing.* Philadelphia, PA: Davis.	*Book:* Nicoll, L. H. (Ed.) (1992). *Perspectives on nursing theory.* New York: J.B. Lippincott.
Chapter in a book: Miller, B. K., Haber J., Byrne, M. (1990). The experience of caring in the teaching-learning process of nursing education: Student and teacher perspectives. In M. Leininger & J. Watson (Eds.), *The caring imperative in education* (pp. 125-135). NY: NLN.	*Chapter in a Book:* Collins, R. M., & Fielder J. H. (1992). Beckstrand's concept of practice theory: A critique. In L. H. Nicoll (Ed.), *Perspectives on nursing theory* (pp. 555-561). New York: J. B. Lippincott.
Document: ANA. (1991). *Standards of clinical nursing practice.* Kansas City, MO: Author.	*Document:* Acute Pain Management Guideline Panel. (1992). *Acute Pain Management: Operative or Medical Procedures and Trauma Practice Guideline* (AHCPR Publication No. 92-0032). MD: Agency for Health Care Policy and Research, Public Health Service, U.S. Department of Health and Human Services.

secondary sources. The Nicoll (1992) book, indicated in the secondary source column, consists of conceptual articles concerning nursing theory, nursing research, and their application to education and practice. Each chapter is written by a nurse author who *did not* develop the theory or carry out the research. These nurse authors write about another nurse's theory or research by summarizing, responding to, or critiquing it in relation to implications for theory verification, practice, education, and/or development of nursing science. This is considered "secondhand" information—hence the term *secondary source*.

The Role of Secondary Sources

There are two general reasons for using secondary sources. One reason is that a primary source is literally unavailable. This is rarely the case in this age of computer searches and interlibrary loan of books and faxing of articles. Another reason, which is more common, is that a secondary source can provide different ways of looking at an issue or problem. Students develop their ability to see things from another person's point of view, which is an essential aspect of critical reading (Paul, 1990). Secondary sources should not be overused, especially for literature reviews. However, secondary sources, as indicated in Table 5-6, have tremendous value for the beginning consumer of research. These sources are generally written by experienced nursing scholars. Such articles usually provide a critical evaluation of or a response to a theory or research study. They usually include implications for practice and/or contributions of the work to the development of the science of nursing. The box on p. 124 lists some specific secondary resources that can serve as effective learning tools for developing the art of critiquing conceptual and data-based literature. However, to learn critiquing skills, the consumer of research must read primary sources and use critiquing criteria.

Pitfalls of Secondary Sources

Students invariably learn some of the limitations of secondary sources through experience. To begin with, unless a source quotes material directly, it is "secondhand" information, regardless of the accuracy of the paraphrasing or interpretation by the writer. In addition, for the author to summarize and perhaps critique a theorist's work and present it in a shortened version, the following may occur:

- All of the theory's concept(s) or aspects of a study and/or definitions may not be fully presented.
- If all the concepts are included, the definitions may be collapsed or paraphrased to such a degree that it no longer represents the theorist's actual work.
- The critique (whether positive or negative) is based on the presentation of incomplete or interpreted data and is therefore less useful to the consumer.

This is not usually the case if an article is retrieved from a refereed journal or reputable edited text. Such articles are written by knowledgeable nurse scholars whose interpretations of the theory and/or related critiques are well done (Marriner-

---

EXAMPLES CONTAINING SECONDARY SOURCES OF RESEARCH STUDIES

JOURNALS

Scholarly Inquiry for Nursing Practice
  In addition to presenting primary data-based or conceptual articles, contains
    commentary critique articles or response articles.
Western Journal of Nursing Research
  In addition to presenting primary data-based or conceptual articles, contains
    brief abstracts—summaries, critiques, and application to practice of research
    articles. Critiques are very useful in assisting the beginning consumer of
    research in developing critiquing skills.

ABSTRACTS

Nursing Scan in Research: Application for Clinical Practice (Publisher: Nursecom,
  Philadelphia, PA)
    Reviews over 1090 nursing and nonnursing national and international journals'
    research articles.
Nursing Abstracts Co. (Forest Hills, New York, Box 295)
  Contains only brief abstract summaries of research articles (authors not
    identified).

Tomey, 1989; Nicoll, 1992). However, the beginning consumer of research should
be aware that sometimes articles may present misconceptions or biased interpretations of a theory or critique of a study. Consulting faculty, advisors, or librarians
about secondary sources is an effective way to secure an appropriate resource.

Secondary Sources of Research Studies: Critique and Response Articles

The box above presents journal and abstract sources of research articles.
These journals also publish secondary source conceptual articles. For instance, *Western Journal of Nursing Research* publishes mainly primary sources of data-based and
some conceptual articles. Many articles are followed by one or two commentary articles (secondary sources). The commentary articles, written by nurse scholars, are
mainly critiques of the primary article. Sometimes the commentary article is followed by a "Response by the Author" article that responds to questions raised by
the commentary article. *Scholarly Inquiry for Nursing Practice* publishes primary
sources of conceptual and data-based articles and includes response articles (i.e., secondary sources). A response article has a slightly different focus from a critique article. Critique articles identify strengths and weaknesses of a study or a theory. A
response generally focuses on a reaction to the scholarly work in terms of its usefulness for the profession, for development of nursing science and theory, and for practice and future research. A response includes the strengths of the work from this

perspective; the weaknesses are not usually addressed directly. Consumers of research can enhance their critical reading skills by reading primary articles, as well as related critique or response (secondary source) articles.

Nursing Scan in Research is a secondary source of data-based material. It contains brief abstracts of research studies with a related critique and application for practice. This publication reviews articles from more than 150 reputable nursing and related health care journals; journals listed in the box on p. 121 are used in their review. It provides a quick way to review a study and keep abreast of the latest information; consumers of research find them useful. However, because these reviews are so brief, it is suggested that one's critical thinking and reading skills would be better enhanced through use of full-length journal articles.

Nursing Abstracts publishes abstracts of articles that are published in at least 77 nursing journals, some of which are listed in the box on p. 121. The writers of these very brief (five- to eight-line) digests are not identified. They are similar in length to a computer search abstract or an abstract published at the beginning of a journal article. This type of abstract may help the reader to decide whether to retrieve an article. Because most data-based computer searches provide an abstract, this type of secondary source has limited use for the consumer of research. It does not provide enough substantive content for the development of critical thinking and reading skills.

Reading Primary and Secondary Sources: Strategies to Enhance Critical Evaluation Skills

The following are recommendations to increase critical evaluation skills. It is suggested that the beginning consumer of research should do the following:
* Read the primary source of a study or theory—not just secondary sources (e.g., nonauthored abstracts or summaries of a study or theory found in an article's review of the literature)
* Seek assistance about the critique from researchers
* Read secondary sources from refereed/peer-reviewed journals that provide a commentary/critique/response by a recognized researcher
* Discuss your response to secondary source articles with your faculty advisor
* Form scholarly reading groups with fellow nursing students or consumer of research nurse colleagues (e.g., all members critically read a research article using the same criteria) and discuss the results with your faculty advisor
* Confer with the reference librarian and faculty advisers about the most useful reputable refereed scholarly journals

CHARACTERISTICS OF A RELEVANT REVIEW OF THE LITERATURE

The box on p. 126 summarizes the important characteristics of a relevant review of the literature. These characteristics can serve as a guide for critiquing the review of the literature and are discussed more formally from this frame of reference

CHARACTERISTICS OF A WRITTEN "RELEVANT" REVIEW OF LITERATURE

Written summary and critique of each reviewed source of information relevant to the project reflects critical thinking and scholarly writing. The content satisfies the following criteria.

Purposes of a literature review were met.

Summary is succinct and adequately represents the reviewed source.

Critiquing (objective critical evaluation) reflects **analysis** and **synthesis** of material:

- Application of accepted "critiquing criteria" to **analyze** for the following:
   Strengths
   Weaknesses or limitations
   Conflicts
   Gaps in information as it relates directly and indirectly to the area of interest
- Evidence of synthesis of the critiques of each source of information. Putting the parts (i.e., each critique) together to form a new whole (Kerlinger, 1986) or connecting link for what is to be studied, replicated, developed, or implemented.

Review consists of **mainly** primary sources.

Sufficient number of sources are used, especially data-based sources.

Summarizes /paraphrases material rather than continually quoting content.

Summaries/critiques of studies are presented in a logical flow ending with a conclusion or synthesis of the reviewed material that reflects why the study, project, or conceptual stand should be taken.

later in the chapter. A discussion of searching and critically reading the literature is essential to carrying out the research consumer role.

Conducting a Search as a Consumer of Research

Most students who are preparing an academic paper read the required course materials, as well as additional library materials. Students often use the term *researching* for this process. In this situation, the student is "searching" the literature to uncover knowledge to prepare an academic term paper on a certain topic rather than to uncover knowledge on a specific topic to carry out a research project. Reviewing the literature for research and nonresearch activities requires the same critical thinking and reading skills. This point is discussed at the beginning of the chapter. From an academic standpoint, depending on the level and type of course, a student's search may be viewed as a minor or major review of the literature. Discovering knowledge is the goal of the "search." A consumer of research needs to know how to search the literature.

Library Activities

Becoming a competent consumer of research requires knowing how to search the literature quickly and efficiently. If the reader is unfamiliar with the process of conducting a computer search, it is strongly recommended that the reference librarian be contacted. Consulting the librarian before proceeding with the computer search is well worth your time. If you are knowledgeable about your library's computer search process, you are ready to begin.

Print Data-Base Resources

Print data bases consist mainly of indexes, card catalogues, and abstract reviews. *Print indexes* are used to find journal sources (periodicals) of data-based and conceptual articles on a variety of topics, as well as publications of professional organizations and various governmental agencies. *Card catalogues* are used to secure books, monographs, conference proceedings, master's theses, and doctoral dissertations. *Abstract reviews* contain summaries of data-based articles and prepared bibliographies. Before the 1980s, a search usually was done by hand using print data bases. This was a tedious and time-consuming process. Examples of the more commonly used print indexes appear in the first box on p. 128. The most relevant and frequently used source for nursing literature was and remains the Cumulative Index to Nursing and Allied Health Literature (CINAHL) (the "Red Books"). CINAHL covers nursing literature from 1956 to the present. The most significant nursing, allied health, and educational print indexes are now available on computer data bases. Print resources are still relied on if a search requires materials before 1983 or if your library does not have computer data bases.

Computer Data-Base Resources

Almost all print data bases are now available through a computer search. Most **computer data bases** are available via software programs such as SilverPlatter or Dialog. These are accessed on-line or via CD-ROM. **CD-ROM** refers to the capability of the computer to use compact disk (CD) information. Most college and university libraries are set up for students to conduct their own computer searches. The computers are CD-ROM-ready for use by the student. These computer data bases are "user-friendly." For instance, the computer's menu usually lists the various data bases available (e.g., **CINAHL, MEDLINE**) and the student simply selects the most appropriate one for the desired search and follows the prompts on the screen. Step-by-step printed guides for the search, as well as search guides for each data base, are usually available. These guides provide information about variables/terms, broadening or narrowing a search, marking or eliminating unwanted records, and printing the citations.

The second box on p. 128 lists several computerized data bases that are available via CD-ROM and On-Line. Many additional data bases are available; many are produced by MEDLARS (e.g., MEDLINE Standard, MEDLINE Express,

---

COMMON DATA-BASE PRINT SOURCES USED BEFORE COMPUTER DATA BASES

INDEXES

1. **CINAHL**   Cumulative Index to Nursing & Allied Health Literature (formerly called Cumulative Index to Nursing Literature); known as the "Red Books"
2. **INI   International Nursing Index** lists published by American Journal of Nursing Company in cooperation with National Library of Medicine (NLM)
3. **Nursing Studies Index**   Developed by Virginia Henderson—nursing literature 1900 to 1959
4. **IM**   Index Medicus—oldest health-related index; first published in 1879
5. **HLI**   Hospital Literature Index—1945 American Hospital Association in cooperation with NLM
6. **CIJE**   Current Index to Journals in Education—first published in 1969 in cooperation with Educational Resources Information Center (ERIC)

CARD CATALOGUES   List books, monographs, theses, dissertations, audiovisuals, and proceedings

ABSTRACT REVIEWS

1. Nursing Abstracts
2. Psychological Abstracts
3. Sociological Abstracts
4. Dissertation Abstracts International
5. Master's Abstracts

COMPUTERIZED DATA BASES: CD-ROM AND ON-LINE*

1. **CINAHL**—Cumulative Index to Nursing & Allied Health Literature†
2. **MEDLINE** Standard—**MED**ical literature analysis and retrieval system on**LINE**
3. **PSYCHLIT**—**PSYCH**ology **LIT**erature
4. **ERIC**—Educational Resources Information Center

*Listed in order of importance and usefulness to nursing.
†Most important for the nurse consumer of research.

MEDLINE on Hard Disk, and MEDLINE Professional). Examples are SOCIOFILE (sociology/social work), GPO (federal government), CATLINE (books), AVLINE (audiovisuals), HealthPLAN (health planning and administration), BIOETHICS-LINE (ethical concerns), and SEDBASE (Meyler's side effects of drugs) (SilverPlatter Fact Sheets, 1993).

ADVANTAGES OF CINAHL FOR THE NURSE CONSUMER OF RESEARCH

1. Uses major nursing subheadings designed especially for nurses rather than medical model terminology
2. Covers literature from over 500 journals (nursing, 13 allied health disciplines, and sciences)
3. Provides full information: journal articles, books, pamphlets, conference proceedings, standards of practice, nursing dissertations, educational software in nursing, chapters of books, and audiovisuals
4. Uses subject headings for many specific types of research variables, content of the study, research methodologies, and instrument used in the study
5. Contains *author* abstracts from over 150 journals
6. Includes extensive abstracts for dissertations, software, and audiovisual records

---

Source: CINAHL. 1992. CINAHL fact sheets 1992. Glendale, CA: CINAHL Information Systems: Glendale, CA.

For most searches in nursing, CINAHL's data base is an excellent way to access relevant information. The box above presents the advantages of CINAHL over the more commonly used data bases. For the consumer of research, an important advantage is that it uses major subject headings specific to nursing (e.g., nursing process terms, NANDA nursing diagnoses, major nursing models and theories). It covers literature from more than 500 journals, including nursing and 13 allied health disciplines and health sciences.

MEDLINE uses medical model terminology rather than nursing terminology; also, it does not cover all the nursing literature. CINAHL reported that of the 534 serials indexed as of March 1992, 176 were not included in MEDLINE. Examples are AORN Journal, AIDS Patient Care, American Journal of Health Promotion, and Harvard Health letter. CINAHL provides easy access to research literature. Subject headings are established for many specific types of research variables, for example, designs, conceptual frameworks, data collection methods, and statistical methods of data analysis. In addition, it provides an instrumentation field that lists all the instruments used in a study (CINAHL, 1992).

Some searches require the use of additional data bases. Review the advantages and disadvantages of each data base before proceeding. It is advisable to review this matter with the reference librarian and/or faculty adviser.

How Many Sources Do I Need?

Questions frequently asked by students are, How many articles do I need? How much is enough? How far back in the literature do I need to go? Often a computer search (e.g., CINAHL data base is from 1983) will yield more than enough materials to complete the purpose of the search.

A general time line for conceptual academic or clinical practice papers/ projects is to go back in the literature from 3 to 5 years; a research project may warrant 10 years or more. With experience you will know when enough is enough. As noted, each computer data base has its own time limitations. If a search requires retrieving materials unavailable through the computer data base, print sources are used for the remainder of the search. Another consideration is the cost of the search if not included in students' tuition fees, the number of entries that can be printed during a search, and, most important, the time line for completing the project.

Each data base usually has a specific search guide, which provides information on the organization of the entries and the terminology used. For instance, CINAHL uses nursing-specific terms, whereas MEDLINE uses medical terminology. Finding the right variables/concepts/terms to "plug in" for a computer search is an important aspect of conducting a search. The reference librarian is the most qualified person to help in this process.

Once the search is completed, the monitor's screen shows the number of retrieved sources. An entry usually consists of the author, title, and source (e.g., book or journal), type (e.g., data-based or conceptual) and may include an abstract. Before printing all the entries (records), it is advisable to browse (scroll) through them and earmark the relevant citations. The searcher can decide this by reviewing the title (TI), author (AU), source (SO), abstract (AB) if available, and document type (DT), if available. Fig. 5-4 provides an example of a typical CINAHL computer search entry. The main focus of this search was on therapeutic nurse-patient relationships. This entry's TI, SO, and AB indicated its usefulness for this purpose. Once the materials are retrieved, most students find it useful to photocopy them. Copying the material allows for organizing the materials for critical reading but can be costly.

Completing the Search

Now the truly important aspects of the search begins—critically reading the retrieved materials. As discussed in Chapter 4, critically reading scholarly material, especially data-based articles, requires several readings and the use of critiquing criteria.

LITERATURE REVIEW FORMAT: WHAT TO EXPECT

Becoming familiar with the format of the literature review assists the research consumer in the task of using critiquing criteria to evaluate the review.

The research question/topic and the retrieved number and type of data-based and conceptual materials usually direct the style in which the review will be organized for a logical presentation. Some reviews are written according to the variables being studied and presented chronologically under each variable. Others present the material chronologically with subcategories or variables discussed within each period; still others present the variables and include subcategories related to the study's types or designs or related subvariables.

SilverPlatter 3.11   <u>**CINAHL (R) 1983 – 10/92**</u>
                                        140 of 244
                                   Marked in Search: 26

TI TITLE: The hybrid model for concept development: its value for the study of
therapeutic alliance
AU AUTHORS (S): Madden-BP
SO SOURCE (BIBLIOGRAPHIC CITATION): Advances-in-Nursing-Science (ANS) 1990
Apr; 12(3); 75-87 (37 ref)
SI SERIAL IDENTIFIER: A55330000
SB JOURNAL SUBSET: Core-Nursing (C); Nursing (N); USA-and Canada (U);
Peer-Reviewed (P)
PY PUBLICATION YEAR: 1990
AB ABSTRACT: Schwartz-Barcott and Kim's hybrid model is used as a research
methodology for the development and analysis of the concept of therapeutic
alliance. Empirical data gathered in a community health setting by field
research techniques are used to compare, to contrast, and to rework exisiting
definitions and related concepts from <u>literature review.</u> The resulting
definitional refinement provides clear distinctions between the concepts of
compliance and therapeutic alliance and assists in selection of appropriate
nursing interventions supportive of clients' health goals.
DE DESCRIPTORS (SUBJECT HEADINGS): *Concept-Formation;
*Nursing-Models-Theoretical; *Patient-Compliance; *Nurse-Patient-Relations;
*Community-Health-Nursing
DE DESCRIPTORS (SUBJECT HEADINGS): Behavior-contracting; Communication-;
Middle-Age; Aged-; Male-; Female-
DT DOCUMENT TYPE: journal; case-study
UD UPDATE CODE: 9005
AN ACCESSION NUMBER: 106776

Fig. 5-4   Example of a Cumulative Index to Nursing and Allied Health
Literature (CINAHL) data base printout entry.

For instance, Krainovich-Miller's (1988) review of the literature for a study
validating the nursing diagnosis of preoperative state anxiety organized the reviewed
material according to various aspects of the anxiety variable under study. It was written from both a chronological historical overview perspective and according to the
clarification of the concept of anxiety from nonnursing and nursing perspectives.
The box on p. 132 illustrates excerpts from the historical aspect of this review; dates
are underlined to denote the chronological presentation. A logical flow was evidenced by presenting various authors' conceptual and data-based literature on the
concept, including signs and symptoms, differentiating fear from anxiety, and methods for validating the diagnosis in a medical/psychiatric and nursing framework.

The study by Grey et al. (1991) (see Appendix B) is a good example of a
literature review that is logically presented according to the variables under study:
"The purpose of the study was to investigate the influence of age, coping behaviors,
and self-care behaviors on psychological, social, and physiologic adaptation in preadolescents and adolescents with diabetes" (p. 144). Although these variables did

KRAINOVICH-MILLER'S (1988) LITERATURE REVIEW:
CHRONOLOGICAL PRESENTATION OF ANXIETY VARIABLE
NOTED BY UNDERLINED PERIOD OR DATES (pp. 16-19)

HISTORICAL OVERVIEW

Although anxiety is accepted as a phenomenon that has existed since the beginning of humankind, the development of the concept of anxiety did not occur until the classical Greek period (McReynolds, 1975). Kierkegaard, the noted theologian and psychologist, was credited in the early 1800s with beginning the major formal work on the development of this concept. His seminal work, *The Concept of Dread*, although published in 1844, was not translated into English until 1944. Kierkegaard (1944) distinguished between two different kinds of anxiety:. . . .

Guislain, a Belgian psychiatrist, initiated a medical model of anxiety in 1826. . . .

In 1895 Freud suggested a new diagnostic category he called anxiety-neurosis. Although Freud recognized the contribution of others concerning the concept of morbid anxiety, no one had presented it as a separate disease (McReynolds, 1975). . . .

During the 30's and 40's, neo-Freudian Harry Stack Sullivan also examined man's experience with anxiety. . . .

In 1950 Rollo May published his classic book *The Meaning of Anxiety*. . . .

The 20th century has been referred to as the age of anxiety (Cattell, 1963; Cohen, 1969). Since the mid-twentieth century there has been a proliferation of published scholarly writings and research, including numerous masters and doctoral studies on the topic of anxiety (May, 1977; McReynolds, 1975; Spielberger et al., 1983).

not appear as subheadings, they were evident in the presented summaries of reviewed studies. The first paragraph of the review primarily presents a number of studies dealing with the psychological adaptation of the preadolescent and adolescent with diabetes. The second through fifth paragraphs present studies investigating adaptation in relation to coping and self-care behaviors. The sixth paragraph reviews studies related to age and developmental status and its effect on adaptation. The final paragraph summarizes the findings of the literature review.

The first box on p. 133 illustrates excerpts for Stewart Fahs and Kinney's (1991) literature review of their study "The Abdomen, Thigh, and Arm as Sites for Subcutaneous Sodium Heparin Injections" (see Appendix A). Literature related to the variables under study was presented chronologically (see underlined dates in the box).

The literature review of a study by Duckett, Henly, and Garvis (1993), "Predicting Breast-Feeding Duration during the Postpartum Hospitalization," organized the review according to predictors and subcategories of the predictors. Studies or conceptual literature related to each predictor and subcategory was chronologically presented. The second box on p. 133 demonstrates how the review was organized.

EXCERPTS FROM STEWART FAHS AND KINNEY'S (1991)
LITERATURE REVIEW: ORGANIZED BOTH
CHRONOLOGICALLY AND ACCORDING TO TECHNIQUE,
NEEDLE SIZE/BRUISING AND PAIN OF HEPARIN, HEPARIN
AND VOLUME, AND TECHNIQUE/HEPARIN/BRUISES OR
HEMATOMAS; DENOTED BY UNDERLINING (p. 204)

LITERATURE REVIEW

Brenner, Wood, and George (1981) studied two injection techniques to
compare angle of injection, aspiration, and massage of tissue. . . .

The effect of three techniques for administering subcutaneous low-dose heparin
on the formation of bruises at the site of injection was investigated by VanBree,
Hollerbach, and Brooks (1984) . . . .

Wooldridge and Jackson (1988) compared two techniques for subcutaneous
heparin injections. . . .

The effect of needle size on bruising and pain of heparin injection was studied
by Coley, Butler, Beck, and Mullane (1987).

Only one study was found in which concentration of heparin and volume of
injectate were reported (Mitchell & Pauszek, 1987 . . . .

The relationship between techniques for administering low-dose heparin and the
formation of bruises or hematomas has been addressed in two review articles
(Hanson, 1987; Schumanln, Bruya, & Henke, 1988). . . .

ORGANIZATION OF DUCKETT, HENLY, AND GARVIS'S
(1993) LITERATURE REVIEW

PREDICTORS OF BREAST-FEEDING DURATION

1. Maternal antecedents (age, education, ethnicity, and parity)
2. Internal resources (reasons for breast-feeding, attitude toward breast-feeding)
3. External resources (encouragement of breast-feeding, sources of breast-feeding
   information)
4. Interferences (discouragement of breast-feeding, problems encountered, and
   in-hospital supplementation) (p. 178)

In contrast to the styles of the previous quantitative studies, the literature reviews' qualitative studies are much shorter or nonexistent. This is because little is
known about the topic under study or the very nature of the qualitative design dic-
tates that a review of the literature be conducted after the study is completed and
compared with the study findings. For example, the introductory section of Beck's
(1992) phenomenological study "The Lived Experience of Postpartum Depression"
states, "What has not been researched, however, is the lived experience of postpar-

tum depression" (p. 166). Although literature on the signs and symptoms of post-partum depression exists, it has not been developed from the perspectives of patients, that is, individuals experiencing the phenomenon. This is the primary reason a phenomenological design was chosen (see Chapter 20).

A similar style is seen in Wilson and Morse's (1991) qualitative grounded theory study "Living with a Wife Undergoing Chemotherapy." The authors begin the first paragraph with the physical and emotional aspects of cancer and the specific purpose of their qualitative study. In the second paragraph they state that the body of literature about a patient's responses to chemotherapy was developed from the health care professional's perspective rather than from the patient and spouse's. The authors conclude in the third paragraph that little is known of the husband's perspective on his wife's undergoing chemotherapy. The researchers chose a grounded theory method "to identify the husband's experience over time and to develop an explanatory model" (p. 79). Consumers of research should be familiar with different literature review styles, so they can knowledgeably evaluate the appropriate presentation of information.

CRITIQUING CRITERIA FOR A REVIEW OF THE LITERATURE

The reader in analyzing the research report must evaluate each step of the research process. The characteristics of a relevant review of the literature (review box, p. 126) and the purposes of the review of the literature (review box, p. 112) provided the framework for the development of literature review evaluation criteria. Difficulties that the consumer of research might have regarding this task and related strategies are presented after a discussion of the critiquing criteria.

Critiquing the literature review of data-based or conceptual reports is a challenging task for the consumer of research. Critiquing criteria have been developed for all aspects of the quantitative research process, for various quantitative designs and qualitative approaches, and for nonresearch projects for the educational and clinical settings. Critiquing criteria for the review of the literature are usually presented from the quantitative research process perspective. Because the focus of this book is on the baccalaureate nurse in the research consumer role, the critiquing criteria for the literature review incorporates this frame of reference.

The important issue is for the reader to determine the overall value of the data-based or conceptual report. Does the review of the literature permeate the report? Does the review of the literature contribute to the significance of the report in relation to nursing theory, research, education, or practice? (Review Fig. 5-1.) The overall question to be answered is, does the review of the literature uncover knowledge? This question is based on the overall purpose of a review of the literature, which is to uncover knowledge (review the box on p. 112). The major goal turns into the question, did the review of the literature provide a strong knowledge base to carry out the reported research or scholarly educational or clinical practice setting project? The box on p. 135 provides critiquing criteria in the form of questions for the consumer of research to ask of a literature review.

CRITIQUING CRITERIA

1. Does the literature review uncover gaps or inconsistencies in knowledge?
2. How does the review reflect critical thinking?
3. Are all the relevant concepts and variables included in the review?
4. Does the summary of each reviewed study reflect the essential components of the study design?
5. Does the critique of each reviewed study include strengths, weaknesses, or limitations of the design; conflicts; and gaps or inconsistencies in information in relation to the area of interest?
6. Were both conceptual and data-based literature included?
7. Were primary sources mainly used?
8. Is there a written summary synthesis of the reviewed scholarly literature?
9. Does the synthesis summary follow a logical sequence that leads the reader to why there is the need for the particular research or nonresearch project?
10. Did the organization of the reviewed studies (i.e., chronologically, or according to concepts/variables, or type/design/level of study) flow logically, enhancing the ability of the reader to evaluate the need for the particular research or nonresearch project?
11. Does the literature review follow the purpose(s) of the study or nonresearch project?

Questions related to the logical presentation of the reviewed articles are somewhat more challenging for the beginning consumer of research. The more students read scholarly articles, the easier this question is to answer. At times the type of question being asked in relation to the particular concept lends itself to presenting the reviewed studies chronologically (i.e., perhaps beginning with early or landmark data-based or conceptual literature). Review the previous discussion on styles or format of literature reviews.

Questions must be asked about whether each explanation of a step of the research process met or did not meet these guidelines (criteria). For instance, the box on p. 112 illustrates the overall purposes of a review of the literature. The second objective listed states that the review of the literature is to determine gaps, consistencies, and inconsistencies in the literature about a subject, concept, or problem. The guide question on Table 19-1 (see Chapter 19, p. 443) is "What gaps in knowledge about the problem are identified, and how does this study intend to fill those gaps?" In this example, the purpose or objective of the literature review became the evaluation question or criterion for critiquing the review of the literature.

Two other important questions to ask are "Were both conceptual and data-based literature included? and "Does the review consist of mainly primary sources?" Other sets of critiquing criteria may phrase these questions differently or more broadly. For instance, the question may be "Does the literature search seem adequate?" or "Does the report demonstrate scholarly writing?" These seem to be difficult questions for a student to answer; however, one place to begin is by determining whether the source is a refereed journal (see box, p. 121). It is reasonable to assume that a scholarly refereed journal publishes manuscripts that are adequately searched, use mainly primary sources, and are written in a scholarly manner. Consultation with a faculty advisor may be necessary to develop skill in answering this question.

Is there a written summary of each reviewed source? Is there a written critique? These questions seem as if they would be easily answered by reading what is reported in the literature review. However, because of style differences and space constraints, summaries are at times every brief and often lack a critique. Further possible reasons for critiques' not being written are discussed earlier in the chapter. Most often the summary includes the purpose, the sample type and size, and the findings. Typically an entire study may be summarized in one or two sentences. Stewart Fahs and Kinney's (1991) study illustrates this point (see Appendix A). The italicized aspects indicate the quantitative research components noted in the italics.

> Wooldridge and Jackson (1988) *compared two techniques for subcutaneous heparin injections* [purpose]. Order of treatment was *randomly assigned* [sample type] for *50 white subjects* [sample size] who served as their own control. *While no difference in number of bruises was found, smaller bruises and fewer and smaller areas of induration were found in the technique employing a larger (3 milliliter) syringe, 0.2 milliliter air bubble, change of needle prior to injection, and sterile dry sponge for applying pressure after the injection* [findings]. (p. 204)

A critique was not apparent in this written report, but it is assumed that Stewart Fahs and Kinney did critique the reported study. Perhaps their evaluation did not seem essential to the review, or page constraints prevented its inclusion.

Another summary and critique of a reviewed study are found in the literature review by Grey et al. (1991; Appendix B). These researchers summarize a study by Burns and colleagues (1986) and conclude with the following critique: "These authors also did not account for the length of time since diagnosis, which may also affect adaptation, since insulin reserves decrease with time (Travis, Brouhard, & Schreiner, 1987)" (p. 145). In addition, this example reflects critical thinking: these researchers identified a weakness of one study through the results of another.

However, it is not enough to present a summary and critique of each source. A literature review requires a complete summary or a synthesis of all reviewed sources. The relationship between and among these studies must be explained. The summary should reflect the putting together of the main points or value of all the sources in relation to the research question. A synthesis of a written review of the literature usually appears at the end of the review section before the research question or hypothesis reporting section. If not labeled as such, it is usually evident in the last paragraph (see Haber & Austin (1992) example noted in Chapter 4, p. 96). A relevant literature review demonstrates synthesis of the reviewed sources (see box, p. 126). Therefore demonstrating synthesis becomes an essential critiquing criterion for the review of the literature.

The literature reviews of the studies found in Appendixes A, B, and C satisfactorily meet critiquing criteria questions, especially in regard to demonstrating synthesis. For example, Stewart Fahs and Kinney (1991; Appendix A) end their literature review with the following:

> Currently many nursing interventions are described in the literature without empirical evidence to support the practices. The use of sites other than the abdomen for subcutaneous heparin injections has not been empirically evaluated. Therefore, the nursing practice of using the abdomen as the only acceptable injection site for low-dose heparin therapy seems to be based on tradition rather than systematic inquiry. (p. 204)

The preceding summary synthesis meets the objective of uncovering knowledge, determining what is known and not known, and finding gaps and inconsistencies in the literature. This synthesis example provides data that support that the literature review reflected critical thinking and scholarly writing and represents the bridge or reason for carrying out the study. This example specifically addresses a number of the questions found in the box on p. 135.

Grey, et al. (1991; Appendix B) conclude their introduction with the statement that "adaptation would be influenced by age, coping behaviors, and self-care behaviors" (p. 144). Although these variables do not appear as subheadings, they are evident in the presented summaries of reviewed studies. The researchers stated the variables to be reviewed. They presented a review of studies related to the variables and ended the review with a summary that supported why they were conducting their particular study. Their summary (synthesis) stated that

> the literature supports the notion that multiple factors influence adaptation to a chronic illness such as diabetes during childhood and adolescence. The relative impact of these factors, however, cannot be determined by existing studies. Thus the present study examined. . . . (p. 145)

Hutchison and Bahr's (1991) qualitative grounded theory study (see Appendix C) is another example of a summary synthesis that meets the critiquing criteria discussed. These researchers did not label the review of the literature as such, but the summary synthesis is unmistakable in the last paragraph:

> Throughout the review of literature, no studies or reports were found that comprehensively focused on ways residents are socially productive through caring acts, or what it means personally to a resident to engage in caring kinds of behaviors. The purpose of this study was to explore and describe the specific types of caring behaviors engaged in by residents and the personal meaning of their involvement in these acts. (p. 85)

Norman, Gadaletta, and Griffin's (1991) study related to an evaluation of blood pressure methods in an acute trauma population provides another well-done summary synthesis example. In this study the review of the literature is labeled "Related Literature." The summary or synthesis is not labeled as such, but it is quite apparent in the last paragraph of the related literature section. These researchers summarized each reviewed study, although a critique as such was not noticeable in the report. (As noted at the beginning of this chapter, this does not mean that critiquing did not occur.) They stated the following:

> Discrepancies occur between direct and indirect methods of blood pressure measurement due to patient physiology, clinician methods, and instrument reliability (Henneman & Henneman, 1989; Rebenson-Piano, Holm & Powers, 1987). Using recommendations from previous work as guidelines, the study was designed to control those factors that could result in extraneous direct and indirect measurement variance. (p. 86)

Whitley's (1992a) conceptual article is an example of a summary synthesis of both conceptual and data-based sources. This article is an analysis of the concept of fear. In one sense a concept analysis could be viewed as an extensive review of the literature that was published in its "long form." Headings and subheadings are labeled for each related variable, and the summary synthesis is labeled "Conclusions." Whitley stated the following:

> During the analysis of the concept of fear, as during the analysis of the concept of anxiety [previously published], the close relationship of these concepts was apparent. The possibility of a fear-anxiety syndrome as discussed by Taylor-Loughlin et al. (1989) does warrant further investigation. It is clear, however, that distinctions between the two concepts are both possible and necessary. By using critical attributes, antecedents, consequences, and empirical referents, these distinctions are accomplished in a theoretically and clinically useful manner. . . . Concept analyses provide the essential initial data to begin tool development for this process. (pp. 160-161)

Another example of a summary synthesis found in a conceptual article is a literature review by Ouellet and Rush (1992). These authors wrote an article entitled "A Synthesis of Selected Literature on Mobility: A Basis for Studying Impaired Mobility." Headings and subheadings facilitate reading the reviewed conceptual and data-based sources. The article concluded with a labeled four-paragraph summary that meets many critiquing criteria questions (see box, p. 135). The reader is invited to use the criteria to critique the following example, taken from the first paragraph of this summary:

> The literature review suggests that a narrow meaning has been ascribed to mobility by nursing and clearly shows that it is rarely discussed within the context of health. On the contrary, it is approached primarily within the confines of immobility and, as such, parallels a disease-oriented model. Yet, health is usually identified as the purpose or goal of nursing. . . . some beginning relationships, between the two have been established by Hogue (1984), Houldin, Salstein, and Ganley (1987), and Mangalam (1968). These works could serve as a departure point for extending the concept of mobility to encompass the various dimensions of health. (p. 72)

Critiquing a review of the literature is an acquired skill. Continue reading and rereading, as well as seeking advice from faculty and seasoned researchers. It is also recommended that the student review at this time the strategies for critically reading the literature, as described in Chapter 4.

KEY POINTS

- The role of the consumer of research for critquing a literature review is based on ANA's (1989) educational guidelines for research activities and ANA's (1991) standards of clinical practice.
- The review of the literature is defined as a broad, comprehensive, in-depth, systematic, and critical review of scholarly publications, unpublished scholarly print materials, audiovisual materials, and personal communications.
- The review of the literature is for research and nonresearch activities.
- The main objectives for the consumer of research in relation to the literature review are to acquire the ability to do the following:
    Efficiently retrieve a sufficient amount of scholarly materials for a literature review
    Critically evaluate data-based and conceptual material based on accepted reviewing criteria
    Critically evaluate a review of the literature based on accepted reviewing criteria.
- Primary resources are essential for literature reviews.
- Secondary sources, from peer reviewed journals, are part of a learning strategy for developing critical evaluation skills.
- There are many advantages for using computer data bases rather than print data bases for retrieving scholarly material.
- Strategies for efficiently retrieving scholarly literature include consulting the reference librarian and using computer data-base software.
- Literature reviews are organized according to variables, as well as chronologically.
- Critiquing criteria for scholarly literature reflect the purposes and characteristics of a relevant literature review and are presented in the form of questions.

REFERENCES

Acute Pain Management Guideline Panel. (1992). *Acute pain management: Operative or medical procedures and trauma practice guideline* (ACHCPR Publication No. 92-0023). Rockville, MD: Agency for Health Care Policy and Research, Public Health Service, U.S. Department of Health and Human Services.

American Nurses Association. (ANA). (1980). *A social policy statement.* Kansas City, MO: Author.

American Nurses Association. (ANA). (1989). *Education for participation in nursing research.* Kansas City, MO: Author.

American Nurses Association. (ANA). (1991). *Standards of clinical nursing practice.* Kansas City, MO: Author.

Avant, K.C. (1990). The art and science in nursing diagnosis development. *Nursing Diagnosis, 1,* 51-56.

Beck, C.T. (1992). The lived experience of postpartum depression: A phenomenological study. *Nursing Research, 41*(2), 166-170.

Bridges, J.M. (1990). Literature review on the images of the nurse and nursing in the media. *Journal of Advanced Nursing, 15,* 850-854.

CINAHL. (1992). *CINAHL fact sheets 1992.* Glendale, CA: CINAHL Information Systems.

Collins, R.M., & Fielder, J.H. (1992). Beckstrand's concept of practice theory: A critique. In L.H. Nicoll (Ed.), *Perspectives on nursing theory* (pp. 555-561). New York: J.B. Lippincott.

Duckett, L., Henly, S.J., & Garvis, M. (1993). Predicting breast-feeding duration during the postpartum hospitalization. *Western Journal of Nursing Research, 15*(92), 177-198.

Glass, E.C. (1991). Importance of research to practice. In M.A. Mateo & K.T. Kirchhoff (Eds.), *Conducting and using nursing research in the clinical setting* (pp. 3-7). Baltimore: Williams & Wilkins.

Grey, M. (1990). The literature review. In G. LoBiondo-Wood & J. Haber (Eds.), *Nursing research: Methods, critical appraisal, and utilization* (pp. 78-88). St. Louis: Mosby.

Grey, M., Cameron, M.E., & Thurber, F.W. (1991). Coping and adaptation in children with diabetes. *Nursing Research, 40*(3), 144-149.

Haber, L.C., & Austin, J.K. (1992). How married couples make decisions. *Western Journal of Nursing Research, 14*(3), 322-342.

Hawks, J.H. (1991). Power: A concept analysis. *Journal of Advanced Nursing, 16,* 754-762.

Hutchison, C.P., & Bahr, R.T. (1991). Types and meanings of caring behaviors among elderly nursing home residents. *Image, 23*(2), 85-88.

Kerlinger, F.N. (1986). *Foundations of behavioral research.* (3rd ed.). New York: Holt, Rinehart & Winston.

Kirchhoff, K.T. (1991). Strategies in research utilization. In M.A. Mateo & K.T. Kirchhoff (Eds.), *Conducting and using nursing in the clinical setting* (pp. 108-112). Baltimore: Williams & Wilkins.

Krainovich-Miller, B. (1988). Clinical validation of the nursing diagnosis of pre-operative state anxiety (Doctoral dissertation. Columbia University Teachers College, 1988). *Dissertation Abstracts International,* 8824404.

LeFort, S.M. (1993). The statistical versus clinical significance debate. *Image, 25*(1), 57-62.

LeMone, P. (1991). Analysis of a human phenomenon: Self-concept. *Nursing Diagnosis, 2*(3), 126-130.

Marriner-Tomey, A. (1989). *Nursing theorists and their work.* (2nd ed.). St. Louis: Mosby.

Miller, B. K., Haber, J., & Byrne, M. (1990). The experience of caring in the teaching-learning process of nursing education: Student and teacher perspectives. In M. Leininger & J. Watson (Eds.), *The caring imperative in education* (pp. 125-135). New York: NLN.

New Webster's Dictionary and Thesaurus. (1991). New York: Book Essentials.

Nicoll, L. H. (1992). *Perspectives on nursing theory.* (2nd ed.). New York: J.B. Lippincott.

Norman, E., Gadaletta, D., & Griffin, C. C. (1991). An evaluation of three blood pressure methods in a stabilized acute trauma population. *Nursing Research, 40*(2), 86-89.

Ouellet, L. L., & Rush, K. L. (1992). A synthesis of selected literature on mobility: A basis for studying impaired mobility. *Nursing Diagnosis, 3*(2), 72-80.

Owens, M. K., & Ehrenreich, D. (1991). Literature review of nonpharmacologic methods for the treatment of chronic pain. *Holistic Nursing Practice, 6*(1), 24-31.

Paul, R. W. (1990). *Critical thinking: What every person needs to survive in a rapidly changing world.* Rohnert Park, CA: Center for Critical Thinking & Moral Critique.

Phillips, J. R. (1992). Research issues: Search in research. *Nursing Science Quarterly, 5*(2), 50-51.

Rogers M. E. (1970). *An introduction to the theoretical basis of nursing.* Philadelphia: F.A. Davis.

Shade, P. (1992). Patient-controlled analgesia: Can client education improve outcomes? *Journal of Advanced Nursing, 17,* 408-413.

SilverPlatter Information. (1993). *1993 Directory of CD-ROM Databases.* Norwood, MA: SilverPlatter Information.

Stepnick, A., McDaniel, R. W., & Bach, C. A. (1991). Nursing research making it easier. *Journal of Nursing Staff Development,* March/April, pp. 61-63.

Stewart Fahs, S., & Kinney, M. R. (1991). The abdomen, thigh, and arm as sites for subcutaneous sodium heparin injections. *Nursing Research, 40*(4), 204-207.

Whitley, G. G. (1992a). Concept analysis of anxiety. *Nursing Diagnosis, 3*(3), 107-116.

Whitley, G. G. (1992b). Concept analysis of fear. *Nursing Diagnosis, 3*(4), 155-160.

Wilson, S., & Morse, J. M. (1991). Living with a wife undergoing chemotherapy. *Image, 23*(2), 78-84.

ADDITIONAL READINGS

American Psychological Association. (APA). (1983). *Publication manual of the American Psychological Association.* (3rd ed.). Washington, DC: Author.

Strunk, W., & White, E. B. (1979). *The elements of style* (3rd ed.). New York: Macmillan.

Tornquist, E. M. (1986). *From proposal to publication: An informal guide to writing about nursing research.* Menlo Park, CA: Addison-Welsey.

CHAPTER

6

The Theoretical Framework

HARRIET R. FELDMAN

LEARNING OBJECTIVES

After reading this chapter the student should be able to do the following:

♦ Identify the purpose and nature of a theoretical framework.
♦ Describe the process involved in developing a theoretical framework.
♦ Differentiate between conceptual and operational definitions.
♦ Describe how a theoretical framework guides research.
♦ Define nursing theory.
♦ Identify the four phenomena of concern to nursing.
♦ Describe the points of critical appraisal used to evaluate the appropriateness, cohesiveness, and consistency of a theoretical framework.

KEY TERMS

concept   proposition
conceptual definition   theoretical framework
construct   theory
hypothesis   variable
operational definition

A theoretical framework is analogous to the frame of a house. Just as the foundation supports a house, a theoretical framework provides a rationale for predictions about the relationships among variables of a research study. This chapter addresses the nature and purpose of a theoretical framework in a research study and shows how to develop and critique a theoretical framework. The following definitions serve as a guide to the ensuing discussion of these topics.

DEFINITION OF THEORY

Theory has been defined in a number of ways. For example, Barnum (1990) states, "A theory is a statement that purports to account for or characterize some phenomenon" and that it "pulls out the salient parts of a phenomenon so that one can separate the critical and necessary factors (or relationships) from the accidental and unessential factors (or relationships)" (p. 1). Chinn and Kramer (1991) say theory is a "systematic abstraction of reality that serves some purpose" (p. 20). They describe each part of the definition as follows: *systematic* implies a specific organizational pattern, *abstraction* means that theory is a representation of reality, and *purposes* include description, explanation, and prediction of phenomena, and control of some reality. According to Meleis (1985), a theory enables us to explain a "maximum number of observable relationships," by setting limits on "what questions to ask and what methods to use to pursue answers to the questions" (p. 30).

Kerlinger's (1986) definition of theory is perhaps the one most widely used in research. It takes a basic view of science, that is, the development of general explanations about natural phenomena via theories. To be more precise, "a theory is a set of interrelated constructs [concepts adapted for a scientific purpose], definitions, and propositions that present a systematic view of phenomena by specifying relations among variables, with the purpose of explaining and predicting the phenomena" (Kerlinger, 1986, p. 9).

Through research, scientists can develop, modify, or evaluate theories. As discussed in Chapter 2, theories are generated by using inductive processes, which lead scientists to *make* predictions about observed phenomena. A deductive approach, however, is used to evaluate and modify existing theory by *testing* predictions about relationships between observed phenomena.

DEFINITION OF A THEORETICAL FRAMEWORK

A *theoretical framework* provides a context for examining a problem, that is, the theoretical *rationale* for developing hypotheses, just as a direction indicator (N-S-E-W) provides a context for using a road map. It is also a frame of reference that is a base for observations, definitions of concepts, research designs, interpretations, and generalizations, much as the frame that rests on a foundation defines the overall design of a house. Finally, a theoretical framework serves as a guide to systematically identifying logical, precisely defined relationships among variables.

Suppose a nurse researcher were interested in studying interventions for reducing postoperative pain in patients with cholecystectomies and found out through a search of the literature that pain perception can be altered by distraction. The nurse might study the use of a distractor (e.g., music) for these patients. Thus the researcher would be studying the relationship between music and postoperative pain. The theoretical framework for this study of the relationship between two variables, music and postoperative pain, is the gate control theory of pain (Melzack & Wall, 1965), which says that pain can be affected by altering such pain-inhibiting mechanisms as a central control system in the cerebral cortex. Distraction can alter this inhibiting mechanism by overriding the competitive sensation of pain. Fig. 6-1 illustrates this theoretical relationship.

An investigator who reports research is obliged to state clearly the theoretical basis for **hypothesis** formulation (which is the researcher's prediction about the outcome of the study), study findings, and outcome interpretations. As in the analogy previously presented, each piece of lumber that the frame of the house comprises must be connected to another piece, as in the relationship between two or more variables. The frame must rest squarely on a solid foundation, just as the relationship between two variables rests firmly on a theoretical framework. The "fit" must be precise, or the house will fall; similarly, the theoretical fit must be precise or the prediction made about the relationship of the variables will in all likelihood not be supported through testing of the hypothesis.

HOW TO USE A THEORETICAL FRAMEWORK AS A GUIDE IN A RESEARCH STUDY

The theoretical framework of a research study places the problem in a theoretical context, bringing meaning to the problem and study findings. It summarizes

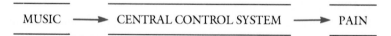

Fig. 6-1   Inventory of relationship between music and pain.

the existing knowledge in the field of inquiry and identifies the linkages among defined concepts, thereby establishing a basis for predicting specific outcomes or generating hypotheses (Fig. 6-2). These linkages or **propositions** spell out how concepts are interrelated and lay a foundation for the development of methods that test the validity and strength of predicted relationships or hypotheses. The examples that follow clarify how theory guides the research process.

Suppose a nurse researcher were interested in alternatives to medication for the treatment of postoperative pain. An examination of the literature might lead to the identification of relaxation training as an intervention. The following questions might be posed:
- On what basis has a linkage between pain and relaxation been established?
- What is the nature of the linkage?
- How can this linkage or relationship be tested?
- What methods can be used for the purpose of testing?

To answer these questions, the researcher must begin by exploring a theoretical framework that is suitable for pursuing the research problem.

Levin, Malloy, and Hyman (1987) examined the relationship between relaxation and postoperative pain in women who were undergoing elective cholecystectomy. In establishing a theoretical explanation for linking these variables, they used the gate control theory of pain, citing two components of the pain experience, physiological and psychological, and the interaction of these components. On the

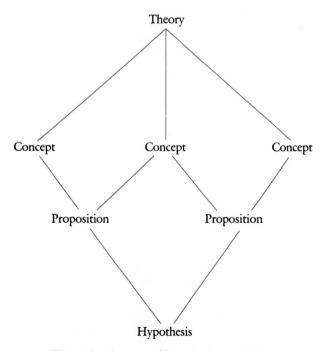

Fig. 6-2   Process of hypothesis generation.

basis of the work of Melzack and Wall (1975), they stated, "The sensation produced by a pain stimulus is modified by motivational-affective and cognitive variables which either block the transmission of neural impulses or allow them through" (p. 464). They further stated, "Anxiety is one motivational-affective variable that has been defined as a state of tension which elicits the stress response" (p. 464) and is incompatible with a state of relaxation. In describing the relaxation response, they referred to both physiological and psychological effects of this technique. They concluded, "If a state of relaxation can be achieved, then anxiety, with its concomitant increased sympathetic activity, is counteracted. A decrease in anxiety has been found to decrease the degree to which a pain stimulus is perceived as distressful" (p. 464).

Fig. 6-3 illustrates the linkage between the independent variable (relaxation) and dependent variable (pain) of this study, showing that by influencing certain psychological and physiological components of the pain experience, that experience can be altered. Taking this rationale a step further, the following hypotheses can be generated:

1. Individuals who practice a relaxation technique will experience reduced intensity of postoperative pain as compared with those who do not practice a relaxation technique.
2. Individuals who practice a relaxation technique will experience reduced postoperative pain distress as compared with those who do not practice a relaxation technique.

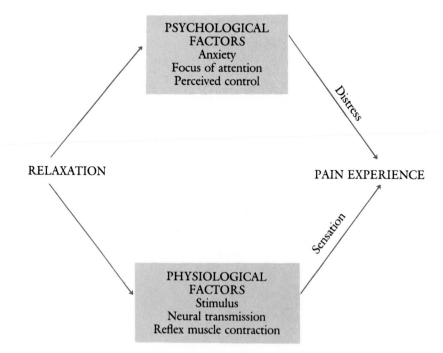

Fig. 6-3   Inventory of relationship between relaxation and pain.

3. Individuals who practice a relaxation technique will report less postoperative anxiety than those who do not practice a relaxation technique.

The first hypothesis evolved from the theoretical linkage between relaxation and physiological factors associated with pain. The second hypothesis evolved from theoretically based psychological factors associated with pain. The third hypothesis evolved from the theoretical linkage between relaxation and psychological factors (anxiety) associated with pain.

Once hypotheses are generated, they are tested. This involves selecting the individual subjects to participate in the study, using instruments that will validly and reliably measure the variables, developing a method of systematically collecting the information needed to test hypothesized relationships, and selecting statistical measures that will determine the extent and meaning or significance of the relationships. Furthermore, the outcomes of the study must be viewed in terms of their support or lack of support of the chosen theoretical rationale.

It is obvious that the theoretical framework plays an important role in guiding the entire process of the research study. If the framework is logically sound and substantiated by previous research studies, there is a strong possibility that the predictions or hypotheses evolving from that framework will be supported; however, if hypotheses are not based firmly on a theoretical rationale, there can be no confidence in the findings. Research consumers must be able to evaluate whether the theoretical framework is consistent with the concepts, definitions, and hypotheses stated by the investigator.

How the theoretical rationale provides a basis for hypothesis development in a research study may not always be made explicit in a research report. For example, although Gift, Moore, and Soeken (1992) hypothesized that patients with a chronic obstructive pulmonary disease (COPD) who were taught progressive muscle relaxation using a taped message would "have greater improvement in their anxiety, dyspnea, and airway obstruction when compared with a control group" (p. 242) who did not receive the tape, they did not explicitly link the variables relaxation, anxiety dyspnea, and airway obstruction. A relationship between anxiety and dyspnea was documented through research that reported higher anxiety during periods of increased dyspnea. Also, other studies are cited that support the relationship between the use of relaxation techniques and anxiety relief and relaxation techniques and improvement in peak expiratory flow rate (an indicator of obstruction). A theoretical relationship, however, was not directly established to show how relaxation reduces anxiety and how anxiety reduction affects airway obstruction and dyspnea. Fig. 6-4 illustrates how this theoretical relationship might have been conceived. Because the study hypothesis was not substantiated through documented presentation of the theoretical rationale, theoretical interpretations are left to the reader.

In some cases, a theoretical rationale is inappropriately used. Examples are (1) a theory designed to explain a particular behavior in infants that may not be appropriate for the study of those behaviors in adults; (2) a theory of management based on observations of male managers that would not be appropriate for the study of management behaviors in females; (3) the theory of power (Barrett, 1988), based on Rogers' (1986) noncausal, holistic model of unitary human beings who are "in

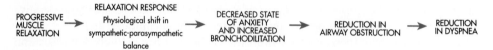

Fig. 6-4 Inventory of relationship between progressive muscle relaxation and reduction in dyspnea.

continuous, mutual process with the environment" (Barrett, 1989, p. 207) that would be inappropriately tested if it used a framework that was based on cause and effect relationships. The inappropriate use of theory, aside from being logically unsound, can lead to erroneous conclusions about the problem being studied and unsubstantiated predictions.

In other cases, the theoretical rationale may be weak. For example, perhaps the theory was not sufficiently tested, the assumptions (see Chapter 2) were incompatible, the concepts were ill defined, or the terms were inconsistent with the theory.

PURPOSE OF HAVING A THEORETICAL FRAMEWORK IN A RESEARCH STUDY

Why is a theoretical framework necessary for a research study? Why can't a researcher just match any two variables that make sense and look at their relationship? As an analogy, consider the first time you traveled by car to an unfamiliar place. How did you get to your destination? Did you use a map? Did you follow someone's directions? Did you stick to the prescribed route, or did you try a shortcut? Did you turn left instead of right because it seemed logical, or did you use known information to make that decision? The map served as a guide to your destination, and when conducting research, a theoretical rationale serves as a guide or map to systematically identifying a logical, precisely defined relationship between variables. Other purposes of a theoretical rationale include providing clear descriptions of variables, suggesting ways or methods to conduct the study, and guiding the interpretation, evaluation, and integration of study findings.

HOW TO DEVELOP A THEORETICAL FRAMEWORK

A research consumer is expected to critique the theoretical framework of research studies. Knowing the basis for and intricacies of developing a theoretical framework will assist the nurse in critiquing this aspect of a research study. Examples are provided to guide consumers in this process.

Selecting Concepts

A concept is an image or symbolic representation of an abstract idea. It is formed by generalizing from particular characteristics. To illustrate, health is a concept formed by generalizing from particular behaviors, for example, being mobile, being free of infection, and communicating appropriately. Other concepts include pain, intelligence, weight, grieving, self-concept, and achievement. Concepts facilitate the delineation of ideas so that systematic inquiry can proceed. Some concepts are directly observable, such as a chair or rain, and others are indirectly observable, for example, anxiety or intelligence. A theoretical framework specifies the relationship between concepts in a study.

Because concepts are the basis for refining ideas and developing theory, it is important to select those concepts that clearly reflect the subject matter being pursued. In evaluating a piece of research, research consumers must consider whether the concepts as defined are examined both in general and specifically in the context of the problem under investigation (see Chapters 7 and 14). Furthermore, one must consider whether they are being measured with the appropriate instruments (see Chapters 14 and 15).

Identifying the Interrelationships Among Concepts

In the process of examining the concepts or variables that guide the research effort, relationships emerge. For example, from a review of the literature in a particular area such as stress, information about related variables can be found (e.g., onset of illness, certain physiological responses, and learning ability). Relationships can also be identified through systematic observation and experience. A relationship may be invariable, tentative, or inconclusive. One type of invariable relationship is a scientific law, for example, Newton's three laws of motion. In this case, no known contradiction has been observed. A tentative or inconclusive relationship is a hypothesis, which expresses a relationship between two or more variables and does not convey truth or falsity. Both laws and hypotheses are types of propositions (see Chapter 2).

The literature review is the part of the research report that generally includes discussion of the theoretical rationale and should explicitly identify propositions in relation to the individual variables described. The hypotheses should express relationships between variables in an unambiguous, precise manner, and they should be based on the propositions that evolved from the theoretical framework (see Chapters 5 and 7).

Formulating Definitions

As stated earlier, concepts are representations of abstract ideas. To develop a theoretical framework that can generate and test hypotheses, concepts must be clearly defined. In thinking back to the earlier illustration about traveling to an unfamiliar place, how do you think you would have arrived if the directions simply read, "First you take one road, then turn at another, and proceed to three more roads?" Without a clear conception of which road, what direction to turn, and how far to proceed, you probably would get lost. The same process applies to any concept. For example, how would you define pain? anxiety? intelligence? In addition to knowing the names of the roads to travel, other specifics are clearly needed, such as what type of vehicle you will use, what town you will travel through, how you will know when you have arrived, and how far you will travel. These parameters delineate the procedure to follow by identifying what *operations* must occur to make the trip. When defining concepts for the purpose of systematic examination, researchers must include both conceptual and operational information.

Conceptual Definitions

Concepts, no matter what their level of abstraction, must be defined as unambiguously as possible, so that they can be easily communicated to others. Even the word *can* is open to various interpretations, for example, a container, being able to, or a commode. A **conceptual definition** conveys the general meaning of the concept, as does a dictionary definition. It reflects the theory used in the study of that concept. The following are several examples of conceptual definitions:

- *Recovery:* the process of healing that takes place after an injury
- *Adaptation:* "the degree to which an individual adjusts psychologically, socially, and physiologically to a long-term illness" (Grey, Cameron, & Thurber, 1991, p. 144)
- *Postoperative pain:* discomfort an individual experiences after a surgical procedure
- *Coping effort:* "amount of physical and/or emotional energy an event or situation requires to adjust to or handle the situation" (Schepp, 1991, p. 44)
- *Perceived uncertainty:* "the individual's perception of a situation as ambiguous" (Wineman, 1990, p. 294)
- *State-anxiety:* "a transitional emotional state aroused in a situation that presents a perceived threat to self-integrity" (Mullooly, Levin, & Feldman, 1988, p. 5)

Because these are general definitions, they do not include an indication of how the concepts will be measured.

Operational Definitions

Operationalization adds another dimension to the conceptual definition by delineating the procedures or operations required to measure the concept. It supplies the information needed to collect data on the problem being studied. Some concepts are easily defined in operational terms; for example, pulse can be measured numerically after finding the radial pulse and counting the number of beats or pulsations for a minute. Other concepts are more difficult to define operationally, such as coping, leaving it up to the investigator to locate and select an instrument that best measures the concept as defined. The following are examples of **operational definitions**:

- *Dyspnea:* "the sensation of difficult breathing" (Gift, Moore, & Soeken, 1992, p. 242), as measured by the Visual Analogue Dyspnea Scale (VADS)
- *Hopelessness:* "the perceptual experience of anticipation of undesirable situations or consequences that are largely beyond one's control, was measured by the Hopelessness Scale" (Abraham, Neundorfer, & Currie, 1992, p. 198)
- *Body attitude:* "individuals' general attitudes about the outward form and appearance of their bodies" (Drake, Verhulst, Fawcett, & Barger, 1988, p. 89), as measured by the Body Attitude Scale

* *Social support:* "a characteristic of the social situation that buffers the effect of stress on the health of the individual" (Northouse, 1988, p. 91), as measured by the Social Support Questionnaire
* *State-anxiety:* "a transitional emotional state aroused in a situation that presents a perceived threat to self-integrity" (Mullooly et al., 1988, p. 5), as measured by the Spielberger State-Trait Anxiety Inventory (Spielberger, Gorsuch & Lushene, 1970)

Each of these examples has a conceptual definition and at least one index of measurement that makes it operational. To summarize, an operational definition provides specificity and direction for constructs to guide the development of the research study. Once a construct is operationalized (made measurable), it is termed a **variable,** and at that point it begins to play a significant role in formulating the theoretical rationale. The research consumer is responsible for evaluating whether variables are clearly defined, both conceptually and operationally. If the meaning of the variable is vague or if the measurement used does not reflect the same meaning as the variable, comparisons of the research with the other investigations will not be valid and the research will be impossible to replicate (see Chapter 7).

Some research reports present conceptual definitions followed by a description of measurement in another section, such as methodology or instrumentation. Other reports present operational definitions; still others may present no definitions, leaving interpretations about the meaning of the variables to the reader. Of course, in the latter instance, it is easy to get lost en route.

FORMULATING THE THEORETICAL RATIONALE

Through the literature review, an investigator becomes aware of or confirms identified theoretical connections between variables. For example, in reviewing the literature on the elderly, Hutchison and Bahr (1991) found that being institutionalized (e.g., in nursing homes) has negative effects on well-being. For example, research showed that nursing home staff discouraged residents from exhibiting helping behaviors toward others and that isolation, apathy, loss of motivation, depression, and similar factors were responsible for deterioration. Other studies showed that some residents tried to reach out to others, thus demonstrating caring. No studies, however, reported on the ways nursing home residents "are socially productive through caring acts, or what it means personally to a resident to engage in caring kinds of behaviors" (Hutchison & Bahr, 1991, p. 85). Their study was designed to describe the types and meanings of caring behaviors of elderly nursing home residents, as well as the personal meanings of these behaviors.

Another example concerns condom use among black women. Jemmott and Jemmott (1991) studied attitudinal and normative influences, and knowledge of acquired immunodeficiency syndrome (AIDS) in black women in relation to AIDS risk behavior, in this case, their intentions to use condoms. The theory of reasoned action (Ajzen & Fishbein, 1980) provided the theoretical framework for the study. The theory "emphasizes highly specific attitudes, subjective norms, intentions and behaviors. According to the theory, behavior is the result of a specific intention . . . a woman's intention to use condoms is a function of her attitude—positive or negative—toward using condoms and her perception of what significant others think she should do" (Jemmott & Jemmott, 1991, p. 228). On the basis of this theory, the purpose of the study was to test hypotheses about women's intentions to use condoms and their attitudes (favorable or unfavorable) and subjective norms (supportive or nonsupportive of condom use). Also studied was knowledge of AIDS in relation to attitudes and intentions.

In the first example, Hutchison and Bahr used an inductive approach to studying types of caring behaviors exhibited by residents in a nursing home and the personal meaning of carrying out these behaviors. They developed a model of types of caring behaviors based on the data obtained during their interviews of nursing home residents. This model can be used to generate hypotheses about caring behaviors and such variables as self-concept, depression, and deterioration. In the second, Jemmott and Jemmott used a deductive approach. Clinical knowledge, past research, and the theory of reasoned action served as the initial impetus for drawing conclusions: that is, generating hypotheses about the attitudes, subjective norms, and knowledge of AIDS in relation to intention to use condoms to address an AIDS risk behavior.

In evaluating the formulation of the theoretical rationale, the internal structures, such as concepts and their definitions, should have clarity and continuity, and the approach to understanding phenomena, whether inductive or deductive, should be logical. For example, the research consumer should evaluate the breadth and depth of the literature review, the presence or absence of unambiguous definitions of concepts and variables, and the advancement of a logical and explicit theoretical rationale firmly based on these structures.

TYPES OF THEORY

Theories may describe a particular phenomenon, explain relationships between or among phenomena, or predict how one phenomenon affects another (Fawcett, 1989, p. 21). Different types of theories are tested by different approaches (see Chapters 8, 9, and 10 for a discussion of research designs). For example, *descriptive theories* "describe or classify specific dimensions or characteristics of individuals, groups, situations, or events by summarizing the commonalities found in discrete observations" (Fawcett, 1989, p. 21). To test descriptive theories, researchers conduct descriptive research studies. Hutchison and Bahr (1991) used a grounded theory approach to describe the types and meanings of caring behaviors in elderly nursing home residents. They observed residents and interviewed them to understand their views of caring. The commonalities that the investigators found led them to develop models of the types of caring behaviors and their meaning as expressed by the residents.

Explanatory theories are those that "specify relations among the dimensions or characteristics of individuals, groups, situations, or events" (Fawcett, 1989, p. 21), and are tested by using correlational research. Grey et al., (1991) conducted a correlational study to determine the influence of age, coping behavior, and self-care on social, psychological, and physiological adaptation in adolescents and preadolescents with diabetes. Through their review of literature, they found that several factors influence adaptation to chronic illness during adolescence; however, the relative impact of these factors had not been determined. They proposed that "adaptation would be influenced by age, coping behaviors, and self-care behaviors" (p. 144), and found differences in these factors among preadolescents and adolescents.

Predictive theories are intended to predict "precise relationships between the dimensions or characteristics of a phenomenon or differences between groups" (Fawcett, 1989, p. 21); they are tested through experimental or quasiexperimental research designs. For example, Gift et al., (1992) used a quasiexperimental design to test the effectiveness of a taped relaxation message in relation to dyspnea and anxiety in patients with chronic obstructive pulmonary disease. Through their research, these investigators sought to make predictions about the use of relaxation in reducing dyspnea and anxiety for future application in practice settings.

THE CONTRIBUTION OF NURSING THEORIES OR FRAMEWORKS TO RESEARCH

When developing a theoretical framework for nursing research studies, knowledge is acquired through two approaches. Either it is developed primarily in disciplines other than nursing and borrowed for the purpose of answering nursing questions, or it is derived by identifying and asking questions about phenomena that are unique to nursing. The contributions made by using borrowed theories are most appropriate when data are related specifically to nursing.

Theories unique to nursing help nursing define how it is different from other disciplines. Nursing theories reflect particular views of the person, health, and other concepts that contribute to the development of a body of knowledge specific to nursing's concerns. But what is *nursing* theory? What are nursing's central phenomena of concern? Where do nursing theories come from if they are not borrowed from other disciplines?

Meleis (1991) defines *nursing theory* as "an articulated and communicated conceptualization of invented or discovered reality (central phenomena and relationships) in or pertaining to nursing for the purpose of describing, explaining, predicting, or prescribing nursing care" (p. 167). She further states that "the primary use of theory is to guide research. Through interaction with practice, guidelines for practice will evolve. Research validates and modifies theory. Theory then guides practice" (p. 168). Fawcett (1989) defines nursing theory as "a relatively specific and concrete set of concepts and propositions that purports to account for or characterize phenomena of interest to the discipline of nursing" (p. 23). The central phenomena of interest (concern) to nursing are persons, their environment, their health, and nursing itself. Therefore theories that deal with these phenomena are termed *nursing* theories. These phenomena, as stated, are not conceptualized or operationalized. Clearly, terms must be defined before relationships among them can be specified.

The next logical question is, How are these phenomena defined? The *person*, for example, can be viewed as active or waiting to be acted upon, as inherently good or inherently bad, as an energy field (Rogers, 1986), or as an integrated whole (Orem, 1990). These definitions come from the "invented or discovered reality" described by Meleis (1991) that is the basis for constructing theories. This reality arises from *conceptual models,* which are abstract umbrellas that provide "a distinctive frame of reference for its adherents, telling them what to look at and speculate about. Most important, a conceptual model determines how the world is viewed . . ." (Fawcett, 1989, p. 3). Thus conceptual models are analagous to the whole map, from which various routes are determined. Travelers may follow various paths in an attempt to find the route that is most suitable (e.g., well paved, without too much traffic, free of tolls) to reaching their destination. Likewise, researchers may test various hypotheses in an attempt to find support for a theory that is framed by a particular conceptual model. As theories are confirmed, the conceptual model is verified (the destination is reached).

There are several well-known nursing theorists whose conceptual models have served as a basis for theory development. Among these are Rogers' (1986) life process interactive person-environment model; King's (1981) model of personal, interpersonal, and social systems; Orem's (1991) model of self-care; Neuman's health care systems model (1988); Johnson's behavioral system model (1980); King's open systems model (1983); and Roy's (1984) adaptation model. Each of these theorists addresses the four phenomena of concern to nursing from a different perspective. For example, Rogers views the person and the environment as energy fields coextensive with the universe; that is, person-environment interactions are mutual and simultaneous. King, however, views the person and the environment as separate, and interactions as cause and effect processes.

How do these conceptual models actually guide the research effort? The following examples of three recent studies based on Orem's work should clarify this process. Conn (1991) studied self-care behaviors of older adults for managing colds and influenza. The interview guide she used contained questions "derived from universal and health deviation self-care requisites" (p. 177), as described by Orem. Self-care actions identified during the interviews were as follows: administer medication, alter fluid intake, alter social interaction, alter rest, alter activity, alter food intake, alter self-care related to breathing, and alter self-care related to elimination. Most study participants (subjects) were found to engage in preventive behaviors and rarely engaged in potentially dangerous self-care practices. In this study, Orem's theory of self-care helped to explain the behaviors of older adults.

Geden and Taylor (1991) developed a measurement instrument to identify perceived capacity to care for self, that is, self-care agency as described by Orem. They state, "The inability to consistently and effectively perform self-care is the situation that validates the requirement for nursing. Hence, nurses need to evaluate patients' capabilities to care for themselves" (p. 47). After initial development of the Self-as-Carer Inventory (SCI) and preliminary testing on a college population, Geden and Taylor (1991) administered the SCI to a more diverse population of men and women from 18 to 94 years of age representing at least six ethnic groups. Initial evaluation of the SCI uncovered four distinct areas related to self-care: (1) knowledge of self, (2) judgment and decisions affecting production of self-care, (3) attention to and awareness of self and self-monitoring, and (4) physical skills and satisfaction with self-care routines. The development of instruments to measure concepts defined by Orem helps researchers to test theories derived from Orem's model of self-care.

A third study, by Wanich, Sullivan-Marx, Gottlieb, and Johnson (1992), examines the effectiveness of selected nursing interventions (nursing staff education, orientation and communication, mobilization, environmental modifications, caregiver education/consultation, medication management, and discharge planning) on acute confusion or delirium in hospitalized elderly. The nursing interventions were based on Orem's self-care deficit theory. "Delirium was considered to be an actual or potential health problem which would interfere with the patient's ability to maintain self-care" (p. 202); it would inhibit patients "from the self-care requisites described by Orem" (p. 202). On the basis of a comprehensive program of intervention designed to address a number of self-care actions, "it was anticipated that delirium would be more appropriately managed and that higher levels of functional status would result" (p. 202). The intervention program resulted in greatly improved functional status in hospitalized patients as compared with patients not exposed to the interventions, irrespective of the person's severity of illness or delirium. In discussing study findings, the investigators stated, "Consistent with the expectations discussed in the theoretical framework, we conclude that activities aimed at maintaining normalcy through mobilization, social interaction, and prevention of hazards result in improved abilities to perform self-care activities" (p. 206).

With this background on what nursing models are, what the phenomena of concern to nursing are, and how nursing theories develop, the contribution of a nursing model to research can be summarized. Chapter 2 focused on the scientific approach to the research process, including the philosophy of science, the sources of human knowledge, and the characteristics of the scientific approach. The development of nursing knowledge was said to depend on both philosophy and science. In addition, the individual researcher's own philosophy of human behavior and other related phenomena was said to guide the intent of the research effort. Similarly a nursing conceptual model serves as the philosophical view of specific phenomena of concern to nursing, from which nursing theories arise. As such it is instrumental in guiding the nursing research effort.

CRITIQUING THE THEORETICAL FRAMEWORK

The criteria for critiquing a theoretical framework are found in a box on p. 156. The theoretical framework provides the context that clarifies and specifies problems, develops and tests hypotheses, evaluates research findings, and makes generalizations. As research consumers, nurses need to know how to critically appraise the theoretical bases for research. The following discussion is intended to assist in this process.

Initially, the research consumer focuses on the concepts being studied. Concepts should clearly reflect the area of investigation; for example, using the general concept of stress when anxiety is more appropriate to the research focus creates difficulties in defining variables and delineating hypotheses.

Next, the consumer must evaluate the completeness and appropriateness of

CRITIQUING CRITERIA

1. Is the theoretical framework clearly identified?
2. Is the theoretical framework consistent with what is being studied?
3. Are the concepts clearly and operationally defined?
4. Was sufficient literature reviewed to support the proposed relationships?
5. Is the theoretical basis for hypothesis formulation clearly articulated? Is it logical?
6. Are the relationships among propositions clearly stated?
7. If the theory is borrowed from a discipline other than nursing, are the data related specifically to nursing?
8. Are the study findings related to the theoretical rationale?

the operational definitions of each concept. Once they are defined, it is important to consider whether the variables are examined in general and specifically in the context of the problem under investigation. The literature review is the source of this kind of discussion.

Finally, it is important to appraise the instruments used to measure the variables in terms of appropriateness; for example, does the instrument measure the variables as defined and is the instrument consistent with the theoretical framework? How do they hold up when compared with other instruments? Are all of the subparts consistently measuring the same characteristics? Are the instruments maintaining their stability when repeatedly used over time (see Chapter 14)?

A second aspect of appraising the theoretical rationale relates to the interrelationships among concepts (hypotheses). Briefly stated, hypotheses should express precisely and unambiguously the relationships between variables. They should be based on the propositions that arise from the theoretical framework and directly answer the research problem identified early in the report. A more detailed discussion of critiquing hypotheses appears in Chapter 7.

When evaluating the theoretical framework itself, it is important to examine both the depth and breadth of the literature review. Has the investigator included sufficient information to substantiate the problem and hypothesis, considering a broad range of possibilities? Is there consistency throughout in terms of the philosophical view of phenomena? Are previous studies sufficiently described so that their validity can be determined? Is there a firm basis for linking the variables and determining the direction of the hypotheses? Can the theory be empirically tested? Does the research contribute to the understanding of the phenomena of interest? Are the findings discussed in relation to the theoretical framework? In summary, the research consumer must evaluate whether the theoretical framework or the map led the researcher to the expected findings or destination in a logical and systematic way.

KEY POINTS

- The use of theory is important as a guide to systematically identifying and studying the logical, precise relationships between variables.
- A construct is an image or symbolic representation of an abstract idea that is adapted for a scientific purpose. Constructs help us refine the ideas that form the basis for developing theory.
- To facilitate the process of refinement, constructs must be clearly defined. In addition, operationalization of the definitions serves to delineate the procedures or operations required to measure the construct.
- One definition of theory is that it is "a set of interrelated constructs, definitions, and propositions that present a systematic view of phenomena by specifying relations among variables, with the purpose of explaining and predicting the phenomena" (Kerlinger, 1986, p. 9).
- A theoretical rationale provides a road map or context for examining problems and developing and testing hypotheses. It gives meaning to the problem and study findings by summarizing existing knowledge in the field of inquiry and identifying linkages among concepts.
- In developing a theoretical framework for nursing, knowledge may be acquired from other disciplines or directly from nursing. In either case, that knowledge is used to answer specific nursing questions.
- Nursing conceptual models provide a context for constructing theories that deal with the central phenomena of concern to nursing, that is, the person, the environment, health, and nursing. They help nursing define how it is different from other disciplines.
- Of significance to the research consumer is the evaluation or critique of the theoretical rationale of a research study. It is important to consider not only the clarity and logic of the theoretical rationale itself, but also whether the operational definitions, measurement instruments, and methods of carrying out collection of data about the variables, hypotheses, and findings are consistent with the theory.

REFERENCES

Abraham, I.L., Neundorfer, M.M., & Currie, L.J. (1992). Effects of group interventions on cognition and depression in nursing home residents. *Nursing Research, 41*(4), 196-202.

Ajzen, I., & Fishbein, M. (1980). *Understanding attitudes and predicting social behavior.* Englewood Cliffs, NJ: Prentice Hall.

Barnum, B.J.S. (1990). *Nursing theory: Analysis, application, evaluation* (3rd ed.). Glenview, IL: Scott, Foresman/Little, Brown Higher Education.

Barrett, E. (1988). Using Rogers' science of unitary human beings in nursing practice. *Nursing Science Quarterly, 1*(2), 50-51.

Barrett, E. (1989). A nursing theory of power for nursing practice: Derivation from Rogers' paradigm. In J.P. Riehl (ed.), *Conceptual models for nursing practice* (3rd ed., pp. 207-217). Norwalk, CT: Appleton & Lange.

Chinn, P., & Kramer, M. (1991). *Theory and nursing: A systematic approach* (2nd ed.). St. Louis: Mosby.

Conn, V. (1991). Self-care actions taken by older adults for influenza and colds. *Nursing Research, 40*(3), 176-181.

Drake, M., Verhulst, D., Fawcett, J., & Barger, D. (1988). Spouses' body image changes during and after pregnancy: A replication in Canada. *Image, 20,* 88-92.

Fawcett, J. (1989). The "what" of theory development. In *Theory development: What, why, how?* New York: National League for Nursing.

Geden, E., & Taylor, S. (1991). Construct and empirical validity of the self-as-carer inventory. *Nursing Research, 40*(1), 47-50.

Gift, A., Moore, T., & Soeken, K. (1992). Relaxation to reduce dyspnea and anxiety in COPD patients. *Nursing Research, 41*(4), 242-246.

Grey, M., Cameron, M.E., & Thurber, F.W. (1991). Coping and adaptation in children with diabetes. *Nursing Research, 40*(3), 144-149.

Hutchison, C.P., & Bahr, Sr. R.T. (1991). Types and meanings of caring behaviors among elderly nursing home residents. *Image, 23*(2), 85-88.

Jemmott, L.S., & Jemmott III, J.B. (1991). Applying the theory of reasoned action to AIDS risk behavior: Condom use among black women. *Nursing Research, 40*(4), 228-234.

Johnson, D.E. (1980). The behavioral system model for nursing. In J.P. Riehl & C. Roy (Eds.), *Conceptual models for nursing practice* (2nd ed., pp. 207-216). New York: Appleton-Century-Crofts.

Kerlinger, F. (1986). *Foundations of behavioral research.* (2nd ed.). New York: Holt, Rinehart & Winston.

King, I. (1981). *A theory for nursing: Systems, concepts, process.* New York: John Wiley & Sons.

King, I.M. (1983). King's theory of nursing. In I.W. Clements & F.B. Roberts (Eds.), *Family health: A theoretical approach to nursing* (pp. 177-188). New York: John Wiley & Sons.

Levin, R.L., Malloy, G.B., & Hyman, R.B. (1987). Nursing management of postoperative pain: Use of relaxation techniques with female cholecystectomy patients. *Journal of Advanced Nursing, 12,* 463-472.

Meleis, A.I. (1991). *Theoretical nursing: Development and progress* (2nd ed.). Philadelphia: J.B. Lippincott.

Melzack, R., & Wall, P. (1965). Pain mechanisms: A new theory. *Science, 150,* 971-979.

Mullooly, V., Levin, R., & Feldman, H. (1988). Music for postoperative pain and anxiety. *Journal of the New York State Nurses Association, 19,* 4-7.

Neuman, B.M. (1988). The Betty Neuman health care systems model: A total person approach to patient problems. In J.P. Riehl & C. Roy (Eds.), *Conceptual models of nursing practice* (3rd ed.) (pp. 119-134). New York: Appleton-Century-Crofts.

Northouse, L. (1988). Social support in patients' and husbands' adjustment to breast cancer. *Nursing Research, 37,* 91-95.

Orem, D. (1991). *Nursing: Concepts of practice.* St. Louis: Mosby.

Rogers, M.E. (1986). Science of unitary human beings. In V.M. Malinski (Ed.), *Explorations on Martha E. Rogers' Science of Unitary Human Beings* (pp. 3-8). Norwalk, CT: Appleton-Century-Crofts.

Roy, C. (1984). *Introduction to nursing: An adaptation model* (2nd ed.). Englewood Cliffs, NJ: Prentice-Hall.

Schepp, K.G. (1991). Factors influencing the coping effort of mothers of hospitalized children. *Nursing Research, 40*(1), 42-46.

Spielberger, C., Gorsuch, R., & Lushene, R. (1970). *Manual for the state-trait anxiety inventory.* Palo Alto, CA: Consulting Psychologists Press.

Wanich, C.K., Sullivan-Marx, E.M., Gottlieb, G.L., & Johnson, J.C. (1992). Functional status outcomes of a nursing intervention in hospitalized elderly. *Image, 24*(3), 201-207.

Wineman, M.W. (1990). Adaptation to multiple sclerosis: The role of social support, functional disability, and perceived uncertainty. *Nursing Research, 39*(5), 294-299.

ADDITIONAL READINGS

Chinn, P.L. (1983). *Advances in nursing theory development.* Rockville, MD: Aspen.

Fawcett, J. (1989). *Analysis and evaluation of conceptual models of nursing* (2nd ed.). Philadelphia: F.A. Davis.

Leddy, S., & Pepper, M. (1985). *Conceptual bases of professional nursing.* Philadelphia: J.B. Lippincott.

Malinski, V.M. (Ed.). (1986). *Explorations on Martha Rogers' Science of Unitary Human Beings.* Norwalk, CT: Appleton-Century-Crofts.

Nicoll, L. (Ed.). (1992). *Perspectives on nursing theory* (2nd ed.). Philadelphia: J.B. Lippincott.

Cody, W.K., & Mitchell, G.J. (1992). Parse's theory as a model for practice: The cutting edge. *Advances in Nursing Science, 15*(2), 52-65.

Silva, M.C., & Sorrell, J.M. (1992). Testing of nursing theory: Critique and philosophical expansion. *Advances in Nursing Science, 14*(4), 12-23.

CHAPTER

7

Research Problems
and Hypotheses

JUDITH HABER

LEARNING OBJECTIVES

After reading this chapter the student should be able to do the following:

* Describe the relationship of the problem statement and hypothesis to the other components of the research process.
* Describe the process of identifying and refining a research problem.
* Identify the criteria for determining the significance of a research problem.
* Identify the characteristics of research problems and hypotheses.
* Describe the advantages and disadvantages of directional and nondirectional hypotheses.
* Compare and contrast the use of statistical versus research hypotheses.
* Discuss the appropriate use of research questions versus hypotheses in a research study.
* Identify the criteria used for critiquing a research problem and hypothesis.
* Apply the critiquing criteria to the evaluation of a problem statement and hypothesis in a research report.

KEY TERMS

conceptual definition   problem statement
dependent variable   research hypothesis
directional hypothesis   research problem
hypothesis   statistical hypothesis
independent variable   testability
nondirectional hypothesis   theory
operational definition   variable
population

Formulation of the research problem and developing hypotheses are key preliminary steps in the research process. The **research problem,** often called a **problem statement,** presents the question that is to be asked in the study. The **hypothesis** attempts to answer the question posed by the research problem.

The first step and one of the most important requirements of the research process is to be able to clearly delineate the study area and state the research problem concisely. Before the study is designed and the hypotheses are formulated, the researcher spends much time narrowing down the broad problem area to a concise and feasible research problem, which provides direction for the study.

Hypotheses can be considered intelligent hunches, guesses, or predictions that assist the researcher in seeking the solution or answer to the research question. Hypotheses are a vehicle for testing the validity of the theoretical framework assumptions and provide a bridge between theory and the real world. In the scientific world, researchers derive hypotheses from theories and subject them to empirical testing. A theory's validity is not directly examined. Instead, it is through the hypotheses that the merit of a theory can be evaluated.

The research consumer often does not see a formal statement of the research problem or hypothesis in research reports or articles because of space constraints or stylistic considerations in such publications. What does appear more often in published articles is a statement of the aims, purpose, or goals of the research study. Nevertheless, it is equally important for both the consumer and producer of research to understand the importance of the problem statement and hypothesis as foundational elements of the research study: elements that set the stage for the development of the research study.

This chapter provides a working knowledge of quantitative research problems and hypotheses, the standards for writing them, and a set of criteria for their evaluation.

DEVELOPING AND REFINING A RESEARCH PROBLEM

A researcher spends a great deal of time refining a research idea into a testable research problem. Unfortunately, the evaluator of a research study is not privy to this creative process, since it occurred during the study's conceptualization. And often, the final problem statement does not appear in the research article unless the study is qualitative rather than quantitative in nature (see Chapter 11). Although this section will not teach you how to formulate a research problem, it is important to provide a glimpse of what the process of developing a research problem may be like for a researcher.

As illustrated in Table 7-1 (pp. 164-165), research problems or topics are not pulled from thin air. Research problems should indicate that practical experience, a critical appraisal of the scientific literature, or interest in untested **theory** has provided the basis for the generation of a research idea. Researchable problems also are generated by professional organization priorities and quality improvement issues (see Chapter 1). The problem statement should reflect a refinement of the researcher's initial thinking. The evaluator of a research study should be able to discern that the researcher has done the following:

1. Defined a specific problem area
2. Reviewed the relevant scientific literature
3. Examined the problem's potential significance to nursing
4. Pragmatically examined the feasibility of studying the research problem

Defining the Problem Area

Researchers generally begin with an interest in some broad topic area, such as pain management, family communication patterns, self-care patterns of elders, or management of urinary incontinence. When nurses ask such questions as "Why are things done this way?" "I wonder what would happen if . . .?" or "What characteristics are associated with . . .?" they are often well on their way to developing a researchable problem.

Usually the research focuses on the *dependent variable* of the study, the variable that will be predicted or explained through its relationship to the independent variable. Brainstorming with teachers, advisors, or colleagues may provide valuable feedback that helps the researcher focus on a specific problem area. Let us consider an example. Suppose a researcher told a faculty advisor that the area of interest was families' relationships with elderly relatives. The advisor may have said, "What is it about the topic that specifically interests you?" Such a conversation may have initiated a chain of thought that resulted in a decision to explore stress in family caregivers of the elderly. Fig. 7-1 illustrates how a broad area of interest (family relationships with elderly relatives) was narrowed to a specific research topic (stress in family caregivers of the elderly).

Beginning the Literature Review

The literature review should reveal that the scientific literature relevant to the problem area has been critically examined. Often concluding sections on recommen-

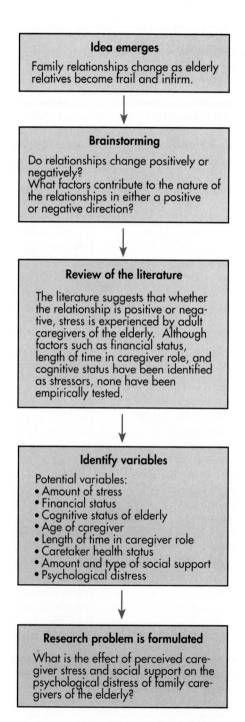

Fig. 7-1   Formulation of a research problem: a process.

Table 7-1   How Practical Experience, Scientific Literature, and Untested Theory Influence the Development of a Research Idea

Area	Influence	Example
Practical experience	Clinical practice provides a wealth of experience from which research problems can be derived. The nurse may observe the occurrence of a particular event or pattern and become curious about why it occurs, as well as its relationship to other factors in the patient's environment.	A nurse working with patients who have chronic obstructive pulmonary disease (COPD) observes that certain patients have more dyspnea than others whose pulmonary status is equally severe. The nurse knows that dyspnea is the most common reason COPD patients seek health care, yet few obtain relief. She also observes that anxiety appears to be closely related to severity of dyspnea in certain patients. Noting the difference in the two groups of dyspneic COPD patients, those who are also anxious and those who are not, the nurse speculates about the effect of progressive muscle relaxation exercises on anxiety, dyspnea, and airway obstruction (Gift, Moore, & Soeken, 1992).
Critical appraisal of the scientific literature	The critical appraisal of research studies that appear in journals may indirectly suggest a problem area by stimulating the reader's thinking. The nurse may observe a conflict or inconsistency in the findings of several related research studies and wonder which findings are most valid.	At a staff meeting where cost-effectiveness was being discussed, a nurse reported that she had read an article indicating that saline flushes were more cost-effective than heparin flushes (saving hospitals up to $1,000,000 per year) and were equally effective in maintaining IV heparin lock patency without increasing the incidence of phlebitis. Another nurse said that other articles they had on file indicated that the heparin flush, although more costly, was more effective. The group agreed that there was a conflict in the data and began a literature review to help them scientifically resolve the discrepancy in the findings and define a problem focus (Goode et al., 1991).
Gaps in the literature	A research idea also may be suggested by a critical appraisal of the literature that identifies gaps in the	A nurse who had just begun working on an oncology unit observed that the concerns and well-being of partners of patients with breast cancer were not a

Table 7-1   How Practical Experience, Scientific Literature, and Untested Theory
Influence the Development of a Research Idea—cont'd

Area	Influence	Example
	literature and suggests areas for future study. Research ideas also can be generated by research reports that suggest the value of replicating a particular study to extend or refine the existing scientific knowledge base.	focus of attention after diagnosis and during treatment of their wife's breast cancer. He wondered whether the partners' emotional and physical concerns and feelings of well-being as predictors of adjustment had even been examined. Where the literature is reviewed relative to this topic, no research studies are identified that would provide a scientific basis for determining factors related to adjustment of breast cancer patients and their partners (Hoskins, 1991).
Interest in untested theory	Verification of an untested nursing theory provides a relatively uncharted territory from which research problems can be derived. Inasmuch as theories themselves are not tested, a researcher may think about investigating a particular concept or set of concepts related to a particular nursing theory. The deductive process would be used to generate the research problem. The researcher would pose questions such as, "If this theory is correct, what kind of behavior would I expect to observe in particular patients and under which conditions?" *or* "If this theory is valid, what kind of supporting evidence would I find?"	A nurse researcher utilizes Roger's Science of Unitary Human Beings model as the basis of a research study designed to verify particular aspects of this conceptual system. A study was designed to test Rogers' theory of accelerating change by investigating the relationships among creativity, actualization, and empathy in persons 18 to 92 years of age (Alligood, 1991).

dations and implications for practice identify remaining gaps in the literature, the need for replication, or the need for extension of the knowledge base about a particular research focus (see Chapter 5). In the previous example of stress in family caregivers of the elderly, the researcher may have conducted a preliminary review of books and journals for theories and research studies regarding factors apparently critical to the families caring for an elderly relative. These factors should be potentially relevant, of interest, and measurable. Possible relevant factors mentioned in the literature include any emotional, social, physical, and financial difficulties associated with caregiving. Other variables, such as demographic characteristics of caregivers and of elders, characteristics of the caregiving situation, and social support, that mediate the effect of caregiver stress also are suggested as important to be considered (Kuhlman, Wilson, Hutchinson & Wallhagen, 1991). This information can then be used by the researcher to further define the research problem. At this point the researcher could write the following tentative problem statement: *What is the effect of stress and social support on the psychological distress of family caregivers of the elderly?* Although the problem statement is not yet in its final form, the reader can envision the interrelatedness of the initial definition of the problem area, the literature review, and the refined problem statement. The person reading a research report examines the end product of this formulation process and thus should have an appreciation of this time-consuming effort.

Significance

Before proceeding to a final formulation of the problem statement, it is crucial for the researcher to have examined the problem's potential significance to nursing. The research problem should have the potential for contributing to and extending the scientific body of nursing knowledge. The problem does not have to be of prize-winning caliber to be significant. However, it should meet the following criteria:

- Patients, nurses, the medical community in general, and society will potentially benefit from the knowledge derived from this study.
- The results will be applicable for nursing practice, education, or administration.
- The results will be theoretically relevant.
- The findings will lend support to untested theoretical assumptions, extend or challenge an existing theory, or clarify a conflict in the literature.
- The findings will potentially formulate or alter nursing practices or policies.

If the research problem has not met any of these criteria, it is wise to extensively revise the problem or discard it. For example, in the previously cited problem statement the significance of the problem includes the following facts:

- The number of elderly in the population will more than double in the next 40 years.
- A decline in federally funded programs for the elderly will place further demands on families for caregiving responsibilities.
- The toll of caregiving on families can be high.
- Previous research studies have been largely exploratory and atheoretical, which makes it difficult to draw conclusions.

Feasibility

The feasibility of a research problem needs to be pragmatically examined. Regardless of how significant or researchable a problem may be, pragmatic considerations such as time; the availability of subjects, facilities, equipment, and money; the experience of the researcher; and any ethical considerations may cause the researcher to decide that the problem is inappropriate because it lacks feasibility (see Chapters 8 and 13).

THE FINAL PROBLEM STATEMENT

A problem may be written in declarative form as illustrated in Table 7-2 or in interrogative form as illustrated in Table 7-3. Both are acceptable formats. The style chosen is largely a function of the researcher's preference. A good problem statement exhibits the following four characteristics:

- It clearly and unambiguously identifies the variables under consideration.
- It clearly expresses the variables' relationship to each other.
- It specifies the nature of the population being studied.
- It implies the possibility of empirical testing.

Because each of these elements is crucial to the formulation of a satisfactory problem statement, the criteria will be discussed in greater detail.

The Variables

Researchers call the properties that they study *variables*. Such properties take on different values. Thus a **variable** is, as the name suggests, something that varies. Properties that differ from each other, such as age, weight, height, religion, and ethnicity, are examples of variables. Researchers attempt to understand how and why differences in one variable are related to differences in another variable. For example, a researcher may be concerned about the variable of pain in postoperative patients. It is a variable because not all postoperative patients have pain or the same

Table 7-2 Problem Statements in Declarative Form

Research focus	Problem statement
Effect of relaxation on anxiety and dyspnea in patients with COPD	This study investigates the effect of relaxation on anxiety and dyspnea in patients with COPD (Gift, Moore, & Soeken, 1992).
Comparison of anxiety symptomatology among Cambodian refugee adolescents before and after resettlement in the United States	Anxiety symptomatology in Cambodian refugee adolescents before and after settlement in the United States had not been compared (Mueck and Sasse, 1992).
Effect of heart transplantation on psychosocial functioning	The study examines the effect of heart transplantation on psychosocial functioning (Bohachick et al., 1992).

Table 7-3 Problem Statements in Interrogative Form

Research focus	Problem statement
Factors that influence adaptation of preadolescents and adolescents with diabetes	What are the influences of age, coping behavior, and self-care on psychological, social, and physiological adaptation in preadolescents and adolescents with insulin-dependent diabetes mellitus (Grey, Cameron & Thurber, 1992)?
Effect of group therapy on cognitive functioning and depression in elderly nursing home residents	What is the effect of group therapy on cognitive functioning and depression in elderly nursing home residents (Abraham, Neundorfer, Currie, 1992)?
Spiritual health, coping responses, and devastating physical illness	What role does spiritual health play in the coping responses of patients to devastating physical illness (Mickley, Soeken, & Belcher, 1992)?

amount of pain. A researcher may also be interested in what other factors can be linked to postoperative pain. It has been discovered that anxiety is associated with pain. Thus anxiety is also a variable, since not all postoperative patients have anxiety or the same amount of anxiety.

When speaking of relationships between variables, the researcher is essentially asking, "Is X related to Y? What is the effect of X on Y? How are X_1 and X_2 related to Y?" The researcher is asking a question about the relationship between one or more **independent variables** and a **dependent variable.** *

An *independent variable,* usually symbolized by X, is the variable that has the presumed effect on the dependent variable. In experimental research studies the independent variable is manipulated by the researcher. For example, a nurse may study how different intramuscular injection sites affect the patient's perception of pain. The researcher may manipulate the independent variable—intramuscular injection sites—by using different injection sites (see Chapter 9). In nonexperimental research the independent variable is not manipulated and is assumed to have occurred naturally before or during the study. For example, the researcher may be studying the relationship between the level of anxiety and the perception of pain. The independent variable—the level of anxiety—is not manipulated; it is just presumed to occur and is observed and measured as it naturally happens (see Chapter 10).

The *dependent variable,* represented by Y, is often referred to as the *consequence* or the presumed effect that varies with a change in the independent variable. The dependent variable is not manipulated. It is observed and assumed to vary with

---

*In cases where there are more than one independent or dependent variables, subscripts are used to indicate the number of variables under consideration.

changes in the independent variable. Predictions are made *from* the independent variable *to* the dependent variable. It is the dependent variable that the researcher is interested in understanding, explaining, or predicting. For example, it might be assumed that the perception of pain—the dependent variable—will vary with changes in the level of anxiety—the independent variable. In this case we are trying to explain the perception of pain in relation to the level of anxiety.

Although variability in the dependent variable is assumed to depend on changes in the independent variable, that does not imply that there is a causal relationship between X and Y or that changes in variable X cause variable Y to change. Let us look at an example where nurses' attitudes toward rape were studied. The researcher discovered that older nurses had a more negative attitude about rape than had younger nurses. The researcher did not conclude that the nurses' attitudes toward rape were *caused* by their age, but at the same time it is apparent that there is a directional relationship between age and attitudes about rape. That is, as the nurses' age increases, their attitudes about rape become more negative. This example highlights the fact that causal relationships are not necessarily implied by the independent and dependent variables. Rather, only a relational statement with possible directionality is proposed.

Although one independent and one dependent variable are used in the examples just given, there is no restriction on the number of variables that can be included in a problem statement. However, remember that problems should not be unnecessarily complex or unwieldy, particularly in beginning research efforts. Problem statements that include more than one independent or dependent variable may be broken down into subproblems that are more concise.

Finally, it should be noted that variables are not inherently independent or dependent. A variable that is classified as independent in one study may be considered dependent in another study. For example, a nurse may review an article about personality factors that are predictive of alcoholism. In this case alcoholism is the dependent variable. When another article about the relationship between alcoholism and marital conflict is reviewed, alcoholism is the independent variable. Whether a variable is independent or dependent is a function of the role it plays in a particular study.

Population

The nature of the **population** being studied needs to be specified in the problem statement. If the scope of the problem has been narrowed to a specific focus and the variables have been clearly identified, the nature of the population will be evident to the reader of a research report. For example, a problem statement that poses the question "Is there a relationship between rooming-in by mothers and preschool childrens' adjustment to hospitalization?" suggests that the population under consideration includes mothers and their hospitalized preschool children. It is also implied that some of the mothers will have had rooming-in, in contrast to other mothers who have not. The researcher or the reader will have an initial idea of the composition of the study population from the outset (see Chapter 12).

Testability

The statement of the research problem must imply that the problem is testable, that is, measurable by either qualitative or quantitative methods. For example, the problem statement "Should nurses work with dying patients?" is incorrectly stated for a variety of reasons; one reason is that it is not testable. It represents a value statement rather than a relational problem statement. A scientific or relational problem must propose a relationship between an independent and a dependent variable and do this in such a way that it indicates that the variables of the relationship can somehow be measured.

Many interesting and important questions are not valid research problems, because they are not amenable to testing.

The question "Should nurses work with dying patients?" could be revised from a philosophical question to a research question that implies **testability**. Two examples of the revised problem statement might be the following:

- Is there a relationship between nurses' attitudes toward dying patients and the quality of nursing care?
- What is the effect of nurses' attitudes about death and dying on empathic communication with terminally ill patients?

These examples illustrate the relationship between the variables, identify the independent and dependent variables, and imply the testability of the research problem.

Now that the elements of the formal problem statement have been presented in greater detail, this information can be integrated by formulating a formal problem statement about stress in families caring for an elderly relative. Earlier in this chapter the following unrefined problem statement is formulated: *What is the effect of stress and social support on the psychological distress of family caregivers of the elderly?* This problem statement was originally derived from a general area of interest—family relationships with elderly relatives. The topic was more specifically defined by delineating a particular problem area—stress in families caring for an elderly relative. The problem crystallized still further after a preliminary literature review and emerged in the unrefined form just given. With the four criteria inherent in a satisfactory problem statement, it is now possible to propose a refined or formal problem statement, that is, one that specifically states the problem in question form and specifies the relationship of the key variables in the study, the population being studied, and the empirical testability of the problem. Congruent with these four criteria, the following problem statement can then be formulated: *What is the effect of perceived caregiver stress and social support on the psychological distress of family caregivers of the elderly?* (Baillie, Norbeck, and Barnes, 1988). Table 7-4 identifies the components of this problem statement as they relate to and are congruent with the four problem statement criteria. Table 7-5 (pp. 172-173) provides additional examples of unrefined problem statements. As column 1 in Table 7-5 is reviewed, the reader will notice that the problem statements suggest the use of different types of research designs; that is, experimental, quasiexperimental, or nonexperimental (see Chapters 9 and 10). It is important to note that the process of moving from the general topic area to the unrefined problem and finally to the refined, formal problem statement often includes several intermediate steps.

Table 7-4   Components of the Problem Statement and Related Criteria

Variables	Population	Testability
Independent variable: perceived caregiver stress and social support	Family caregivers of the elderly	Differential effect of perceived stress and social support on psychological distress
Dependent variable: psychological distress		

STATEMENT OF THE PROBLEM IN PUBLISHED RESEARCH

A formal problem statement is not included in most current research articles. They are, however, used in developing grant proposals, theses, and dissertations when greater detail is required. Used more commonly in articles is a statement of purpose, usually stated in the introductory paragraph or at the beginning or end of the literature review section. As such, it is important for the research consumer to be clear about the difference between these two components of the research process.

As stated earlier, a research problem is a question for which an answer is to be described, explained, or predicted. It is a brief statement of relationships among variables. Downs (1993) highlights the importance of including a statement of the relationships the researcher hopes to establish. Presenting this information early in the article facilitates getting to the point of the study by allowing the researcher, now an author, to produce a diagram of the points that need to be addressed in the article.

The problem is associated with the purpose of the study, but it is not identical. The purpose of the study encompasses the aims or goals the investigator hopes to achieve with the research, not the problem to be solved. For example, a nurse working with rehabilitation patients with bladder dysfunction may be disturbed by the high incidence of urinary tract infections. The nurse may propose the following research question: "What is the optimum frequency of changing urinary drainage bags in patients with bladder dysfunction to reduce the incidence of urinary tract infection?" If this nurse were to design a study, its purpose might be to determine the differential effect of a 1-week and 4-week urinary drainage bag change schedule on the incidence of urinary tract infections in patients with bladder dysfunction. Other examples of purpose statements are illustrated in the box on p. 174.

DEVELOPING THE RESEARCH HYPOTHESES

Like the problem statement, hypotheses are often not stated explicitly in a research article. The evaluator often will find that the hypotheses are embedded in the data analysis, results, or discussion section of the research report. It is then up to the reader to discern the nature of the hypotheses being tested. In light of that stylistic reality, it is important to be acquainted with the components of hypotheses, how they are developed, and the standards for writing and evaluating them.

Table 7-5   Examples of Unrefined and Refined Problem Statements

Type of design suggested	Unrefined problem statement	Critique of problem statement	Refined problem statement
Nonexperimental	Do nurses' attitudes toward patients with acquired immunodeficiency syndrome (AIDS) affect the emotional state of the patient?	Not a concise relational statement Testability is not implied	Is there a relationship between the nurse's attitude toward AIDS and the emotional status of the AIDS patient?
Experimental	How does patient teaching influence maternal anxiety in primiparas after discharge?	Not a concise relational statement Testability is not implied Variables are not clear	The relationship between the amount of patient teaching and the level of anxiety in primiparas after discharge is unknown.
Experimental	To measure the effectiveness of health teaching for hospitalized patients with heart disease in a group setting	Population is not specific	Research has not demonstrated the effect of postcardiac group health teaching on health behaviors of patients after an initial myocardial infarction.
Experimental	Does positioning have an effect on the occurrence of contractures in unconscious patients?	Variables are not clear	What is the difference in the incidence of contractures in comatose patients in relation to frequency of repositioning?

Table 7-5   Examples of Unrefined and Refined Problem Statements—cont'd

Type of design suggested	Unrefined problem statement	Critique of problem statement	Refined problem statement
Experimental	How do nurse-run patient education classes impact on the housebound elderly?	Not a relational statement Population is not defined adequately Variables are not clearly defined Testability is not implied	The effect of nurse-administered educational rehabilitation programs on independent behavior on chronically ill housebound elderly patients has not been determined.
Nonexperimental	How does the mother's feeling of well-being during pregnancy affect how the mother attaches to her baby?	Not a concise relational statement Variables are not clearly defined	Is there a relationship between the physical symptoms of pregnancy and maternal-fetal attachment in primigravidas?
Experimental	Do patients need sexual counseling after hysterectomies?	Not a relational statement Variables are not clearly specified Testability is not implied	Research has not demonstrated the relationship between sexual counseling and the postoperative adjustment of patients after hysterectomy.
Nonexperimental	How does assertiveness relate to feelings of power in depressed women?	Not a clear relational statement Variables are not clearly specified	Is there a relationship between assertive behavior and the perception of power in depressed women?

EXAMPLES OF PURPOSE STATEMENTS

- The purpose of this research was to describe and analyze the relationships among health-promoting behavior, perceived current health status, and life satisfaction in older black adults (Foster, 1992).
- The aim of the present study was to evaluate quantitatively the effect of heart transplantation on psychosocial functioning by comparing postransplanation with pretransplantation functioning (Bohachick et al., 1992).
- The purpose of this study was to evaluate three subcutaneous injection sites for low-dose heparin therapy (Stewart Fahs & Kinney, 1991).
- The goal of this study was to determine (1) the incidence of IV site symptoms and (2) the patient and practice factors associated with the development of these symptoms (Bostrum-Ezrati, Dibble, and Rizzuto, 1990).

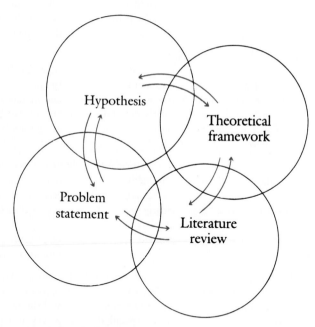

Fig. 7-2 Interrelationships of problem statement, literature review, theoretical framework, and hypothesis.

Hypotheses flow from the problem statement, literature review, and theoretical framework. Fig. 7-2 illustrates this flow. A *hypothesis* is an assumptive statement about the relationship between two or more variables that suggests an answer to the research question. A hypothesis converts the question posed by the research problem into a declarative statement that predicts an expected outcome.

Each hypothesis represents a unit or subset of the research problem. For example, a research problem might pose the question "Is there a relationship among health-promoting behaviors, perceived current health status, and life satisfaction in older black adults?" (Foster et al. 1992). This problem can be broken down into the following two subproblems:

1. Is there a relationship between perceived current health status and life satisfaction in older black adults?
2. Is there a relationship between health-promoting behaviors and life satisfaction in older black adults?

A hypothesis can then be generated for each unit of the research problem—the subproblems. The hypotheses of the research problem already mentioned might be stated in the following way:

Hypothesis 1:   There is a positive relationship between current health status and life satisfaction in older black adults.

Hypothesis 2:   There is a positive relationship between health-promoting activities and life satisfaction in older black adults.

The critiquer of a research report will want to evaluate whether the hypotheses of the study represent subsets of the main research problem as illustrated by the examples just given.

Hypotheses are formulated before the study is actually conducted, because they provide direction for the collection, analysis, and interpretation of data. Hypotheses have three purposes. Their first purpose is to provide a bridge between theory and reality, and in this sense they unify the two domains. Their second purpose is to be powerful tools for the advancement of knowledge, since they enable the researcher to objectively enter new areas of discovery. Their third purpose is to provide direction for any research endeavor by tentatively identifying the anticipated outcome.

Characteristics

Nurses who are conducting research or nurses critiquing published research studies must have a working knowledge about what constitutes a "good" hypothesis. Such knowledge will enable them to have a standard for evaluating their own work or the work of others. The following discussion about the characteristics of hypotheses will present criteria to be used when formulating or evaluating a hypothesis.

The Relationship Statement

The first characteristic of a hypothesis is that it is a declarative statement that identifies the predicted relationship between two or more variables. This implies that there is a systematic relationship between an independent variable and a dependent variable. The direction of the predicted relationship is also specified in this statement. Phrases such as *greater than; less than; positively, negatively,* or *curvilinearly related* (∪- or ∩-shaped); and *difference in* connote the directionality that is proposed in the hypothesis. It is not unusual for a beginning researcher to generate a hypothesis that omits one of the two required variables or that fails to make a prediction about the direction of the relationship. For example, the prediction "Children who have asthma will respond favorably to postural drainage treatments" is not a scientifically acceptable hypothesis. There is only one stated variable, postural drainage treatments. This statement could be revised to make it an acceptable hypothesis containing two variables and a relational statement. The hypothesis would then be stated in the following manner: "Asthmatic children who receive postural drainage treatments (independent variable) will have less bronchial congestion (dependent variable) than have children with no postural drainage." In this hypothesis the two variables are explicitly identified, and the relational aspect of the prediction is contained in the phrase *less than*.

The nature of the relationship, either causal or associative, is also implied by the hypothesis. A causal relationship is one where the researcher is able to predict that the independent variable (X) causes a change in the dependent variable (Y). It is rare in research that one is in a firm enough position to take a definitive stand about a cause-and-effect relationship. For example, a researcher might hypothesize that relaxation training would have a significant effect on the physical and psychological health status of patients who have suffered myocardial infarction. However, it would be difficult for a researcher to predict a strong cause-and-effect relationship because of the multiple intervening variables, such as age, medication, and life-style changes, that might also influence the subject's health status. Variables are more commonly related in noncausal ways; that is, the variables are systematically related but in an associative way. This means that there is a systematic movement in the associated values of the two phenomena. For example, there is strong evidence that asbestos exposure is related to lung cancer. It is tempting to state that there is a causal relationship between asbestos exposure and lung cancer. However, do not overlook the fact that not all of those exposed to asbestos will have lung cancer and not all of those who have lung cancer have had asbestos exposure. Consequently, it would be scientifically unsound to take a position advocating the presence of a causal relationship between these two variables. Rather, one can say only that there is an associative relationship between the variables of asbestos exposure and lung cancer, a relationship where there is a strong systematic association between the two phenomena.

Testability

The second characteristic of a hypothesis is its *testability*. This means that the variables of the study must lend themselves to observation, measurement, and analysis. The hypothesis is either supported or not supported after the data have been collected and analyzed. The predicted outcome proposed by the hypothesis will or will not be congruent with the actual outcome when the hypothesis is tested. Hypotheses advance scientific knowledge by confirming or refuting theories.

Hypotheses may fail to meet the criteria of testability because the researcher has not made a prediction about the anticipated outcome, the variables are not ob-

Table 7-6   Hypotheses That Fail to Meet the Criteria of Testability

Problematic hypothesis	Problematic issue	Revised hypothesis
Anxiety is related to learning.	No predictive statement about the relationship is made; therefore the relationship is not verifiable.	Anxiety is curvilinearly (∩-shaped) related to problem-solving behavior.
Patients who receive preoperative instruction have less postoperative stress than have patients who do not.	The "postoperative stress" variable must be specifically defined so that it is observable or measurable, or the relationship is not testable.	Patients who attend preoperative education classes have less postoperative emotional stress than have patients who do not.
Small-group teaching will be better than individualized teaching for dietary compliance in diabetic patients.	"Better than" is a value-laden phrase that is not objective. Moral and ethical questions containing words such as *should, ought, better than,* and *bad for* are not scientifically testable.	Dietary compliance will be greater in diabetic patients receiving diet instruction in small groups than in diabetic patients receiving individualized diet instruction.
Widowhood causes psychosocial health dysfunction.	Causal relationships are proposed without sufficient evidence. The "widowhood" variable must be specifically defined or the relationship is not testable.	Widowed persons with greater resource strength will have less psychosocial health dysfunction than those with lower resource strength.

servable or measurable, or the hypothesis is couched in terms that are value laden. Table 7-6 illustrates each of these points and provides a remedy for each problem.

Theory Base

A sound hypothesis is consistent with an existing body of theory and research findings. Regardless of whether a hypothesis is arrived at inductively or deductively (see Chapter 2), it must be based on a sound scientific rationale. The reader of a research report should be able to identify the flow of ideas from the problem statement to the literature review, to the theoretical framework, and through the hypotheses (see Chapters 5 and 6). Table 7-7 illustrates this process in relation to the problem statement "What is the effect of perceived caregiver stress and social support on the psychological distress of family caregivers of the elderly?" (Baillie, Norbeck, and Barnes, 1988). In this example it is clear that there is an explicitly developed, relevant body of scientific data that provides the theoretical grounding for the study.

Table 7-7 Flow of Data Among Problem Statement, Literature Review, Theoretical Framework, and Hypothesis

Problem statement	Literature review	Theoretical framework	Hypotheses

What is the effect of perceived caregiver stress and social support on the psychological distress of family caregivers of the elderly?	1. Studies related to emotional, physical, social, and financial difficulties associated with caregiving.
	2. Studies related to antecedent variables related to caregiver strain, burden, or diminished well-being.
	  a. Demographic characteristics of caregivers and of elders.
	  b. Characteristics of the caregiving situation.
	  c. Variables that mediate the effect of caregiver stress, such as social support.
		1. Family caregivers of the elderly experience significant amounts of stress in relation to the burden of caregiving.
		2. The amount of stress varies and is proposed to be a perceptual phenomenon.
		3. Social support is proposed to be a variable that mediates (buffers) stress.
		4. Social support is positively related to coping effectiveness and reduced burden.
		5. Satisfaction with social support is correlated with mental health.
			1. Perceived stress of caregiving will be positively related to psychological distress.
			2. Satisfaction with social support will be negatively related to psychological distress.
			3. Social support will have a buffering effect on the relationship between perceived caregiver stress and psychological distress.

The hypotheses, as stated in Table 7-7, are logically derived from the theoretical framework. However, the research consumer should be cautioned about assuming that the theory-hypothesis link will always be present. In an analysis of nursing practice research from 1977 to 1986, Moody, Wilson, Smyth, Tittle, and Vancott (1988) indicate that only slightly more than half (51%) of the 720 articles analyzed had some type of theoretical perspective.

Wording the Hypothesis

As you read the scientific literature and become more familiar with it, you will observe that there are a variety of ways to word a hypothesis. Regardless of the specific format used to state the hypothesis, the statement should be worded in clear, simple, and concise terms. If this criterion is met, the reader will understand the following:

1. The variables of the hypothesis
2. The population being studied
3. The predicted outcome of the hypothesis

This information may be further clarified by the definition section of a study (see Chapters 6 and 15).

Directional Versus Nondirectional Hypotheses

Hypotheses can be formulated directionally or nondirectionally. A **directional hypothesis** is one that specifies the expected direction of the relationship between the independent and dependent variables. The reader of a directional hypothesis may observe that the existence of a relationship is proposed, as well as the nature or direction of that relationship. The following is an example of a directional hypothesis: "There will be a positive relationship between perceived social support by the mother and attachment between that mother and her infant with Down syndrome" (Quinn, 1991). Examples of directional hypotheses can also be found in Table 7-8 in examples 2 to 5, 7, and 8.

In contrast, whereas a **nondirectional hypothesis** indicates the existence of a relationship between the variables, it does not specify the anticipated direction of the relationship. The following is an example of a nondirectional hypothesis: "There is a relationship between perception of self-competence and breast-feeding behavior." Other examples of nondirectional hypotheses are illustrated in Table 7-8, examples 1 and 6.

Nurses who are learning to critique research studies should be aware that both the directional and nondirectional forms of hypotheses statements are acceptable. However, they should also be aware that there are definite pros and cons pertaining to each one.

Proponents of the nondirectional hypothesis state that this format is more objective and impartial than the directional hypothesis. It is argued that the directional hypothesis is potentially biased, because the researcher, in stating an anticipated outcome, has demonstrated a commitment to a particular position.

On the other side of the coin, proponents of the directional hypothesis argue that researchers naturally have hunches, guesses, or expectations concerning the outcome of their research. It was the hunch, the curiosity, or the guess that initially led them to speculate about the problem. The literature review and the conceptual framework provided the theoretical foundation for deriving the hypothesis. Consequently it might be said that a deductive hypothesis derived from a theory will almost always be directional (see Chapter 2). The theory will provide a critical rationale for proposing that relationships between variables will have particular outcomes. When there is no theory or related research to draw on for rationale or when findings in previous research studies are ambivalent, the nondirectional hypothesis may be appropriate.

In summary, the evaluator of a hypothesis should know that there are several

Table 7-8   Examples of How Hypotheses Are Worded

Hypothesis	Variables*		Type of hypothesis	Type of design suggested
1. There will be a relationship between self-concept and suicidal behavior.	IV:	Self-concept	Nondirectional research	Nonexperimental
	DV:	Suicidal behavior		
2. Synchrony of maternal and newborn sleep rhythms will be negatively related to postpartum blues.	IV:	Synchrony of maternal and newborn sleep rhythms	Directional research	Nonexperimental
	DV:	Postpartum blues		
3. Structured preoperative education is more effective than structured postoperative education in reducing the patient's perception of pain.	IV:	Preoperative education	Directional research	Experimental
	IV:	Postoperative education		
	DV:	Perception of pain		
4. The incidence and degree of severity of subject discomfort will be less after administration of medications by the Z-track intramuscular injection technique than after administration of medications by the standard intramuscular injection technique.	IV:	Z-track intramuscular injection technique	Directional research	Experimental
	IV:	Standard intramuscular injection technique		
	DV:	Subject discomfort		
5. Progressive relaxation will be more effective in reducing indices of physiological arousal than hypnotic relaxation or self-relaxation in patients undergoing cardiac rehabilitation.	IV:	Progressive relaxation	Directional research	Experimental
	IV:	Hypnotic relaxation		
	IV:	Self-relaxation		
	DV:	Physiological arousal indices		
6. There will be a relationship between years of nursing experience and attitude toward patients with human immunodeficiency virus (HIV) disease.	IV:	Years of experience	Nondirectional research	Nonexperimental
	DV:	Attitude toward HIV patients		
7. There will be a positive relationship between trust and self-disclosure in marital relationships.	IV:	Trust	Directional research	Nonexperimental
	DV:	Self-disclosure		
8. There will be a greater decrease in posttest state anxiety scores in subjects treated with noncontact therapeutic touch than in subjects treated with contact therapeutic touch.	IV:	Noncontact therapeutic touch	Directional research	Experimental
	IV:	Contact therapeutic touch		
	DV:	State anxiety		

*IV, Independent variable; DV, dependent variable.

advantages to directional hypotheses, making them appropriate for use in most studies. The advantages are the following:

1. Directional hypotheses indicate to the reader that a theory base has been used to derive the hypotheses and that the phenomena under investigation have been critically thought about and interrelated. The reader should realize that nondirectional hypotheses may also be deduced from a theory base. However, because of the exploratory nature of many studies utilizing nondirectional hypotheses, the theory base may be less well developed.

2. They provide the reader with a specific theoretical frame of reference within which the study is being conducted.

3. They suggest to the reader that the researcher is not sitting on a theoretical fence, and as a result, the analyses of data can be accomplished in a statistically more sensitive way.

The important point for the critiquer to keep in mind regarding directionality of the hypotheses is whether there is a sound rationale for the choice the researcher has proposed regarding directionality.

Statistical Versus Research Hypotheses

Readers of research reports may observe that a hypothesis is further categorized as either a research or a statistical hypothesis. A **research hypothesis,** also known as a scientific hypothesis, consists of a statement about the expected relationship between the variables. A research hypothesis indicates what the outcome of the study is expected to be. A research hypothesis is also either directional or nondirectional. If the researcher obtains statistically significant findings for a research hypothesis, the hypothesis is supported. For example, in a study on AIDS-related risk factors, medical diagnosis, do-not-resuscitate (DNR) orders, and aggressiveness of nursing care, Forrester (1990) hypothesized, "Nurses' attitudes toward aggressiveness of nursing care are reduced in the presence of DNR orders." The author reports statistically significant findings for this hypothesis, and as such, the hypothesis is supported; that is, the predicted outcome was supported by the study findings. The examples in Table 7-8 represent research hypotheses.

A **statistical hypothesis,** also known as a *null hypothesis,* states that there is no relationship between the independent and dependent variables. The examples in Table 7-9 illustrate statistical hypotheses. If in the data analysis a statistically significant relationship emerges between the variables at a specified level of significance, the null hypothesis is rejected. Rejection of the statistical hypothesis is equivalent to acceptance of the research hypothesis. For example, in a study that compared the abdomen, thigh, and arm as sites for subcutaneous sodium heparin injections (Stewart Fahs and Kinney, 1991), a null or statistical hypothesis stated "there is no difference in effectiveness of low-dose heparin therapy, as measured by activated partial thromboplastin time (aPPT), when administered in three different subcutaneous sites." Stewart Fahs and Kinney reported that there was no significant difference in the aPTT time among the three sites of abdomen, thigh, and arm for the subcutaneous low-dose heparin injections. Because the difference between the sites was not

Table 7-9   Examples of Statistical Hypotheses

Hypothesis	Variables*		Type of hypothesis	Type of design suggested
Oxygen inhalation by nasal canula of up to 6 L/min does not affect oral temperature measurement taken with an electronic thermometer.	*IV:* *DV:*	Oxygen inhalation by nasal cannula Oral temperature	Statistical	Experimental
The incidence of pregnancy in adolescent girls attending birth control education classes will not differ from that of girls who do not attend birth control education classes.	*IV:* *DV:*	Birth control education classes Adolescent pregnancy	Statistical	Experimental

*IV, Independent variable; *DV,* dependent variable.

greater than that expected by chance, the null hypothesis was accepted (see Chapter 17).

Some researchers refer to the null hypothesis as a statistical contrivance that obscures a straightforward prediction of the outcome. Others state that it is more exact and conservative statistically, and that failure to reject the null hypothesis implies that there is insufficient evidence to support the idea of a real difference. Readers of research reports will note that, in general, when hypotheses are stated, research hypotheses are more commonly used than statistical hypotheses. It is more desirable to state the researcher's expectation. The reader then has a more precise idea of the proposed outcome. In any study that involves statistical analysis, the underlying null hypothesis is usually assumed without being explicitly stated.

THE RELATIONSHIP BETWEEN THE HYPOTHESIS AND THE RESEARCH DESIGN

Regardless of whether the researcher uses a statistical or a research hypothesis, there is a suggested relationship between the hypothesis and the research design of the study. The type of design, experimental or nonexperimental (see Chapters 9 and 10), will influence the wording of the hypothesis. For example, when an experi-

mental design is utilized, the research consumer would expect to see hypotheses that reflect relationship statements:
- X_1 is more effective than X_2 on Y.
- The effect of X_1 on Y is greater than that of X_2 on Y.
- The incidence of Y will not differ in subjects receiving X_1 and X_2 treatments.
- The incidence of Y will be greater in subjects after X_1 than after X_2.

Such hypotheses indicate that an experimental treatment will be used and that two groups of subjects, experimental and control groups, are being used to test whether the difference predicted by the hypothesis actually exists.

In contrast, hypotheses related to nonexperimental designs reflect associative relationship statements:
- X will be negatively related to Y.
- There will be a positive relationship between X and Y.

Additional examples of this concept are illustrated in Table 7-8.

RESEARCH QUESTIONS

Research studies do not always contain hypotheses. As you become more familiar with the scientific literature, you will notice that exploratory studies usually do not have hypotheses. This is particularly common where there is a dearth of literature or related research studies in a particular area that is of interest to the researcher. The researcher, interested in finding out more about a particular phenomenon, may engage in a fact-finding or relationship-finding mission guided only by research questions. The outcome of the exploratory study may be that data about the phenomenon are amassed and the researcher is then able to formulate hypotheses for a future study. This is sometimes called a *hypothesis-generating study.*

A study by Mass, Buckwalter, and Kelley (1991) examining family members' perceptions of care of institutionalized patients with Alzheimer's disease illustrates how an investigation designed to generate relationships and fill a gap in the literature was guided by research questions. Research questions included the following:
- What are family members' perceptions of care?
- Is there a change in family perceptions of care over time?
- What aspects of care do family members find most and least satisfying?

Because there has been little research on family members after their relatives have been institutionalized, research questions rather than hypotheses are appropriate for this baseline phase of a study to evaluate a special Alzheimer's unit in a long-term care facility. The findings of the study highlighted the need for future hypothesis-testing studies to identify interventions to facilitate family participation as partners in the care of institutionalized relatives with Alzheimer's disease.

Qualitative research studies also are guided by research questions rather than hypotheses. The descriptive findings of qualitative studies also can provide the basis for future hypothesis-testing studies. "What is the lived experience of caring from the perspective of patients and nurses?" is an example of a research question, from a qualitative study by Miller, Haber, and Byrne (1992) that examined perceptions of caring in an acute care hospital setting.

As you can see, research questions tend to be more general than the research problems discussed in the problem statement section of this chapter. However, the more specific they are, the more they provide direction for the study.

In other studies, research questions are formulated in addition to hypotheses to answer questions related to ancillary data. Such questions do not directly pertain to the proposed outcomes of the hypotheses. Rather, they may provide additional and sometimes serendipitous findings that are enriching to the study and valuable in providing direction for further study. Sometimes they are the kernels of new or future hypotheses.

The evaluator of a research study needs to determine whether it was appropriate to formulate a research question rather than a hypothesis, given the nature and context of the study.

CRITIQUING THE RESEARCH PROBLEM AND HYPOTHESES

The care that a researcher takes when developing the problem statement and hypotheses is often representative of the overall conceptualization and design of the study. A methodically formulated research problem provides the basis for hypothesis development. In an empirical research study, the remainder of a study revolves around testing the hypotheses or, in some cases, the research questions. This may be a time-consuming, sometimes frustrating endeavor for the researcher. But in the final analysis, the product, as evaluated by the consumer, most often has been worth the struggle.

Because this text focuses on the nurse as a critical consumer of research, the following sections will pertain primarily to the evaluation of research problems and hypotheses in research reports.

Critiquing the Problem Statement

The box on p. 185 provides several criteria for evaluating this initial phase of the research process—the problem statement. Because the problem statement represents the basis for the study, it is usually introduced at the beginning of the research report. This will indicate the focus and direction of the study to the readers, who will then be in a position to evaluate whether the rest of the study logically flows from its base. Often the author will begin by identifying the general problem area that originally represented some vague discontent or question regarding an unsolved problem. The experiential and scientific background that led to the specific problem is briefly summarized, and the purpose, aim, or goal of the study is identified. Finally, the problem statement and any related subproblems are proposed in those instances that they are used in an article.

The purpose of the introductory summary of the experiential and scientific background is to provide the reader with a glimpse of how the author critically thought about the research problem's development. The introduction to the research problem places the study within an appropriate conceptual framework and sets the stage for the unfolding of the study. This introductory section should also

⬛ CRITIQUING CRITERIA ⬛

THE PROBLEM STATEMENT

1. Was the problem statement introduced promptly?
2. Is the problem stated clearly and unambiguously in declarative or question form?
3. Does the problem statement express a relationship between two or more variables or at least between an independent and a dependent variable, implying empirical testability?
4. Does the problem statement specify the nature of the population being studied?
5. Has the problem been substantiated with adequate experiential and scientific background material?
6. Has the problem been placed within the context of an appropriate theoretical framework?
7. Has the significance of the problem been identified?
8. Have pragmatic issues, such as feasibility, been addressed?
9. Have the purpose, aims, or goals of the study been identified?

THE HYPOTHESES

1. Does the hypothesis directly relate to the research problem?
2. Is the hypothesis concisely stated in a declarative form?
3. Are the independent and dependent variables identified in the statement of the hypothesis?
4. Are the variables measurable or potentially measurable?
5. Is each of the hypotheses specific to one relationship so that each hypothesis can be either supported or not supported?
6. Is the hypothesis stated in such a way that it is testable?
7. Is the hypothesis stated objectively, without value-laden words?
8. Is the direction of the relationship in each hypothesis clearly stated?
9. Is each hypothesis consistent with the literature review?
10. Is the theoretical rationale for the hypothesis explicit?
11. Are research questions appropriately used (i.e., exploratory or qualitative study or in relation to ancillary data analyses)?

include the significance of the study, that is, why the investigator is doing the study. For example, the significance may be to solve a problem encountered in the clinical area and thereby improve patient care; or to resolve a conflict in the literature regarding a clinical issue; or to provide data supporting an innovative form of nursing intervention that is cost-effective.

In reality, the reader often will find that the research problem is not clearly stated at the conclusion of this section. In fact, in some cases it is only hinted at, and the reader is challenged to identify the problem under consideration. In other cases the problem statement is embedded in the introductory text or purpose statement. To some extent, this will depend on the style of the particular journal. Nevertheless the evaluator must remember that the main problem statement should be clearly delineated in the introductory section even if the subproblems are not.

The reader looks for the presence of four key elements that are described and illustrated in an earlier section of this chapter. They are the following:
1. Is the problem stated clearly and unambiguously?
2. Does the problem statement express a relationship between two or more variables, or at least between an independent and dependent variable?
3. Does the problem statement specify the nature of the population being studied?
4. Does the problem statement imply the possibility of empirical testing?

The reader will use these four elements as criteria for judging the soundness of a stated research problem. It is likely that if the problem is unclear in terms of the variables, the population, and the implications for testability, the remainder of the study is going to falter. For example, a research study contained introductory material on anxiety in general, anxiety as it relates to the perioperative period, and the potentially beneficial influence of nursing care in relation to anxiety reduction. The author concluded that the purpose of the study was to determine whether selected measures of patient anxiety could be shown to differ when different approaches to nursing care were used during the perioperative period. The author did not go on to state the research problems. A restatement of the problem in question form might be the following:

$$(Y_1) \qquad\qquad (X_1, X_2, X_3)$$

What is the difference in patient anxiety level in relation to different approaches to nursing care during the perioperative period?

If this process is clarified at the outset of a research study, all that follows in terms of the design can be logically developed. The reader will have a clear idea of what the report should convey and can evaluate knowledgeably the material that follows.

Critiquing the Hypothesis

As illustrated in the box on p. 185, several criteria for critiquing the hypotheses should be used as a standard for evaluating the strengths and weaknesses of the hypotheses in a research report.

1. When reading a research study the research consumer may find the hypotheses clearly delineated in a separate hypothesis section of the research article, after the literature review or theoretical framework section(s). In many cases the hy-

potheses are not explicitly stated and are only implied in the Results or Discussion section of the article. As such, they must be inferred by the critiquer from the purpose statement and the type of analysis used. The reader must be cognizant of this variation and not think that because hypotheses do not appear at the beginning of the article, they do not exist in the particular study. Even when hypotheses are stated at the beginning of an article, they are reexamined in the Results or Discussion section as the findings are presented and discussed. However, the critiquer should expect hypotheses to be appropriately reflected depending on the purpose of the study and format of the article.

2. The hypothesis should directly answer the research problem that was posed at the beginning of the report. Its placement in the research report logically follows the problem statement, the literature review, and the theoretical framework, because the hypothesis should reflect the culmination and expression of this conceptual process. It should be consistent with both the literature review and the theoretical framework. The flow of this process, as depicted in Table 7-8, should be explicit and apparent to the reader. If this criterion is met, the reader feels reasonably assured that the basis for the hypothesis is theoretically sound.

3. As the reader examines the actual hypothesis, several aspects of the statement should be critically appraised. First, the hypothesis should consist of a declarative statement that objectively and succinctly expresses the relationship between an independent and a dependent variable. In wording a complex versus a simple hypothesis, there may be more than one independent *and* dependent variable.

Second, the reader can expect that there may be more than one hypothesis, particularly if there is more than one independent and dependent variable. This will be a function of the type of study being conducted.

Third, the variables of the hypothesis should be understandable to the reader. Often in the interest of formulating a succinct hypothesis statement, the complete meaning of the variables is not apparent. The critiquer must realize that sometimes a researcher is caught between the "devil and the deep blue sea" on that issue. It may be a choice between having a complete but verbose hypothesis paragraph, or a less complete but concise hypothesis. The solution to this dilemma is for the researcher to have a definition section in the research report. The inclusion of **conceptual definitions** and **operational definitions** (see Chapter 6) provides the complete explication of the variables. The critiquer is then able to examine the hypothesis side by side with the definitions and determine the exact nature of the variables under consideration. An excellent example of this process appears in a research article by Woods, Haberman, and Packard (1993), who hypothesized that

> women reporting more direct disease effect demands will report poorer individual adaptation to the illness
>
> and
>
> women reporting more personal disruption demands will report poorer individual adaptation to the illness.

These are appropriately worded hypotheses. However, it is not completely clear what the variables "direct disease effect demands" and "personal disruption demands" imply. It is only when one examines the definitions of these variables, which are included in the literature review section, that the exact nature of the variables becomes clear to the reader:

- Direct disease effect demands: "the physical and psychosocial experience that people attribute directly to the disease with which they live . . . and may include such symptoms as nausea, fatigue, pain, dyspnea, and weakness" (p. 12)
- Personal disruption demands: "represent challenges to one's sense of integrity, continuity, and normalcy" (p. 12)

The context of the variables is now revealed to the evaluator.

Fourth, although a hypothesis can legitimately be nondirectional, it is preferable to indicate the direction of the relationship between the variables in the hypothesis. The reader will find that when there is a dearth of data available for the literature review—that is, the researcher has chosen to study a relatively undefined area of interest—the nondirectional hypothesis may be appropriate. There simply may not be enough information available to make a sound judgment about the direction of the proposed relationship. All that could be proposed is that there will be a relationship between two variables. Essentially, the critiquer wants to determine the appropriateness of the researcher's choice regarding directionality of the hypothesis.

4. The notion of testability is central to the soundness of a hypothesis. One criterion related to testability is that the hypothesis should be stated in such a way that it can be clearly supported or not supported. Whereas the previous statement is very important to keep in mind, the reader should also understand that ultimately neither theories nor hypotheses are ever proved beyond the shadow of a doubt through hypothesis testing. Researchers who claim that their data have "proved" the validity of their hypothesis should be regarded with grave reservation. The reader should realize that, at best, findings that support a hypothesis are considered tentative. If repeated replication of a study yields the same results, greater confidence can be placed in the conclusions advanced by the researchers. An important thing to remember about testability is that although hypotheses are more likely to be accepted with increasing evidence, they are never ultimately proven.

Another point about testability for the consumer to consider is that the hypothesis should be objectively stated and devoid of any value-laden words. Value-laden hypotheses are not empirically testable. Quantifiable words such as *greater than, less than, decrease, increase,* and *positively, negatively,* and *curvilinearly related* convey the idea of objectivity and testability. The reader should be immediately suspicious of hypothesis that are not stated objectively.

5. The evaluator of a research study should be cognizant of the fact that the way that the proposed relationship of the hypothesis is phrased suggests the type of research design that will be appropriate for the study. For example, if a hypothesis proposes that treatment X_1 will have a greater effect on Y than treatment X_2, an experimental or quasiexperimental design is suggested (see Chapter 9). If a hypothesis proposes that there will be a positive relationship between variables X and Y, a nonexperimental design is suggested (see Chapter 10). A review of Table 7-6 provides you with additional examples of hypotheses and the type of research design

that is suggested by each hypothesis. The reader of a research report should evaluate whether the selected research design is congruent with the hypothesis. This factor has important implications for the remainder of the study in terms of the appropriateness of sample selection, data collection, data analysis, interpretation of findings, and ultimately the conclusions advanced by the researcher.

6. If the research report contains research questions rather than hypotheses, the reader will want to evaluate whether this is appropriate to the study. The criterion for making this decision, as presented earlier in this chapter, is whether the study is of an exploratory or qualitative nature. If it is, then it is appropriate to have research questions rather than hypotheses. Ancillary research questions should be evaluated as to whether they answer additional questions secondary to the hypotheses. Sometimes the substance of an additional research question is more appropriately posed as another hypothesis in that it relates in a major way to the original research problem.

KEY POINTS

- Formulation of the research problem and stating the hypothesis are key preliminary steps in the research process. The care with which they are developed is often representative of the overall conceptualization and design of the study.
- The research problem is refined through a process that proceeds from the identification of a general idea of interest to the definition of a more specific and circumscribed topic.
- A preliminary literature review reveals related factors that appear critical to the research topic of interest and aids in further definition of the research problem.
- The significance of the research problem must be identified in terms of its potential contribution to patients, nurses, the medical community in general, and society. Applicability of the problem for nursing practice, as well as its theoretical relevance, must be established. The findings should also have the potential for formulating or altering nursing practices or policies.
- The feasibility of a research problem must be examined in light of pragmatic considerations such as time; availability of subjects, money, facilities, and equipment; experience of the researcher; and ethical issues.
- The final problem statement consists of a statement about the relationship between two or more variables. It clearly identifies the relationship between the independent and dependent variables; it specifies the nature of the population being studied; and it implies the possibility of empirical testing.
- A hypothesis attempts to answer the question posed by the research problem. When testing the validity of the theoretical framework's assumptions, the hypothesis bridges the theoretical and real worlds.
- A hypothesis is a declarative statement about the relationship between two or more variables that predicts an expected outcome. Characteristics of a hypothesis include a relationship statement, implications regarding testability, and consistency with a defined theory base.
- Hypotheses can be formulated in a directional or a nondirectional manner. Hypotheses can be further categorized as either research or statistical hypotheses.

- Research questions may be used instead of hypotheses in exploratory or qualitative research studies. Research questions may also be formulated in addition to hypotheses to answer questions related to ancillary data.
- The critiquing criteria provide a set of guidelines for evaluating the strengths and weaknesses of the problem statement and hypotheses as they appear in a research report.
- The critiquer assesses the clarity of the problem statement, as well as the related subproblems, the specificity of the population, and the implications for testability.
- The interrelatedness of the problem statement, the literature review, the theoretical framework, and the hypotheses should be apparent.
- The appropriateness of the research design suggested by the problem statement is also evaluated.
- The purpose of the study (that is, why the researcher is doing the study) should be differentiated from the problem statement or the research question to be answered.
- The reader evaluates the wording of the hypothesis in terms of the clarity of the relational statement, the implications for testability, and its congruence with a theory base. The appropriateness of the hypothesis in relation to the type of research design suggested by the design also is examined. The appropriate use of research questions is also evaluated in relation to the type of study conducted.

REFERENCES

Abraham, I.L., Neundorfer, M.M., & Currie, L.J. (1992). Effects of group interventions on cognition and depression in nursing home residents. *Nursing Research, 41*(4), 196-202.

Alligood, M.R. (1991). Testing Rogers' theory of accelerating change: The relationships of creativity, actualization and empathy in persons 18 to 92 years of age. *Western Journal of Nursing Research, 13*(1), 84-96.

Baillie, V., Norbeck, J.S., & Barnes, L.A. (1988). Stress, social support, and psychological distress of family caregivers of the elderly. *Nursing Research, 37*, 217-222.

Bohachick, P., Anton, B.B., Wooldridge, P.J., Kormos, R.L., Armitage, J.M., Hardesty, R.L., & Griffith, B.P. (1992). Psychosocial outcome 6 months after heart transplant surgery: A preliminary report. *Research in Nursing & Health, 15*, 165-173.

Bostrum-Ezrati, J., Dibble, S., & Rizzuto, C. (1990). Intravenous therapy management: Who will develop insertion site symptoms? *Applied Nursing Research, 3*(4), 146-152.

Downs, F. (1993). How to get to the point. *Nursing Research, 42*(1), 3.

Forrester, D.A. (1990). AIDS-related risk factors, medical diagnosis, do-not-resuscitate orders and aggressiveness of nursing care. *Nursing Research, 39*(6), 350-354.

Foster, M.F. (1992). Health promotion and life satisfaction in elderly black adults. *Western Journal of Nursing Research, 14*(4), 444-456.

Gift, A.G., Moore, T., & Soeken, K. (1992). Relaxation to reduce dyspnea and anxiety in COPD patients. *Nursing Research, 41*(4), 242-246.

Goode, C.J., Titler, M., Rakel, B., Ones, D.S., Kleiber, C., Small, S., & Triolo, P.K. (1991). A meta-analysis of effects of heparin flush and saline flush: Quality and cost implications. *Nursing Research, 40*(6), 324-330.

Grey, M., Cameron, M.E., & Thurber, F.W. (1991). Coping and adaptation in children with diabetes. *Nursing Research, 40*(3), 144-149.

Hoskins, C. (1991). Patterns of adjustment among breast cancer patients and partners: Preliminary findings. *Proceedings of the International Nursing Conference on Good Nursing Care.* Finland, 140-154.

Kuhlman, G.J., Wilson, H.S., Hutchinson, S., & Wallhagen, M. (1991). Alzheimer's disease and family care giving: Critical syntheses of the literature and research agenda. *Nursing Research, 40*(6), 331-337.

Mass, M.L., Buckwalter, K.C., & Kelley, L.S. (1991). Family members' perceptions of care of institutionalized patients with Alzheimer's disease. *Applied Nursing Research, 4*(3), 135-138.

Mickley, J.R., Soeken, K., & Belcher, A. (1992). Spiritual well-being, religiousness and hope among women with breast cancer. *Image, 24*(4), 267-272.

Miller, B.K., Haber, J., & Byrne, M. (1992). The experience of caring in the acute care setting: Patient's and nurses' perspectives. In D. Gaut (Ed.), *The presence of caring in nursing* (pp. 137-156). New York: National League for Nursing.

Moody, L.E., Wilson, M.E., Smyth, K., Tittle, M., & Vancott, M.L. (1988). Analysis of a decade of nursing practice research: 1977-1986. *Nursing Research, 37,* 374-379.

Mueck, M.A., & Sasse, L. (1992). Anxiety among Cambodian refugee adolescents in transit and resettlement. *Western Journal of Nursing Research, 14*(3), 267-285.

Quinn, M.M. (1991). Attachment between mothers and their Down Syndrome infants. *Western Journal of Nursing Research, 13*(3), 382-396.

Stewart Fahs, P.S., & Kinney, M.R. (1991). The abdomen, thigh, and arm as sites for subcutaneous sodium heparin injections, *Nursing Research, 40*(4), 204-207.

Woods, N.F., Haberman, M.R., & Packard, N.J. (1993). Demands of illness and individual, dyadic, and family adaptation in chronic illness. *Nursing Research, 15*(1), 10-25.

ADDITIONAL READINGS

Campbell, D.T., & Stanley, J.C. (1963). *Experimental and quasi-experimental designs for research.* Chicago: Rand McNally.

Downs, F.S., & Newman, M.A. (1977). *A source book of nursing research.* Philadelphia: F.A. Davis.

Kerlinger, F.N. (1986). *Foundations of behavioral research.* New York: Holt, Rinehart & Winston.

Newman, M.A. (1979). *Theory development in nursing.* Philadelphia: F.A. Davis.

Van Dalen, D.B. (1979). *Understanding educational research.* New York: McGraw-Hill.

LEARNING OBJECTIVES

After reading this chapter the student should be able to do the following:

- Define research design.
- Identify the purpose of the research design.
- Define control as it affects the research design.
- Compare and contrast the elements that affect control.
- Begin to evaluate what degree of control should be exercised in the design.
- Define internal validity.
- Identify the threats to internal validity.
- Define external validity.
- Identify the conditions that affect external validity.
- Evaluate the design using the critiquing questions.

KEY TERMS

constancy   instrumentation
control   internal validity
control group   maturation
experimental group   mortality
external validity   randomization
extraneous variable   reactivity
history   selection bias
homogeneity   testing

The word *design* implies the organization of elements into a masterful work of art. In the world of art and fashion, design conjures up images of processes and techniques that are used to express a total concept. When an individual creates, process and form are employed. The form, process, and degree of adherence to structure depend on the aims of the creator. The same can be said of the research process. The research process and the development of a research design need not be a sterile procedure but one where the researcher develops a masterful work within the limits of a problem and the related theoretical basis. The framework that the researcher creates is the design. When reading a study the research consumer should be able to recognize that the problem statement, purpose, literature review, theoretical framework, and hypothesis all interrelate with, complement, and assist in the operationalization of the design (Fig. 8-1).

Nursing is concerned with a variety of structures that require varying degrees of process and form, such as the administration of holistic and quality patient care, staff organization, student education, and continuing education. When patient care is administered, the nursing process based on assessment, planning, intervention, and evaluation is utilized. Before these four steps can be accomplished, a certain level of knowledge is required. This knowledge is derived from theory, practice, and experience. Validation of these areas is derived from research. To understand and utilize research it is necessary to have knowledge of the process and an equally important in-depth knowledge of the content of the subject area being studied. Previous chapters stress the importance of theory and subject matter knowledge. How a researcher structures, implements, or designs an investigation affects the results of a research project.

For the consumer to understand the implications of research and to utilize research, the central issues in the design of a research project should be understood. This chapter provides an overview of the meaning, purpose, and importance of the

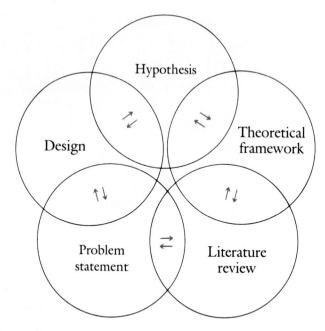

Fig. 8-1   Interrelationships of design, problem statement, literature review, theoretical framework, and hypothesis.

research design in quantitative research, and Chapters 9 and 10 present specific types of designs. Chapter 11 focuses the consumer on the meaning, purpose, and specific types of qualitative designs.

PURPOSE OF RESEARCH DESIGN

The purpose of the research design is to provide the scheme for answering specific research questions. The design in quantitative research then becomes the vehicle for hypothesis testing. The principles of scientific inquiry are utilized to answer research questions. Therefore the design involves a plan, structure, and strategy. These three concepts of design guide a researcher in writing the hypothesis, during the operationalization or the carrying out of the project, and in the analysis and evaluation of the data. The overall purpose of the research design is twofold: to aid in the solution of research questions and to maintain control. All research attempts to answer questions. The design is coupled with the methods and procedures, and together they are the mechanisms for finding solutions to research questions. Control is defined as the measures that the researcher uses to hold the conditions of the investigation uniform. In this way the researcher avoids possible impingement of bias on the dependent variable that may affect the outcome.

A research example that demonstrates how the design can aid in the solution of a research question and maintain control is the landmark study by Brooten et al. (1986; Appendix A). The purpose of the study was to examine whether it is safe and economical to discharge infants of very low birth weight (<1500 g) early if they meet certain conditions. To maintain control the investigators randomly assigned infants to one of two groups. To be included in the study the infants in the control group had to be clinically well and feeding well and had to have had no routine home follow-up care. To maintain further control, the infants in the early discharge group were discharged before they weighed 2200 g. They had to be clinically well, fed by nipple every 4 hours, able to be maintained in an open crib in room air, and have no evidence of serious apnea or bradycardia. The mother or primary caretaker had to demonstrate satisfactory caretaking skills, and the home environment needed to be adequate. By establishing these specific criteria of safety and subject eligibility and by maintaining control, the researchers were able to say what type of infant would benefit most from the early discharge program and extend this outcome study with further research in this and other clinical areas. A variety of considerations, including the type of design chosen, affect the accomplishment of this end. These considerations include objectivity in the conceptualization of the problem, accuracy, economy, control of the experiment, **internal validity,** and **external validity.** There are statistical principles behind the many forms of control, but a clear conceptual understanding is of greater importance for the research consumer.

OBJECTIVITY IN THE PROBLEM CONCEPTUALIZATION

Objectivity in the conceptualization of the problem is derived from a review of the literature and development of a theoretical framework (Fig. 8-1). Using the literature the researcher assesses the depth and breadth of available knowledge concerning the problem. The literature review and theoretical framework should demonstrate to the reader that the researcher reviewed the literature with a critical and objective eye (see Chapters 5 and 6), since this affects the type of design chosen. For example, a question regarding the relationship of the length of a breast-feeding teaching program may suggest either a correlational or an experimental design (see Chapters 9 and 10), whereas a question regarding the physical changes in a woman's body during pregnancy and maternal perception of the unborn child may suggest a survey or case study (see Chapters 10 and 11). Therefore it should be obvious how the researcher's literature review reflects the following:
- When the problem was studied
- What aspects of the problem were studied
- Where it was investigated
- By whom it was investigated
- The gaps or inconsistencies in the literature

The review that incorporates these aspects allows the consumer to judge the objectivity of the problem area and therefore whether the design chosen matches the problem.

ACCURACY

Accuracy in determining the appropriate design is also accomplished through the theoretical framework and review of the literature (see Chapters 5 and 6). Accuracy means that all aspects of a study systematically and logically follow from the identified problem statement. The beginning researcher is wise to answer a question involving few variables that will not require the use of sophisticated designs. The simplicity of a research project does not render it useless or of a lesser value for practice. Although the project is simple, the researcher should not forego accuracy. The consumer should feel that the investigator used the appropriate type of design to answer the research question with a minimum of contamination. The issues of contamination or control are discussed later in this chapter. Also, many clinical problems have not yet been researched. Therefore a preliminary or pilot study would be a wise approach. The key is the accuracy, validity, and objectivity used by the researcher in attempting to answer the question. Accordingly, the researcher should read various levels of studies and assess how and if the criteria for each step of the research process were followed. Research consumers will find that many nursing journals publish not only sophisticated clinical research projects but smaller clinical studies that can also be applied to practice.

An example of a preliminary study that investigated a clinical problem was conducted by Schaaf Treas and Latinis-Bridges (1992). Concerned that a more effective method of maintaining intravenous catheters in neonates is needed to reduce the identified risk factors (phlebitis, septicemia, extravasation) associated with the insertion of intravenous catheters, they conducted a two-group randomized prospective study. The study was designed to test the efficacy of continuous, low-dose heparin infusion as compared with saline solution in prolonging peripheral venous catheter patency in neonates. This study looked at an important clinical problem—prolonging intravenous patency without increasing other potentially harmful risks in neonates in an intensive care unit. The researchers acknowledge the limitations of the study and the need for future research. Although this study does not give nurses all the data to decide whether the use of continuous low-dose heparin has positive results, it does provide a beginning outcome study of the question and suggests avenues of future inquiry for nursing research and utilization in nursing practice.

FEASIBILITY

When critiquing the research design the evaluator also needs to be aware of the pragmatic consideration of feasibility. Sometimes the reality of this does not truly sink in until one does research. It is important to consider feasibility when reviewing a study, including availability of the subjects, timing of the research, time required for the subjects to participate, cost in terms of such items as reproduction, and analysis of the data (Table 8-1). These pragmatic considerations are not presented as a step in the research process as are the theoretical framework or methods, but they do affect every step of the process. As such, the reader of a study should consider these when assessing the investigation. The student researcher may or may not have monies or accessible services. When critiquing an investigation, note the credentials of the author and whether the investigation was part of a student project or part of a fully funded grant project. If the project was a student project, the standards of critiquing are applied more liberally than for a prepared, experienced re-

Table 8-1 Pragmatic Considerations in Determining Feasibility
of a Research Problem

Factor	Pragmatic consideration
Time	The research problem must be one that can be studied within a realistic period of time. All researchers have deadlines for completion of a project. It is essential that the scope of the problem be circumscribed enough to provide ample time for the completion of the entire project. Research studies generally take longer than anticipated to complete.
Subject availability	The researcher needs to determine whether a sufficient number of eligible subjects will be available and willing to participate in the study. If one has a captive audience, like students in a classroom, it may be relatively easy to enlist their cooperation. When a study involves the subjects' independent time and effort, they may be unwilling to participate when there is no apparent reward for doing so. Other potential subjects may have fears about harm or confidentiality and may be suspicious of the research process in general. Subjects with unusual characteristics are often difficult to locate. In general, people are fairly cooperative about participating, but a researcher must consider needing a larger subject pool than will actually participate. At times, when reading a research report the researcher may note how the procedures were liberalized or the number of subjects was altered. This was probably a result of some unforeseen pragmatic consideration.
Facility and equipment availability	All research projects require some kind of equipment. The equipment may be questionnaires, telephones, stationery, stamps, technical equipment, or other apparatus. Most research projects require the availability of some kind of facility. The facility may be a hospital site for data collection or laboratory space or a computer center for data analyses.
Money	Research projects require some expenditure of money. Before embarking on a study the researcher probably itemized the expenses and projected the total cost of the project. This provides a clear picture of the budgetary needs for items like books, stationery, postage, printing, technical equipment, telephone and computer charges, and salaries. These expenses can range from about $100 for a small-scale student project to hundreds of thousands of dollars for a large-scale federally funded project.
Researcher experience	The selection of the research problem should be based on the nurse's realm of experience and interest. It is much easier to develop a research study related to a topic that is either theoretically or experientially familiar. Selecting a problem that is of interest to the researcher is essential for maintaining enthusiasm when the project has its inevitable ups and downs.
Ethics	Research problems that place unethical demands on subjects may not be feasible for study. Researchers must take ethical considerations seriously. The consideration of ethics may affect the choice between an experimental design and a nonexperimental design.

searcher or clinician. Finally, the pragmatic issues raised affect the scope and breadth of an investigation and therefore its generalizability.

CONTROL

A researcher attempts to use a design to maximize the degree of control over the tested variables. **Control** involves holding the conditions of the study constant and establishing specific sampling criteria as described by Brooten et al. (1986). An efficient design can maximize results, decrease errors, and control preexisting or impaired conditions that may affect outcome. To maximize efforts the researcher should maximize control. To accomplish these tasks the research design and methods should demonstrate the researcher's efforts at control.

For example, in a study by Foxall et al. (1992) the researchers attempted to examine the level of loneliness in low-vision adults and to determine whether there was a relationship between loneliness and selected personal and social support factors. Their research questions were the following:

- What is the level of loneliness experienced by low-vision adults?
- Are there relationships between loneliness and personal factors of self-consciousness and optimism of low-vision adults?
- What is the degree to which loneliness can be predicted in low-vision adults by the addition of such factors as social support network and social support satisfaction?

To test these questions and apply control the investigators included in their study individuals who were being seen at two low-vision clinics, and who met the following criteria: (1) had visual acuity of 20/70 or less (up to but not including total blindness) in the better eye, with correction verified by the patient's medical record; (2) had low vision for at least 1 year before data collection, verified by the medical record; (3) were age 19 years or older; (4) were able to speak, hear, and understand English; and (5) lived within a 60-mile radius. Patients who were totally blind (congenital or acquired) were excluded from the study because totally blind persons, compared with persons with low vision, have differences in experiences with blindness. This study illustrates how investigators in one study planned their design to apply controls. Control is important in all designs. When various research designs are critiqued, the issue of control is always raised but with varying levels of flexibility. The issues discussed here will become clearer as you review the various types of designs discussed in later chapters (see Chapters 9 to 11). Control is accomplished by ruling out *extraneous variables* that compete with the independent variables as an explanation for a study's outcome. The **extraneous variable** is one that interferes with the operations of the phenomena being studied, such as age and gender, or as in the previous example of blindness. Means of controlling extraneous variables include the following:

- Use of a homogeneous sample
- Use of consistent data collection procedures
- Manipulation of the independent variable
- Randomization

The following example illustrates and defines these concepts:

> An investigator might be interested in how a new stop-smoking program (independent variable) affects smoking behavior (dependent variable). The independent variable is assumed to affect the outcome or dependent variable. But the investigator needs to be relatively sure that the decrease in smoking is truly related to the stop-smoking program rather than to some other variable, such as motivation. The design of the research study alone does not inherently provide control. But an appropriately designed study with the necessary controls built in can increase the researcher's ability to answer this research question.

Homogeneous Sampling

In the stop-smoking study, extraneous variables may affect the dependent variable. The characteristics of a study's subjects are common extraneous variables. Age, gender, and even newer smoking laws may affect the outcome in the stop-smoking example. These variables may therefore affect the outcome, even though they are extraneous or outside of the study's design. As a control for these and other similar problems, the researcher's subjects should demonstrate **homogeneity** or similarity with respect to the extraneous variables relevant to the particular study (see Chapter 12). These extraneous variables are not fixed but need to be reviewed and decided on, based on the specific problem and its theoretical base. By using a sample of homogeneous subjects, the researcher has used a straightforward step of control.

For example, Jones and Heermann (1992) designed a longitudinal study to explore the relationship of maternal employment to the division of infant caregiving and whether infant characteristics predicted maternal and paternal caregiving during the infant's first year. To assure themselves of a homogenous sample of normal infants, the researchers selected from mothers who had uncomplicated pregnancies and deliveries that resulted in full-term infants with Apgar scores greater than 7 at 5 minutes. Families with planned cesarean deliveries were included. All parents were living together. This control step limits the *generalizability* or the application of the outcomes to other populations when analyzing and discussing the outcomes (see Chapter 18). Results can then be generalized only to a similar population of individuals. You may say that this is limiting. This is not necessarily so because no treatment or program may be applicable to all populations and the consumer or user of research findings needs to take the differences in populations into consideration. It is better to have a "clean" study that can be used to make generalizations about a specific population than a "messy" one that can be used to generalize little or nothing.

If the researcher feels that one of the extraneous variables is important, it may be included in the design. In the smoking example, if individuals are working in an area where smoking is not allowed and this is considered to be important, the researcher could build it into the design and set up a control for it. This can be done by comparing two different work areas—one where smoking is allowed and one where it is not. The important concept to keep in mind is that before the data are collected, the researcher should have identified, planned for, or controlled the important extraneous variables.

Constancy in Data Collection

Another basic, yet critical, component of control is **constancy** in data collection conditions or procedures. *Constancy* refers to the notion that the data collection procedures should reflect to the consumer a cookbook-like recipe of how the researcher controlled the conditions of the study. This means that environmental conditions, timing of data collection, data collection instruments, and data collection procedures used to gain the data are the same for each subject (see Chapter 12). An example of a well-controlled clinical study was done by Caruso et al. (1992). This study was performed to test the effects of four cooling blanket temperatures for time to cool, afterfall (the amount of body temperature fall after removal of cooling blanket), shivering, and self-perceived discomfort among patients receiving antipyretic therapy. To control conditions, the same hypothermia equipment and the same type of hypothermia blanket were used for all subjects. The actual blanket temperature was measured by a Pharmaseal disposable skin surface probe taped to the bottom hypothermia blanket in three places. All equipment was tested before use, and a research assistant remained with the subject during the entire treatment/observation period of the study. Patients were given acetaminophen 650 mg by mouth or rectally. Data were collected from each subject in the same manner and under the same conditions. This type of control aided the researcher's ability to draw conclusions, discuss, and cite the need for further research in this area. For the consumer it demonstrates a clear, consistent, and specific means of data collection. Another method of ensuring constancy of data collection methods is training the data collectors similarly.

Not all of the problems nurses wish to research are amenable to laboratory study. Studies set in clinical settings also need constancy of data collection procedures to demonstrate to the consumer the efforts taken to address the concept of control.

Manipulation of Independent Variable

A third and very effective means of control is manipulation of the independent variable. This refers to administration of a program, treatment, or intervention to only one group within the study but not to the other subjects in the study. The first group is known as the **experimental group,** and the other group is known as the **control group.** In a *control group* the phenomena under study are held at a constant or comparison level. For example, suppose a researcher wants to study the level of infection rates between a new type of surgical dressing and an old type. The older method represents the control group and the new method the experimental group. Experimental designs use manipulation. Nonexperimental designs do not manipulate the independent variable. This does not decrease the usefulness of a nonexperimental design, but the use of a control group in an experimental design is related to the level of the problem and, again, its theoretical framework. But if the problem is amenable to a design that incorporates manipulation of the independent variable, it can increase the theoretical and statistical power of the researcher to draw generalizable results; that is, if all of the other considerations of control are equally addressed (see Chapters 9 and 10). Again the reader should be cautioned that the lack of manipulation of the independent variable does not mean a weaker study. The level of the problem, the amount of theoretical work, and the research that has preceded a project all affect the researcher's choice of a design.

Randomization

Researchers may also choose other forms of control, such as randomization. Randomization is employed when the required number of subjects from the population are obtained in such a manner that each subject in a population has an equal chance of being selected. Randomization eliminates bias, aids in the attainment of a representative sample, and can be employed in various designs (see Chapters 9 and 12). Rice, Mullin, and Jarosz (1992) (see Chapter 19) used one method of randomization when assigning coronary bypass graft patients to preadmission self-instruction or to postadmission instruction by the nurse.

Randomization can also be done with paper-and-pencil–type instruments. By randomly ordering items on the instruments the investigator can assess if there is a difference in response that can be related to the order of the items. This may be especially important in longitudinal studies where bias from giving the same instrument to the same subjects on a number of occasions can be a problem (see Chapters 10 and 15).

QUANTITATIVE CONTROL AND FLEXIBILITY

The same level of control cannot be exercised in all types of designs. The various types of quantitative designs that are introduced to you in Chapters 9 and 10 will fully illuminate the issues that are introduced in this chapter. At times, when a researcher wants to explore a new area where little or no literature on the concept exists, the researcher will probably use an exploratory design. In this type of study the researcher is interested in describing or categorizing a phenomenon in a group of individuals. Rubin's (1967a and 1967b) early work on the development of maternal tasks during pregnancy is an example of exploratory research. In this research she attempted to categorize conceptually the various maternal tasks of pregnancy. Rubin interviewed women throughout their pregnancies and from these extensive interviews developed a framework of the maternal tasks of pregnancy. In critiquing this type of study the issue of control should be applied in a highly flexible manner because of the preliminary nature of the work.

If it is determined from a review of a study that the researcher intended to conduct a correlational study, or a study that looks at the relationship between or among the variables, then the issue of control takes on more importance (see Chapter 10). Control needs to be strictly exercised as much as is possible. At this intermediate level of design it should be clear to the reviewer that the researcher considered the extraneous variables that may have accounted for the outcomes.

All aspects of control are strictly applied to studies that utilize an experimental design (see Chapter 9). The reviewer should be able to locate in the research report how the researcher met the following criteria: the conditions of the research were constant throughout the study, assignment of subjects was random, and an experimental group and control group were utilized. The Caruso et al. (1992) is an example where all the aspects of control were addressed. Because of the control exercised by Caruso et al. the reviewer can see that the highest level of control was applied and that extraneous variables were thereby considered.

INTERNAL AND EXTERNAL VALIDITY

When reading research one needs to feel that the results of a study are valid, based on precision, and faithful to what the researcher wanted to measure. For a study to form the basis of further research, practice, and theory development, it must be believable and dependable. There are two important criteria for evaluating the credibility and dependability of the results: internal validity and external validity. Threats to validity are listed in the box below and discussion follows.

Internal Validity

Internal validity asks whether the independent variable really made the difference. This requires the researcher to rule out other factors or threats as rival explanations of the relationship between the variables. Thus internal validity refers to the causal relationship. Internal validity problems revolve around the issues of control. Six major threats to internal validity are defined by Campbell and Stanley (1966). These should be considered by the researcher in planning the design and by the consumer before implementing results in practice. The consumer of research should note that the threats to internal validity are most clearly applicable to experimental

---

THREATS TO VALIDITY

INTERNAL VALIDITY	EXTERNAL VALIDITY
History	Effects of selection
Maturation	Reactive effects
Testing	Effects of testing
Instrumentation	
Mortality	
Selection bias	

designs, but attention to those factors that can compromise outcomes should be considered to some degree in all quantitative designs. If these threats are not considered, they could negate the results of the research. How these threats may affect specific designs are addressed in Chapters 9 and 10. The following are threats to internal validity:

1. *History.* In addition to the independent variables, another specific event that may have an effect on the dependent variable may occur either inside or outside the experimental setting; this is referred to as **history.** For example, in a study of the effects of a breast-feeding teaching program on the length of time of breast-feeding, an event such as government-sponsored advertisements on the importance of breast-feeding featured on television and newspapers may be a threat of history.

   Another example may be that of an investigator testing the effects of a breast self-examination teaching program on the incidence of monthly breast self-examination. Concurrently, a famous movie star or news correspondent is diagnosed as having breast cancer. The occurrence of this diagnosis in a public figure engenders a great deal of media and press attention. In the course of the media attention medical experts are interviewed widely and the importance of a breast self-examination is supported. If the researcher finds that breast self-examination behavior is improved, the researcher may not be able to conclude that the change in behavior is the result of the teaching program, but it may be the result of the diagnosis given the known figure and the resultant media coverage.

2. *Maturation.* **Maturation** refers to the developmental, biological, or psychological processes that operate within an individual as a function of time and are external to the events of the investigation. For example, suppose one wishes to evaluate the effect of a specific teaching method on baccalaureate students' achievements on a skills test. The investigator would record the students' abilities before and after the teaching method. Between the pretest and posttest the students have grown older and wiser. This growth or change is unrelated to the investigation and may explain differences between the two testing periods rather than the experimental treatment.

   An example of a study in which the investigator took precautions to avoid the threat of maturation is a study conducted by Vessey (1988). Vessey wanted to investigate the relationship between two methods of teaching on children's knowledge of their internal bodies. Posttests of student learning were conducted 1 week after the teaching sessions were completed. This relatively short interval is a strength of the study and allows the investigator to conclude that the results were the result of the design of the study and not maturation in a population of children who are learning new skills rapidly.

3. *Testing.* **Testing** is defined as the effect of taking a pretest on the score of a posttest. The effect of taking a pretest may sensitize an individual and

improve the score of the posttest. Individuals generally score higher when they take a test a second time regardless of the treatment. The differences between posttest and pretest scores may not be a result of the independent variable but rather of the experience gained through testing.

An example in which testing might have accounted for the results was in a study conducted by Lowe and Roberts (1988). The study was designed to assess the congruence between in-labor report and postpartum recall of labor pain. The researchers measured labor pain on several occasions during labor and the postpartum period. They found that postpartal women tended to devalue early labor pain and inflate transitional labor pain when compared with their in-labor report. The researchers noted in discussing the results that the bias of repeated measures of pain during labor may have primed the postpartum responses and that the practice of reporting pain repeatedly on the same instrument during labor and memory may have influenced the results.

4. *Instrumentation.* **Instrumentation** threats are changes in the measurement of the variables or observational techniques that may account for changes in the obtained measurement. The use by Caruso, et al. (1992) of the same equipment and procedures for each data collection session is an example of how researchers took steps to avoid the threat of instrumentation.

Noll et al. (1992) used the Oximetix Opticath pulmonary artery catheter, Oximeter 3 computer, and printer (Abbott Critical Care Division, Mountain View, Calif.) to determine fluctuation in mixed oxygen saturation in critically ill medical patients during a period of rest. To control for accuracy and reliability the researchers validated the calibrations before data collection. The researchers noted also that the values of $S\bar{v}o_2$ obtained by the Opticath correlate well ($r = 0.90$ to 0.97) with values obtained directly by a co-oximeter at a range of 24% to 85%. This is also an example of how researchers took steps to prevent the threat of instrumentation.

Another example that fits into this area is related to techniques of observation. If an investigator has several raters collecting observational data, all must be trained in a similar manner. If they are not similarly trained, a lack of consistency may occur in their ratings and therefore a major threat to internal validity will occur.

At times, even though the researcher takes steps to prevent problems of instrumentation, this threat may still occur. In a study by Lipson (1992) that was designed to explore the health and adjustment processes of Iranian immigrants, the investigator in English and two highly qualified research assistants who were Iranian and therefore spoke Persian conducted semistructured interviews with the study's subjects. The researcher notes that when the interviewer was an Iranian, the subjects described the political nature of their immigration responses to the Iranian interviewers, but when the interviewer was an American, they did not. This is a problem that would be difficult to prevent because of the delicate political circumstances of the immigrants. When a critiquer finds such a threat, it needs to be evaluated within the total context of the study, as, in fact, the researcher did in this study.

5. *Mortality.* **Mortality** is the loss of study subjects from the first data collection point (pretest) to the second data collection point (posttest). If the subjects who remain in the study are not similar to those who dropped out, the results could be affected. In a study of how a media campaign affects the incidence of breast-feeding, if most dropouts were non-breast-feeding women, the perception given could be that exposure to the media campaign increased the number of breast-feeding women, whereas it was the effect of experimental mortality that led to the observed results.

   An example of a study in which the results may be due to subject mortality is that conducted by Murphy (1988). The study used a longitudinal design to examine the relationships between stress, potential mediators of stress, and health outcomes. Data were collected over a 3-year period. A number of the subjects did not participate at the second data collection. Murphy (1988), citing her earlier research (1986) and that of Green et al. (1983), believed that possibly some of the bereaved who continued in the study were worse off than those who dropped out. She further concluded that it is unknown whether individuals who are more distressed participate in follow-up studies more frequently than those who perceive their emotional distress to be lower.

6. *Selection bias.* If the precautions are not used to gain a representative sample, a bias of subjects could result from the way the subjects were chosen. Selection effects are a problem in studies where the individuals themselves decide whether to participate in a study. Suppose an investigator wishes to assess if a new breast-feeding program contributes to the incidence and length of time of breast-feeding. If the new program is offered to all, chances are that women who are more motivated to learn about breast-feeding will take part in the program. Assessment of the effectiveness of the program is problematic, because the investigator cannot be sure if the new program increased the number of women who breast-fed their newborns or if only highly motivated individuals joined the program. The way to avoid **selection bias** in this case is to randomly assign the women to either the new teaching method group or a control group that receives a different type of instruction. In the study by Rice et al. (1992) (see Chapter 19) the researchers controlled for selection bias by establishing selection criteria and by randomly assigning subjects to one of the two study groups.

External Validity

External validity deals with possible problems of generalizability of the investigation's findings to additional populations and to other environmental conditions. External validity questions under what conditions and with what types of subjects the same results can be expected to occur. The goal of the researcher is to select a design that maximizes both internal and external validity. This is not always possible; if this is the case, the researcher needs to establish a minimum requirement of meeting the criteria of external validity.

The factors that may affect external validity are related to selection of subjects, study conditions, and type of observations. These factors are termed *effects of selection, reactive effects,* and *effects of testing.* The reader will notice the similarity in names of the factors of selection and testing and those of threats to internal validity. When considering them as internal threats the consumer assesses them as they relate to the independent and dependent variables *within* the study, and when assessing them as external threats the consumer considers them in terms of the generalizability or utility *outside the study* to other populations and settings. Problems of internal validity are generally easier to control. Generalizability issues are more difficult to deal with, because it means that the researcher is assuming that other populations are similar or like the one being tested. A discussion of each of the external validity factors follows:

1. *Effect of selection.* Selection refers to the generalizability of the results to other populations. An example of the effects of selection occurs when the researcher is not able to attain the ideal sample population. At times, numbers of available subjects may be low or not accessible to the researcher; the researcher may then need to choose a nonprobability method of sampling over a probability method (see Chapter 12). Therefore the type of sampling method utilized and how subjects are assigned to research conditions affect the generalizability to other groups or the external validity.

   An example of the effect of selection is depicted with the following example. Aaronson (1989) studied perceived and received social support during pregnancy and its effects on health behavior practices during pregnancy. The sample consisted of 529 pregnant women who responded to questionnaires and a phone interview. In the discussion of the findings she cautions the reader to avoid extensive generalizations. The investigator states:

   One note of caution, however, is necessary. The findings and conclusions of this study are based on a relatively homogenous, middle class sample. Consequently, the findings cannot be generalizations to more ethnically diverse groups or to those of lower socioeconomic status. (p. 7)

   Her remarks caution the reader to avoid extensive generalizations and let the reader know that there are limitations of the findings.

2. *Reactive effects.* **Reactivity** is defined as the subjects' responses to being studied. Subjects may respond to the investigator not because of the study procedures, but merely as an independent response to being studied. This is also known as the *Hawthorne effect,* named after Western Electric Corporation's Hawthorne plant, where a study of working conditions was conducted. The researchers developed several different working condi-

tions (i.e., turning up the lights, piping in music loudly or softly, and changing work hours). They found that no matter what was done, the workers' productivity increased. They concluded that production increased as a result of the workers' knowing that they were being studied rather than because of the experimental conditions.

A threat to internal validity can also be a threat to external validity. An example where this can be found is in the study conducted by Lipson (1992) on the Iranian immigrants. The reaction to the interviewer in this study is a threat to instrumentation and is also reactivity and therefore a threat to the generalizability of the findings. It should be noted that even though this is a problem in the study, the study is excellent because it points out the many needs of immigrants related to health care and to health care providers. Chrisman (1992), a reviewer, noted that the immigrants demonstrated concerns related to language and different ways of expression and explanation of their illnesses. Yet Chrisman notes also that more research in this area is needed so that nurses can better assess and intervene with immigrants. This study is a good example of how a researcher took an interest in a relevant nursing care issue, developed a study to explore the issue, dealt with the real problems of research in the area, and is also developing an area of specialty that will ultimately improve patient care.

3. *Effect of testing.* Administration of a pretest in an experimental situation affects the generalizability of the findings to other populations. Just as pretesting affects the posttest results within a study, pretesting affects the posttest results and generalizability outside the study. For example, suppose a researcher wants to conduct a study with the aim of changing attitudes toward acquired immunodeficiency syndrome (AIDS). To accomplish this an education program on the risk factors for AIDS is incorporated. To test whether the education program changes attitudes toward AIDS, tests are given before and after the teaching intervention. The pretest on attitudes allows the subjects to examine their attitudes regarding AIDS. The subjects' responses on follow-up testing may be different from those of individuals who were given the education program and who did not see the pretest. Therefore when a study is conducted and a pretest is given, it may prime the subjects and affect their ability to generalize to other situations.

There are other threats to external validity that depend on the type of design and methods of sampling utilized by the researcher, but these are beyond the scope of this textbook. Detailed coverage of the issues related to internal and external validity is offered by Campbell and Stanley (1966).

CRITIQUING THE RESEARCH DESIGN

Criteria for critiquing the research design are given in the box on p. 208.

Critiquing the design of a study requires one to first have knowledge of the overall implications that the choice of a particular design may have for the study as a

CRITIQUING CRITERIA

1. Is the type of design employed appropriate?
2. Does the researcher use the various concepts of control that are consistent with the type of design chosen?
3. Does the design used seem to reflect the issues of economy?
4. Does the design used seem to flow from the proposed research problem, theoretical framework, literature review, and hypothesis?
5. What are the threats to internal validity?
6. What are the controls for the threats to internal validity?
7. What are the threats to external validity?
8. What are the controls for the threats to external validity?

whole. The concept of the research design is an all-inclusive one that parallels the concept of the theoretical framework. The research design is similar to the theoretical framework in that it deals with a piece of the research study that affects the whole. For one to knowledgeably critique the design in the light of the entire study, it is important to understand the factors that influence the choice and the implications of the design. In this chapter the meaning, purpose, and importance factors of design choice, as well as the vocabulary that accompanies these factors, have been introduced.

Several criteria for evaluating the design can be drawn from the preceding chapter. One should remember that these criteria are applied differently with various designs. Different application does not mean that the consumer will find a haphazard approach to design. It means that each design has particular criteria that allow the evaluator to classify the design as to type, such as experimental or nonexperimental. These criteria need to be met and addressed in conducting an experiment. The particulars of specific designs are addressed in Chapters 9 and 10. The following discussion pertains primarily to the overall evaluation of a research design.

The research design should reflect that an objective review of the literature and the establishment of a theoretical framework guided the choice of the design. There is no explicit statement regarding this in a research study. A consumer can evaluate this by critiquing the theoretical framework (see Chapter 6) and literature review (see Chapter 5). Is the problem new and not researched extensively? Has a great deal been done on the problem, or is it a new or different way of looking at an old problem? Depending on the level of the problem, certain choices are made by the investigators. Rice et al. (1992) (see Chapter 19) conducted a study to compare the effects of two approaches to teaching postoperative therapeutic exercise (preadmission self-instruction and postadmission instruction by a nurse) to CABG patients on postadmission indicators such as mood state, exercise performance behaviors, teaching time postadmission, analgesia needs, and length of hospitalization. They used theory, their previous research, and others' previous research to design their study and extend the research in this area as objectively and as accurately as possible. The study was intended to build on previous research and fill a gap through replication and extension and to explore the mood of patients, which had not been studied previously.

The consumer should be alert for the means used by investigators to maintain control, such as homogeneity in the sample, consistent data collection procedures, how or if the independent variable was manipulated, and whether randomization was used. As the reader can see in Chapter 9 all of these criteria must be met for an experimental design. As the reader begins to understand the types of designs and levels of research, namely, quasiexperimental and nonexperimental designs such as survey and interrelationship designs, the reader will find that these concepts are applied in varying degrees, or, as in the case of a survey study, the independent variable is not manipulated at all (see Chapter 10). The level of control and its applications presented in Chapters 9 to 10 provide the remaining knowledge to fully critique the aspects of the design in a study.

Once it has been established whether the necessary control or uniformity of conditions has been maintained, the evaluator needs to determine whether the study is believable or valid. The evaluator should ask whether the findings are the result of the variables tested and internally valid or whether there could be another explanation. To assess this aspect the threats to internal validity should be reviewed. If the investigator's study was systematic, was well grounded in theory, and followed the criteria for each of the processes, the reader will probably conclude that the study is internally valid.

In addition, the critical reader needs to know whether a study has external validity or generalizability to other populations or environmental conditions. External validity can be claimed only after internal validity has been established. If the credibility of a study (internal validity) has not been established, a study could not be generalized (external validity) to other populations. Determination of external validity goes hand in hand with the sampling frame (see Chapter 12). If the study is not representative of any one group or phenomena of interest, external validity may be limited or not present at all. The evaluator will find that establishment of internal and external validity needs not only knowledge of the threats to internal and external validity, but also a knowledge of the phenomena being studied. A knowledge of the phenomena being studied allows critical judgments to be made regarding the linkage of theories and variables for testing. The critical reader should find that the design follows from the theoretical framework, literature review, problem statement, and hypotheses. The evaluator should feel, on the basis of clinical knowledge as well as the knowledge of the research process, that the investigators in a study are not comparing apples to oranges.

KEY POINTS

- The purpose of the design is to provide the format of a masterful and creative piece of research. There are many types of designs. No matter which type of design the researcher uses, the purpose always remains the same.
- The consumer of research should be able to locate within the study a sense of the question that the researcher wished to answer. The question should be proposed with a plan or scheme for the accomplishment of the investigation. Depending on the question, the consumer should be able to recognize the steps taken by the investigator to ensure control.
- The choice of the specific design depends on the nature of the problem. To specify the nature of the problem requires that the design reflects the investigator's attempts to maintain objectivity, accuracy, pragmatic considerations, and, most important, control.
- Control not only affects the outcome of a study, but also its future use. The design should also reflect how the investigator attempted to control threats to both internal and external validity. Internal validity needs to be established before external validity can be. Both are considered within the sampling structure.
- No matter which design the researcher chooses, it should be evident to the reader that the choice was based on a thorough examination of the problem within a theoretical framework.
- The design, problem statement, literature review, theoretical framework, and hypothesis should all interrelate to demonstrate a woven pattern.
- The choice of the design is affected by pragmatic issues. At times, two different designs may be equally valid for the same problem.

REFERENCES

Aaronson, L.S. (1989). Perceived and received support: Effects on health behavior during pregnancy. *Nursing Research, 38,* 4-9.

Brooten, D., Kumar, S., Brown, L.P., Butts, P., Finkler, S.A., Bakewell-Sachs, S., Gibbons, A., & Delivoria-Papadopoulos, M. (1986). A randomized clinical trial of early hospital discharge and home follow-up of very-low-birth-weight infants. *The New England Journal of Medicine, 315,* 934-939.

Campbell, D., Stanley, J. (1966). *Experimental and quasi-experimental designs for research.* Chicago: Rand McNally.

Caruso, C.C., Hadley, B.J., Shukla, R., Frame, P., & Khoury, J. (1992). Cooling effects and comfort of four cooling blanket temperatures in humans with fever. *Nursing Research, 41,* 68-72.

Chrisman, N.J. (1992). Review of the health and adjustment of Iranian immigrants [Commentary]. *Western Journal of Nursing Research, 14,* 27-28.

Foxall, M.J., Barron, C.R., Von Dollen, K., Jones, P.A., & Shull, K.A. (1992). Predictors of loneliness in low-vision adults. *Western Journal of Nursing Research, 14,* 86-99.

Green, B.L., Grace, M.C., Lindy, J.D., Titchener, J.L., & Lindy, J.G. (1983). Levels of functional impairment following a civilian disaster: The Beverly Hills Supper Club fire. *Journal of Consulting and Clinical Psychology, 51,* 573-580.

Jones, L.C., & Heermann, J.A. (1992). Parental division of infant care: Contextual influences and infant characteristics. *Nursing Research, 41,* 228-235.

Lipson, J.G. (1992). The health and adjustment of Iranian immigrants. *Western Journal of Nursing Research, 14,* 10-24.

Lowe, N.K., & Roberts, J.E. (1988). The convergence between in-labor report and postpartum recall of parturition pain. *Research in Nursing & Health, 11,* 11-22.

Murphy, S.A. (1986). Stress, coping and mental health outcomes following a natural disaster: Bereaved family members and friends compared. *Death Studies, 10,* 411-429.

Murphy, S.A. (1988). Mental distress and recovery in a high-risk bereavement sample 3 years after untimely death. *Nursing Research, 37,* 30-35.

Noll, M.L., Fountain, R.L., Duncan, C.A., Weaver, L., Osmanski, V.P., & Halfmann, S. (1992). Fluctuation in mixed venous oxygen saturation in critically ill medical patients: A pilot study. *American Journal of Critical Care, 1,* 102-106.

Rice, V.H., Mullin, M.H., & Jarosz, P. (1992). Preadmission self-instruction effects on postadmission and post-operative indicators in CABG patients: Partial replication and extension. *Research in Nursing & Health, 15*(4), 253-259.

Rubin, R. (1967a). Attainment of the maternal role: 1. Processes. *Nursing Research, 16,* 237-245.

Rubin, R. (1967b). Attainment of the maternal role: 2. Models and referents. *Nursing Research, 16,* 342-346.

Schaaf Treas, L., & Latinis-Bridges, B. (1992). Efficacy of heparin in peripheral venous infusion in neonates. *Journal of Obstetric, Gynecologic and Neonatal Nursing, 21*(4), 214-219.

Vessey, J.A. (1988). Comparison of two teaching methods on children's knowledge of their internal bodies. *Nursing Research, 37,* 262-267.

ADDITIONAL READINGS

Cook, T.D., & Campbell, D.T. (1979). *Quasi-experimentation: Design analysis issues for field settings.* Boston: Houghton-Mifflin.

Judd, C.M., & Kenny, D.A. (1981). *Estimating the effects of social interventions.* Cambridge: Cambridge University Press.

Kerlinger, F.N. (1986). *Foundations of behavioral research* (3rd ed.). New York: Holt, Rinehart & Winston.

LEARNING OBJECTIVES

After reading this chapter the student should be able to do the following:

- List the criteria necessary for inferring cause-and-effect relationships.
- Distinguish the differences between experimental and quasiexperimental designs.
- Define internal validity problems associated with experimental and quasiexperimental designs.
- Describe the use of experimental and quasiexperimental designs for evaluation research.
- Critically evaluate the findings of selected studies that test cause-and-effect relationships.

KEY TERMS

after-only design   intervening variable
after-only nonequivalent   manipulation
control group design   nonequivalent control group
antecedent variable   design
control   quasiexperimental design
dependent variable   randomization
evaluation research   Solomon four-group design
experimental design   time series design
independent variable   true experiment

One of the fundamental purposes of scientific research in any profession is to determine cause-and-effect relationships. In nursing, for example, we are concerned with developing effective approaches to maintaining and restoring wellness. Testing such nursing interventions to determine how well they actually work—that is, evaluating the outcomes in terms of efficacy and cost-effectiveness—is accomplished by using experimental and quasiexperimental designs. These designs differ from nonexperimental designs in one important way: the researcher actively brings about the desired effect and does not passively observe behaviors or actions. In other words, the researcher is interested in making something happen, not merely observing customary patient care. Experimental and quasiexperimental studies also are important to consider in relation to research utilization. It is the findings of such studies that provide the validation of clinical practice and rationale for changing specific aspects of practice (see Chapter 3).

Experimental designs are particularly suitable for testing cause-and-effect relationships because they help to eliminate potential alternative explanations for the findings. To infer causality requires that the following three criteria be met: the causal variable and effect variable must be associated with each other, the cause must precede the effect, and the relationship must not be explainable by another variable. When the reader critiques studies that use experimental and quasiexperimental designs, the primary focus will be on the validity of the conclusion that the experimental treatment, or the **independent variable,** caused the desired effect on the outcome, or **dependent variable.** The validity of the conclusion depends on just how well the researcher has controlled the other variables that may explain the relation-

SUMMARY OF EXPERIMENTAL AND QUASIEXPERIMENTAL
RESEARCH DESIGNS

I. EXPERIMENTAL DESIGNS

True experiment (pretest-posttest control group) design
Solomon four-group design
After-only design

II. QUASIEXPERIMENTAL DESIGNS

Nonequivalent control group design
After-only nonequivalent control group design
Time series design

ship studied. Thus the focus of this chapter is to explain how the various types of experimental and quasiexperimental designs control extraneous variables.

It should be made clear, however, that most research in nursing is not experimental. This is because nursing, unlike the physical sciences, is still identifying the content and theory that are the exclusive province of nursing science. In addition, an experimental design requires that all of the relevant variables have been defined so that they can be manipulated and studied. In most problem areas in nursing this requirement has not been met. Therefore nonexperimental designs used in identifying variables and determining their relationship to each other often need to be done before experimental studies are performed.

The purpose of this chapter is to acquaint you with the issues involved in interpreting studies that use **experimental design** and **quasiexperimental design**. The designs discussed are listed in the box above.

THE TRUE EXPERIMENTAL DESIGN

An *experiment* is a scientific investigation that makes observations and collects data according to explicit criteria. True experiments have three identifying properties—randomization, control, and manipulation. These properties allow for other explanations of the phenomenon to be ruled out and thereby provide the strength of the design for testing cause-and-effect relationships.

Random Assignment to Group

Random assignment to group involves the distribution of subjects to either the experimental group or the control group on a purely random basis. That is, each subject has an equal and known probability of being assigned to any group. Random assignment may be done individually or by groups (Conlon & Anderson, 1990; Hauck et al., 1991). Random assignment to groups allows for the elimination of any systematic bias in the groups with respect to attributes that may affect the dependent variable being studied. The procedure for random assignment assumes that any important intervening variables will be equally distributed between the groups and, as discussed in Chapter 8, minimizes variance. Note that random assignment to groups is different from random sampling discussed in Chapter 15.

Control

By **control** we mean the introduction of one or more constants into the experimental situation. Control is acquired by manipulating the causal or independent variable, by randomly assigning subjects to a group, by very carefully preparing experimental protocols, and by using comparison groups. In experimental research the comparison group is the control group, or the group that receives the usual treatment, rather than the innovative experimental one.

Manipulation

We have said that experimental designs are characterized by the researcher "doing something" to at least some of the involved subjects. This "something," or the independent variable, is *manipulated* by giving it to some participants in the study and not to others or by giving different amounts of it to different groups. The independent variable might be a treatment, a teaching plan, or a medication. It is the effect of this **manipulation** that is measured to determine the result of the experimental treatment.

The concepts of control, **randomization,** and manipulation and their application to experimental design are sometimes confusing for students. To see how these properties allow researchers to have confidence in the causal inferences they make by allowing them to rule out other potential explanations, the use of these properties are examined in one report. O'Sullivan and Jacobson (1992) used a clinical randomized experiment to study the effects of a special health care program for adolescent mothers and their infants. Mothers aged 17 years or younger and their infants were randomly assigned to one of two groups after the mothers consented to participate in the study. This means that all of the mothers had an equal chance of being assigned to the control or the experimental group. The use of random assignment to group helps to assure that the two study groups are comparable on preexisting factors that might affect the outcome of interest, such as maternal age, length of prenatal care, and complications of pregnancy. Note that the researcher checks statistically whether the procedure of random assignment did in fact produce groups that are similar.

The two study groups were a routine well-baby care group and a group that received routine care and special services, such as rigorous follow-up care, discussions with the mother about plans to return to school and use of family planning, and extra health teaching. The degree of control exerted over the experimental conditions is illustrated by the detailed description in the report of the special care program. This helps to ensure that all members of the experimental group receive similar treatment. The control group provides a comparison against which the experimental group can be judged.

In this study, the type of well-baby care—routine or the special program—was manipulated. Mothers and infants in the experimental group received the special care program, and those in the control group received routine well-baby care. All of the participants had outcomes measured at 12 and 18 months of infant age.

The use of the experimental design allowed the researchers to rule out many of the potential threats to internal validity of the findings, such as selection, history, and maturation (see Chapter 8). By exerting clear and careful control over the experimental special care program, the investigators were able to make the assertion that the special care program was effective in decreasing repeat pregnancies, increasing the percentage of infants who were fully immunized, and decreasing the use of the emergency room for infant care.

The strength of the true experimental design lies in its ability to help the researcher and the reader to control the effects of any extraneous variables that might constitute threats to internal validity. Such extraneous variables may be either antecedent or intervening. The **antecedent variable** occurs before the study but may affect the dependent variable and confuse the results. Factors such as age, gender, socioeconomic status, and health status might be important antecedent variables in nursing research, because they may affect dependent variables such as recovery time and ability to integrate health care behaviors. Antecedent variables that might affect the dependent variables in the O'Sullivan and Jacobson (1992) study might include mother's health status, drug use, infant gestational age, and socioeconomic status. Random assignment to groups helps to assure that groups will be similar on these variables so that differences in the dependent variable may be attributed to the experimental treatment. It should be noted, however, that the researcher should check and report how the groups actually compared on such variables. The **intervening variable** occurs during the course of the study and is not part of the study, but it affects the dependent variable. An example of an intervening variable that might affect the outcomes of this study (O'Sullivan & Jacobson, 1992) is a change in health care financing to increase prenatal care for pregnant adolescents. Certainly, if care provided to pregnant adolescents changed in any major way while the study was being implemented, the study would be affected.

Types of Experimental Designs

There are several different experimental designs (Campbell & Stanley, 1966). Each is based on the classic design called the **true experiment** diagrammed in Fig. 9-1, *A*. In this figure, you will note that subjects have been assigned randomly to the experimental or the control group. The experimental treatment is given only to those in the experimental group, and the pretests and posttests are those measurements of the dependent variables that are made before and after the experimental treatment is performed. All true experimental designs have subjects randomly assigned to groups, have an experimental treatment introduced to some of the sub-

Comparison of Experimental Designs

A TRUE OR CLASSIC EXPERIMENT

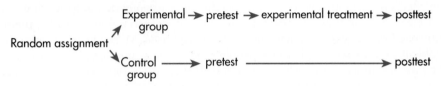

B SOLOMON FOUR-GROUP DESIGN

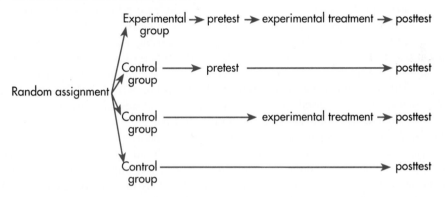

C AFTER-ONLY EXPERIMENTAL DESIGN

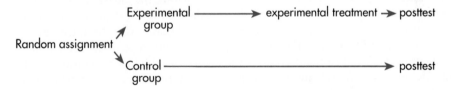

Fig. 9-1   Comparison of experimental designs. **A,** True or classic experiment; **B,** Solomon four-group design; **C,** after-only experimental design.

jects, and have the effects of the treatment observed. Designs vary primarily in the number of observations that are made.

As shown, subjects are randomly assigned to the two groups, experimental and control, so that antecedent variables are controlled. Then pretest measures or observations are made so that the researcher has a baseline for determining the effect of the independent variable. The researcher then introduces the experimental variable to one of the groups and measures the dependent variable again to see whether it has changed. The control group gets no experimental treatment but is also measured later for comparison with the experimental group. The degree of difference between the two groups at the end of the study indicates the confidence the researcher has that a causal link exists between the independent and dependent variables. Because random assignment and the control inherent in this design minimize the effects of many threats to internal validity, it is a strong design for testing cause-and-effect relationships. However, the design is not perfect. Some threats cannot be controlled in true experimental studies (see Chapter 8). Mortality effects are often a problem in such studies, because people tend to drop out of studies that require their participation over an extended period. If there is a difference in the number of people who drop out of the experimental group from that of the control group, a mortality effect might explain the findings. When reading such a work, it is important to examine the sample and the results carefully to see if deaths occurred. Testing is also a problem in these studies, because the researcher is usually giving the same measurement twice, and subjects tend to score better the second time just by learning the test. Researchers can get around this problem in one of two ways: they might use different forms of the same test for the two measurements, or they might use a more complex experimental design called the *Solomon four-group design*.

The **Solomon four-group design,** shown in Fig. 9-1, *B*, has two groups that are identical to those used in the classic experimental design, plus two additional groups, an experimental after-group and a control after-group. As the diagram shows, all four groups have randomly assigned subjects as with experimental studies, but the addition of these last two groups helps to rule out testing threats to internal validity that the before and after groups may experience. Suppose a researcher is interested in the effects of some counseling on chronically ill patients' self-esteem, but just taking a measure of self-esteem may influence how the subjects report themselves. For example, the items might make the subjects think more about how they view themselves so that the next time they fill out the questionnaire, their self-esteem might appear to have improved. In reality, however, their self-esteem may be the same as it was before; it just looks different because they took the test before. The use of this design with the two groups that do not receive the pretest allows for evaluating the effect of the pretest on the posttest in the first two groups. Although this design helps to evaluate the effects of testing, the threat of mortality remains a problem as with the classic experimental design.

Another frequently used experimental design is the **after-only design,** shown in Fig. 9-1, *C*. This design, which is sometimes called the *posttest only control group design,* is composed of two randomly assigned groups, but unlike in the true experimental design, neither group is pretested or measured. Again, the independent variable is introduced to the experimental group and not to the control group. The process of randomly assigning the subjects to groups is assumed to be sufficient to ensure a lack of bias so that the researcher can still determine whether the treatment created significant differences between the two groups. This design is particularly useful when testing effects are expected to be a major problem and the number of available subjects is too limited to use a Solomon four-group design. This was the design used by O'Sullivan and Jacobson (1992) because it was inappropriate to measure infant outcomes before the birth of the infant. Stewart Fahs and Kinney (1991; Appendix A) studied the use of three different injection sites for low-dose heparin therapy. Subjects were randomly assigned to three groups—those who received injections in either the abdomen, arm, or thigh. The authors did measure activated partial thromboplastin time before and after the heparin injections, but the measurements of bruising were taken only at 60 and 72 hours post injection. The assumption is that there is no bruising present before the injection so it is not necessary to measure before the injection. The authors then demonstrated that there were no differences in bruising or efficacy of the heparin by injection site, and a common nursing practice was found to have no scientific support.

Field and Laboratory Experiments

Experiments also can be classified by setting. Field experiments and laboratory experiments share the properties of control, randomization, and manipulation, and they use the same design characteristics, but they are conducted in various environments. Laboratory experiments take place in an artificial setting that is created specifically for the purpose of research. In the laboratory the researcher has almost total control over the features of the environment, such as temperature, humidity, noise level, and subject conditions. On the other hand, field experiments are exactly what the name implies—experiments that take place in some real, existing social setting such as a hospital or clinic where the phenomenon of interest usually occurs. Because most experiments in the nursing literature are field experiments and control is such an important element in the conduction of experiments, it should be obvious that studies conducted in the field are subject to treatment contamination by factors specific to the setting that the researcher cannot control. However, studies conducted in the laboratory are by nature "artificial," because the setting is created for the purpose of research. Thus laboratory experiments, although stronger in relationship to internal validity questions than field work, suffer more from problems with external validity. For example, a subject's behavior in the laboratory may be quite different from the person's behavior in the real world—a dichotomy that presents problems in generalizing findings from the laboratory to the real world. When research reports are read, then, it is important to consider the setting of the experiment and what impact it might have on the findings of the study.

Consider the study of a strategy to promote night sleep in hospitalized children (White et al., 1990). This study could have been done in a sleep laboratory, which would have allowed complete control over the external environment of the study, a variable that might be important in studying sleep. However, there is no guarantee that the results found in a study in a sleep laboratory would be applicable to children in hospital settings, so the study would lose some external validity.

Advantages and Disadvantages of the Experimental Design

As we have said, experimental designs are the most appropriate for testing cause-and-effect relationships. This is because of the design's ability to control the experimental situation. Therefore it offers better corroboration than if the independent variable is manipulated in a certain way, *then* certain consequences can be expected to ensue. Such studies are important because one of nursing's major research priorities is documenting outcomes to provide a basis for changing or supporting current nursing practice (see Chapter 1). In the study by Stewart Fahs and Kinney (1991; Appendix A), the authors were able to conclude from their study that there were no differences in the amount of bruising by site of injection used for subcutaneous heparin injections. Their study helps to debunk nursing practices that are not based in scientific reality. Similarly, in the classic study by Brooten et al. (1986), the authors were able to conclude that infants with low birth weight who were discharged early and received follow-up care from nurse-specialists had outcomes that were as good as or better than those of infants who received routine care. These studies and others like them allow nurses to anticipate in a scientific manner the outcomes of their actions and provide the basis for effective high-quality care strategies.

Still, experimental designs are not the ones most commonly used. There are several reasons that most nursing research studies are not experimental. First, experimentation assumes that all of the relevant variables involved in a phenomenon have been identified. For many areas of nursing research this simply is not the case, and descriptive studies need to be completed before experimental interventions can be applied. Second, there are some significant disadvantages to these designs.

One problem with an experimental design is that many variables important in predicting outcomes of nursing care are not amenable to experimental manipulation. It is well known that health status varies with age and socioeconomic status. No matter how careful a researcher is, no one can assign subjects randomly by age or a certain level of income. In addition, some variables may be technically manipulable, but their nature may preclude actually doing so. For example, the ethics of a researcher who tried to randomly assign groups for a study of the effects of cigarette smoking and asked the experimental group to smoke two packs of cigarettes a day would be seriously questioned. It is also potentially true that such a study would not work, since nonsmokers randomly assigned to the smoking group would be unlikely to comply with the research task.

Another problem with experimental designs is that they may be difficult or impractical to perform in field settings. It may be quite difficult to randomly assign patients on a hospital floor to different groups when they might talk to each other about the different treatments. Experimental procedures may also be disruptive to the usual routine of the setting. If several nurses are involved in administering the experimental program, it may be impossible to ensure that the program is administered in the same way to each subject.

Finally, just being studied may influence the results of a study. This is called the *Hawthorne effect*. As discussed in Chapter 8, this effect means that merely because subjects know that they are subjects in a study, they may answer questions or perform differently.

Because of these problems in carrying out true experiments, researchers frequently turn to another type of research design to evaluate cause-and-effect relationships. Such designs, because they look like experiments but lack some of the control of the true experimental design, are called *quasiexperiments.*

QUASIEXPERIMENTAL DESIGNS

In a quasiexperimental design full experimental control is not possible. *Quasiexperiments* are research designs where the researcher initiates an experimental treatment but where some characteristic of a true experiment is lacking. Control may not be possible because of the nature of the independent variable or the nature of the available subjects. Usually what is lacking in a quasiexperimental design is the element of randomization. In other cases the control group may be missing. However, like experiments, quasiexperiments involve the introduction of an experimental treatment.

Compared with the true experimental design, quasiexperiments are similar in their utilization. Both types of designs are used when the researcher is interested in testing cause-and-effect relationships. However, the basic problem with the quasiexperimental approach is a weakened confidence in making causal assertions. Because of the lack of some controls in the research situation, quasiexperimental designs are subject to contamination by many, if not all, of the threats to internal validity discussed in Chapter 8.

Types of Quasiexperimental Designs

There are many different quasiexperimental designs. We discuss only the ones most commonly used in nursing research. Again we use the notations introduced earlier in the chapter.

Refer back to the true experimental design shown in Fig. 9-1 and compare it with the **nonequivalent control group design** shown in Fig. 9-2, *A.* You should

A <u>NONEQUIVALENT CONTROL GROUP DESIGN</u>

Experimental group ⟶ pretest ⟶ experimental treatment ⟶ posttest

Control group ⟶ pretest ⟶ posttest

B <u>AFTER-ONLY NONEQUIVALENT CONTROL GROUP DESIGN</u>

Experimental group ⟶ experimental treatment ⟶ posttest

Control group ⟶ posttest

C <u>TIME SERIES DESIGN</u>

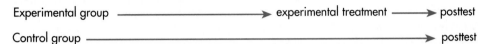

Experimental group ⟶ pretest ⟶ pretest ⟶ experimental treatment ⟶ posttest ⟶ posttest

Control group ⟶ pretest ⟶ pretest ⟶ posttest ⟶ posttest

Fig. 9-2 Comparison of quasiexperimental designs. **A,** Nonequivalent control group design; **B,** after-only nonequivalent control group design; **C,** time series design.

note that this design looks exactly like the true experiment except that subjects are not randomly assigned to groups. Suppose a researcher is interested in the effects of a new diabetes education program on the physical and psychosocial outcome of newly diagnosed patients. If conditions were right, the researcher might be able to randomly assign subjects to either the group receiving the new program or the group receiving the usual program, but for any number of reasons, that design might not be possible. For example, nurses on the unit where patients are admitted might be so excited about the new program that they cannot help but include the new information for all patients. So the researcher has two choices—to abandon the experiment or to conduct a quasiexperiment. To conduct a quasiexperiment the researcher might find a similar unit that has not been introduced to the new program and study the newly diagnosed diabetic patients who are admitted to that unit as a comparison group. The study would then involve this type of design.

The nonequivalent control group design is commonly used in nursing research studies conducted in field settings. The basic problem with the design is the weakened confidence the researcher can have in assuming that the experimental and comparison groups are similar at the beginning of the study. Threats to internal validity, such as selection, maturation, testing, and mortality, are possible with this design. However, the design is relatively strong, because the gathering of the data at the time of the pretest allows the researcher to compare the equivalence of the two groups on important antecedent variables before the independent variable is introduced. In our example the motivation of the patients to learn about their diabetes might be important in determining the effect of the new teaching program. The researcher could include in the measures taken at the outset of the study some measure of motivation to learn. Then differences between the two groups on this variable can be tested, and if significant differences exist, they can be controlled statistically in the analysis. Nonetheless the strength of the causal assertions that can be made on the basis of such designs depends on the ability of the researcher to identify and measure or control possible threats to internal validity.

Now suppose that the researcher did not think to measure the subjects before the introduction of the new treatment (or she or he was hired after the new program began) but later decided that it would be useful to have data demonstrating the effect of the program. Perhaps, for example, a third party asks for such data to determine whether the extra cost of the new teaching program should be paid. The study that could be conducted would look like the **after-only nonequivalent control group design,** shown in Fig. 9-2, *B.*

This design is similar to the after-only experimental design, but randomization is not used to assign subjects to group. This design makes the assumption that the two groups are equivalent and comparable before the introduction of the independent variable. Thus the soundness of the design and the confidence that we can put in the findings depend on the soundness of this assumption of preintervention comparability. Often it is difficult to support the assertion that the two nonrandomly assigned groups are comparable at the outset of the study, because there is no way of assessing its validity. In the example of the teaching program for newly diagnosed diabetic patients, measuring the subjects' motivation after the teaching program would not tell us whether their motivations differed before they received the program, and it is possible that the teaching program would motivate individuals to learn more about their health problem. Therefore the researcher's conclusion that the teaching program improved physical status and psychosocial outcome would be subject to the alternative conclusion that the results were an effect of preexisting motivations (selection effect) in combination with greater learning in those so motivated (selection-maturation interaction). Nonetheless this design is frequently used in nursing research, because there often are limited opportunities for data collection and because it is particularly useful when testing effects may be problematic. Consider again the example of the experiment conducted by O'Sullivan and Jacobson (1992). Suppose that they had not randomly assigned the new mothers to groups. The study would then be an example of an after-only nonequivalent control group design. Had the authors chosen to conduct the study with this design and if they had found the same results, they would have been less confident of the results, since selection effects may have been stronger.

One approach that is used by researchers when only one group is available is to study that group over a longer period. This quasiexperimental design is called a **time series design,** and it is pictured in Fig. 9-2, *C.* Time series designs are useful for determining trends. Jones, Robertson, and Pieper (1992) studied the impact of legal drinking age on pedestrian fatalities by examining death rates using data from the National Highway Traffic Safety Administration for several years before and after the legal changes. By showing that the trends changed from the time that the legal drinking age was 18 years to the time that it was 21, the authors demonstrated that raising the legal drinking age to 21 resulted in lower pedestrian death rates. This study is considered a quasiexperiment because the authors were interested in determining the effect of the change in legal drinking age on pedestrian fatalities. However, they could not assign states to change their drinking ages randomly, so they examined trends over time and were able to determine that the change to age 21 had a positive effect.

To rule out some alternative explanations for the findings of a one-group pretest-posttest design, researchers can measure the phenomenon of interest over a longer period and introduce the experimental treatment sometime during the course of the data collection period. Even with the absence of a control group, the broader range of data collection points help to rule out such threats to validity as history effects. Obviously our problem related to the earlier example of teaching diabetic patients will not lend itself to this design, because we do not have access to the patients before the diagnosis.

An example of how a time series design would strengthen causal conclusions is provided by Gardner (1991), who compared primary and team nursing by studying units using team nursing and after conversion to primary nursing. Data on quality of care, impact on nursing staff, and cost were collected once before the transition and twice after. There were no comparison units that were not changing, so that there was no control group. It is difficult to be confident that the outcomes described are the result of the change in nursing care delivery rather than the development of the profession or changes in patient mix. If the author had more data from before the transition, showing that there was not a trend, it would strengthen the conclusion that the increased quality of care and decreased cost were caused by the change in nursing delivery systems. The use of a time series design would weaken the alternative explanation that the changes occurred because of something else that happened during the study period. However, the testing threat to validity looms large in these designs, since measures are repeated so many times (see Chapter 8).

Advantages and Disadvantages of Quasiexperimental Designs

Given the problems inherent in interpreting the results of studies using quasiexperimental designs, you may be wondering why anyone would use them. Quasiexperimental designs are used frequently because they are practical, feasible, and generalizable. These designs are more adaptable to the real-world practice setting than the controlled experimental designs. In addition, for some hypotheses these designs may be the only way to evaluate the effect of the independent variable of interest.

The weaknesses of the quasiexperimental approach involve mainly the inability to make clear cause-and-effect statements. However, if the researcher can rule out any plausible alternative explanations for the findings, such studies can lead to furthering knowledge about causal relationships. Researchers have several options for ferreting out these alternative explanations. They may control them a priori by design or control them statistically, or in some cases, common sense or knowledge of the problem and the population can suggest that a particular explanation is not plausible. Nonetheless it is important to replicate such studies to support the causal assertions developed through the use of quasiexperimental designs.

The literature on cigarette smoking is an excellent example of how findings from many studies, experimental and quasiexperimental, can be linked to establish a causal relationship. A large number of well-controlled experiments with laboratory animals randomly assigned to smoking and nonsmoking conditions have documented that lung disease will develop in smoking animals. Whereas such evidence is suggestive of a link between smoking and lung disease in humans, it is not directly transferable because animals and humans are different. But we cannot randomly assign humans to smoking and nonsmoking groups for ethical and other reasons. So researchers interested in this problem have to use quasiexperimental data to test their hypotheses about smoking and lung disease. Several different quasiexperimental designs have been used to study this problem, and all had similar results—that there is a causal relationship between cigarette smoking and lung disease. Note that the combination of results from both experimental and quasiexperimental studies led to the conclusion that smoking causes cancer, since the studies together meet the causal criteria of relationship, timing, and lack of an alternative explanation. Nonetheless, the tobacco industry has taken the stand that because the studies on humans are not true experiments, there may be another explanation for the relationships that have been found. For example, they suggest that the tendency to smoke is linked to the tendency for lung disease to develop and smoking is merely an unimportant intervening variable. The reader needs to study the evidence from studies to determine whether the cause-and-effect relationship that is postulated is believable.

EVALUATION RESEARCH AND EXPERIMENTATION

As the science of nursing expands and the cost of health care rises, nurses and others have become increasingly concerned with the ability to document the costs and the benefits of nursing care (see Chapter 1). This is a complex process, but at its heart is the ability to evaluate or measure the outcomes of nursing care. Such studies are usually associated with quality assurance and evaluation. Studies of evaluation or quality assurance do exactly what the name implies: such studies are concerned with the determination of the quality of nursing and health care and with assurance that the public is receiving high-quality care.

Quality assurance in nursing is in its infancy. We are just beginning to apply techniques of experimentation to the study of the delivery of nursing care. Many early quality assurance studies documented whether nursing care met predetermined standards. These were important studies, but they do not allow us to evaluate different ways of providing care.

Evaluation research is the utilization of scientific research methods and procedures to evaluate a program, treatment, practice, or policy; it uses analytic means to document the worth of an activity. Such research is not a different design. Evaluation research uses both experimental and quasiexperimental designs (as well as nonexperimental) for the purpose of determining the effect or outcomes of a program. Bigman (1961) listed the purposes and uses of evaluation research:

1. To discover whether and how well the objectives are being fulfilled
2. To determine the reasons for specific successes and failures
3. To direct the course of experiment with techniques for increasing effectiveness
4. To uncover principles underlying a successful program
5. To base further research on the reasons for the relative success of alternative techniques
6. To redefine the means to be used for attaining objectives and to redefine subgoals, in light of research findings

Evaluation studies may be either formative or summative. *Formative evaluation* refers to assessment of a program as it is being implemented; usually the focus is on evaluation of the process of a program rather than the outcomes. *Summative evaluation* refers to the assessment of the outcomes of a program that is conducted after completion of the program. An example of a study using both formative and summative evaluation with experimental design is found in the study by Abraham, Neundorfer, and Currie (1992). The authors studied the effects of cognitive-behavioral group therapy, focused visual imagery group therapy, and education-decision groups on cognition, depression, hopelessness, and dissatisfaction with life in depressed nursing home residents. Data were collected before the interventions, 8 and 20 weeks after treatment initiation, and 4 weeks after treatment termination. At the data collection points midway through the intervention period, the authors were collecting data about the formative aspects of the program; they were interested in both the implementation of the interventions and the outcomes. They also measured the outcomes of the program at the end, representing a summative evaluation. The study by O'Sullivan and Jacobson (1992) that evaluated the effectiveness of a health care program for first-time adolescent mothers and their infants is another example of the experimental design applied to summative evaluation.

The use of experimental and quasiexperimental designs in quality assurance and evaluation studies allows for the determination not only of whether care is adequate, but also which method of care is best under certain conditions. Further, such studies can be used to determine whether a particular type of nursing care is cost-effective: that is, that the care not only does what it is intended to do, but also does it at less or equivalent cost. The study by Brooten et al. (1986) was very important to nursing, as well as the health care in general, because the authors were able to demonstrate that the intervention was safe and efficacious and that there was a significant cost savings because of early discharge from the hospital with follow-up care by clinical nurse specialists. That model has now been expanded to other clinical areas, such as gerontological nursing (Naylor, 1990). In an era of health care reform and cost containment for health expenditures, it has become increasingly important to evaluate the relative costs and benefits of new programs of care. Relatively few studies in nursing and medicine have done so, but in terms of outcomes, measuring costs and cost savings will be important to future studies.

CRITIQUING EXPERIMENTAL AND QUASIEXPERIMENTAL DESIGNS

We have said that various designs for research studies differ in the amount of control the researcher has over the antecedent and intervening variables that may impact the results of the study. True experimental designs offer the most possibility for control, and preexperimental designs offer the least. Quasiexperimental designs lie somewhere between. Research designs must balance the needs for internal validity and external validity to produce useful results. In addition, judicious use of design requires that the chosen design be appropriate to the problem, free of bias, and capable of answering the research question.

Questions that the reader should pose when reading studies that test cause-and-effect relationships are listed in the box on p. 227. All of these questions should help the reader to judge whether it can be confidently believed that a causal relationship exists.

For studies where either experimental or quasiexperimental designs are used, first try to determine the type of design that was used. Often a statement describing the design of the study appears in the abstract and in the Methods sections of the paper. If such a statement is not present, the reader should examine the paper for evidence of the following three characteristics: control, randomization, and manipulation. If all are discussed, the design is probably experimental. On the other hand, if the study involves the administration of an experimental treatment but does not involve the random assignment of subjects to groups, the design is quasiexperimental.

Then try to identify which of the various designs within these two types of

CRITIQUING CRITERIA

1. What design is used in the study?
2. Is the design experimental or quasiexperimental?
3. Is the problem one of a cause-and-effect relationship?
4. Is the method used appropriate to the problem?
5. Is the design suited to the setting of the study?

EXPERIMENTAL DESIGNS

1. What experimental design is used in the study, and is it appropriate?
2. How are randomization, control, and manipulation applied?
3. Are there any reasons to believe that there are alternative explanations for the findings?
4. Are all threats to validity, including mortality, addressed in the report?
5. Whether the experiment was conducted in the laboratory or a clinical setting, are the findings generalizable to the larger population of interest?

QUASIEXPERIMENTAL DESIGNS

1. What quasiexperimental design is used in the study, and is it appropriate?
2. What are the most common threats to the validity of the findings of this design?
3. What are the plausible alternative explanations, and have they been addressed?
4. Are the author's explanations of threats to validity acceptable?
5. What does the author say about the limitations of the study?
6. Are there other limitations related to the design that are not mentioned?

EVALUATION RESEARCH

1. Does the study identify a specific problem, practice, policy, or treatment that it will evaluate?
2. Are the outcomes to be evaluated identified?
3. Is the problem analyzed and described?
4. Is the program to be analyzed described and standardized?
5. Is measurement of the degree of change (outcome) that occurs identified?
6. Is there a determination of whether the observed outcome is related to the activity or to some other causes?

designs was used. Determining the answer to these questions gives you a head start, because each design has its inherent threats to validity and this step makes it a bit easier to critically evaluate the study. The next question to ask is whether the researcher required a solution to a cause-and-effect problem. If so, the study is suited to these designs. Finally, think about the conduct of the study in the setting. Is it realistic to think that the study could be conducted in a clinical setting without some contamination?

The most important question to ask yourself as your read experimental studies is "What else could have happened to explain the findings?" Thus it is important that the author provide adequate accounts of how the procedures for randomization, control, and manipulation were carried out. The paper should include a description of the procedures for random assignment to such a degree that the reader could determine just how likely it was for any one subject to be assigned to a particular group. The description of the independent variable should also be detailed. The inclusion of this information helps the reader to decide if it is possible that the treatment given to some subjects in the experimental group might be different from what was given to others in the same group. In addition, threats to validity, such as testing and the occurrence of deaths, should be addressed. Otherwise there is the potential for the findings of the study to be in error and less believable to the reader.

This question of potential alternative explanations or threats to internal validity for the findings is even more important when critically evaluating a quasiexperimental study, because quasiexperimental designs cannot possibly control many plausible alternative explanations. A well-written report of a quasiexperimental study will systematically review potential threats to the validity of the findings. Then the reader's work is to decide if the author's explanations make sense.

When critiquing evaluation research, the reader should look for a careful description of the program, policy, procedure, or treatment being evaluated. In addition, the reader may need to determine the design used to evaluate the program and assess the appropriateness of the design for the evaluation. Once the design has been determined, the reader assesses threats to validity for the appropriate design in determining the appropriateness of the authors' conclusions related to the outcomes. As with all research, studies using these designs need to be generalizable to a larger population of people than those actually studied. Thus it is important to decide whether the experimental protocol eliminated some potential subjects and whether this affected not only internal validity but also external validity.

KEY POINTS

- Two types of design commonly used in nursing research to test hypotheses about cause-and-effect relationships are experimental and quasiexperimental designs. Both are useful for the development of nursing knowledge, because they test the effects of nursing actions and lead to the development of prescriptive theory.
- True experiments are characterized by the ability of the researcher to control extraneous variation, to manipulate the independent variable, and to randomly assign subjects to research groups.

- Experiments conducted either in clinical settings or in the laboratory provide the best evidence in support of a causal relationship because the following three criteria can be met:
  1. The independent and dependent variables are related to each other.
  2. The independent variable chronologically precedes the dependent variable.
  3. The relationship cannot be explained by the presence of a third variable.
- Researchers frequently turn to quasiexperimental designs to test cause-and-effect relationships because there are many times when experimental designs are impractical or unethical.
- Quasiexperiments may lack either the randomization or comparison group characteristics of true experiments, or both of these factors. Their usefulness in studying causal relationships depends on the ability of the researcher to rule out plausible threats to the validity of the findings, such as history, selection, maturation, and testing effects.
- The overall purpose of critiquing such studies is to assess the validity of the findings and to determine whether these findings are worth incorporating into the nurse's personal practice.

REFERENCES

Abraham, I.L., Neundorfer, M.M., & Currie, L.J. (1992). Effects of group interventions on cognition and depression in nursing home residents. *Nursing Research, 41*(4), 196-202.

Bigman, S.K. (1961). Evaluating the effectiveness of religious programs. *Review of Religious Research, 2,* 99-110.

Brooten, D., Kumar, S., Brown, L.P., Butts, P., Finkler, S., Bakewell-Sachs, S., Gibbons, A., & Delivoria-Papadopoulos, M. (1986). A randomized clinical trial of early hospital discharge and home follow-up of very-low-birth-weight infants. *New England Journal of Medicine, 315,* 934-939.

Campbell, D., & Stanley, J. (1966). *Experimental and quasiexperimental designs for research.* Chicago: Rand-McNally.

Conlon, M., & Anderson, G.C. (1990). Three methods of random assignment: Comparison of balance achieved on potentially confounding variables. *Nursing Research, 39*(6), 376-378.

Gardner, K. (1991). A summary of findings of a five-year comparison study of primary and team nursing. *Nursing Research, 40*(2), 113-117.

Hauck, W.W., Gilliss, C.L., Donner, A., & Gortner, S. (1991). Randomization by cluster. *Nursing Research, 40*(6), 356-358.

Jones, N.E., Robertson, L., & Pieper, C. (1992). *American Journal of Public Health, 82,* 112-115.

Naylor, M. (1990). Comprehensive discharge planning for hospitalized elderly: A pilot study. *Nursing Research, 39,* 156-161.

O'Sullivan, A.O., & Jacobson, B.J. (1992). A randomized trial of a health care program for first-time adolescent mothers and their infants. *Nursing Research, 41*(4), 210-215.

Stewart Fahs, P.S., & Kinney, M.R. (1991). The abdomen, thigh, and arm as sites for subcutaneous sodium heparin injections. *Nursing Research, 40*(4), 204-207.

White, M.A., Williams, P.D., Alexander, D.J., Powell-Cope, G.M., & Conlon, M. (1990).

Sleep onset latency and distress in hospitalized children. *Nursing Research, 39*(3), 134-139.

ADDITIONAL READINGS

Atwood, J.R., & Taylor, W. (1991). Regression discontinuity design: Alternative for nursing research. *Nursing Research, 40*(5), 312-315.

Cook, T.D. (1990). The generalization of causal connections: Multiple theories in search of clear practice. In L. Sechrest, E. Perrin, & J. Bunker (Eds.), *AHCPR Conference Proceedings: Research methodology: Strenthening causal interpretations of nonexperimental data* (pp. 9-31), Rockville, MD: Agency for Health Care Policy and Research.

Cook, T.D., & Campbell, D.T. (1979). *Quasi-experimentation: Design and analysis issues for field settings.* Chicago: Rand-McNally.

Given, B.A., Keilman, L.J., Collins, C., & Given, C.W. (1990). Strategies to minimize attrition in longitudinal studies. *Nursing Research, 39*(3), 184-186.

Given, C.W., Given, B.A., & Coyle, B.W. (1985). Prediction of patient attrition from experimental behavioral interventions. *Nursing Research, 34,* 293-298.

Hinshaw, A.S., Gerber, R.N., Atwood, J.R., & Allen, J.R. (1983). The use of predictive modeling to test nursing practice outcomes. *Nursing Research, 32,* 35-42.

Jacobson, B.S., & Meininger, J.C. (1990). Seeing the importance of blindness. *Nursing Research, 39,* 54-57.

Polivka, B.J., & Nickel, J.T. (1992). Case-control design: An appropriate strategy for nursing research. *Nursing Research, 41,* 250-253.

Strickland, O.L., & Waltz, C.F. (1988). *Measurement of nursing outcomes: Measuring client outcomes* (Vol. 1). New York: Springer.

Suchman, E.A. (1967). *Evaluative research.* New York: Russell Sage Foundation.

Waltz, C.F., & Strickland, O.L. (1988). *Measurement of nursing outcomes: Measuring client outcomes* (Vol. 2). New York: Springer.

CHAPTER
10

Nonexperimental Designs

GERI LoBIONDO-WOOD
JUDITH HABER

LEARNING OBJECTIVES

After reading this chapter the student should be able to do the following:

- Describe the overall purpose of nonexperimental designs.
- Describe the characteristics of descriptive/exploratory survey and interrelationship designs.
- Define the differences between descriptive/exploratory survey and interrelationship designs.
- List the advantages and disadvantages of surveys and each type of interrelationship design.
- Identify methodological and metaanalysis types of research.
- Identify the purposes of methodological and metaanalysis types of research.
- Discuss relational inferences versus causal inferences as they relate to nonexperimental designs.
- Identify the criteria used to critique nonexperimental research designs.
- Apply the critiquing criteria to the evaluation of nonexperimental research designs as they appear in research reports.

KEY TERMS

correlational study   metaanalysis
cross-sectional study   methodological research
descriptive/exploratory   nonexperimental research
surveys   prediction study
developmental study   prospective study
ex post facto study   psychometrics
interrelationship study   retrospective data
longitudinal study   retrospective study

Nonexperimental research designs are used in studies where the researcher wishes to construct a picture of a phenomenon or make account of events as they naturally occur. In experimental research the independent variable is manipulated; in nonexperimental research it is not. In nonexperimental research the independent variables have already occurred, so to speak, and the investigator cannot directly control them by manipulation. Thus in an experimental design the researcher actively manipulates one or more variables, but in a nonexperimental design the researcher explores relationships.

The reader of research reports will find that most of the studies that are conducted and reported use a nonexperimental design. Many phenomena that are of interest and relevant to nursing do not lend themselves to an experimental design. For example, nurses studying the phenomena of pain may be interested in the amount of pain, variations in the amount of pain, and patient responses to postoperative pain. The investigator would not design an experimental study that would potentially intensify a patient's pain just to study the pain experience from any one of these perspectives. Instead, the researcher would perhaps examine the factors that contribute to the variability in a patient's postoperative pain experience. A nonexperimental research design would then be used to help answer such questions.

Nonexperimental research also requires a clear, concise problem statement that is based on a theoretical framework. Even though the researcher does not actively manipulate the variables, the concepts of control introduced in Chapter 8 should be followed as much as possible. Following the phases of research utilization as conceptualized by Stetler (in press), several nonexperimental studies examining the same concepts can be used as the basis for cognitive, instrumental, or symbolic application of findings (see Chapter 3).

Researchers are not in agreement on how to classify nonexperimental studies.

SUMMARY OF NONEXPERIMENTAL RESEARCH DESIGNS

   I. Descriptive/exploratory survey studies
  II. Interrelationship studies
      A. Correlational studies
      B. Ex post facto studies
      C. Prediction studies
      D. Developmental studies
         1. Cross-sectional and longitudinal studies
         2. Retrospective and prospective studies

For purposes of discussion this chapter will divide nonexperimental designs into **descriptive/exploratory survey studies** and **interrelationship studies** as illustrated in the box above. An overall schema of quantitative research design is presented in Fig. 10-1. These categories are somewhat flexible, and other sources may classify nonexperimental studies in a different way. Some studies fall exclusively within one of these categories, whereas other studies have characteristics of more than one category. This chapter will introduce the reader to the various types of nonexperimental designs, the advantages and disadvantages of nonexperimental designs, the use of nonexperimental research, the issues of causality, and the critiquing process as it relates to nonexperimental research.

DESCRIPTIVE/EXPLORATORY SURVEY STUDIES

The broadest category of nonexperimental designs is the survey study. Survey studies are also further classified as descriptive or exploratory research designs. The reader of research will find that survey or exploratory/descriptive survey studies can meet the aims of a researcher in several different ways. Descriptive/exploratory survey studies collect detailed descriptions of existing variables and use the data to justify and assess current conditions and practices or to make more intelligent plans for improving health care practices. The reader of research will find that the terms *exploratory, descriptive,* and *survey* are used either alone, interchangeably, or together to describe the design of a study. Investigators use this design to search for accurate information about the characteristics of particular subjects, groups, institutions, or situations or about the frequency of a phenomenon's occurrence. The types of variables of interest can be classified as opinions, attitudes, or facts. An example of a study whose aim was to explore an opinion or attitude variable was conducted by Cole and Slocumb (1993). They studied whether nurses possessed differing attitudes toward acquired immunodeficiency syndrome (AIDS) patients depending on how the patients acquired the virus and found significant differences among the attitudes toward AIDS patients relative to the mode of acquiring the virus. Studies such as this provide the basis for further exploration into this area and also for the develop-

NONEXPERIMENTAL ⟶ QUASIEXPERIMENTAL ⟶ EXPERIMENTAL

Fig. 10-1   Continuum of quantitative research design.

ment of educational programs for nurses that will promote positive care for AIDS patients.

Examples of facts include attributes of individuals that are a function of their membership in society, such as gender, income level, political and religious affiliations, ethnicity, occupation, and educational level. An example of a study that explored facts was conducted by Mason, Jensen, and Boland (1992). In this study the researchers noted that health care risks in homeless men were quite high. To begin to study this problem in the geographic location where the researchers resided they explored the health behaviors and health risks in homeless men in Utah. The researchers noted that the significance of this study would be that nurses could target health promotion/illness prevention programs focused on the needs of the homeless, thereby decreasing health risks and costs among Utah's homeless male population.

Another example of an exploratory survey was conducted by Schneider and LoBiondo-Wood (1992). Appropriate assessment and intervention of children's responses to various health care procedures are important parts of nursing care. An exploratory study was conducted to assess whether there were differences among a group of subjects regarding childrens' pain perceptions. This study assessed whether children, their parents, and their nurses differ in their perception of pain associated with a health care procedure (immunization). This study, like the two previously discussed, does not manipulate variables but assesses perceptions of children's pain in order to provide data for future nursing intervention studies.

Data in survey research can be collected by either a structured questionnaire or a structured or unstructured interview (see Chapter 14). Survey researchers study either small or large samples of subjects drawn from defined populations. The units of analysis can be either broad or narrow and can be made up of people or institutions. For example, if a primary care rehabilitation unit based on a case management model were to be established in a hospital, a survey might be taken of the prospective applicant's attitudes with regard to case management before the staff of the unit are selected. In a broader example, if a hospital were contemplating converting all patient care units to a case management concept, a survey might be conducted to determine attitudes of a representative sample of nurses in hospital X toward case management. The data might provide the basis for projecting in-service needs of nursing regarding case management. The scope and depth of a survey are a function of the nature of the problem.

Surveys are descriptive and exploratory in nature. In descriptive/exploratory surveys, investigators attempt only to relate one variable to another; they do not attempt to determine causation.

There are both advantages and disadvantages of survey research. Two major advantages are that a great deal of information can be obtained from a large population in a fairly economical manner and that survey research information can be surprisingly accurate. If a sample is representative of the population (see Chapter 12), a relatively small number of respondents can provide an accurate picture of the target population.

There are several disadvantages of descriptive/exploratory survey studies. First, the information obtained in a survey tends to be superficial. The breadth rather than the depth of the information is emphasized. Second, conducting a survey requires a great deal of expertise in a variety of research areas. The survey investigator must know sampling techniques, questionnaire construction, interviewing, and data analysis to produce a reliable and valid study. Third, large-scale surveys can be time-consuming and costly, although the use of on-site personnel can reduce costs.

Research consumers should recognize that a well-constructed descriptive/exploratory survey can provide a wealth of data about a particular phenomenon of interest even though relationships between variables are not being examined.

INTERRELATIONSHIP STUDIES

In contrast to investigators who use survey research, other investigators who use nonexperimental designs endeavor to trace interrelationships between variables that will provide a deeper insight into the phenomenon of interest. These studies can be classified as interrelationship studies. The following types of interrelationship studies will be discussed: **correlational studies, ex post facto studies, prediction studies,** and **developmental studies.**

Correlational Studies

The research consumer will find that an investigator uses a correlational design to examine the relationship between two or more variables. The researcher is not testing whether one variable causes another variable but whether the variables covary; that is, as one variable changes, does a related change occur in the other variable? The researcher using this design is interested in quantifying the magnitude or strength of the relationship between the variables. The positive or negative direction of the relationship is also a central concern of the researcher (see Chapter 17 for a complete explanation of the correlation coefficient). For example, Redeker (1992) conducted a correlation study whose purposes were to examine the relationships between uncertainty and coping and to describe the changes in these relationships between 1 and 6 weeks after coronary artery bypass surgery (CABS). The researcher noted that recovery from coronary artery bypass surgery is widely recognized as a stressful experience. She also used a conceptual/theoretical framework that was consistent with the operational definitions used in the study. An analysis of the data showed that there were significant and positive relationships between most of the uncertainty and coping variables; that the correlations among the coping subscales were all statistically significant except for one of the subscales; and that the relationships among the uncertainty variables were mixed. The significant correlations found in this study suggest that there is a positive relationship between uncertainty and coping.

It should be remembered that the researchers were not testing a cause-and-effect relationship. All that is known is that the researchers found a relationship and that one variable (uncertainty) varied in a consistent way with another variable (coping) for the particular sample studied. When reviewing a correlational study it is important to remember what relationship the researcher is testing and to notice whether the researcher implied a relationship that is consistent with the theoretical framework and hypotheses being tested. Correlational studies offer researchers and research consumers the following advantages:

- An increased flexibility when investigating complex relationships among variables
- An efficient and effective method of collecting a large amount of data about a problem area
- A potential for practical application in clinical settings
- A potential foundation for future, more rigorous research studies
- A possible framework for investigating the relationship between variables that are inherently not manipulable

The reader will find that the correlational design has a quality of realism about it and is particularly appealing because it suggests the potential for practical solutions to clinical problems. The following are disadvantages of correlational studies:

- The variables of interest are beyond the researcher's control
- The researcher is unable to manipulate the variables of interest
- The researcher does not employ randomization in the sampling procedures because of dealing with preexisting groups, and therefore generalizability is decreased
- The researcher is unable to determine a causal relationship between the variables because of the lack of manipulation, control, and randomization

One of the most common misuses of a correlational design is the researcher's conclusion that a causal relationship exists between the variables. In the Redeker (1992) study the investigator appropriately concluded that a relationship exists between the variables, not that coping caused uncertainty. The investigator also appropriately concluded that the ability to generalize from this study is limited by the demographic characteristics of the sample (predominantly white male) and clinical delimitations (severity of illness and use of one setting). The report of the study also concludes with some very thoughtful recommendations for future clinical studies in this area. This study is a good example of a clinical study that uses a correlation design well. The inability to draw causal statements should not lead the research consumer to conclude that a nonexperimental correlational study uses a weak design. It is a very useful design for clinical research studies, because many of the phenomena of clinical interest are beyond the researcher's ability to manipulate, control, and randomize. For instance, a researcher interested in studying the grief experiences of women who have recently miscarried could not randomly assign subjects to grief and nongrief groups. Also, the experience of a miscarriage is a naturally occurring process and, as such, cannot be manipulated.

Table 10-1   Paradigm for the Ex Post Facto Design

Groups (not randomly assigned)	Independent variable (not manipulated by investigator)	Dependent variable
Exposed group Cigarette smokers	X Cigarette smoking	Y_E Lung cancer
Control group Nonsmokers		Y_C No lung cancer

Ex Post Facto Studies

When scientists wish to explain causality or the factors that determine the occurrence of events or conditions, they prefer to employ an experimental design. However, they cannot always manipulate the independent variable X or use random assignments. In cases where experimental designs cannot be employed, ex post facto studies may be used. *Ex post facto* literally means "from after the fact." Ex post facto studies are also known as causal-comparative studies or comparative studies. As we discuss this design further, the reader will see that many elements of ex post facto research are similar to quasiexperimental designs (Campbell and Stanley, 1963).

In ex post facto studies the consumer will find that the researcher hypothesizes, for instance, that X (cigarette smoking) is related to and a determinant of Y (lung cancer), but X, the presumed cause, is not manipulated and subjects are not randomly assigned to groups. Rather, a group of subjects who have experienced X (cigarette smoking) in a normal situation is located and a control group of subjects who have not is chosen. The behavior, performance, or condition (lung tissue) of the two groups is compared to determine whether the exposure to X had the effect predicted by the hypothesis. Table 10-1 illustrates a paradigm for ex post facto design. Examination of Table 10-1 reveals that although cigarette smoking appears to be a determinant of lung cancer, the researcher is still not in a position to conclude that there is a causal relationship between the variables, because there has been no manipulation of the independent variable or random assignment of subjects to groups.

The advantages of the ex post facto design are similar to those inherent in the correlational design. The additional benefit of the ex post facto design is that it offers a higher level of control than the correlational studies. For example, in the cigarette smoking study a group of nonsmokers' lung tissue samples are compared with samples of smokers' lung tissue. This comparison enables the researcher to establish that there is a differential effect of cigarette smoking on lung tissue. However, the researcher remains unable to draw a causal linkage between the two variables, and this inability is the major disadvantage of the ex post facto design.

Another disadvantage of ex post facto research is the problem of an alternative hypothesis being the reason for the documented relationship. If the researcher obtains data from two existing groups of subjects, such as one that has been exposed to X and one that has not, and the data support the hypothesis that X is related to Y, the researcher cannot be sure whether X or some extraneous variable is the real cause of the occurrence of Y. Finding naturally occurring groups of subjects who are similar in all respects except for their exposure to the variable of interest is very difficult. There is always the possibility that the groups differ in some other way, such as exposure to some other lung irritants such as asbestos, which can affect the findings of the study and produce spurious results. Consequently, the critiquer of such a study needs to cautiously evaluate the conclusions drawn by the investigator.

Prediction Studies

Researchers in education and management positions at times want to make a forecast or prediction about how successful individuals will be in a particular setting, field of specialty, or circumstance. In this case *prediction studies* are employed. For example, in a study conducted by Mills et al. (1992), first-time nurse candidates from a 4-year baccalaureate nursing program were examined to identify predictors of success on NCLEX-RN examinations. Retrospective data from student records (examples of record data were gender, high school GPA, ACT scores, and cumulative GPA for nursing courses) and NCLEX-RN scores reported by the state board of nursing were the data sources. The researchers stated that having this information would enable faculty to recognize students at risk for NCLEX-RN failure. The goal of the study was to identify preexisting characteristics of the individual that were predictive of a relationship to the dependent variable, success on the state board examinations.

In another example, in a study conducted by Johansen, Bowles, and Haney (1988, p. 375) an attempt was made to pilot test a statistical forecasting model and to illustrate its use in "(a) estimating the number of cancer and myocardial infarction patients who are likely to need intermittent skilled home nursing services after discharge; (b) estimating the statewide costs of providing these services after discharge; and (c) incorporating change patterns of hospital length of stay and severity of illness, and reflecting these changes in the estimates of number of patients and costs."

To test the model that the researchers developed they used only objectively recorded patient variables; examples are age, marital status, number of critical care days (for patients with myocardial infarction), number of procedures undertaken during hospitalization (for patients with cancer), and number of secondary diagnoses. Variables chosen were based on the literature and clinical experience. The goals of the study were to (1) demonstrate how a model could produce estimates of need and cost and (2) allow simulation of changes in the health care delivery system to assess how these changes are reflected in the estimates. In this study the researchers also used retrospective data from two patient groups to forecast needs. It was also hoped that other researchers could use the model to forecast home care needs for other types of patient groups.

The research consumer will find that prediction studies use retrospective data from one group to make predictions about a similar group. This type of design generally employs sophisticated statistical techniques when exploring relationships among variables in one group to make predictions about the behavior of another group.

The major advantage of predictive studies is that they facilitate intelligent decision making, because objective criteria are available to guide the process. This can be particularly important in situations where critical choices, such as student selection, are made. The major disadvantage or limitation of prediction studies is that the design does not imply a cause-and-effect relationship between the chosen independent predictor variables and the dependent criterion variable. In addition, if the predictor variables were not chosen with a sound rationale, a study may not be valid.

Developmental Studies

There are also classifications of nonexperimental designs that use a time perspective. Investigators who use *developmental studies* are concerned not only with the existing status and interrelationship of phenomena but also with changes that result from elapsed time. The following four types of developmental study designs will be discussed: cross-sectional, longitudinal, retrospective, and prospective.

Cross-sectional and Longitudinal Studies

Cross-sectional studies examine data at one point in time; that is, the data are collected on only one occasion with the same subjects rather than on the same subjects at several points in time. An example of a cross-sectional study is Koniak-Griffin's (1988) study, which focused on the relationship between maternal-fetal attachment, social support, and self-esteem in a group of culturally divergent pregnant adolescents. The adolescents filled out three questionnaires at one point in time during their pregnancy. The questionnaires measured the adolescents' perceptions of self-worth, social support, and maternal-fetal attachment.

Another cross-sectional study approach is to simultaneously collect data on the variables of interest from different cohort groups. For example, if an investigator wishes to look at the development of maternal-fetal attachment in relationship to quickening in primiparas, the designated data collection periods may be the 12th, 24th, and 36th weeks of pregnancy. The researcher would then select equivalent groups of primiparas who are at each respective point in their pregnancy. The data from each group would then be compared by use of statistical measures.

An excellent example of a cross-sectional study with different age cohort groups is the one conducted by Grey, Cameron, and Thurber (1991; Appendix A). This study focused on comparing the influence of age, coping behavior, and self-care on psychological, social, and physiological adaptation in preadolescents and adolescents with diabetes. Children with insulin-dependent diabetes mellitus between 8 and 18 years of age and their parents participated in the study and filled out several questionnaires at one point in time measuring the study's variables. Differences between preadolescent and adolescent groups were analyzed by dividing the subjects by Tanner's stages of sexual maturation.

In contrast to the cross-sectional design, **longitudinal studies** collect data from the same group at different points in time. For instance, the investigator conducting the same maternal-fetal attachment study could elect to use a longitudinal design. In that case the investigator would test the same group of primiparas at each data collection point. By collecting data from each subject at the 12th, 24th, and 36th weeks of pregnancy, a longitudinal perspective of the attachment process is accomplished (LoBiondo-Wood, 1985).

There are many advantages and disadvantages to both designs. When assessing the appropriateness of a cross-sectional study versus a longitudinal study, the research consumer should first assess what the goal of the researcher was in light of the theoretical framework. In the example of the maternal-fetal attachment study, the researcher is looking at a developmental process; therefore a longitudinal design seems more appropriate. However, the disadvantages inherent in a longitudinal design must also be considered. Data collection may be of long duration because of the time it takes for the subjects to progress to each data collection point. In the attachment study it would take each woman 24 weeks to complete the data collection process. It would take the investigator 6 months to complete the data collection *if* all of the subjects were obtained at one time. This does not even account for intervening variables, such as attrition, miscarriage, or complications of pregnancy, that might occur after the study has begun. The internal validity threat of mortality is also ever-present and unavoidable in a longitudinal study.

These realities make a longitudinal design costly in terms of time, effort, and money. There is also a chance of confounding variables that could affect the interpretation of the results. Subjects in such a study may respond in a socially desirable way that they believe is congruent with the investigators' expectations. This is similar to the Hawthorne effect discussed in Chapters 8. However, despite the pragmatic constraints imposed by a longitudinal study, the researcher should proceed with this design if the theoretical framework supports a longitudinal developmental perspective.

The advantages of a longitudinal study are that each subject is followed separately and thereby serves as his or her own control; increased depth of responses can be obtained; and early trends in the data can be investigated. The researcher can assess changes in the variables of interest over time.

In contrast, cross-sectional studies are less time-consuming, less expensive, and thus more manageable for the researcher. Because large amounts of data can be collected at one point, the results are more readily available. In addition, the confounding variable of maturation, resulting from the elapsed time, is not present. However, the economic accomplishments are sacrificed in terms of the investigator's lessened ability to establish an in-depth developmental assessment of the interrelationships of the phenomena being studied. Thus the researcher is unable to determine whether the change that occurred is related to the change that was predicted by the hypothesis, because the same subjects were not followed over a period of time. In other words, the subjects are unable to serve as their own controls (see Chapter 8).

In summary, it is important for the consumer to realize that longitudinal studies begin in the present and end in the future. Cross-sectional studies look at a broader perspective of a cross section of the population at a specific point in time.

Retrospective and Prospective Studies

Retrospective studies are essentially the same as ex post facto studies. The term *retrospective* is mainly used by epidemiologists, whereas the term *ex post facto* is preferred by social scientists. In either case, the dependent variable has already been affected by the independent variable, and the investigator attempts to link present events to events that have occurred in the past. An example of a retrospective study is one in which a researcher conducted a retrospective chart review comparing patients who had received heparin with patients who had not received heparin in normal saline injection for maintenance of intermittent intravenous sites to assess efficacy of the two methods for site patency.

The investigator would begin with a theoretical framework that was derived from a systematic retrospective search to identify the factors related to the development of intermittent intravenous site maintenance. The findings of such retrospective studies can provide the basis for further investigation and require additional research information.

In another example of a retrospective study Shannahan and Cottrell (1985) studied the effect of delivering in a birth chair on the duration of the second stage of labor, fetal outcome (Apgar scores), and maternal blood loss. To conduct the study within a retrospective design, the researchers conducted a retrospective chart review of 60 primiparous women at 37 to 41 weeks' gestation within a 2-month period in one hospital setting. All subjects had a normal pregnancy, spontaneous labor, no augmentation of labor, and admission and postpartum hemoglobin and hematocrit determinations. The data collected from each chart included type of delivery, episiotomy, laceration, anesthesia, analgesia, Apgar scores, blood test results, and the duration of the second stage of labor. The researchers found that the birth chair offered no untoward effects on the infant's status, but the mothers who gave birth in birth chairs did have significantly lower hemoglobin and hematocrit values than the mothers who delivered on tables.

The researchers identified a number of areas for future research in this area. They also noted that they were doing further research and assessing the same variables using a prospective design. This is an excellent example of how researchers develop and expand clinical knowledge by conducting follow-up studies that further test variables.

Prospective studies explore presumed causes or presumed relationships and then move forward in time to the presumed effect. As such, they are much like longitudinal studies; they start in the present and end in the future. They are also commonly used by epidemiologists. For example, a researcher might want to test the incidence of alcohol consumption during pregnancy in relation to resulting low-birth-weight infants. To test this hypothesis the investigator would draw a sample of pregnant women, some who regularly consumed alcohol during their pregnancy and others who did not. The occurrence of low-birth-weight infants in both groups would then be analyzed. These data would allow the investigator to assess whether regular alcohol consumption during pregnancy was related to the birth weight of the infant.

In another situation the researcher may wish to study the development of a particular health outcome. In this type of study the investigator selects the participants from a population known to be free of the health outcome under study and classifies the participants according to whether they have one or more factors (independent variables) presumably related to the outcome. These participants, who are frequently referred to as a *cohort,* are then studied over a period, ranging from months to years, to determine who develops the health outcome. The Framingham heart study examined the effect of blood pressure, cholesterol levels, smoking, exercise, and other variables on the development of coronary artery disease in a cohort of healthy men. The subjects were studied at specified intervals over a period of years.

An example of a prospective study was conducted by Schraeder (1993). The aim of this study was to compare the ability of three types of preschool developmental assessment tools available for use by pediatric nurse practitioners to predict school success in the primary grades, kindergarten through second, in a group of very-low-birth-weight (VLBW) infants (birth weight <1500 g). The original sample size in the study was 41 children who were VLBW and who were 4 years of age when they entered the study. The final sample consisted of 35 children who were tested at intervals from kindergarten through second grade.

When reading the study by Schraeder (1993), the reader will note that Schraeder classifies the study's design as prospective and longitudinal. This is correct, and the consumer of research will find this often when reading research reports because studies often reflect aspects of more than one design label, as in this case.

Prospective studies are less common than retrospective studies. This may be explained by the fact that it can take a long time for the phenomenon of interest to become evident in a prospective study. For example, if researchers were studying pregnant women who regularly consume alcohol, it would take 9 months for the effect of low birth weight in the subjects' infants to become evident. The problems inherent in a prospective study are therefore similar to those of a longitudinal study. However, prospective studies are considered to be stronger than retrospective studies because of the degree of control that can be imposed on extraneous variables that might confound the data.

CAUSALITY IN NONEXPERIMENTAL RESEARCH

A great concern of nurses when they are conducting research is the issue of causality. Scientists are interested in explaining cause-and-effect relationships. Historically researchers have said that only experimental research can support the concept of causality. For example, nurses are interested in discovering what causes anxiety in many settings. If we can uncover the causes, we could perhaps develop interventions that would prevent or decrease the anxiety. Causality makes it necessary to order events chronologically; that is, if we find in a randomly assigned experiment that event 1 (stress) occurs before event 2 (anxiety) and that those in the stressed group were anxious whereas those in the unstressed group were not anxious, we can say that the hypothesis of stress causing anxiety is supported by these empirical observations. If these results were found in a nonexperimental study where some subjects underwent the stress of surgery and were anxious and others did not have surgery and were not anxious, we would say that there is an association or relationship between stress (surgery) and anxiety. But on the basis of the results of a nonexperimental study we could not say that the stress of surgery *caused* the anxiety.

There are also many variables like anxiety that nurse researchers wish to study that cannot be manipulated, nor would it be wise to try to manipulate them. Yet there is a need to have studies that can assert a causal sequence; in light of this need, many nurse researchers are using several analytical techniques that can explain the relationships among variables to establish causal links. These techniques are called *causal modeling* and *associated causal analysis techniques* (Asher, 1976; Ferketich & Verran, 1984; Verran & Ferketich, 1984). The reader of research will also find the terms *path analysis, LISREL, analysis of covariance structures,* and *structural equation modeling* (SEM) used to describe these techniques (Pedhazur & Schmelkin, 1991). An example of a study that used causal modeling was conducted by Mercer, Ferketich, and DeJoseph, (1993). In this study the researchers assessed the partner relationships of a sample of women hospitalized for high-risk pregnancy, their partners, and a sample of women who were experiencing a low-risk pregnancy and their partners to determine risk status (effects of antepartal stress) or gender differences at different points during the pregnancy and during early infancy. The periods studied were pregnancy, the postpartal hospitalization, and 1, 4, and 8 months after birth. The researchers developed a theoretical model from earlier research and in this study tested the model to study partner relationships longitudinally during the transition to parenthood in couples who were experiencing a high-risk pregnancy. The study found some differences between the low-risk and high-risk groups, as well as between the genders. The researchers point to the need for further research into the antecedents and mediators of the partner relationships during high-risk pregnancy and for the need for further model testing. The researchers' recommendations of further research also point to the fact that no matter which type of design or which statistical procedure is used, there is a need for future testing and refinement of the principles that guide nursing care.

A full description of the techniques and principles of causal modeling is beyond the scope of this text. A review of the additional references will provide the reader with the basic assumptions and principles of these techniques.

ADDITIONAL TYPES OF DESIGNS

Other types of designs that complement the science of research exist that use a different perspective to collect, analyze, and interpret data. These additional types of designs are valid and useful and may be considered for special areas of investigation. They provide another means of viewing and interpreting phenomena that gives further breadth and knowledge to nursing science and practice. These additional types of research are important links in the development of nursing research. The additional types are *methodological* and *metaanalysis.* Methodological research is the development of data collection instruments; metaanalysis is the synthesis of research studies in a specific area.

Methodological Research

Methodology is a general term and has many meanings. It may mean different ways of doing research for different purposes, ways of stating hypotheses, methods of data collection and measurement, and techniques of data analysis. Methodology also includes aspects of the philosophy of science as an overall critical approach to research (Kerlinger, 1986). As you will find in succeeding chapters (see Chapters 14 and 15), methodology influences research strongly. **Methodological research** is the controlled investigation of the theoretical and applied aspects of mathematics, statistics, measurement, and the means of gathering and analyzing data (Kerlinger, 1986).

The most significant and critically important aspect of methodological research that is addressed in measurement and statistics is called **psychometrics.** Psychometrics deals with the theory and development of measurement instruments or measurement techniques through the research process. Psychometrics thus deals with the measurement of a concept, such as anxiety or interpersonal conflict, with reliable and valid tools (see Chapter 15 for a discussion of reliability and validity). Psychometrics is a critical issue for nurse researchers. Many of the tools used by nurse researchers have been developed by other disciplines, such as psychology and sociology, and may not necessarily be totally appropriate for nursing's use. Since nurses have become more sophisticated in their investigations and knowledge of research, the development of appropriate tools to measure phenomena of interest has increased. Methodological research is critical to the reliability and validity of a study. For example, Klein (1983) conducted a study on the use of contraceptives in women seeking abortion and their perception of the chance and ability to conceive. Although the study's purpose and problems were clear, the tool that was developed and used by the author exhibited various psychometric problems. When studies have inherent psychometric problems, they render the findings questionable or limited.

The main problem for nurse researchers is locating appropriate measurement tools. In the Klein study an important concept, risk-taking behavior, may impinge on contraceptive use and thereby clinical practice, and so it needed to be measured. The appropriate tool was lacking, so the author developed one. Many of the phenomena of interest to nursing practice and research are intangible, such as interpersonal conflict and maternal-fetal attachment. The intangible nature of various phenomena, yet the recognition of the need to measure them, places methodological research in an important position.

Methodological research differs from other designs of research. First, it does not include all of the research process steps as discussed in Chapter 4. Second, to implement its techniques the researcher must have a sound knowledge of psychometrics or must consult with a researcher knowledgeable in psychometric techniques. The methodological researcher is not interested in the interrelationship of the independent variable and dependent variable or in the effect of an independent variable on a dependent variable. The methodological researcher is interested in identifying an intangible construct and making it tangible with a paper-and-pencil tool or observation protocol.

Basically a methodological study includes the following steps:
1. Defining the construct or behavior to be measured
2. Formulating the items
3. Developing instructions for users and respondents
4. Testing the tool's reliability and validity

These steps require a sound, specific, and exhaustive literature review to identify the theories underlying the construct. The literature review provides the basis of item formulation. Once the items have been developed, the researcher assesses the tool's reliability and validity (see Chapter 15). Various aspects of these procedures may differ according to the tools's use, purpose, and stage of development.

Examples of methodological research can be found in the classic studies done by Bergstrom et al. (1987) and by Braden and Bergstrom (1987). In these studies the researchers identified the construct of pressure sore etiology and defined it conceptually and operationally. Common considerations that researchers incorporate into methodological research are outlined in Table 10-2. Many more examples of methodological research can be found in nursing research literature (Frank-Stromberg, 1992; Waltz & Strickland, 1988; Strickland & Waltz, 1988). Psychometric or methodological studies are found primarily in journals that report research. The specific procedures of methodological research are beyond the scope of this book, but the reader is urged to look closely at the tools used in studies. References of psychometric or methodological research are provided in the Additional Readings list in this chapter.

METAANALYSIS

Metaanalysis is not a design per se but a research method that takes the results of many studies in a specific area and synthesizes their findings to draw conclusions regarding the state of the art in the area of focus. The synthesis of the data can be accomplished in several different ways (Glass, McGaw, & Smith, 1981; Hunter & Schmidt, 1990). The consumer of research should note that a researcher who conducts a metaanalysis does not conduct the original analysis of data in the area but rather takes the data from already published studies and synthesizes the information by following a set of controlled and systematic steps. Metaanalysis can be used to synthesize both descriptive and experimental research studies (Reynolds, Timmerman, Anderson, & Sabol Stevenson, 1992). Only recently have studies of this nature become more prevalent in nursing research. An example of a nursing metaanalysis was conducted by Brown (1992). Brown took data from 73 studies on diabetes patient education literature and used mataanalysis techniques to determine the influence of study/subject characteristics, such as study quality and age of subjects, on patient outcomes, such as patient knowledge and self-management skills, weight loss, glycosylated hemoglobin level, and psychological outcomes.

Another example of a metaanalysis was conducted by Brown and Grimes (1993). This study conducted for the American Nurses Association analysized 38 studies of nurse practitioners and 15 studies of certified nurse midwives, using phy-

Table 10-2   Common Considerations in the Development
of Measurement Tools

Consideration	Example
The well-constructed scale, test, interview schedule, or other form of index should consist of an objective, standardized measure of samples of a behavior that has been clearly defined. Observations should be made on a small but carefully chosen sampling of the behavior of interest, thus permitting us to feel confident that the samples are representative.	In their study of pressure sore risk, Bergstrom et al. (1987) selected six factors that were assessed as being representative of "pressure sore risk" as it had been defined. The basis for the decision was findings from a thorough review of previous theoretical and research literature.
The tool should be *standardized;* that is, a set of uniform items and response possibilities that are uniformly administered and scored.	In the studies by Bergstrom et al. (1987) the evaluation of pressure sore risk consisted of objective assessment by research nurses in various settings. Without specific criteria and ratings for the observed behaviors, the evaluations would be based on the nurses' subjective impressions, which may have varied significantly between observers and conditions.
The items of a measurement tool should be unambiguous; they should be clear-cut, concise, exact statements with only one idea per item. Negative stems or items with negatively phrased response possibilities result in a double negative and ambiguity in meaning and scoring.	In constructing a tool to measure job satisfaction, a nurse-scientist writes the following items, "I never feel that I don't have time to provide good nursing care." The response format consists of "Agree," "Undecided," and "Disagree." It is very likely that a response of "Disagree" will not reflect the respondent's true intent because of the confusion that is created by the double negatives.
The type of items used in any one test or scale should be restricted to a limited number of variations. Subjects who are expected to shift from one kind of item to another may fail to provide a true response as a result of the distraction of making such a change.	Mixing true-or-false items with questions that require a yes-or-no response and items that provide a response format of five possible answers is conducive to a high level of measurement error.
Items should not provide irrelevant clues. Unless carefully constructed, an item may furnish an indication of the expected response or answer. Furthermore the correct answer or expected response to one item should not be given by another item.	An item that provides a clue to the expected answer may contain value words that convey cultural expectations, such as, "A good wife enjoys caring for her home and family."

Table 10-2   Common Considerations in the Development
of Measurement Tools—cont'd

Consideration	Example
The items of a measurement tool should not be made difficult by requiring unnecessarily complex or exact operations. Furthermore, the difficulty of an item should be appropriate to the level of the subjects being assessed. Limiting each item to one concept or idea helps to accomplish this objective.	A test constructed to evaluate learning in an introductory course in research methods may contain an item that is inappropriate for the designated group, such as, "A nonlinear transformation of data to linear data is a useful procedure before testing a hypothesis of curvilinearity."
The diagnostic, predictive, or measurement value of a tool depends on the degree to which it serves as an indicator of a relatively broad and significant area of behavior known as the *universe of content* for the behavior. As already emphasized, a behavior must be clearly defined before it can be measured. The definition is developed from the universe of content; that is, the information and research findings that are available for the behavior of interest. The items should reflect that definition. To what extent the test items appear to accomplish this objective is an indication of the validity of the instrument.	Two nurse researchers, A and B, are studying the construct of patient satisfaction. Each has defined this construct in a different way. Consequently, the measurement tool that each nurse devises will include different questions. The questions on each tool will reflect the universe of content for patient satisfaction as defined by each researcher.
The instrument should also adequately cover the defined behavior. The primary consideration is whether the number and nature of items in the sample are adequate. If there are too few items, the accuracy or reliability of the measure must be questioned. In general, there should be a minimum of 10 items for each independent aspect of the behavior of interest.	Very few people would be satisfied with an assessment of such traits as intelligence if the scales were limited to three items.
The measure must prove its worth empirically through tests of reliability and validity.	A researcher should demonstrate to the reader that scale is accurate and measures what it purports to measure (see Chapter 15).

sician care as the standard for comparison. In the area of clinical outcomes, nurses achieved equivalent outcomes or scored more favorably than physicians on many variables explored. Studies like the two examples can provide nurses with a synthesis and integration of research findings in an area and provide indicators of future research needs.

CRITIQUING NONEXPERIMENTAL DESIGNS

Criteria for critiquing nonexperimental designs are presented in the box on p. 249. When critiquing nonexperimental research designs the consumer should keep in mind that such designs offer the researcher the least amount of control. The first step in critiquing nonexperimental research is to determine which type of design was used in the study. Often a statement describing the design of the study appears in the abstract and in the methods section of the report. If such a statement is not present, the reader should closely examine the paper for evidence of which type of design was employed. The reader should be able to discern that either a survey or interrelationship design was used, as well as the specific subtype. For example, the reader would expect an investigation of self-concept development in children from birth to 5 years of age to be an interrelationship study using a longitudinal design.

Next, the critiquer should evaluate the theoretical framework and underpinnings of the study to determine if a nonexperimental design was the most appropriate approach to the problem. For example, the numerous mother-infant attachment studies discussed throughout this text are all theoretically suggestive of a nonmanipulable interrelationship between attachment and any of the independent variables under consideration. As such, a nonexperimental correlational, longitudinal, or cross-sectional design is suggested by these studies. Investigators will use one of these designs to examine the relationship between the variables in naturally occurring groups. Sometimes the reader may think that it would have been more appropriate if the investigators had used an experimental or quasiexperimental design. However, the reader must recognize that pragmatic or ethical considerations may also have guided the researchers in their choice of design (see Chapters 8 and 13).

Then the evaluator should assess whether the problem is at a level of experimental manipulation. Many times researchers merely wish to examine if relationships exist between variables. Therefore when one critiques such studies, the purpose of the study should be determined. If the purpose of the study does not include describing a cause-and-effect relationship, the researcher should not be criticized for not looking for one. However, the evaluator should be wary of a nonexperimental study in which the researcher suggests a cause-and-effect relationship in the findings.

Finally, the factor(s) that actually influence changes in the dependent variable are often ambiguous in nonexperimental designs. As with all complex phenomena, multiple factors can contribute to variability in the subjects' responses. When an experimental design is not used for controlling some of these extraneous variables that can influence results, the researcher must strive to provide as much control of them as possible within the context of a nonexperimental design. For example, when it

CRITIQUING CRITERIA

1. Which nonexperimental design is utilized in the study?
2. Based on the theoretical framework, is the rationale for the type of design evident?
3. How is the design congruent with the purpose of the study?
4. Is the design appropriate for the research problem?
5. Is the design suited to the data collection methods?
6. Does the researcher present the findings in a manner that is congruent with the utilized design?
7. Does the research go beyond the relational parameters of the findings and erroneously infer cause-and-effect relationships between the variables?
8. Are there any reasons to believe that there are alternative explanations for the findings?
9. Where appropriate, how does the researcher discuss the threats to internal and external validity?
10. How does the author deal with the limitations of the study?

has not been possible to randomly assign subjects to treatment groups as an approach to controlling an independent variable, the researcher may use a strategy of matching subjects for identified variables. For example, in a study of infant birth weight, pregnant women could be matched on variables such as weight, height, smoking habits, drug use, and other factors that might influence birthweight. The independent variable of interest, such as the type of prenatal care, would then be the major difference in the groups. The reader would then feel more confident that the only real difference between the two groups was the differential effect of the independent variable, because the other factors in the two groups were theoretically the same. However, the consumer should remember also that there may be other influential variables that were not matched, such as income, education, and diet. Rival factors represent a major influence on the interpretation of a nonexperimental study because they impose limitations on the generalizability of the results.

If the consumer is critiquing one of the additional types of research discussed, it is important first to identify the type of research used. Once the type of research is identified, its specific purpose and format need to be understood. The format and methods of methodological and metaanalysis vary; knowing how they vary allows a consumer to assess whether the process was applied appropriately.

Some of the basic principles of these methods were presented. The specific criteria for evaluating these designs are beyond the scope of this text, but the references provided will assist in this process. Even though the format and methods vary, it is important to remember that all research has a central goal: to answer questions scientifically.

KEY POINTS

- Nonexperimental research designs are used in studies that construct a picture or make an account of events as they naturally occur. The major difference between nonexperimental and experimental research is that in nonexperimental designs the independent variable is not actively manipulated by the investigator.
- Nonexperimental designs can be classified as either survey studies or interrelationship studies.
  - Survey research collects detailed descriptions of existing phenomena and uses the data either to justify current conditions and practices or to make more intelligent plans for improving them. Survey studies and interrelationship studies are both descriptive and exploratory in nature.
  - Interrelationship studies endeavor to explore the interrelationships between variables that provide deeper insight into the phenomena of interest.
- Correlational, ex post facto, prediction, and developmental studies are examples of interrelationship studies. Developmental studies are further broken down into categories of cross-sectional, longitudinal, retrospective, and prospective studies.
- Methodological and metaanalysis are examples of other means of adding to the body of nursing research. The advantages and disadvantages of each type of design must be considered by the researcher and critiquer when evaluating the merits of nonexperimental design.
- Nonexperimental research designs do not enable the investigator to establish cause-effect relationships between the variables. Consumers must be wary of nonexperimental studies that make causal claims about the findings unless a causal modeling technique is used.
- Nonexperimental designs also offer the researcher the least amount of control. Rival factors represent a major influence on the interpretation of a nonexperimental study because they impose limitations on the generalizability of the results and as such should be fully assessed by the critical reader.
- The critiquing process is directed toward evaluating the appropriateness of the selected nonexperimental design in relation to factors such as the research problem, theoretical framework, hypothesis, methodology, and the data analysis and interpretation.

REFERENCES

Asher, H.B. (1983). *Causal modeling* (2nd ed.). Beverly Hills, CA: Sage.
Bergstrom, N., Braden, B.J., Laguzza, A., & Holman, V. (1987). The Braden scale for predicting pressure sore risk. *Nursing Research, 36,* 205-210.

Brown, S.A. (1992). Meta-analysis of diabetes patient education research: Variations in intervention effects across studies. *Research in Nursing and Health, 15,* 409-420.

Brown, S.A., & Grimes, D. (1993). Study shows nurse practitioner care may rival physician primary care. *The American Nurse,* Jan/Feb, p. 3.

Campbell, D.T., & Stanley, J.C. (1963). *Experimental and quasi-experimental designs for research.* Chicago: Rand McNally.

Cole, F.L., & Slocumb, E.M. (1993). Nurse's attitudes toward patients with AIDS. *Advances in Nursing Science, 18,* 1112-1117.

Ferketich, S.L. & Verran, J.A. (1984). Residual analysis for causal model assumptions. *Western Journal of Nursing Research, 6*(1), 41-60.

Frank-Stromberg, M.F. (Ed.). (1992). *Instruments for clinical nursing research.* Boston: Jones and Bartlett.

Glass, G., McGaw, B., & Smith, M. (1981). *Meta-analysis in social research.* Newbury Park, CA: Sage.

Grey, M., Cameron, M.E., & Thurber, F.W. (1991). Coping and adaptation in children with diabetes. *Nursing Research, 40,* 144-149.

Hendrix, M.J., Sabritt, D., McDaniel, A., & Field, B. (1988). Perceptions and attitudes toward nursing impairment. *Research in Nursing & Health, 10,* 323-334.

Hunter, J.E., & Schmidt, F.L. (1990). *Methods of meta-analysis.* Newbury Park, CA: Sage.

Johansen, S., Bowles, S., & Haney, G. (1988). A model for forecasting intermittent skilled home nursing needs. *Research in Nursing & Health, 11,* 375-382.

Kerlinger, F.H. (1986). *Foundations of behavioral research* (3rd ed.). New York: Holt, Rinehart & Winston.

Klein, P.M. (1983). Contraceptive use and perceptions of chance and ability of conceiving in women electing abortion. *Journal of Obstetrics and Gynecology, 12,* 167-171.

Koniak-Griffin, D. (1988). The relationship between social support, self-esteem, and maternal-fetal attachment in adolescents. *Research in Nursing & Health, 11,* 269-278.

LoBiondo-Wood, G. (1985). The progression of physical symptoms in pregnancy and the development of maternal-fetal attachment. *Dissertation Abstracts International, 46,* 2625-B. (University Microfilms No. 85-21, 973.)

Mason, D.J., Jensen, M., & Boland, D.L. (1992). Health behaviors and health risks among homeless males in Utah. *Western Journal of Nursing Research, 14,* 775-787.

Mercer, R.T., Ferketich, S.L., & DeJoseph, J.E. (1993). Predictors of partner relationships during pregnancy and infancy. *Research In Nursing & Health, 16,* 45-46.

Mills, A.C., Sampel, M.E., Pohlman, V.C., & Becker, A.M. (1992). The odds for success on NCLEX-RN by nurse candidates from a four-year baccalaureate nursing program. *Journal of Nursing Education, 31*(9), 403-408.

Newman, M.A., & Gaudiano, J.K. (1984). Depression as an explanation for decreased subjective time in the elderly. *Nursing Research, 33,* 137-139.

Pedhazur, E.J., & Schmelkin, L.P. (1991). *Measurement, design, and analysis,* Hillsdale, NJ: Lawrence Erlbaum Associates.

Redeker, N.S. (1992). The relationship between uncertainty and coping after coronary bypass surgery. *Western Journal of Nursing Research, 14,* 48-60.

Reynolds, N.R., Timmerman, G., Anderson, J., & Sabol Stevenson, J. (1992). Meta-analysis for descriptive research. *Research in Nursing and Health, 15,* 467-476.

Schneider, E.M., & LoBiondo-Wood, G. (1992). Perceptions of procedural pain: Parents, nurses, and children. *Children's Health Care, 21,* 157-162.

Schraeder, B.D. (1993). Assessment of measures to detect preschool academic risk in very-low-birth-weight children. *Nursing Research, 42,* 17-21.

Shannahan, M.D., and Cottrell, B.H. (1985). Effect of the birth chair on duration of second-stage labor, fetal outcome and maternal blood loss, *Nursing Research, 34:* 89-92.

Stetler, C.B. (in press). Refinement of the Stetler/Marram model for application of research findings to practice, *Nursing Outlook.*

Strickland, O.L., and Waltz, C.F. (1988). *Measurement of nursing outcomes: measuring client outcomes,* vol. 1, New York, Springer Publishing Co.

Verran, J.A. & Ferketich, S.L. (1984). Residual analysis for statistical assumptions of regression equations. *Western Journal of Nursing Research. 6,* 1, 27-40.

Waltz, C.F., and Strickland, O.L. (1988). *Measurement of nursing outcomes: measuring client outcomes,* vol. 2, New York, Springer Publishing Co.

ADDITIONAL READINGS

Anastasi, A. (1988). *Psychological Testing* (6th ed.). New York: Macmillan Publishing Company.

Huck, S.W., and Sandler, H.M. (1979). *Rival hypotheses.* New York: Harper & Row.

Miller, D. (1991). *Handbook of Research Design and Social Measurement.* (5th ed.). Newbury CA.: Sage.

Waltz, C.F., and Bausell, R.B. (1991). *Nursing research: design, statistics and computer analysis.* Philadelphia: F.A. Davis.

11

Qualitative Approaches to Research

PATRICIA R. LIEHR
MARIANNE TAFT MARCUS

LEARNING OBJECTIVES

After reading this chapter the student should be able to do the following:

- Distinguish the characteristics of qualitative research from those of quantitative research.
- Recognize the uses of qualitative research for nursing.
- Identify the processes of phenomenological, grounded theory, ethnographic, and historical methods.
- Recognize nursing phenomena that lend themselves to use of case study methodology.
- Identify research methodology emerging from nursing theory.
- Discuss significant issues that arise in conducting qualitative research in relation to such topics as ethics, criteria for judging scientific rigor, combination of qualitative and quantitative approaches, and use of computer software to assist data management.
- Apply the critiquing criteria to evaluate a report of qualitative research.

KEY TERMS

axial coding	historical research method
bracketing	internal criticism
case study method	key informants
constant comparative method	life context
data saturation	lived experience
domains	phenomenological method
emic	primary sources
ethnographic method	qualitative research
etic	secondary sources
external criticism	symbolic interaction
grounded theory method	theoretical sampling

Nursing is both a science and an art. **Qualitative research** combines the scientific and artistic natures of nursing to enhance understanding of the human health experience. It is a general term encompassing a variety of philosophical underpinnings and research methods. Boyd (1990) provides a comprehensive definition: "Qualitative research involves broadly stated questions about human experiences and realities, studied through sustained contact with people in their natural environments, generating rich, descriptive data that help us to understand their experiences" (p. 183).

Over recent years, there has been heightened interest in qualitative research methods as recorded by an increasing number of reports of qualitative research in professional nursing journals. A review of four journals, *Advances in Nursing Science, Image, Nursing Research,* and *Research in Nursing and Health,* indicated that from 1988 until 1992, reports of qualitative research more than tripled (Fig. 11-1). This count included only full research reports (not abstracts or briefs) that were conducted by using inductive strategies. In Chapter 20, Streubert cites several other journals that significantly contribute to the growing number of qualitative research reports. So, this count does not conclusively reflect the total amount of qualitative research being done by nurses. It is offered merely as an example of an upward trend in established nursing publications.

According to Leininger (1992), there are more than 20 identified qualitative research methods. This chapter focuses on four methods most commonly used by nurses: **phenomenological, grounded theory, ethnographic,** and **historical.** Each of these methods, although distinct from the others, also shares characteristics that

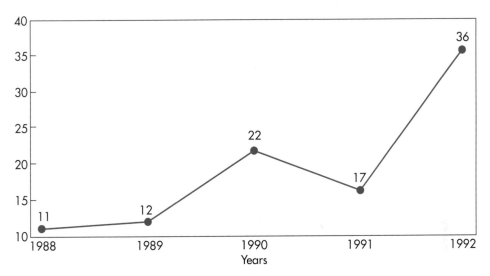

Fig. 11-1   Number of qualitative nursing research articles published in four journals *(Advances in Nursing Science, Image, Nursing Research,* and *Research in Nursing and Health)* from 1988 to 1992.

identify it as a method within the qualitative research approach. Some of the basic tenets distinguishing the qualitative from the quantitative approach are reviewed to establish a foundation before discussing qualitative methodologies. Use of the qualitative approach requires different beliefs, different research activities, and different questions from the use of the quantitative research approach. Table 11-1 (p. 256) compares the researcher's beliefs, activities, and questions when using the quantitative and qualitative approaches.

QUANTITATIVE AND QUALITATIVE RESEARCH APPROACHES
Beliefs

Chapter 2 introduces the reader to the quantitative approach in nursing research. Quantitative approaches are grounded by beliefs that humans are a composite of many body systems that can be objectively measured, one at a time or in combination. As one reads and critiques quantitative studies, it is often apparent that the researcher has focused on measuring one or more human characteristics (e.g., psychological, physiological, social), striving to isolate the characteristics of interest and gain a clear, context-free picture of what is studied. A context-free picture is achieved by eliminating or controlling variables that may interfere with the variables being studied.

In contrast, qualitative approaches embrace the wholeness of humans, focusing on human experience in naturalistic settings. The researcher using this approach believes that unique humans attribute meaning to their experiences and experiences

Table 11-1   Comparison of Researcher Beliefs, Activities, and Questions When Using Quantitative and Qualitative Approaches

	Quantitative	Qualitative
Researcher beliefs	• Humans are biopsychosocial beings, known by their biological, psychological, and social characteristics. • Truth is objective reality that can be experienced with the senses and measured by the researcher.	• Humans are complex beings who attribute unique meaning to their life situations. They are known by their personal expressions. • Truth is the subjective expression of reality as perceived by the participant and shared with the researcher. Truth is context-laden.
Researcher activities	• Researcher selects a representative (of population) sample and determines size before collecting data. • Researcher uses an extensive approach to collect data. • Questionnaires and measurement devices are preferably administered in one setting by an unbiased individual to control for extraneous variables. • Reliability and validity of instruments and internal and external validity permit judgment of scientific rigor. • Primarily deductive analysis is used, generating a numerical summary that allows the researcher to reject or accept the null hypothesis.	• Researcher selects participants who are experiencing the phenomenon of interest and collects data until saturation is reached. • Researcher uses an intensive approach to collect data. • Researcher conducts interviews and participant or nonparticipant observation in environments where participants usually spend their time. Researcher bias is acknowledged and set aside. • Creditability, auditability, fittingness, and conformability permit judgment of scientific rigor. • Primarily inductive analysis is used, leading to a narrative summary, which synthesizes participant information, creating a description of human experience.
Research questions	• What is the relationship between the incidence of maternity blues during the first week after birth and postpartum depression in primiparas at 1, 6, and 12 weeks postpartum? • What are the differences in the incidence and severity of maternity blues and postpartum depression for women experiencing early hospital discharge and those with customary lengths of hospital stay? (Beck, Reynolds & Rutowski, 1992)	• What is the essential structure of the lived experience of postpartum depression? (Beck, 1992)

evolve from life context. **Life context** is the matrix of human—human-environment relationships emerging over the course of day-to-day living. From this perspective, one person's experience of pain is distinct from another's and can be known by the individual's subjective description of it.

The researcher interested in studying the lived experience of pain for the adolescent with rheumatoid arthritis will spend time in the adolescent's natural settings, such as home and school, to uncover the meaning of pain as it extends beyond the facts of the number of medications taken or a rating on a Likert scale. This approach is grounded in the belief that factual objective data do not capture the human experience. Rather, the meaning of the adolescent's pain emerges within the context of personal history, current relationships, and future plans as the individual lives daily life in dynamic interaction with environment. That is, the experience of pain is believed to be a unique personal experience that is context-laden.

Research Activities

The activities of the researcher using the quantitative approach are discussed throughout Part 2 of this book. Table 11-1 contrasts some of these familiar activities with those used in the qualitative approach. Rather than determining sample size before initiation of the study, data collection is terminated when saturation is reached. **Data saturation** occurs when the information being shared with the researcher becomes repetitive. That is, the ideas conveyed by the participant have been shared before by other participants; inclusion of additional participants does not result in new ideas. Generally, the number of participants, when using the qualitative approach, is smaller than the number of subjects needed when using the quantitative approach. Fewer subjects are intensively studied (qualitative) as compared with a larger number extensively studied (quantitative).

The research activities of each approach reflect the previously discussed beliefs about the importance of context. Whereas quantitative approaches strive to eliminate extraneous variables, qualitative approaches explore all dimensions of human uniqueness that may aid the researcher in understanding the meaning of the experience for the participant. The researcher is the major instrument, conducting interviews, observing, and gathering data. The researcher's unique interaction in the participant's setting contributes to the meaning uncovered. It is the researcher's responsibility to recognize personal biases and set them aside. Researcher bias will color what is learned by covertly directing observation and interview, as well as shading interpretation of the data. The researcher goes where the data lead.

In spite of this rigorous attention to the researcher as an instrument, what a participant shares with one researcher may not be exactly what would be shared with another. This subjective expression cocreated by researcher and participant is in contrast to the objective measurement valued by quantitative approaches.

The researcher using the qualitative approach begins collecting bits of information and piecing them together, building a mosaic or a picture of the human experience being studied. As with a mosaic, when one steps away from the work, the whole picture emerges. This whole picture transcends the bits and pieces and cannot be known from any one bit or piece. In presenting the narrative summary, the researcher strives to capture the human experience and present it so that others can understand it. This inductive analysis contrasts with the primarily deductive analysis used in quantitative approaches. Deductive analysis begins with a picture and seeks to explore pieces of the picture by testing the relationship of one piece with another.

Research Questions

The choice to use either quantitative or qualitative methods is guided by the research question. Generally, questions that suggest a test of relationship or difference are addressed through a quantitative approach. Questions that suggest an exploration of a human experience are addressed through a qualitative approach. The questions noted in Table 11-2 were posed by the same researcher, Cheryl Tatano Beck, about postpartum depression. When using a quantitative approach, Beck, Reynolds, and Rutowski (1992) raised a question of relationship between variables (maternity blues and postpartum depression) and a question of difference between groups (early discharge versus customary discharge). In contrast, when using a qualitative approach, Beck (1992) was interested in the lived experience of postpartum depression. Table 11-2 compares the two studies, highlighting the previously discussed differences in quantitative and qualitative approaches.

In each of these studies, Beck used a different research approach to study the same topic, postpartum depression. She was guided by her research questions. In each instance, she embraced a different set of values and activities to add to the body of nursing knowledge of postpartum depression. Clearly, no nurse is either a quantitative or a qualitative researcher. Although most nurse researchers tend to use one or the other research approach repeatedly, their choice of approach is guided by their questions.

THE QUALITATIVE APPROACH AND NURSING SCIENCE

Qualitative research is particularly well suited to study the human experience of health, a central concern of nursing science. Because qualitative methods focus on the whole of human experience and the meanings ascribed by individuals living the experience, these methods permit broader understanding and deeper insight into complex human behaviors than what might be obtained from surveys or other linear measures of perceptions (Lincoln, 1992). Two examples are cited to emphasize the capacity of qualitative methods to guide nursing practice and to contribute to instrument and theory development.

Morgan and Laing (1991) explored the meaning of a diagnosis of Alzheimer's disease for caregiving spouses. This was done through a series of unstructured and semistructured interviews carried out in the participants' homes. Two major themes, grief and role strain, emerged to illuminate the lived world of these individuals. In-depth exploration of the themes revealed that the caregivers' past relationship with their spouse influenced their attitudes toward caregiving. Spouses whose marriages had been intimate and stable mourned the loss of that re-

Table 11-2 Comparison of Two Studies Examining Postpartum Depression: The Quantitative and Qualitative Approaches

	Maternity blues and postpartum depression	The lived experience of postpartum depression: a phenomenological study
Subjects	$n = 49$ primiparous American-born women who had uncomplicated pregnancies and vaginal deliveries	$n = 7$ mothers who attended a local postpartum depression support group; 4 were primaparous, and 3 were multiparous; 4 had vaginal and 3 had cesarean deliveries
Data collectors	Four trained research assistants who had no health-related education to "ensure that they would not become confounding variables"	The researcher was the data collector (see Instruments)
Instruments	Stein's Maternity Blues Scale, a 13-symptom self-rated scale with acceptable reliability and validity; Beck Depression Inventory, measuring 21 categories of symptoms and attitudes and reporting well-established reliability and validity	Researcher interviewed the subjects and scheduled follow-up interviews to be sure that participants agreed with her interpretation of their experiences; before each interview the researcher recalled and transcended her biases to capture the participant's reality
Analysis/summary	Deductive analysis was accomplished through inferential statistics: "No significant differences were found at 1, 6, and 12 weeks postpartum in the mean depression scores for mothers who were discharged after the customary length of hospital stay"	Inductive analysis was conducted by using the phenomenological method; the meaning of participants' descriptions was distilled and synthesized into 11 themes, including loneliness, obsessive thoughts of being a bad mom, fear and guilt over pondering harming infant, inability to concentrate, and insecurity leading to a need to be mothered herself

lationship with their partner. Those whose previous relationship had not been stable experienced a high level of distress and strain in their new caregiving role. Although grief and role strain are not new concepts when thinking about individuals and families experiencing Alzheimer's disease, their relationship to the historical context of the marriage provides new insight into the meaning of caregiving.

The results of Morgan and Laing's work (1991), or of any study of individuals living with health changes, may effectively communicate insights that contribute to high-quality nursing care. Thus qualitative nursing studies generate rich, descriptive data and promote increased sensitivity to the health experiences of others. Information obtained from in-depth qualitative studies may also provide the researcher with descriptive categories that can be used to construct a quantitative instrument—one that is based on subjects' actual experiences rather than the judgment of outsiders.

Qualitative studies also may serve the purpose of conceptualization or theory development. Hutchinson (1986) used the grounded theory method to generate a substantive theory that explains the process by which nurses become chemically dependent. Data collection was extensive and included interviewing nurses in recovery, reading case histories of nurses who had been required to appear before the board of nursing, attending board of nursing hearings, observing meetings of nurses in a self-help group, and accompanying a nurse investigator on her rounds to do urine checks on nurses in recovery. After this protracted period of data collection, Hutchinson constructed a theory that describes a trajectory of self-annihilation taken by nurses who become chemically dependent in the midst of living with pain.

Qualitative methods have direct relevance to nursing practice in that they move beneath the surface of outcomes, such as chemical dependency, to uncover life processes that contributed to the outcome. A knowledge of these life processes increases understanding and provides a basis for intervention that may enhance quality of life (Munhall, 1992). For instance, description of the life processes that precede the use of such substances as alcohol and other drugs could provide valuable information to guide nursing intervention.

FOUR QUALITATIVE RESEARCH METHODS

Thus far an overview distinguishing the quantitative from the qualitative research approach has been presented. The contribution of qualitative study to nursing science has been introduced. These topics provide a foundation for examining the four qualitative methods discussed in this chapter. The phenomenological, grounded theory, ethnographic, and historical methods are briefly contrasted in Table 11-3. More detailed comparison of these methods is provided for the consumer of nursing research throughout this chapter. Parse, Coyne, and Smith (1985) suggested that research methods, whether quantitative or qualitative, include five basic elements:
1. Identifying the phenomenon
2. Structuring the study
3. Gathering the data
4. Analyzing the data
5. Describing the findings (p. 16)

Each qualitative method is defined, followed by a discussion of these five basic elements. The factors that distinguish the methods are highlighted, and research examples are presented, providing critiquing direction for the beginning research consumer.

Table 11-3 Comparison of Qualitative Methods: Essence, Foundation, and Questions

Method	Essence of method	Foundation	Example questions from published studies
Phenomenological	Description of the "lived experience"	Philosophy	What is it like to be a provider of care in the NICU? (Swanson, 1990) What are the essential features of self-transcendence in women with advanced breast cancer? (Coward, 1990)
Grounded theory	Systematic set of procedures used to arrive at theory about basic social processes	Symbolic interaction and the social sciences	How do caregivers of family members with Alzheimer's disease experience bereavement? (Jones & Martinson, 1992) How do patients with AIDS manage their illness? (Ragsdale, Kotorba, & Morrow, 1992)
Ethnographic	Descriptions of cultural groups or subgroups	Cultural anthropology	How do nurses from various health care settings perceive collaboration between indigenous and cosmopolitan health care systems? (Uphall, 1992) What is the meaning of wellness to aging individuals? What factors contribute to wellness and aging? (Miller, 1991)
Historical	Systematic compilation of data to describe some past event	Philosophy, art, and science	How did philosophy, training methods, and settings establish the foundation of nursing education in America? (Davis, 1991) How did nurses actively influence the development of ICUs through observation and triage, as well as seeking out necessary knowledge? (Fairman, 1992)

Phenomenological Method

The **phenomenological method** is a process of learning and constructing the meaning of human experience through intensive dialogue with persons who are living the experience. According to Powers and Knapp (1990), phenomenology is a way of thinking about what life experiences are like for people. It is an investigation of the lived experience.

Phenomenology has its roots in philosophy. Breatano (Powers & Knapp, 1990) planted the seeds, which were cultivated by his student, Husserl. Husserl (Jennings, 1986) developed the phenomenological method of inquiry, in part as a response to the popular philosophers of the time who believed that experimental methods could be used to study all human phenomena. These philosophers focused on objectivity and what could be observed as a basis for establishing truth. Husserl was driven to establish a rigorous science that found truth in the lived experience.

Identifying the Phenomenon

Because the focus of the phenomenological method is the lived experience, the researcher is likely to choose this method when studying some dimension of day-to-day existence for a particular group of individuals. For instance, the nurse may be interested in the experience of hope for the patient who has cancer or the experience of anger for persons who have heart disease. Sowell, Bramlett, Gueldner, Gritzmacher, and Martin (1991) studied the lived experience of survival and bereavement after the death of a lover from acquired immunodeficiency syndrome (AIDS). Their research report is used to guide the reader's understanding of the phenomenological method.

Structuring the Study

For the purpose of describing structuring, the following topics are addressed: the research question, the researcher's perspective, and sample selection. The issue of human subjects' protection has been suggested as a dimension of structuring (Parse et al., 1985); this issue is discussed generally with ethics in a subsequent section of the chapter.

Research question. Research questions that warrant the use of the phenomenological method are those that query the lived experience, such as "What is the experience of hope for persons who have cancer?" or "How do persons who have heart disease experience anger?" When the question is asked of the participant, it frequently takes the form of a statement. For instance, Sowell et al. (1991) phrased their request for information in this way: "Please describe your experience of losing a lover to AIDS. Describe events and feelings which you experienced both prior to and after the death of your lover" (p. 91).

Researcher's perspective. When using the phenomenological method, the researcher's perspective is **bracketed.** That is, the researcher identifies personal biases about the phenomenon of interest to clarify how personal experience and beliefs may color what is heard and reported. The researcher is expected to set aside personal biases—to bracket them—when engaged with the participants. By becoming aware of personal biases, the researcher is more likely to be able to pursue issues of importance introduced by the participant, rather than leading the participant to issues deemed important by the researcher.

According to their review of literature, Sowell et al. (1991) concluded that the loss of a lover affected the health of the survivor. They presented theories of grief and bereavement that established a basis for the study and influenced their ideas. Thus they made their values explicit, allowing the reader to identify how their perspective may influence the study.

Sample selection. The reader of a phenomenological study report will find that the selected sample will be living the experience the researcher is querying. Sowell and colleagues recruited participants from community groups who provided services to persons with AIDS and their significant others. Sometimes the experience of interest will have occurred in the participant's past. Because phenomenologists believe that each individual's history is a dimension of the present, a past experience will exist in the present moment. For instance, the participants in the Sowell et al. study had experienced the death of their lover in the past. The researchers asked participants to recall events and feelings before and after the death of their lover. The critiquer will notice that the researcher using the phenomenological method is collecting remembered information from the participant.

Data Gathering

Written or oral data may be collected when using the phenomenological method. The researcher may pose the query in writing and ask for a written response or may schedule a time to interview the participant and tape record the interaction. In either case the researcher may return to ask for clarification of written or tape recorded transcripts. To some extent, the particular data collection strategy is guided by the choice of specific analysis technique. If the van Kaam technique is used, a large number of written descriptions will be collected; if the Colaizzi technique is used, a small number of interviews will be transcribed (Boyd, 1990).

Sowell et al. (1991) used the Colaizzi technique. They taped interviews, which were then transcribed for analysis. A unique approach to data collection was included by allowing each participant to select his or her interviewer from a list that identified the gender and geographic location of the researcher. This selection encouraged comfortable disclosure by the participant.

Data Analysis

There are several techniques for data analysis when using the phenomenological method. For detailed information about specific techniques, the critiquer is referred to original sources (Spiegelberg, 1976; van Kaam, 1969; Colaizzi, 1978; Giorgi et al., 1975). Although the techniques are slightly different from each other, there is a general pattern of moving from the participant's description to the researcher's synthesis of all participants' descriptions. The steps generally include the following:

1. Thorough reading and sensitive presence with the entire transcription of the participant's description

2. Identification of shifts in participant thought resulting in division of the transcription into thought segments
3. Specification of the significant phrases in each thought segment, using the words of the participant
4. Distillation of each significant phrase to express the central meaning of the segment in the words of the researcher
5. Preliminary synthesis of central meanings of all thought segments for each participant with a focus on the essence of the phenomenon being studied
6. Final synthesis of the essences that have surfaced in all participants' descriptions, resulting in an exhaustive description of the **lived experience**

Sowell et al. (1991) began with the words of their participants about losing their lover. An example of a participant's significant phrase was "Well, it's just not real. It's not happening; it's just motion, and if you do enough motion you stay real busy and you go to sleep" (p. 91). The central meaning of the phrase was distilled by the researchers: "The individual feels discomfort from the meaning, grasping only the mechanical reality of the activities" (p. 91). The essences of the phenomenon were presented as themes and included "disconnectedness from self" as one of several. All themes were synthesized to describe the dimensions of the lived experience of losing a lover to AIDS: isolation/disconnectedness, emotional confusion, and acceptance/denial.

Describing the Findings

When using the phenomenological method, the researcher provides the reader with a path of information leading from the research question, through samples of participant's significant phrases, researcher's interpretation, and leading to the final synthesis that elaborates the lived experience. One paragraph from the Sowell et al. paper exemplifies the synthesis relating the lived experience.

> The individual who loses a lover to AIDS experiences intense and ambivalent feelings and emotions. They are faced with the potential of isolation and disconnection from their friends, their family, their lover's family and even from themselves. This isolation frequently becomes a reality. They may be unsure of their support system and often feel removed even from themselves by going through the motions of life, yet feeling no connection to it. (p. 93)

When reading the report of a phenomenological study, the critiquer will find that detailed descriptive language is used to convey the complex meaning of the lived experience.

Grounded Theory Method

The critiquer who is assessing a study that uses the **grounded theory method** finds an inductive approach that implements a systematic set of procedures to arrive at theory about basic social processes. The emergent theory is based on, or connected to, observations and perceptions of the social scene (Crabtree & Miller, 1992). The aim of the grounded theory approach is to discover underlying social forces that shape human behavior (Thorne, 1991). This method is used to construct theory where no theory exists or in situations when existing theory fails to explain a set of circumstances.

Symbolic interaction is the theoretical base for grounded theory. Symbolic interactionist tradition holds that the relationship between self and society is an ongoing process of symbolic communication, whereby individuals create a social reality. George Herbert Mead, social psychologist, is credited with originating this tradition in the early twentieth century (Powers & Knapp, 1990).

Glaser and Strauss (1967) developed the systematic approach to the study of interactions, known as the *grounded theory method,* to bridge a perceived gap between theory and research and the consequent undervaluing of qualitative studies. In this method, theory remains closely connected to data through descriptive examples that provide direct empirical evidence that the theory fits the phenomenon under investigation. Theory generated in this manner may then serve as a conceptual framework on which to base a testable hypothesis and subsequent quantitative studies (Powers & Knapp, 1990).

Developed originally as a sociologist's tool to investigate interactions in social settings, the grounded theory method, or procedure, is not bound to that discipline. Investigators from different disciplines may study the same phenomenon from varying perspectives (Strauss & Corbin, 1990). As an example, in an area of study such as chronic illness, a nurse might be interested in coping patterns within families, a psychologist in personal adjustment, and a sociologist in group behavior in health care settings (Strauss & Corbin, 1990). Theory generated by each discipline will reflect the discipline and will serve the discipline in explaining the phenomenon.

Identifying the Phenomenon

Researchers typically use the grounded theory method when they are interested in social processes from the perspective of human interactions. The basic social process, or core category that is the foundation of a theory, is often expressed as a gerund, indicating change across time as social reality is negotiated. For example, Bright (1992) studied *making place,* or the evolutionary process that occurs when a newborn receives recognition in an intergenerational family context. Price's study, which began as an investigation of uncertainty during chronic illness, will be elaborated as a way of introducing the research consumer to the grounded theory method.

Structuring the Study

Research question. Research questions appropriate for the grounded theory method are those that question a basic social process. They tend to be action- or change-oriented, such as "How does the family as an intergenerational system respond to the birth of the first grandchild?" (Bright, 1992, p. 81). In a grounded theory study, the research question can be a statement or a broad question that permits in-depth explanation of the phenomenon. For instance, the reader will recognize Price's question implied in the statement that her study addressed: "How patients learn self management through applying diabetes information and how they adapt it to their lives" (Price, 1993, p. 32).

Researchers' perspective. The grounded theorist is interested in providing a study of the processes that occur as individuals interact with others in the social setting in response to life circumstances. The researcher will bring some knowledge of the literature to the study, but the critiquer will notice that an exhaustive literature review is not done. This allows theory to emerge directly from data. For example, Price (1993) notes that other studies of self-management of diabetes use a priori models related to compliance, behavior modification, or cognitive style to explain and predict patient behaviors. However, the current study (Price, 1993) provides a description of factors and processes that emerge as diabetes self-management is learned. Price (1993) indicates that self-management was examined from the patients' perspective, but such factors as social circumstances and doctors' orders are investigated to provide sufficient depth for theory generation. Thus grounded theory is more likely to be sensitive to contextual values and not merely to the researcher's values (Lincoln & Guba, 1985).

Another important aspect of the researcher's perspective is concern that theory remain connected to or "grounded in" the data. As noted, Price (1993) initially intended to study the concept of uncertainty within chronic illness as experienced by adults in an outpatient setting. However, as the data emerged, the concept of uncertainty was found to be subsumed by the broader central theme, learning self-management.

Sample selection. Sample selection involves choosing participants who are experiencing the circumstance, and selecting events and incidents related to the social process under investigation. Price recruited adult diabetics through a diabetes newsletter distributed in the area. Enrollment criteria required that the participants be diagnosed with diabetes mellitus for at least 1 year but no longer than 10 years. All of the 18 subjects required two or more injections of insulin daily, and all were monitoring their own blood glucose level. Thus the participants had a period for learning and they had specific activities or tasks that were required for self-management. Price also describes other factors or variables, such as age, education, marital status, and whether the participants were involved in support groups or had attended formal diabetes education classes.

Data Gathering

In the grounded theory method, the critiquer will find that data are collected through interviews and through skilled observations of individuals interacting in a social setting. Interviews are audiotaped and then transcribed, and observations are recorded as field notes. Open-ended questions are used initially to identify concepts.

Price (1993) interviewed each participant twice for approximately 2 hours each time. Most of the interviews were in the participants' homes. The interview questions were based on the researcher's clinical experience and focused on aspects of uncertainty. Questions were developed "to probe the areas of diagnosis, treatment, prognosis, and perceived disruptions of body changes and social interactions due to chronic disease" (p. 34). Examples of questions include the following:

- "What about diabetes worries you the most?"
- "What about diabetes is/remains puzzling or confusing? Are those things *always* confusing or puzzling?"

- "Are there other areas of uncertainties or unknowns that you often have to deal with that we have not talked about?" (p. 34)

Data Analysis

A major feature of the grounded theory method is that data collection and analysis occur simultaneously. The process requires systematic, detailed record keeping using field notes and transcribed interview tapes. Hunches about emerging patterns in the data are noted in memos, and the researcher directs activities in the field by pursuing these hunches. This technique, called **theoretical sampling,** is used to select experiences that will help the researcher test ideas and gather complete information about developing concepts. The researcher begins by noting indicators or actual events, actions, or words in the data. Concepts, or abstractions, are developed from the indicators (Strauss, 1987).

The initial analytic process is called *open coding* (Strauss, 1987). Data are examined carefully line by line, broken down into discrete parts, and compared for similarities and differences (Strauss & Corbin, 1990). Data are compared with other data continuously as they are acquired during research. This is a process called the **constant comparative method.** Codes in the data are clustered to form categories. The categories are expanded and developed or collapsed into one another. Theory is constructed through this systematic process. As a result, data collection, analysis, and theory generation have a direct reciprocal relationship (Strauss & Corbin, 1990).

Related literature, both technical and nontechnical, is reviewed continuously throughout data collection and analysis. All literature is treated as data and is compared with the researchers' developing theory as it progresses. When critiquing a study using grounded theory, expect to find, at the end of the report, the researcher's grounded theory formally related to and incorporated with existing knowledge.

Price (1993) described data analysis in her study. Phrases, or indicators, in the data included the following:

- "I *trust my body* about 90% of the time."
- "I feel like I am fairly *well tuned in* to *my body.*"
- "I am always *listening,* running checks on how I feel; there is *never a time that I am not thinking about it.*" (p. 35)

These phrases were coded as "body trust" and "body listening." Through an intense coding process around a single theme called **axial coding,** "body listening" was developed in depth. The researcher noted when "body listening" occurred and what physical cues were monitored. The theme "body listening" was central to the process under investigation and was elevated to the status of a category, "experiencing body changes through 'body listening' " Through the next process, selective coding, 11 categories were collapsed into 4 major categories: personal considerations, monitoring, cognitive skills, and control. Through this rigorous process and further consultation with the subjects, the core category was identified as "learning self-management of diabetes." A model depicting the sequential steps in the process was described, and the four factors were found to be operative at each stage of the model and to be important to the direction of movement between the stages.

Describing the Findings

Grounded theory studies are reported in sufficient detail to provide the reader with the steps in the process and the logic of the method. Price (1993) takes the reader through the steps of data collection, theoretical sampling, constant comparisons, and three levels of coding to a schematic model that depicts the process. Reports of grounded theory studies use descriptive language to assure that the theory reported in the findings remains connected to the data.

Ethnographic Method

The **ethnographic method** focuses on scientific descriptions of cultural groups. The critiquer should know that the goal of the ethnographer is to understand the natives' view of their world or the **emic** view. The emic, or insiders', view is contrasted to the **etic,** or outsiders', view obtained when the researcher uses quantitative analyses of behavior (Parse et al., 1985; Powers & Knapp, 1990). The ethnographic approach requires that the researcher enter the world of the study participants to watch what happens, listen to what is said, ask questions, and collect whatever data are available (Boyle, 1991). The term *ethnography* is used to mean both the research technique and the product of that technique, the study itself (Hughes, 1992).

Sanday (1989) notes that ethnography is at least as old as the work of Herodotus, the ancient Greek ethnographer, who recorded the infinite variety and strangeness he saw in other cultures. Modern ethnographic tradition is based in cultural anthropology and the works of Malinowski (1922), Mead (1928), and Boas (1948). Thorne (1991) indicates that nurses have used the method to study cultural variations in health and to study patient groups as subcultures within larger social contexts.

Identifying the Phenomenon

The critiquer may expect that the phenomenon in an ethnographic study will vary in scope from a long-term study of a very complex culture, such as that of the Aborigines, to a shorter-term study of a phenomenon within subunits of cultures, such as promoting wellness in aged persons (Miller, 1991), nursing collaboration with indigenous healers in Swaziland (Uphall, 1992), the expanded role of first-line nurse managers (Everson-Bates, 1992), or the health experience of Afghan refugees in Northern California (Lipson, 1991). Kleinman (1992) notes the clinical utility of ethnography in describing the "local world" of groups of patients who are experiencing a particular phenomenon, such as suffering (p. 127). The local worlds of patients have cultural, political, economic, institutional, and social-relational dimensions in much the same way that larger complex societies have these units of analysis. Mayo's (1992) study of the phenomenon of lifelong patterns of physical activity among African-American women is used as an example throughout the presentation of ethnography.

Structuring the Study

The research question. When reviewing the report of ethnographic research, notice that questions are asked about lifeways or particular patterns of behavior within the social context of a culture or subculture. Culture is viewed as the system of knowledge and linguistic expressions used by social groups that allows the researcher to interpret or make sense of their world (Aamodt, 1991). Ethnographic nursing studies address questions that concern how cultural knowledge, norms, values, and other contextual variables influence one's health experience. Uphall (1992, p. 27) asked, "How do nurses from various health care settings (government, private, missions, industrial and nongovernmental organizations) perceive collaboration between indigenous and cosmopolitan health care systems?" Other possible ethnographic questions include "What does comforting mean in Hispanic families?" "What are patient and nurse roles like in intensive care units?" "What are the meanings of health and illness care to migrant workers?" Often the research question is implied in the purpose statement. As an example, Mayo (1992) constructed her study to ask, "What are the lifelong patterns of physical activity among black working women?"

Researchers' perspective. When using the ethnographic method, the researcher's perspective is that of an interpreter entering an alien world and attempting to make sense of that world from the insider's point of view (Agar, 1986). Like phenomenologists and grounded theorists, ethnographers make their own beliefs explicit and bracket, or set aside, their personal biases as they seek to understand the world view of others (Parse et al., 1985). Mayo (1992) identifies the cultural-ecological orientation as the frame of reference for her study of the physical activity practices of African-American working women. This perspective holds that definitions of health are derived by cultural groups using scientific information, common sense, and personal experience (Kleinman, 1980). Mayo (1992) further notes, "Despite the widespread availability of information about the health promoting benefits of physical activity more than one half of all American women and two thirds of African-American women are sedentary" (p. 318).

Sample selection. The ethnographer selects a cultural group who are living the phenomenon under investigation (Parse et al., 1985). The researcher gathers information from general informants and from key informants. **Key informants** are individuals who have special knowledge, status, or communication skills, and who are willing to teach the ethnographer about the phenomenon (Crabtree & Miller, 1992). Mayo (1992) initiated contact with potential informants through personal directors, occupational health nurses, and professional acquaintances. She conducted 51 unstructured interviews and identified a study group of 24 African-American working women.

Data Gathering

Ethnographic data gathering involves participant observation or immersion in the setting, informant interviews, and interpretation by the researcher of cultural patterns (Crabtree & Miller, 1992). According to Boyle (1991), ethnographic research in nursing as in other disciplines always involves "face-to-face interviewing, with data collection and analysis taking place in the natural setting" (p. 276). Thus field work is a major focus of the method. Other techniques may include obtaining life histories and collecting material items reflective of the culture. Photographs and films of the informants in their world can be used as data sources. Spradley (1979) identified three categories of questions for ethnographic inquiry: *descriptive,* or broad, open-ended questions; *structural,* or in-depth questions that expand and verify the unit of analysis; and *contrast,* or questions that further clarify and provide criteria for exclusion.

Through participant observation, Mayo (1992) gathered information about the physical activity practices of a subsample of 13 women during such activities as aerobic dance, walking, jogging, weight lifting, and floor exercises. Interview questions ranged from the open-ended "Tell me about your physical activity, starting at whatever age you want; describe your experiences, and what you have done in the past or do now in terms of activity" to the specific "What things, such as people, your own feelings, the time of year, facility availability, or finances, help or block your participation in physical activity?"

Data Analysis

As with the grounded theory method, data are collected and analyzed simultaneously. Data analysis proceeds through several levels as the researcher looks for the meaning of cultural symbols in the informants' language. Analysis begins with a search for **domains** or symbolic categories that include smaller categories. Language is analyzed for semantic relationships, and structural questions are formulated to expand and verify data. Mayo (1992) used the biomedical labels *cardiorespiratory, muscular,* and *metabolic* to group the emic criteria for physical fitness supplied by the informants. For example, such terms as *conditioned, better balance, better shape all over, in good shape,* and *flexible* constituted the category of muscular. Analysis proceeds through increasing levels of complexity and includes taxonomic analysis or in-depth verification of domains, componential analysis or analysis for contrasts among categories, and theme analysis or uncovering of cultural themes. The data, grounded in the informants' reality and synthesized by the researcher, lead eventually to hypothetical propositions about the cultural phenomenon under investigation. Mayo (1992) proceeded through the levels of analysis to conceptualize the idea that physical activity behaviors among American black women reflect a process of nongenetic adaptation to social and physical environmental conditions. The management of physical activity was further described by Lazarus and Folkman's (1984) concept of coping. The reader is encouraged to consult Spradley (1979), Leininger (1985), or Parse, Coyne, and Smith (1985) for detailed descriptions of the ethnographic analysis process.

Describing the Findings

Ethnographic studies yield large quantities of data amassed as field notes of observations, interview transcriptions, and other artifacts, such as photographs. When critiquing, be aware that the report of findings usually provides examples from data, thorough description of the analytic process, and statements of the hypothetical propositions and their relationship to the ethnographer's frame of reference. Complete ethnographies may be published as monographs.

Historical Method

LoBiondo-Wood (1990) defined the **historical research method** as "the systematic compilation of data and the critical presentation, evaluation and interpretation of facts regarding people, events and occurrences of the past" (p. 212). One of the goals of the researcher using historical methodology is to shed light on the past so that it can guide the present and the future.

The historical method is embedded in philosophy, art, and science (Cramer, 1992). Nursing's focus on historical methodology was led by Teresa E. Christy, who established it as a legitimate method of inquiry more than a decade ago (Schweer, 1982). Christy elaborated the method (1975) and the need (1981) for historical research long before most nurse scholars accepted it as a legitimate research method. Since 1990, issues of *Nursing Research* have included a short paper dedicated to "Moments in Nursing History." This inclusion documents the increasing acceptance of historical methods of nursing research.

Historical methodology can emerge from within the quantitative or qualitative approach. However, the nature of history is fundamentally narrative (qualitative) rather than numerical (quantitative).

Identifying the Phenomenon

The historical method requires that the phenomenon of interest is a past event that can be circumscribed to permit distinction from other events. Baer's (1992) study of the Illinois Training School's search for university status is cited to highlight for the critiquer the process of using historical methods. The paper provides information about how nursing can get caught between shifting social priorities; the phenomenon has been labeled "unattained aspirations" by Baer (1992). By focusing on the Illinois Training School from 1880 to 1959, Baer delineated her inquiry of unattained aspirations to one nursing school during a critical period in its history.

Structuring the Study

Research question. When critiquing, expect to find the research question embedded in the phenomenon to be studied. The question is implicitly rather than explicitly stated. In Baer's study (1992), the researcher questioned how nursing gets caught in shifting social priorities. Baer described the process of being caught with unattained aspirations, using the Illinois Training School experience.

Researcher's perspective. Christy (1975) notes that the researcher's first responsibility is to understand the information being acquired without imposing his or her own interpretation. The researcher does this by being aware of personal biases that may color the interpretation. The report of historical research provides no documentation of this step of the research process.

Sample selection. In historical research, sample selection is accomplished by identifying data sources (Sarnecky, 1990). The more clearly a researcher delineates the phenomenon, the more specifically data sources can be identified. All possible sources of data will be listed by the researcher. Data may include written or video documents, interviews with persons who witnessed the phenomenon, photographs, and any other artifacts that shed light on the phenomenon. Once again, the research report does not reveal all the data sources that were explored.

Gathering the Data

Once a list of possible data sources has been composed, the researcher will begin the process of learning what is available. Sometimes pivotal information cannot be retrieved and must be eliminated from the list of possible sources. To determine which data sources were used when reviewing a published study, the reader will look at the reference list. Baer (1992) used official university documents, diaries, newspapers and personal letters, to name only a few. She may have wanted to talk with some individuals who had lived through the Training School experience she was studying, but sources who can recall the significant events and engage in dialogue are not always available.

Sources of data may be primary or secondary. **Primary sources** are eyewitness accounts provided by original documents, films, letters, diaries, records, artifacts, periodicals, or tapes (LoBiondo-Wood, 1990). In contrast, **secondary sources** provide a view of the phenomenon from another's perspective.

Analyzing the Data

Data will be analyzed first for importance and then for validity and reliability. To judge importance, the researcher separates what is (1) of clear value from (2) the "mildly interesting" and (3) the unimportant (Sarnecky, 1990). The unimportant will be discarded as data sources and data of clear value are included. Mildly interesting data require further review before they are included or discarded.

Validity of documents is established by external criticism; reliability is established by internal criticism. **External criticism** judges the authenticity of the data source. The researcher seeks to ensure that the data source is what it seems to be. For instance, if the researcher is reviewing a handwritten letter of Florence Nightingale, some of the validity issues are the following:
• Are the ink, paper, and wax seal on the envelope representative of Nightingale's time?
• Is the wax seal one that Nightingale used in other authentic data sources?
• Is the writing truly Nightingale's?

Only if the data source passes the test of external criticism does the researcher begin internal criticism. **Internal criticism** concerns the reliability of information within the document (Christy, 1975). To judge reliability, the researcher must familiarize herself or himself with the time in which the data emerged. A sense of the context and language of the time is essential to understanding a document. The meaning of a word in one era may not be equivalent to the meaning in another era. Knowing the language, customs, and habits of the historical period is critical for judging reliability.

The researcher assumes that a primary source provides a more reliable account than a secondary source (Christy, 1975). The further a source moves from providing an eyewitness account, the more questionable is its reliability. The researcher using historical methods attempts to establish fact, probability, or possibility

---

ESTABLISHING FACT, PROBABILITY, AND POSSIBILITY WITH THE HISTORICAL METHOD

FACT

Two independent primary sources that agree with each other

or

One independent primary source that receives critical evaluation *and* one independent secondary source that is in agreement and receives critical evaluation *and* no substantive conflicting data

PROBABILITY

One primary source that receives critical evaluation *and* no substantive conflicting data

or

Two primary sources that disagree about particular points

POSSIBILITY

One primary source that provides information but is not adequate to receive critical evaluation

or

Only secondary or tertiary sources.

Modified from "The Methodology of Historical Research: A Brief Introduction by T.E. Christy, 1975, *Image: Journal of Nursing Scholarship, 24,* (3), pp. 189-192.

(see the box above). The critiquer should not expect a report of data analysis. It is not reported by the researcher using historical methods; rather, a description of the findings is presented.

Describing the Findings

The findings of an historical study are presented as a well-synthesized chronicle. The entire manuscript is the description of findings. "If the synthesis is successful, the reader thinks the research and the writing have been effortless. The reader is never aware of the painstaking work, the careful attention to detail, nor the arduous pursuit of clues endured by the writer of history" (Christy, 1975, p. 192).

THE QUALITATIVE APPROACH: NURSING METHODOLOGY

The qualitative methodologies that are elaborated throughout this chapter are derived from other disciplines, such as sociology, anthropology, and philosophy. The discipline of nursing borrowed these methodologies to conduct research. However, as the discipline matured, methodology based on nursing ontology (belief system) emerged. Madeleine Leininger (1985; 1988) and Rosemarie Rizzo Parse (1992; 1990) are examples of nurse theorists who have created research methods specific to their theories. Table 11-4 compares the methodology of these theorists. Each method was developed over years and tested by other researchers. Each attempts to advance nursing knowledge through inquiry that is congruent with their theory.

Table 11-4   Nursing Research Methodology

	Leininger	Parse
Theory	Cultural Care Diversity and Universality	Human Becoming
Research methodology	Ethnonursing is the study and analysis of the local or indigenous peoples' viewpoints, beliefs, and practices about nursing care behavior and processes of designated cultures. (Leininger, 1978, p. 15)	Parse's research methodology is the study of universal health experiences through true presence both with participants sharing life stories and with transcribed data to uncover meaning. Study findings are meshed with the concepts of the theory of human becoming. (Parse, 1992)
Example of research question(s)	What are the meanings and expressions of health to older Greek-Canadian widows? What Greek folk health and illness care beliefs and practices are prevalent with Greek-Canadian widows? (Rosenbaum, 1991)	What is the structure of the lived experience of grieving a personal loss? (Cody, 1991)

ISSUES IN QUALITATIVE RESEARCH
Case Study Methodology: Underused but Promising

The **case study method** focuses on a selected contemporary phenomenon over time to provide an in-depth description of its essential dimensions and processes. In the health sciences, case studies have been used primarily for teaching. Patient stories have been related to highlight an unusual case or present a typical case example. Recent nursing literature has affirmed the value of nurse-patient stories for many purposes (Sandelowski, 1991), including distinguishing the novice from the expert nurse (Benner, Tanner, & Chesla, 1992), developing meaningful nursing ethics (Parker, 1990), and providing evidence to encourage political action (Sullivan, 1992). Benner (1984; 1991) described the value of sharing paradigm cases, narrative accounts that chronicle nursing practice and advance understanding of the discipline.

These "case study" references are distinct from case study methodology used for research purposes. According to Yin (1989), "as a research endeavor, the case study contributes uniquely to our knowledge of individual, organizational, social and political phenomena" (p. 14). Although case study methodology has been endorsed by nurses (Sterling & McNally, 1992; Munro, 1992), there are currently few

Table 11-5 Characteristics of Qualitative Research Generating Ethical Concerns

Characteristics	Ethical concerns
Naturalistic setting	Some researchers using methods that rely on participant observation may believe that consent is not always possible or necessary.
Researcher-participant interaction	Relationships developed between the researcher and participant may allow the participant to expect other than research behaviors.
Researcher as instrument	The researcher is the study instrument, collecting data and interpreting the participant's reality.
Emergent nature of design	Planning for questioning and observation emerges over the time of the study. So it is difficult to inform the participant precisely of potential threats before he or she agrees to participate.

examples of nursing studies that use case study methodology. The methodology often is used in historical research, but in these instances it focuses on past rather than contemporary events.

Many of the phenomena of interest to nursing are contemporary events that unfold over time, easily lending themselves to case study methodology. The experience of becoming a parent, living through a natural disaster such as a hurricane, or living with a chronic illness are some examples. Case study methodology promises to offer another qualitative avenue for nursing investigation in the future.

Ethics

Inherent in all research is the demand for the protection of human subjects. This demand exists for both quantitative and qualitative research approaches. Human subjects' protection as applicable to the quantitative approach is discussed in Chapter 13. These basic tenets hold true for the qualitative approach. However, several characteristics of qualitative methodologies outlined in Table 11-5 generate unique concerns and necessitate an expanded view of protecting human subjects.

Naturalistic Setting

The concerns that arise when research is conducted in naturalistic settings focus on the issue of the need to gain consent. Some fieldwork models allow that the researcher collect data without informing participants (Johnson, 1992). For nurses, this circumstance is most likely to occur when collecting data in public settings, where the researcher can easily gain entry as an accepted member of the community without explanation. Ramos (1989) distinguishes public from private behaviors. She indicates that public behaviors are not personal disclosures, but private behaviors, which are not socially disclosed, require "clearance" to be used in a public manner. Johnson addressed the issue of forgoing consent. He notes, "Many research ethical committees would automatically fail to grant access to studies where the proposed sample will not be able to choose between being included or excluded from the investigation" (p. 218).

Controversy exists regarding the appropriateness of collecting data without consent. Even when situations permit it, Munhall (1988) suggests that participants be informed after the study and given an opportunity to read, question, and validate the research report.

Researcher-Participant Interaction

The nature of the researcher-participant interaction over time introduces the possibility that the research experience becomes a therapeutic one. Wilde (1992) proposed that there is merit in routinely including other nursing roles (clinician, counselor, therapist, teacher) in researcher-participant interactions, but this idea generally is not accepted. It is useful for the researcher to be mindful of the role and gently guide participants to focus on the purpose of the researcher-participant experience. However, the "therapeutic imperative of nursing (advocacy) takes precedence over the research imperative (advancing knowledge) if conflict develops" (Munhall, 1988, p. 151). That is, the nurse researcher will never choose to pursue knowledge when aware that participant health is threatened by this pursuit.

Researcher as Instrument

The responsibility to remain true to the data, interpreting findings in a way that accurately reflects the participant's reality, is a serious ethical obligation for the researcher (Munhall, 1988; Ramos, 1989). To accomplish this, the researcher may return to the subjects at critical interpretive points and ask for clarification or validation.

Emergent Nature of Design

The emergent nature of the research design creates a need for ongoing negotiation of consent with the participant. In the course of a study, situations change and what was agreeable at the beginning may become intrusive. Sometimes, as data collection proceeds and new information emerges, the study shifts direction in a way that is not acceptable to the participant. For instance, if the researcher was present in a family's home during a time that marital discord arose, the family may choose to renegotiate the consent. The opportunity to renegotiate consent establishes a relationship of trust and respect characteristic of the ethical conduct of research.

Credibility, Auditability, Fittingness

Quantitative studies use reliability and validity of instruments, as well as internal and external validity criteria, as measures of scientific rigor (see Table 11-1, p. 256), but these are not appropriate for qualitative work. The rigor of qualitative methodology is judged by unique criteria appropriate to the research approach. Credibility, auditability, fittingness, and confirmability are scientific rigor criteria proposed by Guba and Lincoln (1981) and elaborated for nursing research by San-

Table 11-6   Criteria for Judging Scientific Rigor: Credibility, Auditability, Fittingness, and Confirmability

Criteria	Criteria characteristics
Credibility	Truth of findings as judged by participants and others within the discipline
Auditability	Accountability as judged by the adequacy of information leading the reader from the research question and raw data through various steps of analysis to the interpretation of findings
Fittingness	Faithfulness to everyday reality of the participants, described in enough detail so that others in the discipline can evaluate importance for their own practice, research, and theory development
Confirmability	Findings that reflect implementation of creditability, auditability, and fittingness standards

delowski (1986). Although lists of specific criteria vary slightly (Lincoln & Guba, 1985; Strauss & Corbin, 1990), the general themes of credibility, auditability, and fittingness persist as criteria for judging the scientific rigor of qualitative research. The meaning of credibility, auditability, fittingness, and confirmability is briefly explained in Table 11-6. As can be seen, confirmability is assured when the other criteria have been met (Sandelowski, 1986). Lincoln and Guba (1985) and Sandelowski (1986) provide detailed activities that may be undertaken to achieve credibility, auditability, and fittingness.

Combining Qualitative and Quantitative Approaches

There has been ongoing debate about combining qualitative and quantitative approaches (Boyd, 1990). Leininger (1992) offers two principles to guide the researcher in this matter:
- The quantitative and qualitative approaches are very different in their belief systems and their purposes; and
- The researcher should not mix research methods across approaches because it violates the integrity of the approach; it is acceptable and desirable to mix methods within one approach. (p. 395)

Leininger believes that any one study should be conducted with one or the other approach. The fundamental differences cited in Table 11-1 suggest the confusion a researcher may experience with one foot in qualitative and one in quantitative approaches for a single study. Leininger does concede that findings from the two approaches may complement each other. Beck's studies (Table 11-2, p. 259) of postpartum depression highlight this point.

In a recent report using grounded theory method to study postpartum depression, Beck (1993) has further expanded understanding of the phenomenon and posed a theory of postpartum depression, "teetering on the edge." In the research report, Beck (1993) discussed how the combination of phenomenological and grounded theory methods contributed to the development of her theory of postpartum depression.

Morse (1991) provided another view distinct from Leininger's in its suggestion that methods from the two approaches may be combined. This combination of methods is labeled *simultaneous* or *sequential triangulation*. Simultaneous triangulation is the combination of qualitative and quantitative methods in one study at the same time. In sequential triangulation, one approach precedes the other. Each combination is made for distinct reasons (Table 11-7). Morse is like Leininger in her emphasis that findings from each approach complement each other. She discusses the importance of keeping the quantitative and qualitative data sets separate and meeting the criteria of each approach to derive complementary findings successfully. Morse (1991) provides a systematic, thoughtful structure (Table 11-7), which supports selective combination to "strengthen research results and contribute to theory and knowledge development" (p. 122).

The debate regarding ways to combine methods is far from finished. There is an intrinsic drive for nurses to substantiate the description of lived experience with hard data—or perhaps, it is a mandate to substantiate hard data with descriptions of lived experience. In our current health care climate, with its focus on patient outcomes, the individual meaning ascribed to health has increasing value. Who is best prepared to identify desirable outcomes? What research models can most effectively be used to accomplish this task? Nursing is challenged to create unique research models capable of addressing the complexity of humans, while maintaining the integrity of its belief systems.

Computer Management of Qualitative Data

At the completion of data collection, the qualitative researcher is faced with volumes of data requiring sorting, coding, and synthesizing. The researcher reports may use one of the computer programs that are available to assist with the task of data management. Unlike computer programs used with quantitative data, these programs do not analyze data. Data analysis is the task of the researcher. However, data can be managed by computers. Reid (1992) distinguishes three data management functions (pp. 125-126):

1. Data preparation: entry of data from field notes, interviews, and various other sources; cleaning of data to assure that spelling is correct and data are easy to evaluate
2. Data identification: dividing data into meaningful segments for analysis/synthesis
3. Data manipulation: searching for particular words or phrases and sorting them from the text

Tesch (1991) presents an overview of five personal computer programs (QUALPRO; Ethnograph; Textbase Alpha; Text Analysis Package; HyperQual) commonly used to manage qualitative data. She provides detailed information that would permit the reader to select the program most suitable for specific needs. Morse and Morse (1989) suggest the use of QUAL, a mainframe program, when

Table 11-7   Simultaneous and Sequential Combinations of Quantitative and Qualitative Research Methods: Rationale and Examples

Combination	Rationale	Example
SIMULTANEOUS		
Qualitative + quantitative	There is a qualitative foundation, and quantitative methods are used to provide complementary information.	The researcher is interested in the experience of feeling depressed after the loss of a spouse. Phenomenological methods could be used to address the research question; administration of a depression scale would provide complementary information.
Quantitative + qualitative	There is a quantitative foundation, and qualitative methods are used to provide complementary information.	The researcher is testing hypotheses about depression after the death of a spouse. The phenomenological method is used to uncover the experience for a select group who acknowledge feelings of depression.
SEQUENTIAL		
Qualitative → quantitative	Findings from qualitative investigation lead to use of the quantitative approach.	The researcher has described the experience of feeling depressed after the death of a spouse. The themes emerging from the data are used to create a depression scale. The scale is tested for reliability and validity.
Quantitative → qualitative	Findings from quantitative investigation lead to use of the qualitative approach.	The researcher has tested hypotheses linking the death of a spouse with depression and found no significant relationships. A qualitative study is undertaken to uncover the experience of living through the death of one's spouse in an effort to let the data lead to common thoughts and feelings.

Modified from "Approaches to Qualitative-Quantitative Methodological Triangulation" by J.M. Morse, 1991, *Nursing Research, 40*(1), pp. 120-123.

CRITIQUING CRITERIA

IDENTIFYING THE PHENOMENON

1. Is the phenomenon focused on human experience within a natural setting?
2. Is the phenomenon relevant to nursing and/or health?

STRUCTURING THE STUDY

Research Question

3. Does the question specify a distinct process to be studied?
4. Does the question identify the context (participant group/place) of the process that will be studied?
5. Does the choice of a specific qualitative method fit with the research question?

Researcher's Perspective

6. Are the biases of the researcher reported?
7. Do the researchers provide a structure of ideas that reflect their beliefs?

Sample Selection

8. Is it clear that the selected sample is living the phenomenon of interest?

DATA GATHERING

9. Are data sources and methods for gathering data specified?
10. Is there evidence that participant consent is an integral part of the data gathering process?

DATA ANALYSIS

11. Can the dimensions of data analysis be identified and logically followed?
12. Does the researcher paint a clear picture of the participant's reality?
13. Is there evidence that the researcher's interpretation captured the participant's meaning?
14. Have other professionals confirmed the researcher's interpretation?

DESCRIBING THE FINDINGS

15. Are examples provided to guide the reader from the raw data to the researcher's synthesis?
16. Does the researcher link the findings to existing theory or literature?

the size of data sets exceeds the limits of personal computers. The critiquer of qualitative research is referred to these sources for detailed information about software capabilities.

CRITIQUING QUALITATIVE RESEARCH

Although general criteria for critiquing qualitative research are proposed in the box on p. 280, each qualitative method has unique characteristics that influence what the research consumer may expect in the published research report. The proposed general criteria are most useful for critiquing studies using the phenomenological, grounded theory, and ethnographic methods. They are less relevant for critiquing research using the historical method.

The criteria for critiquing are formatted to evaluate the selection of the phenomenon, the structure of the study, data gathering, data analysis, and description of the findings. Each question of the criteria focuses on factors that are discussed throughout the chapter. The credibility (criteria 13 and 14), auditability (criteria 15), and fittingness (criteria 12) of the study are addressed by specific criteria (also see Chapter 20 for additional discussion of critiquing qualitative research).

KEY POINTS

- "Qualitative research involves broadly stated questions about human experiences and realities, studied through sustained contact with people in their natural environments, generating rich, descriptive data that help us to understand their experiences" (Boyd, 1990, p. 183).
- Qualitative research studies are guided by research questions.
- Data saturation occurs when the information being shared with the researcher becomes repetitive.
- Qualitative research methods include five basic elements: identifying the phenomenon, structuring the study, gathering the data, analyzing the data, and describing the findings.
- The phenomenological method is a process of learning and constructing the meaning of human experience through intensive dialogue with persons who are living the experience.
- The grounded theory method is an inductive approach that implements a systematic set of procedures to arrive at theory about basic social processes.
- The ethnographic method focuses on scientific descriptions of cultural groups.
- The historical method is the systematic compilation of data and the critical presentation, evaluation, and interpretation of facts regarding people, events, and occurrences of the past.
- The case study method focuses on a selected contemporary phenomenon over time to provide an in-depth description of its essential dimensions and processes.
- Ethical issues in qualitative research involve issues related to the naturalistic setting, researcher-participant interaction, researcher as instrument, and the emergent nature of the design.

- Credibility, auditability, fittingness, and confirmability are criteria for judging the scientific rigor of a qualitiative research study.
- Triangulation is a research method that combines qualitative and quantitative research methods.
- Qualitative research data can be managed through the use of specific computer software programs.

REFERENCES

Aamodt, A.A. (1991). Ethnography and epistemology: Generating nursing knowledge. In J.M. Morse (Ed.), *Qualitative nursing research: A contemporary dialogue* (pp. 40-53).

Agar, M.H. (1986). *Speaking of ethnography.* Beverly Hills, CA: Sage.

Alexander, J.C. (1987). *Twenty lectures: Sociological theory since World War II.* New York: Columbia University Press.

Baer, E.D. (1992). Aspirations unattained: The story of the Illinois Training School's search for university status. *Nursing Research, 41*(1), 43-48.

Beck, C.T. (1993). Teetering on the edge: A substantive theory of postpartum depression. *Nursing Research, 42*(1), 42-48.

Beck, C.T. (1992). The lived experience of postpartum depression: A phenomenological study. *Nursing Research, 41*(3), 166-170.

Beck, C.T., Reynolds, M.A., & Rutowski, P. (1992). Maternity blues and postpartum depression. *Journal of Obstetric, Gynecologic and Neonatal Nursing, 21*(4), 287-293.

Benner, P. (1991). The role of experience, narrative and community in skilled ethical comportment. *Advances in Nursing Science, 14*(2), 1-12.

Benner, P., Tanner, C., & Chesla, C. (1992). From beginner to expert: Gaining a differentiated clinical world in critical care nursing. *Advances in Nursing Science, 14*(3), 13-28.

Boas, F. (1948). Race, language, and culture. New York: MacMillan.

Boyd, C.O. (1990). Qualitative approaches to research. In G. LoBiondo-Wood & J. Haber (Eds.), *Nursing research: Methods, critical appraisal and utilization* (pp. 181-210). St. Louis: Mosby–Year Book.

Boyle, J.S. (1991). Field research: A collaborative model for practice and research. In J.M. Morse (Ed.), *Qualitative nursing research: A contemporary dialogue* (pp. 273-299). Newbury Park, CA: Sage.

Bright, M.A. (1992). Making place: The first birth in an intergenerational family context. *Qualitative Health Research, 2*(1), 75-98.

Christy, T.E. (1975). The methodology of historical research: A brief introduction. *Image: Journal of Nursing Scholarship, 24*(3), 189-192.

Christy, T.E. (1981). The need for historical research in nursing. *Image: Journal of Nursing Scholarship, 4,* 227-228.

Cody, W.K. (1991). Grieving a personal loss. *Nursing Science Quarterly, 4*(2), 61-68.

Colaizzi, P. (1978). Psychological research as the phenomenologist views it. In R.S. Valle & M. King (Eds.), *Existential phenomenological alternatives for psychology* (pp. 48-71). New York: Oxford University Press.

Coward, D.D. (1990). The lived experience of self-transcendence in women with advanced breast cancer. *Nursing Science Quarterly, 3*(4), 162-169.

Crabtree, B.F., & Miller, W.L. (Eds.). (1992). *Doing qualitative research.* Newbury Park, CA: Sage.

Cramer, S. (1992). The nature of history: Meditations on Clio's craft. *Nursing Research, 41*(1), 4-7.

Davis, A.T. (1991). America's first school of nursing: The New England Hospital for Women and Children. *Journal of Nursing Education, 30*(4), 158-161.

Everson-Bates, S. (1992). First-line nurse managers in the expanded role: An ethnographic analysis. *Journal of Nursing Administration, 22*(3), 32-37.

Fairman, J. (1992). Watchful vigilance: Nursing care, technology, and the development of intensive care units. *Nursing Research, 41*(1), 56-58.

Giorgi, A. Fischer, C.L., & Murray, E.L. (Eds.). (1975). *Duquesne studies in phenomenological psychology.* Pittsburgh: Duquesne University Press.

Glaser, B.G., & Strauss, A.L. (1967). *The discovery of grounded theory: Strategies for qualitative research.* Chicago: Aldine.

Guba, E., & Lincoln, Y. (1981). *Effective evaluation.* San Francisco: Jossey-Bass.

Hughes, C.C. (1992). "Ethnography": What's in a word—process? product? promise? *Qualitative Health Research, 2*(4), 439-450.

Hutchinson, S. (1986). Chemically dependent nurses: The trajectory toward self-annihilation. *Nursing Research, 35*(4), 196-201.

Jennings, J.L. (1986). Husserl revisited: The forgotten distinction between psychology and phenomenology. *American Psychologist, 41*(11), 1231-1240.

Johnson, M. (1992). A silent conspiracy? Some ethical issues of participant observation in nursing research. *International Journal of Nursing Studies, 29*(2), 213-223.

Jones, P.S., & Martinson, I.M. (1992). The experience of bereavement in caregivers of family members with Alzheimer's disease. *Image, 24*(3), 172-176.

Kleinman, A. (1980). *Patients and healers in the context of culture.* Berkeley: University of California Press.

Kleinman, A. (1992). Local worlds of suffering: An interpersonal focus for ethnographies of illness experience. *Qualitative Health Research, 2*(2), 127-134.

Lazarus, R., & Folkman, S. (1984). *Stress appraisal, and coping.* New York: Springer.

Leininger, M.M. (1978). *Transcultural nursing: Concepts, theories and practices.* New York: John Wiley & Sons.

Leininger, M.M. (1985). Ethnography and ethnonursing: Models and modes of qualitative data analysis. In M.M. Leininger (Ed.), *Qualitative research methods in nursing* (pp. 33-72). Orlando: Grune & Stratton.

Leininger, M.M. (1985). *Qualitative research methods in nursing.* New York: Grune & Stratton.

Leininger, M.M. (1988). Leininger's theory of nursing: Cultural care diversity and universality. *Nursing Science Quarterly, 1*(4), 152-160.

Leininger, M.M. (1992). Current issues, problems, and trends to advance qualitative paradigmatic research methods for the future. *Qualitative Health Research, 2*(4), 392-415.

Lincoln, Y.S., & Guba, E.G. (1985). *Naturalistic inquiry.* Newbury Park, CA: Sage.

Lincoln, Y.S. (1992). Sympathetic connections between qualitative methods and health research. *Qualitative Health Research, 2*(4), 375-391.

Lipson, J.G. (1991). Afghan refugee health: Some findings and suggestions. *Qualitative Health Research, 1*(3), 349-369.

LoBiondo-Wood, G. (1990). Additional types of research. In G. LoBiondo-Wood & J. Haber (Eds.), *Nursing research: Methods, critical appraisal and utilization* (2nd ed.) (pp. 211-226). St. Louis: Mosby–Year Book.

Malinowski, B. (1922) 1961. *Argonauts of the Western Pacific.* New York: E.P. Dutton.

Mayo, K. (1992). Physical activity practices among American Black working women. *Qualitative Health Research, 2*(3), 318-333.

Mead, M. (1928) 1949. *Coming of age in Samoa.* New York: New American Library, Mentor Books.

Miller, M.P. (1991). Factors promoting wellness in the aged person: An ethnographic study. *Advances in Nursing Science, 13*(4), 38-51.

Morgan, D.G., & Laing, G.P. (1991). The diagnosis of Alzheimer's disease: Spouse's perspectives. *Qualitative Health Research, 1*(3), 370-387.

Morse, J.M. (1991). Approaches to qualitative-quantitative methodological triangulation. *Nursing Research, 40*(1), 120-123.

Morse, J.M., & Morse, R.M. (1989). QUAL: A mainframe program for qualitative data analysis. *Nursing Research, 38*(2), 188-189.

Munhall, P.L. (1992). Holding the Mississippi River in place and other implications for qualitative research. *Nursing Outlook, 40*(6), 257-262.

Munhall, P.L. (1988). Ethical considerations in qualitative research. *Western Journal of Nursing Research, 10*(2), 150-162.

Munro, B.H. (1992). How many subjects are enough? *Clinical Nurse Specialist, 6*(1), 20.

Parker, R.S. (1990). Nurses' stories: The search for a relational ethic of care. *Advances in Nursing Science, 13*(1), 31-40.

Parse, R.R., Coyne, A.B., & Smith, M.J. (1985). *Nursing research: Qualitative methods.* Bowie, MD: Brady.

Parse, R.R. (1990). Parse's research methodology with an illustration of the lived experience of hope. *Nursing Science Quarterly, 3*(1), 9-17.

Parse, R.R., (1992). Human becoming: Parse's theory of nursing. *Nursing Science Quarterly, 5*(1), 35-42.

Parse, R.R., Coyne, A.B., & Smith, M.J. (1985). *Nursing research: Qualitative methods.* Bowie, MD: Brady.

Powers, B.A., & Knapp, T.R. (1990). *A dictionary of nursing theory and research.* Newbury Park, CA: Sage.

Price, M.J. (1993). An experiential model of learning diabetes self-management. *Qualitative Health Research, 3*(1), 29-54.

Ragsdale, D., Kotarba, J.A., & Morrow, J.R. (1992). Quality of life of hospitalized persons with AIDS. *Image, 24*(4), 259-265.

Ramos, M.C. (1989). Some ethical implication of qualitative research. *Research in Nursing and Health, 12,* 57-63.

Reid, A.O. (1992). Computer management strategies for text data. In B.F. Crabtree & W.L. Miller (Eds.), *Doing qualitative research* (pp. 125-145). Newbury Park, CA: Sage.

Rosenbaum, J.N. (1991). The health meanings and practices of older Greek-Canadian widows. *Journal of Advanced Nursing, 16,* 1320-1327.

Sandelowski, M. (1991). Telling stories: Narrative approaches in qualitative research. *Image: Journal of Nursing Scholarship, 23*(3), 161-166.

Sanday, R.R. (1989). The ethnographic paradigm(s). In J. Van Maanen (Ed.), *Qualitative Methodology* (pp. 19-36). Newbury Park, CA: Sage.

Sarnecky, M.T. (1990). Historiography: A legitimate research methodology for nursing. *Advances in Nursing Science, 12*(4), 1-10.

Schweer, K.D. (1982). Lessons from nursing's historian: A tribute to Teresa E. Christy, Ed.D., F.A.A.N. (1927-1982). *Image: Journal of Nursing Scholarship, 14*(3), 66.

Sowell, R.L., Bramlett, M.H., Gueldner, S.H., Gritzmacher, D., & Martin, G. (1991). The lived experience of survival and bereavement following the death of a lover from AIDS. *Image: Journal of Nursing Scholarship, 23*(2), 89-94.

Spiegelberg, H. (1976). *The phenomenological movement.* Vols I and II. The Hague: Martinus Nijhoff.

Spradley, J.P. (1979). *The ethnographic interview.* New York: Holt, Rinehart & Winston.

Sterling, Y.M., & McNally, J.A. (1992). Single subject research for nursing practice. *Clinical Nurse Specialist, 6*(1), 21-26.

Strauss, A.L. (1987). *Qualitative analysis for social scientists.* New York: Cambridge University Press.

Strauss, A., & Corbin, J. (1990). Basics of qualitative research: Grounded theory procedures and techniques. Newbury Park, CA: Sage.

Sullivan, E.M. (1992). Nurse practitioners and reimbursement. *Nursing and Health Care, 13*(5), 236-241.

Swanson, K.M. (1990). Providing care in the NICU: Sometimes an act of love. *Advances in Nursing Science, 13*(1), 60-73.

Tesch, R. (1991). Computer programs that assist in the analysis of qualitative data: An overview. *Qualitative Health Research, 1*(3), 309-325.

Thorne, S.E. (1991). Methodological orthodoxy in qualitative research: Analysis of the issues. *Qualitative Health Research, 1*(2), 178-199.

Uphall, M.J. (1992). Nursing perceptions of collaboration with indigenous healers in Swaziland. *International Journal of Nursing Studies, 29*(1), 27-36.

van Kaam, A. (1969). *Existential foundations in psychology.* New York: Doubleday.

Wilde, V. (1992). Controversial hypotheses on the relationship between researcher and informant in qualitative research. *Journal of Advanced Nursing, 17,* 234-242.

Yin, R.K. (1989). *Case study research: Design and methods.* Newbury Park, CA: Sage.

CHAPTER
12
Sampling

JUDITH HABER

LEARNING OBJECTIVES

After reading this chapter the student should be able to do the following:

- Identify the purpose of sampling.
- Define population, sample, and sampling.
- Compare and contrast a population and a sample.
- Discuss the eligibility criteria for sample selection.
- Define nonprobability and probability sampling.
- Identify the types of nonprobability and probability sampling strategies.
- Compare the advantages and disadvantages of specific nonprobability and probability sampling strategies.
- Discuss the factors that influence determination of sample size.
- Discuss the procedure for drawing a sample.
- Identify the criteria for critiquing a sampling plan.
- Use the critiquing criteria to evaluate the sampling section of a research report.

KEY TERMS

cluster sampling	quota sampling
convenience sampling	random selection
data saturation	representative sample
delimitation	sample
element	sampling
eligibility criteria	sampling frame
matching	sampling interval
multistage (cluster) sampling	sampling unit
network sampling	simple random sampling
nonprobability sampling	snowballing
population	stratified random sampling
probability sampling	systematic sample
purposive sampling	

Sampling is the process of selecting representative units of a population for study in a research investigation. Although sampling is a complex process, it is a familiar one. In our daily lives we gather knowledge, make decisions, and formulate predictions based on sampling procedures. For example, nursing students may make generalizations about the overall quality of nursing professors as a result of their exposure to a **sample** of nursing professors during their undergraduate programs. Patients may make generalizations about a hospital's food during a one-week hospital stay. It is apparent that limited exposure to a limited portion of these phenomena forms the basis of our conclusions and so much of our knowledge and decisions are based on our experience with samples.

Scientists also derive knowledge from samples. Many problems in scientific research cannot be solved without employing sampling procedures. For example, when testing the effectiveness of a medication for patients with cancer, the drug is administered to a sample of the population for whom the drug is potentially appropriate. The scientist must come to some conclusions without administering the drug to every known patient with cancer or every laboratory animal in the world. But because human lives are at stake, the scientist cannot afford to arrive casually at conclusions that are based on the first dozen patients available for study. The consequences of arriving at erroneous conclusions or making inaccurate generalizations from a small, nonrepresentative sample are much more severe in scientific investigations than in everyday life. Consequently, research methodologists have expended considerable effort to develop sampling theories and procedures that produce accurate and meaningful information. Essentially, researchers sample representative segments of the population, because it is rarely feasible or necessary to sample the entire population of interest to obtain relevant information.

This chapter will familiarize the research consumer with the basic concepts of sampling as they primarily pertain to the principles of quantitative research design, nonprobability and probability sampling, sample size, and the related critiquing process. Sampling issues that relate to qualitative research designs are discussed mainly in Chapter 11.

SAMPLING CONCEPTS
Population

A **population** is a well-defined set that has certain specified properties. A population can be composed of people, animals, objects, or events. For example, if a researcher is studying undergraduate nursing students, the type of educational preparation of the population must be specified. In this instance the population consists of undergraduate students enrolled in a generic baccalaureate nursing program. Examples of other possible populations might be all male patients admitted for a first myocardial infarction in hospital ABC during the year 1992, all children with Down's syndrome in the state of New York, or all men and women with a diagnosis of unipolar depression in the United States. These examples illustrate that a population may be broadly defined and potentially involve millions of people or narrowly specified to include only several hundred people.

The reader of a research report should consider whether the researcher has identified the population descriptors that form the basis for the **eligibility criteria** that are used to select the sample from the array of all possible units, be they people, objects, or events. Let us consider the population previously defined as undergraduate nursing students enrolled in a generic baccalaureate program. Would this population include part-time as well as full-time students? Would it include students who had previously attended another nursing program? How about foreign students? Would freshmen through seniors qualify? Insofar as it is possible, the researcher must demonstrate that the exact criteria used to decide whether an individual would be classified as a member of a given population have been specifically delineated. The population descriptors that provide the basis for eligibility criteria should be evident in the sample; that is, the characteristics of the population and the sample should be congruent. The degree of congruence is evaluated to assess the representativeness of the sample. For example, if a population was defined as full-time, American-born, senior nursing students enrolled in a generic baccalaureate nursing program, the sample would be expected to reflect these characteristics.

Eligibility criteria may also be viewed as **delimitations,** or those characteristics that restrict the population to a homogeneous group of subjects. Examples of delimitations include the following: gender, age, marital status, socioeconomic status, religion, ethnicity, level of education, age of children, health status, and diagnosis. In a study evaluating the repeatability of the urine stream interruption test and its relationship to other measures of pelvic strength (Sampselle & DeLancey, 1992), the researchers established several of the following delimitations:

- Females who were either nulliparous, primiparous, or secundiparous
- Females who were not currently pregnant
- Females who were at least 1 year past giving birth vaginally, if in either parous group
- Females who had no history of urinary dysfunction
- Females who had no history of gynecological surgery
- Females who had no underlying neuromuscular disease

These delimitations were selected because their potential effect on the performance of urine stream interruption would limit the validity of the findings, as well as the ability to generalize about the findings. Let us consider the criterion of not being currently pregnant. If pregnant and nonpregnant women were grouped together in the sample, the researchers would have two groups whose ability to perform urine stream interruption may be very different because of the pregnancy variable and hence the accuracy of the findings may be distorted. Heterogeneity of this sample group would inhibit the researchers' ability to interpret the findings meaningfully and make generalizations. It is much wiser to study only one homogeneous group or include specific groups as distinct subsets of the sample and study the groups comparatively. In this study, Sampselle and DeLancey recruited 75 women between the ages of 18 and 35 and divided them into subsample groups of 25 subjects each, according to level of parity: that is, nulliparous, primiparous, and secundiparous. This provided distinct subject subsets that they could study comparatively. You should remember that delimitations are not established in a casual or meaningless way, but they are established to control for extraneous variability or bias. Each delimitation should have a rationale, presumably related to a potential contaminating effect on the dependent variable. The careful establishment of sample delimitations will increase the precision of the study and contribute to the accuracy and generalizability of the findings (see Chapter 8).

The population criteria establish the *target population:* that is, the entire set of cases about which the researcher would like to make generalizations. A target population might include all undergraduate nursing students enrolled in generic baccalaureate programs in the United States. It often is not feasible, because of time, money, and personnel, to pursue using a target population. An *accessible population,* one that meets the population criteria and that is *available,* is used instead. For example, an accessible population might include all full-time generic baccalaureate students attending school in Pennsylvania. Pragmatic factors must also be considered when identifying a potential population of interest.

It is important to know that a population is not restricted to human subjects. It may consist of hospital records; blood, urine, or other specimens taken from patients at a clinic; historical documents; or laboratory animals. For example, a population might consist of all the urine specimens collected from patients in the Crestview Hospital antepartum clinic or all of the patient charts on file at the Day Surgery

Center. It is apparent that a population can be defined in a variety of ways. The important point to remember is that the basic unit of the population must be clearly defined, since the generalizability of the findings will be a function of the population criteria.

Samples and Sampling

Sampling is a process of selecting a portion of the designated population to represent the entire population. A **sample** is a set of elements that make up the population, and an **element** is the most basic unit about which information is collected. The most common element in nursing research is individuals, but other elements, such as places or objects, can form the basis of a sample or population. A **sampling unit** is the element or set of elements used for selecting the sample. Sometimes the sampling unit and the element represent the same thing, and other times it is more efficient to use a unit larger than the element for sampling purposes. For example, a researcher was planning a study that compared the effectiveness of different nursing interventions on the healing rate of decubitus ulcers. Four hospitals, each using a different treatment protocol, were identified as the sampling units rather than the nurses themselves or the treatment alone.

The purpose of sampling is to increase the efficiency of a research study. The novice reviewer of research reports must realize that it would not be feasible to examine every element or unit in the population. When sampling is properly done it allows the researcher to draw inferences and make generalizations about the population without examining each unit in the population. Sampling procedures that entail the formulation of specific criteria for selection ensure that the characteristics of the phenomena of interest will be, or are likely to be, present in all of the units being studied. The researcher's endeavors to ensure that the sample is representative of the target population put the researcher in a stronger position to draw conclusions from the sample findings that are generalizable to the population.

Evaluators of research studies will find that samples and sampling procedures vary in terms of merit. The foremost criterion in evaluating a sample is its representativeness. A **representative sample** is one whose key characteristics closely approximate those of the population. If 70% of the population in a study of child-rearing practices consisted of women and 40% were full-time employees, a representative sample should reflect these characteristics in the same proportions.

It must be understood that there is no way to guarantee that a sample is representative without obtaining a data base about the entire population. Because it is difficult and inefficient to assess a population, the researcher must employ sampling strategies that minimize or control for sample bias. If an appropriate sampling strategy is used, it almost always is possible to obtain a reasonably accurate understanding of the phenomena under investigation by obtaining data from a sample.

TYPES OF SAMPLES

Sampling strategies are generally grouped into two categories: **nonprobability sampling** and **probability sampling.** In *nonprobability* sampling, elements are chosen by nonrandom methods. The drawback of this strategy is that there is no way of estimating the probability that each element has of being included in the samples. Essentially there is no way of ensuring that every element has a chance for inclusion in the nonprobability sample. *Probability sampling* uses some form of random selection when choosing the sample units. This type of sample enables the researcher to estimate the probability that each element of the population will be included in the sample. Probability sampling is the more rigorous type of sampling strategy, and it is more likely to result in a representative sample. The remainder of this section is devoted to a discussion of different types of nonprobability and probability sampling strategies. A summary of sampling strategies appears in Table 12-1. You may wish to refer to this table as the various nonprobability and probability strategies are discussed in the following sections.

Nonprobability Sampling

The nonprobability sampling strategy is less rigorous than the probability sampling strategy, and it tends to produce less accurate and less representative samples. However, most samples, not only in nursing research but in other disciplines as well, are nonprobability samples. Although such samples are more feasible for the researcher to obtain, the use of nonprobability samples does limit the ability of the researcher to make generalizations about the findings. The three major types of nonprobability sampling are the following: convenience, quota, and purposive sampling strategies.

Convenience Sampling

Convenience sampling is the use of the most readily accessible persons or objects as subjects in a study. The subjects may include volunteers, the first 25 patients admitted to hospital X with a particular diagnosis, all people who enrolled in program Y during the month of September, or all students enrolled in course Z at a particular university during 1993. The subjects are convenient and accessible to the researcher and are so called a *convenience sample*. For example, a researcher studying marital communication patterns used a convenience sample of the first 200 couples meeting the sample criteria and who volunteered to participate in the study. Another researcher studying the effect of group patient education on cardiac rehabilitation used all patients transferred from the coronary care unit to the intermediate coronary care unit in hospital X between September and December 1992.

The advantage of a convenience sample is that it is easier for the researcher to obtain subjects. The researcher may have to be concerned only with obtaining a sufficient number of subjects who meet the same criteria.

The major disadvantage of a convenience sample is that the risk of bias is greater than in any other type of sample (see Table 12-1). The problem of bias is related to the fact that convenience samples tend to be self-selecting; that is, the researcher ends up obtaining information only from the people who volunteer to participate. In this case the following questions must be raised: What motivated some of the people to participate and others to not participate? What kind of data would I have obtained if nonparticipants had also responded? How representative are the

Table 12-1   Summary of Sampling Strategies

Sampling strategy	Ease of drawing sample	Risk of bias	Representativeness of sample
NONPROBABILITY			
Convenience	Very easy	Greater than any other sampling strategy	Because samples tend to be self-selecting, representativeness is questionable
Quota	Relatively easy	Contains unknown source of bias that affects external validity	Builds in some representativeness by using knowledge about the population of interest
Purposive	Relatively easy	Bias increases with greater heterogeneity of the population; conscious bias is also a danger	Very limited ability to generalize because sample is handpicked
PROBABILITY			
Simple random	Laborious	Low	Maximized; probability of nonrepresentative-ness decreases with increased sample size
Stratified random	Time-consuming	Low	Enhanced
Cluster	Less time-consuming than simple or stratified	Subject to more sampling errors than simple or stratified	Less representative than simple or stratified
Systematic	More convenient and efficient than simple, stratified, or cluster sampling	Bias in the form of nonrandomness can be inadvertently introduced	Less representative if bias occurs as a result of coincidental nonrandomness

people who did participate in relation to the population? For example, a researcher may stop people on a street corner to ask their opinion on some issue; place advertisements in the newspaper; or place signs in local churches, community centers, or supermarkets indicating that volunteers are needed for a particular study. For example, in a study examining the self-care behaviors that older adults use to manage colds and influenza episodes, subjects were recruited from volunteer organizations,

Table 12-2   Numbers and Percentages of Students in Strata of a Quota Sample of 5000 Graduates of Nursing Programs in City X

	Diploma graduates	Associate degree graduates	Baccalaureate graduates
Population	2000(40%)	2000(40%)	1000(20%)
Strata	200	200	100

community groups, religious organizations, older adult congregate meal sites, older adult apartment buildings, senior centers, and shopping malls (Conn, 1991).

The evaluator of a research report should recognize that the convenience sample is the weakest form of sampling strategies with regard to generalizability. Its use should be avoided whenever possible. When a convenience sample is used, caution should be exercised in analyzing and interpreting the data. When critiquing a research study that has employed this sampling strategy, the reviewer will be justifiably skeptical about the external validity of the findings (see Chapter 8).

Quota Sampling

Quota sampling refers to a form of nonprobability sampling in which knowledge about the population of interest is used to build some representativeness into the sample (see Table 12-1). A quota sample identifies the strata of the population and proportionally represents the strata in the sample. For example, the data in Table 12-2 reveal that 40% of the 5000 nurses in city X are diploma graduates, 40% are associate degree graduates, and 20% are baccalaureate graduates. Each stratum of the population should be proportionately represented in the sample. In this case the researcher used a proportional quota sampling strategy and decided to sample 10% of a population of 5000, or 500 nurses. Based on the proportion of each stratum in the population, 200 diploma graduates, 200 associate degree graduates, and 100 baccalaureate graduates were the quotas established for the three strata. The researcher recruited subjects who met the eligibility criteria of the study until the quota for each stratum was filled. In other words, once the researcher obtained the necessary 200 diploma, 200 associate degree, and 100 baccalaureate graduates, the sample was complete.

The researcher systematically ensures that proportional segments of the population are included in the sample. The quota sample is not randomly selected—that is, once the proportional strata have been identified, the researcher obtains subjects until the quota for each stratum has been filled—but it does increase the representativeness of the sample. This sampling strategy addresses the problem of over-representation of underrepresentation of certain segments of a population in a sample.

The characteristics chosen to form the strata are selected according to a researcher's judgment based on knowledge of the population and the literature review. The criterion for selection should be a variable that would reflect important differences in the dependent variables under investigation. Age, gender, religion, ethnicity, medical diagnosis, socioeconomic status, level of completed education, and occupational rank are among those variables that are likely to be important stratifying variables in nursing research investigations.

The critiquer of a research study seeks to determine whether the sample strata appropriately reflect the population under consideration and whether the stratifying variables are homogeneous enough to ensure a meaningful comparison of differences among strata. Even when the preceding factors have been addressed by the researcher, the evaluator must remember that as a nonprobability sample, the quota strategy contains an unknown source of bias that affects external validity.

A researcher may even offer to pay the participants for their time. The problem is that those who choose to participate may not be typical of the population with regard to the variables being measured. The older adults in the Conn (1991) study were found to be very active self-care agents with regard to managing colds and influenza. But because of the volunteer nature of the sample, it is impossible to determine whether the 160 volunteer subjects were representative of older adults in terms of cold and influenza self-care. There is no way to assess the biases that may be operating. In cases where the phenomena under investigation are relatively homogeneous within the population, the risk of bias may be minimal. However, in heterogeneous populations the risk of bias is great.

Purposive Sampling

Purposive sampling is a strategy in which the researcher's knowledge of the population and its elements is used to handpick the cases to be included in the sample. The researcher usually selects subjects who are considered to be *typical* of the population. For example, in a qualitative research study by Beck (1992) examining the lived experience of postpartum depression, a purposive sample of mothers who had attended a postpartum depression support group and were diagnosed as having postpartum depression was used, since they were typical of the population under consideration and could illuminate the phenomenon being studied (see Chapters 11 and 20).

A purposive sample is used also when a highly unusual group is being studied, such as a population with a rare genetic disease such as Tay-Sachs disease. In this case the researcher would describe the sample characteristics precisely to ensure that the reader will have an accurate picture of the subjects in the sample.

In another situation the researcher may wish to interview individuals who reflect different ends of the range of a particular characteristic. For example, a researcher investigates the psychosocial needs in individuals who test positive for the human immunodeficiency virus (HIV) but have no symptoms, in comparison with individuals who have active acquired immunodeficiency syndrome (AIDS).

The researcher who uses a purposive sample assumes that errors of judgment in overrepresenting or underrepresenting elements of the population in the sample will tend to balance out. However, there is no objective method for determining the validity of this assumption. The evaluator must be aware of the fact that the more heterogeneous the population, the greater the chance of bias being introduced in the selection of a purposive sample. As indicated in Table 12-1, conscious bias in the selection of subjects remains a constant danger. As such, the findings from a study using a purposive sample should be regarded with caution. As with any nonprobability sample, the ability to generalize is very limited. The following are several instances when a purposive sample may be appropriate:

1. The effective pretesting of newly developed instruments with a purposive sample of divergent types of people
2. The validation of a scale or test with a known-groups technique
3. The collection of exploratory data in relation to an unusual or highly specific population, particularly when the total target population remains an unknown to the researcher
4. The collection of descriptive data as in qualitative studies that seek to describe the lived experience of a particular phenomenon, such as postpartum depression, caring, hope, or surviving suicide.

Even when the use of a purposive sample is appropriate, the researcher, as well as the critiquer, should be cognizant of the limitations of this sampling strategy.

Probability Sampling

The primary characteristic of probability sampling is the **random selection** of elements from the population. *Random selection* occurs when each element of the population has an equal and independent chance of being included in the sample. Four commonly used probability sampling strategies are **simple random sampling, stratified random sampling, cluster sampling,** and **systematic sampling.**

Random selection of sample subjects should not be confused with *random assignment* of subjects. The latter, as discussed in Chapter 9, refers to the assignment of subjects to either an experimental or a control group on a purely random basis.

Simple Random Sampling

Simple random sampling is a laborious and carefully controlled process. Because the more complex probability designs incorporate the principles of simple random sampling in their procedures, the principles of this strategy are presented.

The researcher defines the population (a set), lists all of the units of the population (a **sampling frame**), and selects a sample of units (a subset) from which the sample will be chosen. For example, if American hospitals specializing in respiratory problems are the sampling unit, a list of all such hospitals would be the sampling frame. If certified clinical specialists constituted the accessible population, a list of those nurses would be the sampling frame.

Once a list of the population elements has been developed, the best method of selecting a sample is to employ a table of random numbers containing columns of digits, such as the one appearing in Fig. 12-1. Such tables can be generated by computer programs. After assigning consecutive numbers to units of the population, the researcher starts at any point on the table of random numbers and reads consecutive numbers in any direction (horizontally, vertically, or diagonally). When a number is read that corresponds with the written unit on a card, that unit is chosen for the

1000 Random Integers Between 0 and 99

```
40  23   0  29  10  94  17  58  12  85  13  25  80  84  72  74  54  63  55  31
32  98  49  23  74  97  51  42  21  87  48  64  54  38  84  68  14  17  35  48
84  34  84  14  53  65  67  37   2  45  84  21  71  34  10  80  72  27  11  13
86  37  24  89  23   4  44  40  72  81  44  69  25  44  34  34  34  75  50  50
50  58  85   8  22  24  73  20  63  35  60  87  91  92  96  80  19  22  87  24
 1  87  43  82   9  31  40  88  33  28  82  73  18   6  48  64  59  45  34   3
21  19  42  76  84  67  29  68   8  66  93  89  96  28  12  14  38  47  52  65
32  66  33  21  81  97  39  76  67  27  97  22  76  89  41  11  91  29   6  66
16  82  42  75  35  42  92  90  77  24  21   8  36  16   5  54  89  51  57  85
74  32  63  65  93  96  18  36  82  72  39  69  37  97  51  17  36  71  38  30
50  94   4  66  17  37  10  53   8  29  67  74  88  38  11  59  60  91  56  17
71  47  81  18  53  98   7  87  29  37  22  93  13   6  95   7  95  71  14   6
71  93  48  16  33  19  46  21  60  44  52  91  52  58  10   9  41  31  35  18
20  94  13  99  45   6  53  54   1  25  79  28   1  48  36  26  68  37  59   7
75  22  69  56  62  40  64  45  40  99  94  14  98  84  22  38  24  87  43  71
16  87  41   0  88  83  11  37  71  78  22  39  43  37  75  84  84  11  55  58
92  90  80   2  30  37  85  55  56  50   3  71  24  13  62  74  82  44  90  32
96  89  31  32  37  45  70  67  80  55  58   9  55  60  61  55  86  44  27  77
38  29  36  94  65  39  56  29  29  65  88  13  71  38  71   8  81  66  31  44
20   6  61  66  90  13  70  60  92  53  87  49  34  42  14  47  75  33  26   9
63  44  94  21  14  13  41  80  39  72  29   3  25  89  44  88  13  49  18  58
13  32  93  90  31  75  86  95  18  51  61  59  84  95  67  54  40  30  29  63
26  35  48  81  19  24  36  36  76  16  46   5  93  41  97  46  79  54  95  49
89  74  96  95  94  69  31  60  16  69  76  42  28  71  69  34  46  55  20  42
50  39  28  64  20  68  60  33  92  82  61  70   5  68  95  88  12  85  18  94
55  86   5  96  87  69  75  93  54  79   0  57  45   8  86  59  25  21   9  29
75  35   1   2  86  62  70  83  85  13  97  37  13  73  16  38  36  23  54  11
74  50   1  77  87  92  68  87  57  36  17  47   0  97  78  72  72  45  54  51
34  24  35  13  26  42  22  75  47   2  34  87  15  50  65  27   5  72  28  68
73  33  42  65  91  24  44  84  71  55  70   1  27  30   8  61  65  61  18  92
 7  55  12   6  61  17  23  95  91  58  60  30  35  61  34  27  75  44  35  64
10  94  18   4   3  19  21  37  28  55  76  25  10  29  80  64   8  81  20  32
20  48  92  87  95  58  57  73  42   1  12  81  94  85  63  97  24  19  93  51
81  10  92  49  70  15  76   4  36  92  62  99  78  32  86  74  43  22  98  46
66  67  82  94  67  75  16  88  84  98   0  52  37   0  43   9   0  51   2  62
64  92  36  11   3  52  44  65  45  67  97  86  92   2  50   5  93  66  73  40
36  29  98  46  88  23  28  44   8  71  69  43  53  16  87  21  56  23  37  24
15  11  82  30  59  94  23  30  40  25  87  26  24  30  44  53  33  65  72  55
89  57  49  79  83  88  42  45  41  93  38  24  15  80  97  18  61  12  13  42
23  36  65   9  64  26  93  37  26  44  42  17  45  68  27  77  74  56  49  34
 9  93  90  61  45  40  75  85  64  66  36  89  72  43  99  90  92  10  10  85
53  94  30  31  62  92  82  30  94  56  40   4  50  53   9  74  87   2  36  36
18  69  77  38  89  78  30  68  71  92  22  93  91  74  52   1  97  69  71  42
50  20  76  36   6  20  75  56  36   5  14  70   9  78  23  33  91  33  25  72
30  46   1  10  16  72  69  26  94  39  80  36  36  68  92  74  22  74  41  42
59  47   7  92  77  55   2  12   5  24   0  30  25  62  83  36  92  96  36  75
93  22   3  20  82  44  16  69  98  72  30  57  77  15  90  29  32  38   3  48
 9  55  27  41  40  94  77  14  54  10  25  75   1  74  72  15  69  80  33  58
70   8   3   5  46  89  28  86  40   6  25  40  81  26  63  97  87  48  26  41
19   6  89  31  80  60  13  89  17  69  38  93  58  55  54  69  74  33   8  55
```

Fig. 12-1 A table of random numbers.

sample. The investigator continues to read until a sample of the desired size is drawn. The advantages of simple random sampling are the following:

1. The sample selection is not subject to the conscious biases of the researcher.
2. The representativeness of the sample in relation to the population characteristics is maximized.
3. The differences in the characteristics of the sample and the population are purely a function of chance.
4. The probability of choosing a nonrepresentative sample decreases as the size of the sample increases.

Simple random sampling was used in a study examining the relationship between nursing care requirements and nursing resource consumption in home health care using both an intensity index and nursing diagnoses. Using a table of random numbers, a random sample of 306 patient records was drawn from patients dismissed during a 6-month period who received at least three nursing visits at home from a specific home health care agency.

Consumers must remember that despite the utilization of a carefully controlled sampling procedure that minimizes error, there is no guarantee that the sample will be representative. Factors such as sample heterogeneity and subject dropout may jeopardize the representativeness of the sample despite the most stringent random sampling procedure.

The major disadvantage of simple random sampling is that it is a time-consuming and inefficient method for obtaining a random sample. Consider the task of listing all of the baccalaureate nursing students in the United States. In addition, it may be impossible to obtain an accurate or complete listing of every element in the population. Imagine trying to obtain a list of all completed suicides in New York City for the year 1993. It often is the case that although suicide may have been the cause of death, another cause, such as cardiac failure, appears on the death certificate. It would be difficult to estimate how many elements of the target population would be eliminated from consideration. The issue of bias would definitely enter the picture despite the researcher's best efforts. Thus the evaluator of a research report must exercise caution in generalizing from reported findings, even when random sampling is the stated strategy, if the target population has been difficult or impossible to list completely.

Stratified Random Sampling

Stratified random sampling requires that the population be divided into strata or subgroups. The subgroups or subsets that the population is divided into are homogeneous. An appropriate number of elements from each subset are randomly selected, on the basis of their proportion in the population. This strategy's goal is to achieve a greater degree of representativeness. Stratified random sampling is similar to the proportional stratified quota sampling strategy discussed earlier in the chapter. The major difference is that stratified random sampling uses a random selection procedure for obtaining sample subjects. Fig. 12-2 provides an example that illustrates the use of stratified random sampling.

Entire population

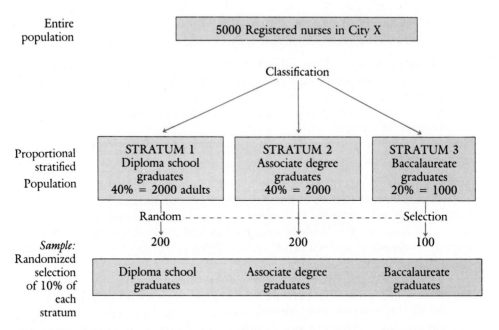

Fig. 12-2 Subject selection using a proportional stratified random sampling strategy.

The population is stratified according to any number of attributes, such as age, gender, ethnicity, religion, socioeconomic status, or level of completed education. The variables selected to make up the strata should be adaptable to homogeneous subsets with regard to the attributes being studied.

The following criteria can be used for decision making in the selection of a stratified sample:
1. Is there a critical variable or attribute that provides a logical basis for stratifying the sample?
2. Does the population list contain sufficient information about the attributes that will be used to divide the sample into subsets?
3. Is it appropriate for each subset to be equal in size, or is it more appropriate for each subset to be proportionally stratified based on the proportion of each subset in the population?
4. If proportional sampling is being used, is there a sufficient number of subjects in each subset for basing meaningful comparisons?
5. Once the subset comparison has been determined, are random procedures used for selection of the sample?

As illustrated in Table 12-1, there are several advantages to a stratified sampling strategy: (1) the representativeness of the sample is enhanced; (2) the researcher has a valid basis for making comparisons among subsets if information on the critical variables has been available; and (3) the researcher is able to oversample a disproportionately small stratum to adjust for their underrepresentation, statistically weigh the data accordingly, and continue to be able to make legitimate comparisons.

The obstacles encountered by a researcher using this strategy include the following: (1) the difficulty of obtaining a population list containing complete critical variable information; (2) the time-consuming effort of obtaining multiple enumerated lists; and (3) the time and money involved in carrying out a large-scale study using a stratified sampling strategy. The critiquer needs to question the appropriateness of this sampling strategy to the problem under investigation. For example, if the reader refers to Fig. 12-2, it is clear that the study population consisted of diploma, associate degree, and baccalaureate degree nurses—three distinct strata. It is appropriate for the researcher to strive to represent all three strata proportionately in the study sample. This strategy would not be necessary if the researcher were studying only one of the three subsets, unless that subset were being logically divided into strata based on other attributes.

Multistage Sampling (Cluster Sampling)

Multistage sampling involves a successive random sampling of units (clusters) that progress from large to small and meet sample eligibility criteria. The first stage sampling unit consists of large units or "clusters." The second stage sampling unit consists of smaller units or "clusters." Third stage sampling units are even smaller. For example, if a sample of clinical specialists is desired, the first sampling unit would be a random sample of hospitals, obtained from an American Hospital Association list, who meet the eligibility criteria (e.g., size, type). The second stage sampling unit would consist of a list of clinical nurse specialists (CNSs) practicing at each hospital selected in the first stage—the list obtained from the vice president for nursing at each hospital. The criteria for inclusion in the list of CNSs were (1) certified CNS with at least 2 years experience as a CNS; (2) at least 50% of the CNS's time must be spent in providing direct patient care; and (3) full-time employment at the hospital. The second stage sampling strategy called for random selection of two CNSs from each hospital and who meet the just-mentioned eligibility criteria.

When multistage sampling is used in relation to large national surveys, states are used as the first stage sampling unit, proceeding to successively smaller units like counties, cities, districts, and blocks as the second stage sampling unit, and then households as the third stage sampling unit.

Sampling units or clusters can be selected by simple random or stratified random sampling methods. Suppose that the hospitals, described in the example above, were grouped into four strata according to size (number of beds): (1) 200 to 299; (2) 300 to 399; (3) 400 to 499; and (4) 500 or more. Stratum 1 comprised 25% of the population; stratum 2 comprised 30% of the population; stratum 3 comprised 20% of the population; and stratum 4 comprised 25% of the population. This means that either a simple random or a proportional, stratified sampling strategy is used to randomly select hospitals that would proportionately represent the population of hospitals in the American Hospital Association list.

The main advantage of cluster sampling, as illustrated in Table 12-1, is that it is considerably more economical in terms of time and money than other types of probability sampling, particularly when the population is large and geographically dispersed or when a sampling frame of the elements is not available. There are two major disadvantages: (1) more sampling errors tend to occur than with simple random or stratified random sampling; and (2) the appropriate handling of the statistical data from cluster samples is very complex.

The reader who is evaluating a research report will need to consider whether the use of cluster sampling is justified in light of the research design, as well as other pragmatic matters, such as economy.

Systematic Sampling

Systematic sampling refers to a sampling strategy that involves the selection of every "kth" case drawn from a population list at fixed intervals, such as every tenth member listed in the directory of the American Association of Critical Care Nurses. Systematic sampling might be used to sample every "kth" person to enter a hospital lobby or to be hospitalized with a diagnosis of acquired immunodeficiency syndrome (AIDS) in 1993. When systematic sampling is used, the population must be narrowly defined as consisting, for example, of all those people entering or leaving in order for the sample to be considered as a probability sample. If senior citizens were sampled systematically on entering a hospital lobby, the resulting sample would not be called a *probability sample*, since not every senior citizen would have a chance of being selected. As such, systematic sampling can sometimes represent a nonprobability sampling strategy.

However, systematic sampling strategies can be designed to fulfill the requirements of a probability sample. First, the listing of the population (sampling frame) must be random in relation to the variable of interest. For example, subjects were being selected from every tenth hospital room for a study on patient satisfaction with nursing care. Every tenth room happens to be a private room in the hospital where the study is being conducted. It is possible that the responses of patients in private rooms with regard to patient satisfaction might be different from those of patients in semiprivate rooms. Because of the nonrandom arrangement of the rooms, bias may have been introduced.

Second, the first element or member of the sample must be selected randomly. In this case the researcher, who has a population list or sampling frame, first divides the population (N) by the size of the desired sample (n) to obtain the sampling interval width (k). The sampling interval is the standard distance between the elements chosen for the sample. For example, to select a sample of 50 family nurse practitioners from a population of 500 family nurse practitioners, the sampling interval would be as follows:

$$k = \frac{500}{50} = 10$$

Essentially, every tenth case on the family nurse practitioner list would be sampled. Once the sampling interval has been determined, the researcher uses a table of random numbers (see Fig. 12-1) to obtain a starting point for the selection of the 50 subjects. If the population size is 500 and a sample size of 50 is desired, a number between 1 and 500 is randomly selected as the starting point. In this instance, if the first number is 51, the family nurse practitioners corresponding to numbers 51, 61, 71, and so forth, would be included in the sample of 50. Another procedure recommended in many texts is to randomly select the first element from within the first sampling interval. If the sampling interval is 5, a number between 1 and 5 would be selected as the random starting point. For example, the number 3 is randomly chosen. Keeping in mind the sampling interval of 5, the next elements selected would correspond to the numbers 8, 13, 18, and so on, until the sample was obtained. Although this latter procedure is technically correct, choosing a random starting point from across the total population of elements is more attractive because every element has a chance to be chosen for the sample during the first selection step.

Systematic and simple random sampling are essentially the same type of procedure. The advantage of systematic sampling is that the results are obtained in a more convenient and efficient manner (see Table 12-1). The disadvantage of systematic sampling is that bias in the form of nonrandomness can inadvertently be introduced to the procedure. This problem may occur if the population list is arranged so that a certain type of element is listed at intervals that coincide with the sampling interval. Let us say that if every tenth nursing student on a population list of all types of nursing students in New York State were a baccalaureate student and the sampling interval were 10, baccalaureate students would be overrepresented in the sample. Cyclical fluctuations are also a factor. For example, if a list is kept of nursing students using the college library each day, a biased sample will probably be obtained if every seventh day is chosen as the sampling interval, because fewer and perhaps different nursing students probably study in the library on Sundays than on weekdays. Therefore caution must be exercised about departures from randomness as they affect the representativeness of the sample and, as a result, affect the external validity of the study.

The critiquer will want to note whether a satisfactory random selection procedure was carried out. If randomization was not used, the systematic sampling may have become a nonprobability quota sample. It is important to be cognizant of this issue, because the implications related to interpretation and generalizability are drastically altered if the evaluator is dealing with a nonprobability sample.

Special Sampling Strategies

Several special sampling strategies are used in nonprobability sampling. **Matching** is a special strategy used to construct an equivalent comparison sample group by filling it with subjects who are similar to each subject in another sample group in relation to such preestablished variables as age, gender, level of education, medical diagnosis, or socioeconomic status. Theoretically, any variable other than the independent variable that could affect the dependent variable should be matched. In reality, the more variables matched, the more difficult it is to obtain an adequate sample size. For example, matching was used in a study examining satisfaction with breast-feeding. Each group was matched in relation to parity and previous breast-feeding experience to obtain two equivalent groups with respect to those variables.

Networking sampling, sometimes referred to as **snowballing,** is a strategy used for locating samples difficult or impossible to locate in other ways. This sampling strategy takes advantage of social networks and the fact that friends tend to have characteristics in common. When a researcher has found a few subjects with the needed eligibility criteria, they are asked for their assistance in getting in touch with others with similar criteria. For example, Lipson (1992) used networking and snowballing to obtain the names of Iranian immigrants to San Francisco, the site of a study examining the health and adjustment of Iranian immigrants.

SAMPLE SIZE

There is no single rule that can be applied to the determination of a sample's size. When arriving at an estimate of sample size, many factors, such as the following, must be considered:
1. The type of design used
2. The type of sampling procedure used
3. The type of formula used for estimating optimum sample size
4. The degree of precision required
5. The heterogeneity of the attributes under investigation
6. The relative frequency of occurrence of the phenomenon of interest in the population; that is, a common versus a rare health problem
7. The projected cost of using a particular sampling strategy

The sample size should be determined before the study is conducted. A general rule of thumb is always to use the largest sample possible. The larger the sample, the more representative of the population it is likely to be; smaller samples produce less accurate results.

The exception to this principle occurs when using certain qualitative designs. In this case, sample size is not predetermined. Sample sizes in qualitative research tend to be small because of the large volume of verbal data that must be analyzed and because this type of design tends to emphasize intensive and prolonged contact with subjects (Sandelowski, 1986). Subjects are added to the sample until **data saturation** is reached: that is, new data no longer emerge during the data collection process. Fittingness of the data is a more important concern than representativeness of subjects (see Chapter 11).

The principle of "larger is better" holds true for both probability and non-probability samples. Results based on small samples (under 10) tend to be unstable—the values fluctuate from one sample to the next. Small samples tend to increase the probability of obtaining a markedly nonrepresentative sample. As the sample size increases, the mean more closely approximates the population values and thus introduces less sampling error.

An example of this concept is illustrated by a study in which the average monthly sleeping pill consumption is being investigated for patients on a rehabilitation unit after a cerebrovascular accident. The data in Table 12-3 indicate that the population consists of 20 patients whose average consumption of sleeping pills is 15.15 per month. Two simple random samples with sample sizes of 2, 4, 6, and 10

Table 12-3 Comparison of Population and Sample Values and Averages in Study of Sleeping Pill Consumption

Number in group	Group	Number of sleeping pills consumed (values expressed monthly)	Average
20	Population	1, 3, 4, 5, 6, 7, 9, 11, 13, 15, 16, 17, 19, 21, 22, 23, 25, 27, 29, 30	15.15
2	Sample 1A	6, 9	7.5
2	Sample 1B	21, 25	23.0
4	Sample 2A	1, 7, 15, 25	12.0
4	Sample 2B	5, 13, 23, 29	17.5
6	Sample 3A	3, 4, 11, 15, 21, 25	13.3
6	Sample 3B	5, 7, 11, 19, 27, 30	16.5
10	Sample 4A	3, 4, 7, 9, 11, 13, 17, 21, 23, 30	13.8
10	Sample 4B	1, 4, 6, 11, 15, 17, 19, 23, 25, 27	14.8

have been drawn from the population of 20 patients. Each sample average in the right-hand column represents an estimate of the population average, which is known to be 15.15. In most cases the population value is unknown to the researchers, but because the population is so small, we could calculate it. As we examine the data in Table 12-3, we note that with a sample size of 2, the estimate might have been wrong by as much as 8 sleeping pills in sample 1B. As the sample size increases, the averages get closer to the population value and the differences in the estimates between samples A and B get smaller as well. Large samples permit the principles of randomization to work effectively, that is, to counterbalance, in the long run, atypical values.

It is possible to estimate the sample size with the use of a statistical procedure known as *power analysis* (Cohen, 1977). It is beyond the scope of this chapter to describe this complex procedure in great detail, but a simple example will illustrate its use. A researcher wants to determine the effect of nurse preoperative teaching on patient postoperative anxiety. Patients are randomly assigned to an experimental group or a control group. How many patients should be used in the study? When using power analysis the researcher must estimate how large a difference will be observed between the groups; that is, the difference in the mean amount of postoperative anxiety after the experimental preoperative teaching program. If a small difference is expected, the sample would need to be large (in this case 196 patients in each group) to ensure that the differences will actually be revealed in a statistical analysis. If a medium-sized difference is expected, the total sample size would be 128—64 in each group. When expected differences are large, it does not take a very large sample to ensure that differences will be revealed through statistical analysis.

Power analysis is an advanced statistical technique that is used increasingly by researchers and is a requirement for external funding (Polit & Sherman, 1990). When it is not used, research studies may be based on samples that are too small.

When samples are too small, the researcher may have unsupported hypotheses and may commit a type I error of rejecting a null hypothesis when it should have been accepted (see Chapter 17). A researcher may also commit a type II error of accepting a null hypothesis when it should have been rejected if the sample is too small (see Chapter 17).

Despite the principles related to determining sample size that have been identified, the consumer should be aware that large samples do not ensure representativeness or accuracy. A large sample cannot compensate for a faulty research design. The proportion of the population that is sampled does not provide a guarantee of accurate results. It is often possible to obtain accurate results from only a small fraction of a large population. For example, a 10% probability sample of a population containing 1500 elements will yield more precise results than a nonprobability 0.01% sample of a population with 100,000 elements.

The critiquer should evaluate the sample size in terms of whether it adequately represents the elements and subsets of the population. Unless representativeness is ensured, all the data in the world become inconsequential.

SAMPLING PROCEDURES

Criteria for drawing a sample vary according to the sampling strategy. Regardless of which strategy is used, it is important that the procedure be systematically organized. This will eliminate the bias that occurs when sample selection is carried out inconsistently. Bias in sample representativeness and generalizability of findings are important sampling issues that have generated national concern. Many of the landmark adult health studies, such as the Framingham heart study and the Baltimore longitudinal study on aging historically excluded women as subjects. Despite the all-male samples, the findings of these studies were generalized from males to *all* adults despite the lack of female representation in the samples. Consequently, careful identification of the target population is a crucial step in the process. If a researcher wants to be able to draw conclusions about psychosocial stressors related to *all* patients with a first-time myocardial infarction, then both males *and* females must be included in the target population. Sometimes the target population has to be gender-specific, as when studying breast or prostate cancer or aspects of pregnancy or menopause.

Several general steps, as illustrated in Fig. 12-3, can be identified that will ensure a consistent approach by the researcher. Initially the target population must be identified; that is, the entire group of people or objects about whom the researcher wants to draw conclusions or make generalizations. The target population may consist of all male patients with a first-time myocardial infarction, all children with acute leukemia, all pregnant teenagers, or all doctoral students in the United States. Next, the accessible portion of the target population must be delineated. An accessible population might consist of all clinical specialists in the state of California, or all male patients with acquired immunodeficiency syndrome (AIDS) admitted to hospital X during 1992, or all pregnant teenagers in a specific prenatal clinic, or all children with acute leukemia under care at a specific hospital specializing in oncology. Then, a sampling plan or a protocol for actually selecting the sample from the

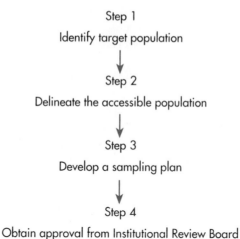

Step 1

Identify target population

Step 2

Delineate the accessible population

Step 3

Develop a sampling plan

Step 4

Obtain approval from Institutional Review Board

Fig. 12-3   Summary of general sampling procedure.

accessible population is formulated. The researcher makes decisions about how subjects will be approached, how the study will be explained, and who will select the sample—the researcher or a research assistant. Regardless of who implements the sampling plan, consistency in how it is done is of paramount importance. The reader of a research study will want to find a description of the sample, as well as the sampling procedure, in the report. On the basis of the appropriateness of what has been reported, the critiquer is able to make judgments about the soundness of the sampling protocol, which of course will affect the interpretations made about the findings. Finally, once the accessible population and sampling plan have been established, permission is obtained from the institution's research board. This permission provides free access to the desired population.

When an appropriate sample size and sampling strategy have been used, the researcher can feel more confident that the sample is representative of the accessible population; however, it is more difficult to feel confident that the accessible population is representative of the target population. Are clinical specialists in California representative of all clinical specialists in the United States? It is impossible to be sure about this. Researchers must exercise judgment when assessing typicality. Unfortunately there are no guidelines for making such judgments, and there is even less basis for the critiquer to make such decisions. The best rule of thumb to use when evaluating the representativeness of a sample and its generalizability to the target population is to be realistic and conservative about making sweeping claims relative to the findings.

CRITIQUING THE SAMPLE

The criteria for critiquing the sampling technique of a study are presented in the box on p. 306. The research consumer approaches the sample section of a research report with a different perspective than does the researcher. The consumer

CRITIQUING CRITERIA

1. Have the sample characteristics been completely described?
2. Can the parameters of the study population be inferred from the description of the sample?
3. To what extent is the sample representative of the population as defined?
4. Are criteria for eligibility in the sample specifically identified?
5. Have sample delimitations been established?
6. Would it be possible to replicate the study population?
7. How was the sample selected? Is the method of sample selection appropriate?
8. What kind of bias, if any, is introduced by this method?
9. Is the sample size appropriate? How is it substantiated?
10. Are there indications that rights of subjects have been ensured?
11. Does the researcher identify the limitations in generalizability of the findings from the sample to the population? Are they appropriate?
12. Does the researcher indicate how replication of the study with other samples would provide increased support for the findings?

must raise two questions. The first question asks, "If this study were to be replicated, would there be enough information presented about the nature of the population, the sample, the sampling strategy, and sample size for another investigator to carry out the study?" The second question asks, "Are the previously mentioned factors appropriate in light of the particular research design, and if not, which factors require modification, especially if the study is to be replicated?"

Sampling is considered to be one important aspect of the methodology of a research study. As such, data pertaining to the sample usually appear in the methodology section of the research report. The sampling content presented should reflect the outcome of a series of decisions based on sampling criteria appropriate to the design of the study, as well as the options and limitations inherent in the context of the investigation. The following discussion will highlight several sampling criteria that the research consumer will want to consider when evaluating the merit of a sampling strategy as it relates to a specific research study.

Initially the parameters or attributes of the study population should clearly specify to what population the findings may be generalized. Generally the target population of the study is not specifically identified by the researcher, but the nature of it is implied in the description of the accessible population and/or the sample. For example, if a researcher states that 100 subjects were randomly drawn from a population of married primiparas who vaginally delivered full-term infants at hospital L during 1993, the critiquer is able to specifically evaluate the parameters of the population. Demographic characteristics of the sample, such as age, gender, diagnosis, ethnicity, religion, and marital status, should also be presented in either a tabled or a narrative summary, since they provide further explication about the nature of the sample and enable the critiquer to evaluate the sampling procedure more accurately. For example, in a study by Dilorio, Faherty, and Manteuffel (1992) titled "Self-Efficacy and Social Support in Self-Management of Epilepsy," the authors present detailed data summarizing demographic variables of importance. These data are reproduced as follows:

> The respondents ranged from 17 to 66 years of age, with a mean age of 35.5 years. Over half (52%) of the respondents were female; 73.5% were White, 22.4% were Black, 1% were of other ethnic backgrounds, and 3.1% chose not to respond to this item. Almost 90% of the respondents held high school diplomas, and 56.1% had attended at least some college. Half (50%) of the participants were employed full time, 9.2% worked part time, 34.7% were unemployed at the time of the survey, and 6.1% chose not to respond to this item. Approximately 25% held professional or managerial positions. The mean age when seizures began was 15.6 years, with a range from birth to 55 years. The respondents had suffered from seizures from 1 to 46 years, with an average of 20.2 years. Approximately 56% reported that they suffered generalized seizures, 28.6% suffered petit mal seizures, 27.6% experienced complex partial seizures, and 17.3% had partial seizures. Atonic (6.1%) and myoclonic (1%) seizures were also reported. These percentages include those subjects who reported having more than one type of seizure. The median number of seizures experienced by the respondents during the previous year was three; 60% of the respondents reported five or fewer seizures. The median number of medications taken was one, with a range of one to four. (p. 296)

This example illustrates how a detailed description of the sample provides the critiquer with a frame of reference about the study population and sample and generates questions to be raised. For instance, the reader will note subjects experienced six types of seizures. However, type of seizure was not a factor in grouping subjects who were examined as one group. The evaluator who has this demographic sample information available is able to question a sampling strategy that does not also consider the differential effect of type of seizure on self-management in epilepsy. It would seem logical that there might be a difference in self-management if one has generalized versus petit mal seizures.

It is also helpful if the researcher has presented a rationale for having elected to study one type of population versus another. For example, why did the previously cited study focus only on married primiparas who vaginally delivered full-term infants, as opposed to unmarried women or women who had had cesarean births? In a research study that uses a nonprobability sampling strategy, it is particularly important to fully describe the population and the sample in terms of who the study subjects are, how they were chosen, and why they were chosen. If these criteria are adhered to, the degree of heterogeneity or homogeneity of the sample can be determined. The use of a homogeneous sample minimizes the amount of sampling error introduced, a problem particularly common in nonprobability sampling.

Next, the defined representativeness of the population should be examined. Probability sampling is clearly the ideal sampling procedure for ensuring the representativeness of a study population. Use of random selection procedures, such as simple random, stratified, cluster, or systematic sampling strategies, minimizes the occurrence of conscious and unconscious biases, which, of course, would affect the researcher's ability to generalize about the findings from the sample to the population. The evaluator should be able to identify the type of probability strategy used and to determine whether the researcher adhered to the criteria for a particular sampling plan. In experimental and quasiexperimental studies the evaluator must know also whether or how the subjects were assigned to groups. If the criteria have not been followed, the reader would have a valid basis for being cautious about the proposed conclusions of the study.

Although random selection is the ideal in establishing the representativeness of a study population, more often realistic barriers, such as institutional policy, inaccessibility of subjects, lack of time or money, and current state of knowledge in the field, necessitate the use of nonprobability sampling strategies. Many important research problems that are of interest to nursing do not lend themselves to experimental design and probability sampling. This is particularly true with qualitative research designs. A well-designed, carefully controlled study using a nonprobability sampling strategy can yield accurate and meaningful findings that make a significant contribution to nursing's scientific body of knowledge. The critiquer needs to ask a philosophical question: "If it is not possible or appropriate to conduct an experimental or quasiexperimental investigation that uses probability sampling, should the study be abandoned?" The answer usually suggests that it is better to carry out the investigation and be fully aware of the limitations of the methodology than to lose the knowledge that can be gained. The researcher is always able to move on to subsequent studies that either replicate the study or use more stringent design and sampling strategies to refine the knowledge derived from a nonexperimental study.

The greatest difficulty in nonprobability sampling stems from the fact that not every element in the population has an equal chance of being represented in the sample. Therefore it is likely that some segment of the population will be systematically underrepresented. If the population is homogeneous on critical characteristics, systematic bias will not be very important. However, few of the attributes that researchers are interested in are sufficiently homogeneous to render sampling bias an irrelevant consideration.

Next, the sampling plan's suitability to the research design should be evaluated. Experimental and quasiexperimental designs use some form of random selection or random assignment of subjects to groups (see Chapter 9). The critiquer evaluates whether the researcher adhered to the principles of random selection and assignment. Lack of adherence to such principles compromises the representativeness of the sample and the external validity of the study. The following are questions the evaluator might pose relative to this issue:

1. Has a random selection procedure been identified, such as a table of random members?
2. Has the appropriate random sampling plan been selected; that is, has a proportional stratified sampling plan been selected instead of a simple random sampling plan in a study where there are three distinct occupational levels that appear to be critical variables for stratification?
3. Has the particular random sampling plan been carried out appropriately; that is, if a cluster sampling strategy was used, did the sampling units logically progress from the largest to the smallest?

Random sampling should not be looked on as a cure-all. Sometimes bias is inadvertently introduced even when the principle of random selection is used.

Nonexperimental designs often use nonprobability sampling strategies. In this instance the question that can be raised by the critiquer is whether a nonexperimental design and a related nonprobability sampling plan were most appropriate for this study. It is sometimes true that if the researcher had used another type of design or sampling plan, he or she could have constructed a stronger study that would have allowed greater confidence to be placed in the findings and greater generalizability. However, the critiquer is rarely in a position to know what factors entered into the decision to plan one type of study versus another.

When critiquing qualitative research designs, the evaluator would apply criteria related to sampling strategies that are relevant for a particular type of qualitative study. In general, sampling strategies are purposive, since the study of specific phenomena in their natural setting is emphasized; any subject belonging to a specified group is considered to represent that group. For example, when a qualitative study such as "Living with a Wife Undergoing Chemotherapy" (Wilson & Morse, 1991) is conducted, the specified group is husbands whose wives are undergoing chemotherapy. The goal of the researcher is to establish the meaning of their slices of life: that is, the typicality or atypicality of the observed events, behaviors, or responses in the lives of the husbands (see Chapter 11).

Then the evaluator should determine whether the sample size is appropriate and whether its size is justifiable. It no longer is unusual for the researcher to indicate in a research article how the sample size was arrived at; this is also seen commonly in doctoral dissertations. The method of arriving at the sample size and the rationale should be briefly mentioned. For example, a researcher may state in a very detailed way:

> The sample size was set on the basis of a significance level of 0.05, a medium effect of 0.13, and a power of 0.95 in multiple regression analysis (Cohen, 1977). This sample size, $N = 168$, is larger than required for nine predictors with a conventional power of 0.80 ($N = 110$). The sample size was expanded to allow for the shrinkage of R^2.

The importance of this example lies not in understanding every technical word cited, but rather in understanding that this type of statement or some abbreviated form of it meets the criteria stated at the beginning of the paragraph and should be evident on the research report.

Other considerations with respect to sample size, especially where the sample size appears to be small or inadequate and there is no stated rationale for the size, are the following:

- How will the sample size affect the accuracy of the results?
- Are any subsets or cells of the sample overrepresented or underrepresented?
- Are any of the subsets so small as to limit meaningful comparisons?
- Has the researcher examined the effect of attrition or dropouts on the results?
- Has the researcher recognized and identified any limitations posed by the size of the sample?

Essentially, these criteria demand that the critiquer carefully scrutinize several important elements pertaining to sample size that have implications for the generalizability of the findings. Keep in mind that qualitative studies will not discuss predetermining sample size or methods for arriving at sample size. Rather, sample size will tend to be small and a function of data saturation (see Chapter 11).

Finally, evidence that the rights of human subjects have been protected should appear in the sample section of the research report. The critiquer will evaluate whether permission was obtained from an institutional review board that reviewed the study relative to the maintenance of ethical research standards (see Chapter 3). For example, the review board examines the research proposal to determine whether the introduction of an experimental procedure may be potentially harmful and therefore undesirable. The critiquer also examines the report for evidence of informed consent of subjects, as well as protection of confidentiality or anonymity. It is highly unusual for research studies not to demonstrate evidence of having met these criteria. Nevertheless, the careful evaluator will want to be certain that ethical standards that protect sample subjects have been maintained.

It is evident that there are many factors to consider when critiquing the sample section of a research report. The type and appropriateness of the sampling strategy become crucial elements in the analysis and interpretation of data, in the conclusions derived from the findings, and in the generalizability of the findings from the sample to the population. As stated earlier in this chapter, the major purpose of sampling is to increase the efficiency of a research study by using a sample that is representative of the particular population so that every element need not be studied, and yet generalizing the findings from the sample to the population. The critiquer needs to justify that the sampling strategy used provided a valid basis for feeling confident of the findings and their generalizability.

KEY POINTS

- *Sampling* is a process that selects representative units of a population for study. Researchers sample representative segments of the population, because it is rarely feasible or necessary to sample entire populations of interest to obtain accurate and meaningful information.

- A *population* is a well-defined set that has certain specified properties. A population may consist of people, objects, or events.
- Researchers establish *eligibility criteria;* these are descriptors of the population and provide the basis for selection into a sample. Eligibility criteria, also referred to as *delimitations,* include the following: age, gender, socioeconomic status, level of education, religion, and ethnicity.
- The researcher must identify the *target population;* that is, the entire set of cases about which the researcher would like to make generalizations. However, because of pragmatic constraints, the researcher usually utilizes an *accessible population,* one that meets the population criteria and is available.
- A *sample* is a set of elements that make up the population.
- A *sampling unit* is the element or set of elements used for selecting the sample. The foremost criterion in evaluating a sample is the *representativeness* or congruence of characteristics with the population.
- Sampling strategies consist of nonprobability and probability sampling.
    - In *nonprobability sampling* the elements are chosen by nonrandom methods. Types of nonprobability sampling include convenience, quota, and purposive sampling.
    - *Probability sampling* is characterized by the random selection of elements from the population. In *random selection* each element in the population has an equal and independent chance of being included in the sample. Types of probability sampling include simple random, stratified random, cluster, and systematic sampling.
- Sample size is a function of the type of sampling procedure being used, the degree of precision required, the type of sample estimation formula being used, the heterogeneity of study attributes, the relative frequency of occurrence of the phenomena under consideration, and cost.
- Criteria for drawing a sample vary according to the sampling strategy. Systematic organization of the sampling procedure minimizes bias. The target population is identified, the accessible portion of the target population is delineated, permission to conduct the research study is obtained, and a sampling plan is formulated.
- The critiquer of a research report evaluates the sampling plan for its appropriateness in relation to the particular research design. Completeness of the sampling plan is examined in light of potential replicability of the study. The critiquer evaluates whether the sampling strategy is the strongest plan for the particular study under consideration.
- An appropriate systematic sampling plan will maximize the efficiency of a research study. It will increase the accuracy and meaningfulness of the findings and enhance the generalizability of the findings from the sample to the population.

REFERENCES

Beck, C.T. (1992). The lived experience of postpartum depression: A phenomenological study, *Nursing Research, 41* (3), 166-170.

Cohen, J. (1977). *Statistical power analysis for the behavioral sciences* (rev. ed.). New York, Academic Press.

Conn, V. (1991). Self-care actions taken by older adults for influenza and colds. *Nursing Research, 40* (3), 176-181.

Dilorio, C., Faherty, B., & Manteuffel, B. (1992). Self-efficacy and social support in self-management of epilepsy, *Western Journal of Nursing Research, 14* (3), 292-307.

Lipson, J.G. (1992). The health and adjustment of Iranian immigrants. *Western Journal of Nursing Research. 14* (1), 10-24.

Polit, D.F., and Sherman, R.E. (1990). Statistical power in nursing research. *Nursing Research, 39* (6), 365-368.

Sampselle, C.M., and DeLancey, J.O.L. (1992). The urine stream interruption test and pelvic muscle function. *Nursing Research, 41* (2), 73-77.

Sandelowski, M. (1986). The problem of rigor in qualitative research. *Advances in Nursing Science, 8* (3), 27-37.

Wilson, S., and Morse, J.M. (1991). Living with a wife undergoing chemotherapy. *Image, 23* (2), 78-84.

ADDITIONAL READINGS

Downs, F.S., and Newman, M.A. (1977). *A source book of nursing research*. Philadelphia: F.A. Davis.

Floyd, J.A. (1993). Systematic sampling: Theory and clinical methods. *Nursing Research, 42* (5), 290-293.

Kerlinger, F.N. (1986). *Foundations of behavioral research*. New York: Holt, Rinehart & Winston.

Levey, P.S., and Lemeshow, S. (1980). *Sampling for health professionals*. New York: Lifetime Learning.

Stewart Fahs, P., and Kinney, M.R. (1991). The abdomen, thigh, and arm as sites for subcutaneous sodium heparin injections. *Nursing Research, 40* (4), 204-207.

Volicer, B.J. (1984). *Multivariate statistics for nursing research*. Orlando, FL: Grune & Stratton.

Yarandi, H.N. (1991). Planning sample sizes: comparison of factor level means. *Nursing Research, 40* (1), 57-58.

CHAPTER
13

Legal and Ethical Issues

BETTIE S. JACKSON

LEARNING OBJECTIVES

After reading this chapter the student should be able to do the following:

- Describe the historical background that led to the development of ethical guidelines for the use of human subjects in research.
- Identify the essential elements of an informed consent form.
- Evaluate the adequacy of an informed consent form.
- Describe the institutional review board's role in the research review process.
- Identify populations of subjects who require special legal and ethical research considerations.
- Appreciate the nurse researcher's obligations to conduct and report research in an ethical manner.
- Describe the nurse's role as patient advocate in research situations.
- Discuss the nurse's role in assuring that FDA guidelines for testing of medical devices are followed.
- Discuss animal rights in research situations.
- Critique the ethical aspects of a research study.

KEY TERMS

animal rights	informed consent
anonymity	institutional review board
assent	justice
beneficence	product testing
benefits	respect for persons
confidentiality	risk-benefit ratio
consent	risks
ethics	

Listen, Martin. I am aware that the technique of experimenting on humans without their consent is against any traditional concept of medical ethics. But I believe the results justify the methods. Seventeen young women have unknowingly sacrificed their lives. That is true. But it has been for the betterment of society and the future guarantee of the defense superiority of the United States. From the point of view of two hundred million Americans, it is a very small one. Think of how many young women willfully take their lives each year, or how many people kill themselves on the highways, and to what end? Here these seventeen women have added something to society, and they have been treated with compassion. (Cook, 1981, p. 292)

"When people rely on rules to protect them from harm, they are not interested in pieces of paper, but in the conduct of the people who are supposed to be governed by the rules" (Hanks, 1984a, p. 1). It is not just rules and regulations dealing with the involvement of human subjects in research that assure that research will be conducted legally and ethically. Researchers themselves and caregivers providing care to patients, who also happen to be research subjects, must be fully committed to the tenets of informed consent and patients' rights. The principle "the ends justify the means" must never be tolerated. Researchers and caregivers of research subjects must take every precaution to protect people being studied from physical or mental harm or discomfort. It is not always clear what constitutes harm or discomfort.

The focus of this chapter is the legal and ethical considerations that must be addressed before, during, and after the conduct of research. Informed consent, institutional review boards, and research involving vulnerable populations—the elderly, pregnant women, children, prisoners, persons with AIDS, and animals—are discussed. The nurse's role as patient advocate, whether functioning as researcher, caregiver, or research consumer, is addressed.

ETHICAL AND LEGAL CONSIDERATIONS IN RESEARCH: AN HISTORICAL PERSPECTIVE

Ethical and legal considerations with regard to research first received attention after World War II. When the then U.S. Secretary of State and Secretary of War learned that the trials for war criminals would focus on justifying the atrocities committed by Nazi physicians as "medical research," the American Medical Association was asked to appoint a group to develop a code of ethics for research that would be used as a standard for judging the medical atrocities committed by physicians on concentration camp prisoners.

The 10 rules included in what was called the *Nuremberg Code* appear in the box below. Its definitions of the terms *voluntary, legal capacity, sufficient understanding,* and *enlightened decision* have been the subject of numerous court cases and presidential commissions involved in setting ethical standards in research (Creighton, 1977). The code that was developed requires informed consent in all cases but makes no provisions for any special treatment of children, the elderly, or the mentally incompetent. Several other international standards have followed, the

---

ARTICLES OF THE NUREMBERG CODE

1. The voluntary consent of the human subject is absolutely essential.
2. The study should be such as to yield fruitful results for the good of society, unprocurable by other means of study, and not random and unnecessary in nature.
3. The experiment should be so designed and based on the results of animal experimentation and knowledge of the natural history of the disease or other problems under study that the anticipated results will justify the performance of the experiment.
4. The experiment should be conducted to avoid all unnecessary physical and mental suffering and injury.
5. No experiment should be conducted where there is a prior reason to believe that death or disabling injury will occur.
6. The degree of risk to be taken should never exceed that determined by the humanitarian importance of the problem to be solved by the experiment.
7. Proper preparations should be made and adequate facilities provided to protect the subject against . . . injury, disability, or death.
8. The experiment should be conducted only by scientifically qualified persons.
9. The human subject should be at liberty to bring the experiment to an end.
10. During the experiment, the scientist . . . if he has probable cause to believe that a continuation of the experiment is likely to result in injury, disability or death to the experimental subject . . . will bring it to a close.

Modified from *Experimentation with human beings* (pp. 289-290) by J. Katz, 1972, New York: Russell Sage Foundation.

Table 13-1   Highlights of Unethical Research Studies Conducted in the United States

Research study	Year	Focus of study	Ethical principle violated
Hyman vs. Jewish Chronic Disease Hospital case	1965	Doctors injected aged and senile patients with live cancer cells to study their rejection response.	Informed consent was not obtained, and there was no indication that the study had been reviewed and approved by an ethics committee. The two physicians claimed that they did not wish to evoke emotional reactions or refusals to participate by informing the subjects of the nature of the study (Hershey & Miller, 1976).
Milledgeville, Georgia, case	1969	Investigational drugs were used on mentally disabled children without first obtaining the opinion of a psychiatrist.	There was no review of the study protocol or institutional approval of the program before implementation (Levine, 1986).
Tuskegee, Alabama, syphillis study	1932-1973	For 40 years the United States Public Health Service conducted a study using two groups of poor black male sharecroppers. One group consisted of those who had untreated syphillis; the other group was judged to be free of the disease. Treatment was withheld from the group having syphillis even after penicillin became generally available and accepted as effective treatment in the 1950s. Steps were taken to prevent the subjects from obtaining it. The researchers wanted to study the untreated disease.	Many of the subjects who consented to participate in the study were not informed about the purpose and procedures of the research. Others were unaware that they were subjects. The degree of risk outweighed the potential benefit. Withholding of known effective treatment violates the subjects' right to fair treatment and protection from harm (Levine, 1986).

Research study	Year	Focus of study	Ethical principle violated
San Antonio contraceptive study	1969	In a study examining the side effects of oral contraceptives, 76 impoverished Mexican-American women were randomly assigned to an experimental group receiving birth control pills or a control group receiving placebos. Subjects were not informed about the placebo and attendant risk of pregnancy. Eleven subjects became pregnant, 10 of whom were in the placebo control group.	Principles of informed consent were violated; full disclosure of potential risk, harm, results, or side effects was not evident in the informed consent document. The potential risk outweighed the benefits of the study. The subjects' right to fair treatment and protection from harm was violated (Levine, 1986).
Willowbrook Hospital	1972	Mentally incompetent children ($n = 350$) were not admitted to Willowbrook Hospital, a residential treatment facility, unless parents consented to their children being subjects in a study examining the natural history of infectious hepatitis and the effect of gamma globulin. The children were deliberately infected with the hepatitis virus under various conditions; some received gamma globulin; others did not.	Principle of voluntary consent was violated. Parents were coerced to consent to their children's participation as research subjects. Subjects or their guardians have a right to self-determination: that is, they should be free of constraint, coercion, or undue influence of any kind. Many subjects feel pressured to participate in studies if they are in powerless, dependent positions (Rothman, 1982).

BASIC ETHICAL PRINCIPLES RELEVANT TO THE CONDUCT OF RESEARCH

Respect for Persons	People have the right to self-determination and to treatment as autonomous agents. Thus they have the freedom to participate or not participate in research. Persons with diminished autonomy are entitled to protection.
Beneficence	An obligation to do no harm and maximize possible benefits. Persons are treated in an ethical manner when their decisions are respected, they are protected from harm, and efforts are made to secure their well-being.
Justice	Human subjects should be treated fairly. An injustice occurs when benefit to which a person is entitled is denied without good reason or when a burden is imposed unduly.

most notable of which was the Declaration of Helsinki, which was adopted in 1964 by the World Medical Assembly and then later revised in 1975 (Levine, 1979).

In the United States, federal guidelines for the ethical conduct of research involving human subjects were not developed until the 1970s. Some of the most atrocious, and hence memorable, examples of unethical research studies took place in the United States as recently as the 1970s. These examples are highlighted in Table 13-1 (pp. 316–317). They are sad reminders of our own tarnished research heritage and illustrate the human consequences of not adhering to ethical research standards.

The conduct of harmful, illegal research made additional controls necessary. In 1973 the Department of Health, Education and Welfare published the first set of proposed regulations on the protection of human subjects. The most important provision was a regulation mandating that an institutional review board (IRB) functioning in accordance with specifications of the department must review and approve all studies. The National Research Act, passed in 1974 (Public Law 93-348), created the National Commission for the Protection of Human Subjects of Biomedical and Behavioral Research. A major charge of the Commission was to identify the basic principles that should underlie the conduct of biomedical and behavioral research involving human subjects and develop guidelines to assure that research is conducted in accordance with those principles (Levine, 1986). Three ethical principles were identified as relevant to the conduct of research involving human subjects: the principles of **respect for persons, beneficence,** and **justice.** They are defined in the box above. Included in a report issued in 1979, called the *Belmont Report,* these principles provided the basis for regulations affecting research sponsored by the federal government. The Belmont Report also served as a model for many of the ethical codes developed by scientific disciplines (National Commission, 1978).

In 1980 the Department of Health and Human Services developed a set of regulations in response to the Commission's recommendations. These regulations were published in 1981 and revised in 1983 (Department of Health and Human Services, 1983). These regulations include the following:
• General requirements for informed consent
• Documentation of informed consent
• Institutional review board (IRB) review of research proposals
• Exempt and expedited review procedures for certain kinds of research
• Criteria for IRB approval of research
These regulations are discussed in the sections on informed consent and institutional review later in this chapter.

Current and Future Ethical Dilemmas in Research

On a national level, the ethical dilemmas in research for the present and twenty-first centuries will be in the area of biotechnology and the use of animals for research. In 1993 the U.S. Government ended a 5-year moratorium and began approving animal patents. Patents have been issued to organizations for the development of "transgenic" or genetically engineered animals suited to research in humans (Andrews, 1993). Another use of animals for research is in the area of xenograft transplantation. In 1992 three liver transplants were done using two baboons and one pig. Several centers have obtained approval from their institutional review boards to perform xenograft transplants. The **ethics,** as well as the risks and benefits of this type of human/animal research, are still in question; the issue is very controversial.

Other areas of research that engender much discussion and controversy are fetal tissue research and use of women who are of childbearing potential as subjects in drug/therapeutic studies. In 1993 an executive order lifted the government's ban on fetal tissue research. This allows the resumption of research into the testing of fetal tissue for use in the treatment of such diseases as Parkinson's.

In the past, women of childbearing potential were denied access to participation as subjects in drug or potentially therapeutic studies because of the unknown potentially harmful effects of drugs and other therapies that were in various stages of testing on fetuses. This policy has led to the exclusion of women from many important drug and research studies over the years. Currently researchers seeking funds from the National Institutes of Health have to justify excluding women from such studies (Burd, 1993).

Over the next decade many questions and controversies will arise in relation to the risks and benefits of the just-mentioned areas of research and as a result of ever-increasing technology in health care in areas that have not been defined as yet. Though these areas of research may seem far removed from nursing research and patient care, they will affect the type of patients nurses will care for and the type of clinical research nurses will conduct.

EVOLUTION OF ETHICS IN NURSING RESEARCH

The evolution of ethics in nursing research can be traced back to 1897 and the constitution of the Nurses' Associated Alumnae Organization. One of the first purposes of this organization was to establish a code of ethics for the nursing profession. In 1900 Isabel Hampton Robb wrote *Nursing Ethics: For Hospital and Private Use.* In describing moral laws by which people must abide, she states:

> Etiquette, speaking broadly, means a form of behavior or manners expressly or tacitly required on particular occasions. It makes up the code of polite life and includes forms of ceremony to be observed, so that we invariably find in societies that a certain etiquette is required and observed either tacitly or by expressed agreement.

Clearly, Hampton Robb's comments reflect the norms of Victorian society. However, they highlight a historical concern for ethical actions by nurses as health care providers (Robb, 1900).

In 1967 the American Nurses' Association (ANA) charged its Committee on Research Studies with the task of developing guidelines for the nurse researcher in clinical research. In 1968 the ANA Board of Directors approved the statement titled, "The Nurse in Research: ANA Guidelines on Ethical Values." Not only were basic principles regarding the use of human subjects endorsed, but the role of the nurse as investigator, as well as practitioner, was described.

The ANA established the Commission on Nursing Research in 1970. By doing so, it publicly affirmed nursing's obligation to support the advancement of scientific knowledge and reflected a commitment to support two sets of human rights: (1) the rights of qualified nurses to engage in research and have access to resources necessary for implementing scientific investigation and (2) the rights of all persons who are participants in research performed by investigators whose studies impinge on the patient care provided by nurses. The ANA emphasized human rights in terms of three domains: (1) right to freedom from intrinsic risk or injury, (2) right to privacy and dignity, and (3) right to anonymity.

The American Nurses' Association's *Human Rights Guidelines for Nursing in Clinical and Other Research,* published in 1975, reflects the nursing profession's code of ethics for research. The box on p. 321 provides a summary of this document, one that helps ensure that research maintains ethical, as well as scientific, rigor. This document is relevant for *all* nurses; the nurse as a researcher or caregiver must assure patients that their human rights will be safeguarded. In fact, nurses, when interviewing for potential employment, should ask what is expected of them in terms of research responsibilities. For example, nurses might ask:

* Are nurses required to collect data or administer medications or treatments in double-blind clinical trials?
* Are written research protocols available as references?
* Has the IRB ruled on each protocol?
* Are nurses free to decline to participate without jeopardizing their position?
* What channels exist for addressing ethical concerns with regard to research being conducted?

Clearly, ignorance and naivete vis a vis ethical and legal guidelines for the conduct of research must never be an excuse for a nurse's failure to be familiar with and act on

AMERICAN NURSES' ASSOCIATION HUMAN RIGHTS GUIDELINES FOR NURSES IN CLINICAL AND OTHER RESEARCH

Guideline 1: Right to Self Determination

Implementation: Where research participation is a condition of employment, nurses must be informed in writing of the nature of the activity involved in advance of employment. If nurses are not so informed, they must be given the opportunity of not participating in the research.

Potential of risk to others must be clarified in relation to the types of risk involved, the ways of recognizing when risk is present, and the ways in which to counteract potential and unnecessary danger.

Guideline 2: Right to Freedom from Risk or Harm

Implementation: Investigators must ensure freedom of risk from harm by estimating the potential physical or emotional risk and benefit involved. Vulnerable and captive subjects, such as students, patients, prisoners, mentally incompetent, children, the elderly, and the poor, must be carefully monitored for sources of potential risk of injury so they can be protected.

Guideline 3: Scope of Application

Implementation: Guidelines for protection of human rights apply to all individuals, that is, subjects involved in research activities. The use of subjects with limited civil freedom can usually be justified only when there is benefit to them or others in similar circumstances.

Guideline 4: Responsibility to Support Knowledge Development

Implementation: Nurses have an obligation to support the development of knowledge that expands the depth and breadth of the scientific knowledge or base of nursing practice.

Guideline 5: Informed Consent

Implementation: The right to self-determination is protected when informed consent is obtained from the prospective subject or legal guardian.

Guideline 6: Participation on Institutional Review Boards

Implementation: As professionals accountable to the public who are the consumers of health care, nurses have an obligation to support the inclusion of nurses on institutional review boards (IRBs). Nurses also have an obligation to serve on IRBs to review ethical implications of proposed and ongoing research. All studies involving data collection from humans, animals, or records should be reviewed by a review board of health professionals and community representatives who ensure the protection of subject rights.

From *Guidelines for Nurses in Clinical and Other Research* by American Nurses' Association, 1975, Kansas City, MO: Author.

behalf of the patients whose human rights must, at all times, be safeguarded. Nurse researchers are often among the most responsible and conscientious investigators when it comes to respecting the rights of human subjects. All nurses should be aware that the tenets of the American Nurses Association's *Code for Nurses* (1985) are integral with the ANA *Human Rights Guidelines for Nursing in Clinical and Other Research* mentioned earlier.

Fowler (1988), a nurse ethicist, calls for an international code of ethics for nursing research. She raises many ethical questions that nurses around the world need to address now and in the future. Davis (1990) supports the concept of shared values among all nurses, stating that many of nursing's shared values are found in their professional codes. Some countries have their own code; others use the International Council of Nurses (ICN) Code for Nurses.

PROTECTION OF HUMAN RIGHTS

Human rights are the claims and demands that have been justified in the eyes of an individual or by a group of individuals. The term refers to five rights outlined in the ANA (1985) guidelines:
1. Right to self-determination
2. Right to privacy and dignity
3. Right to anonymity and confidentiality
4. Right to fair treatment
5. Right to protection from discomfort and harm

These rights apply to everyone involved in a research project, including research team members who may be involved in data collection, practicing nurses involved in the research setting, as well as the subjects participating in the study. As consumers of research read a research article, they must realize any issues highlighted in Table 13-2 should have been addressed and resolved before a research study is approved for implementation.

Procedures for Protecting Basic Human Rights
Informed Consent

Informed consent illustrated by the ethical principles of respect and its related right to self-determination already have been outlined in the box on p. 318 and Table 13-2. Nurses need to understand elements of informed consent so that they are knowledgeable participants in obtaining informed consents from patients and/or in critiquing this process as it is presented in research articles.

Informed consent is the legal principle that, at least in theory, governs the patient's ability to accept or reject individual medical interventions designed to diagnose or treat an illness. It is also the doctrine that determines and regulates participation in research (Dubler, 1987). The Code of Federal Regulations (1983) defines the meaning of *informed consent:*

> The knowing consent of an individual or his/her legally authorized representative, under circumstances that provide the prospective subject or representative sufficient opportunity to consider whether or not to participate without undue inducement or any element of force, fraud, deceit, duress, or other forms of constraint or coercion. (pp. 9–10)

No investigator may involve a human being as a research subject before obtaining the legally effective informed consent of a subject or legally authorized representative.

ELEMENTS OF INFORMED CONSENT

1. A statement that the study involves research.
2. An explanation of the purposes of the research, delineating the expected duration of the subject's participation.
3. A description of the procedures to be followed, and identification of any procedures which are experimental.
4. A description of any reasonably foreseeable risks or discomforts to the subject.
5. A description of any benefits to the subject or to others that may reasonably be expected from the research.
6. A disclosure of appropriate alternative procedures or course of treatment, if any, that might be advantageous to the subject.
7. A statement describing the extent to which anonymity and confidentiality of the records identifying the subject will be maintained.
8. For research involving more than minimal risk, an explanation as to whether any medical treatments are available if injury occurs and, if so, what they consist of, or where further information may be obtained.
9. An explanation about who to contact for answers to questions about the research and researcher subjects' rights, and who to contact in the event of a research-related injury to the subject.
10. A statement that participation is voluntary, that refusal to participate will not involve any penalty or less benefit to which the subject is otherwise entitled, and the subject may discontinue participation at any time without penalty or loss of otherwise entitled benefits.

From "Protection of Human Subjects" in *Code of Federal Regulations, OPRR Reports,* March 8, 1983.

Prospective subjects must have time to decide whether to participate in a study. The researcher must not coerce the subject into participating. The language of the consent form must be understandable. For example, the reading level should be no greater than eighth grade for adults and the use of technical research language should be avoided (Rempusheski, 1991). According to the Code of Federal Regulations, subjects in no way should be asked to waive their rights or release the investigator from liability for negligence.

The elements that need to be contained in an informed consent are listed in the box above. It is important to note that many institutions require additional elements. A sample of an informed consent form is presented in Fig. 13-1.

Most investigators obtain consent through personal discussion with potential subjects. This process allows the person to obtain immediate answers to questions. However, consent forms, written in narrative or outline form, highlight elements that both inform and remind subjects of the nature of the study and their participation (Rempusheski, 1991).

Assurance of **anonymity**, and **confidentiality**, defined in Table 13-2 (see pp. 324–327), is usually conveyed in writing. This is sometimes difficult in unique

Table 13-2 Protection of Human Rights

Basic human right	Definition
Right to self-determination	Based on the ethical principle of respect for persons; people should be treated as autonomous agents who have the freedom to choose without external controls. An autonomous agent is one who is informed about a proposed study and is allowed to choose to participate or not to participate (Brink, 1992); and Subjects have the right to withdraw from a study without penalty. Subjects with diminished autonomy are entitled to protection. They are more vulnerable because of age, legal or mental incompetence, terminal illness, or confinement to an institution. Justification for use of vulnerable subjects must be provided.
Right to privacy and dignity	Based on the principle of respect, privacy is the freedom of a person to determine the time, extent, and circumstances under which private information is shared or withheld from others.
Right to anonymity and confidentiality	Based on the principle of respect, **anonymity** exists when the subject's identity cannot be linked, even by the researcher, with his or her individual responses (ANA, 1985). **Confidentiality** means that individual identities of subjects will not be linked to the information they provide and will not be publicly divulged.

Violation of basic human right	Example
A subject's right to self-determination is violated through the use of coercion, covert data collection, and deception. • Coercion occurs when an overt threat of harm or excessive reward is presented to ensure compliance. • Covert data collection occurs when people become research subjects and are exposed to research treatments without knowing it. • Deception occurs when subjects are actually misinformed about the purpose of the research. • Potential for violation of the right to self-determination is greater for subjects with diminished autonomy; they have decreased ability to give informed consent and are vulnerable.	Subjects may feel that their care will be adversely affected if they refuse to participate in research. The Jewish Chronic Disease Hospital Study (Table 13-1) is an example of a study in which patients and their doctors did not know that cancer cells were being injected. In the Milgrim (1963) Study, subjects were deceived when asked to administer electric shocks to another person; the person was really an actor who pretended to feel the shocks. Subjects administering the shocks were very stressed by participating in this study though they were not administering shocks at all. The Willowbrook Study (Table 13-1) is an example of how coercion was used to obtain parental consent of vulnerable mentally retarded children who would not be admitted to the institution unless the children participated in a study in which they were deliberately injected with the hepatitis virus.
The Privacy Act of 1974 was instituted to protect subjects from such violations. These occur most frequently during data collection when invasive questions are asked that might result in loss of job, friendships, or dignity or might create embarrassment and mental distress. It also may occur when subjects are unaware that information is being shared with others.	Subjects may be asked personal questions such as "Were you sexually abused as a child?" "Do you use drugs?" "What are your sexual preferences?" When questions are asked using hidden microphones or hidden tape recorders, the subjects' privacy is invaded because they have no knowledge that the data are being shared with others. Subjects also have a right to control access of others to their records.
Anonymity is violated when the subjects' responses can be linked with their identity. Confidentiality is breached when a researcher, by accident or by direct action, allows an unauthorized person to gain access to study data which contain information about subject identity or responses that create a potentially harmful situation for subjects.	Subjects are given a code number instead of using names for identification purposes. Subjects' names are never used when reporting findings. Breaches of confidentiality with regard to sexual preference, income, drug use, prejudice, or personality variables can be harmful to subjects. Data are analyzed as group data so that individuals cannot be identified by their responses.

Continued.

Table 13-2   Protection of Human Rights—cont'd

Basic human right	Definition
Right to fair treatment	Based on the ethical principle of justice, people should be treated fairly and should receive what they are due or owed. Fair treatment is equitable selection of subjects and their treatment during the research study. This includes selection of subjects for reasons directly related to the problem studied versus convenience, compromised position, or vulnerability. It also includes fair treatment of subjects during the study, including fair distribution of risks and benefits regardless of age, race, or socioeconomic status.
Right to protection from discomfort and harm	Based on the ethical principle of beneficence, people must take an active role in promoting good and preventing harm in the world around them, as well as in research studies. Discomfort and harm can be physical, psychological, social, or economic in nature. There are five categories of studies based on levels of harm and discomfort: 1. No anticipated effects 2. Temporary discomfort 3. Unusual level of temporary discomfort 4. Risk of permanent damage 5. Certainty of permanent damage

Violation of basic human right	Example
Injustices with regard to subject selection have occurred as a result of social, cultural, racial, and gender biases in society. Historically, research subjects often have been obtained from groups of people who were regarded as having less "social value," the poor, prisoners, slaves, the mentally incompetent, and the dying. Often subjects were treated carelessly, without consideration of physical or psychological harm.	The Tuskegee Syphillis Study (1973), the Jewish Chronic Disease Study (1965), the San Antonio Conctraceptive Study (1969), and the Willowbrook Study (1972) (Table 13-1) all provide examples related to unfair subject selection. Investigators should not be late for data collection appointments, terminate data collection on time, not change agreed upon procedures or activities without consent, and provide agreed upon benefits such as a copy of the study findings or a participation fee.
Subjects' right to be protected is violated when researchers know in advance that harm, death, or disabling injury will occur and thus the benefits do not outweigh the risk.	Temporary physical discomfort involving minimal risk include fatigue or headache; emotional discomfort includes the expense involved in traveling to and from the data collection site. Studies examining sensitive issues, such as rape, incest, or spouse abuse, might cause unusual levels of temporary discomfort by opening up current and/or past traumatic experiences. In these situations, researchers assess distress levels and provide debriefing sessions during which the subject may express feelings, and ask questions. The researcher has the opportunity to make referrals for professional intervention. Studies having the potential to cause permanent damage are more likely to be medical rather than nursing in nature. A recent clinical trial of a new drug, a monoclonal antibody endotoxin (Centocor), was suspended when preliminary findings revealed a higher mortality rate for the treatment group versus the placebo group. Evaluation of the data led to termination of the trial. In some research, such as the Tuskegee Syphillis Study or the Nazi medical experiments, subjects experienced permanent damage or death.

Informed Consent

The Caldwell Medical Center
Code No. _____

I understand that I am being treated with the drug *cis*-platin, which may cause the unpleasant side effects of nausea and vomiting. Treatment to control these side effects includes using various medications, reducing the intake of food and fluids before chemotherapy, maintaining a quiet environment, and accepting support from others. In addition, I understand that using various coping strategies is helpful to persons in similar situations.

I understand that the purpose of this study is to help clients learn some coping techniques and evaluate how their use affects the occurrence of nausea and vomiting after *cis*-platin is administered. If I agree to participate in this research study, I understand that I will be randomly assigned to one of the following three nursing treatment programs:

1. I will meet with one of the investigators before I receive my chemotherapy. We will discuss my experience and the methods that other clients and I have found helpful.

or

2. I will meet with one of the investigators before I receive my chemotherapy. I will follow directions for practicing a technique that produces, under my own control, a state of altered consciousness called *self-hypnosis.* I will be asked to practice this technique during and after receiving my chemotherapy. I will be expected to practice this technique daily so that I may learn to use it without being directed by another person.

or

3. I will be given the customary nursing care that is rendered to every client taking the drugs that I am receiving.

In addition, if necessary, I will receive only the medication Reglan to control nausea and vomiting.

I understand that in no case will I receive less than the usual standard and expected level of nursing care that I am already receiving.

I understand that if I am selected to be in Group 2, a simple test to determine my susceptibility to this technique will be performed. Most people are susceptible, but if I am not and I wish to continue in the study, I will be randomly assigned to one of the two remaining groups.

I understand that this research study has been discussed with my physician and that he or she is aware of my participation. The treatments prescribed to control the side effects of nausea and vomiting will not be altered if I participate in this study.

Fig. 13-1   Example of an informed consent form.

Informed Consent — cont'd

I understand that a nurse investigator will be in my room while my chemotherapy is ending and for 4 hours after the treatment. I understand that nursing care will be provided by the nurses on the unit and not by the nurse-investigator. The research nurse will be taking notes on my reactions to the chemotherapy. Once an hour she will ask me to rate my nausea. I can expect that this will take only a few minutes of my time and that, if I am sleeping, I will not be awakened.

I have been told that this routine will be followed for three courses of chemotherapy, during three separate hospitalizations.

I understand that the benefits from this treatment are that I may experience less nausea and vomiting or fewer of the feelings of being sick to my stomach that often occur with *cis*-platin. There are no side effects or risks from my participation.

My participation is voluntary and I may choose to not participate or to withdraw at any time without jeopardizing my future treatment.

My identity will not be revealed in any way. My name will be encoded so that I will remain anonymous.

I also understand that if I believe I have sustained an injury as a result of participating in this research study, I may contact the investigators, Ms. B. J. Simon at 608-0011 or B. A. Smith at 124-6142, or the Office of the Institutional Review Board at 124-2500 so that I can review the matter and identify the medical resources that may be available to me.

I understand the following statements:

1. The Caldwell Medical Center will furnish whatever emergency medical care that the medical staff of this hospital determine to be necessary.
2. I will be responsible for the cost of such emergency care personally, through my medical insurance, or by another form of coverage.
3. No monetary compensation for wages lost as a result of an injury will be paid to me by The Caldwell Medical Center.
4. I will receive a copy of this consent form.

_____	_____
Date	Patient
_____	_____
Witness	Investigator

The Institutional Review Board of the Caldwell Medical Center has approved the solicitation of subjects for participation in this research proposal.

Fig. 13-1—cont'd   For legend see opposite page.

research situations that capture the public's attention, for example, that involving Dr. Barney Clark, the first recipient of an artificial heart.

The consent form must be signed by the subject and dated. The presence of witnesses is not always necessary but does constitute evidence that the subject concerned actually signed the form. In cases where the subject is a minor or is physically or mentally incapable of signing the consent, the legal guardian or representative must sign. The investigator also signs the form to indicate commitment to the agreement.

Generally the signed informed consent form is given to the subject. The researcher should keep a copy also. Some research, such as a retrospective chart audit, may not require informed consent—only institutional approval. Or in some cases, where minimal risk is involved, the investigator may have to provide the subject only with an information sheet and verbal explanation. In other cases, such as a volunteer convenience sample, completion and return of research instruments provide evidence of consent. The IRB will help to advise on exceptions to these guidelines, cases in which the IRB might grant waivers or amend its guidelines in other ways. The IRB makes the final determination as to the most appropriate documentation format. Research consumers should note whether and what kind of evidence of informed consent has been provided in a research article.

The Institutional Review Board

Institutional review boards (IRBs) are boards that review research projects to assess that ethical standards are met in relation to the protection of the rights of human subjects. The National Research Act (1974) requires that such agencies as universities, hospitals, and other health agencies applying for a grant or contract for any project or program that involves the conduct of biomedical or behavioral research involving human subjects must submit with their application assurances that they have established an institutional review board, sometimes called a *human subjects committee,* which reviews the research projects and protects the rights of the human subjects (Federal Code, 1983). At agencies where no federal grants or contracts are awarded, there is usually a review mechanism similar to an IRB process, such as a research advisory committee.

The National Research Act requires that the IRB have at least five members of various backgrounds to promote complete and adequate project review. The members must be qualified by virtue of their expertise and experience and reflect professional, gender, racial, and cultural diversity. Membership must include one member whose concerns are primarily nonscientific (lawyer, clergy, ethicist) and at least one member from outside the agency.

The IRB is responsible for protecting subjects from undue risk and loss of personal rights and dignity. The board reviews the study's protocol to ensure that it meets the requirements of ethical research that appear in the box on p. 331. Most boards provide guidelines or instructions for researchers that include steps to be taken to receive IRB approval. For example, guidelines for writing a standard consent form or criteria for qualifying for an expedited rather than a full IRB review

CODE OF FEDERAL REGULATIONS FOR IRB APPROVAL OF RESEARCH STUDIES

To approve research, the IRB must determine that the following Code of Federal Regulations has been satisfied:

1. The risks to subjects are minimized.
2. The risks to subjects are reasonable in relation to anticipated benefits.
3. The selection of the subjects is equitable.
4. Informed consent, in one of several possible forms, must be and will be sought from each prospective subject or the subject's legally authorized representative.
5. The informed consent form must be properly documented.
6. Where appropriate, the research plan makes adequate provision for monitoring the data collected to ensure subject safety.
7. Where appropriate, there are adequate provisions to protect the privacy of subjects and the confidentiality of data.
8. Where some or all of the subjects are likely to be vulnerable to coercion or undue influence, such as persons with acute or severe physical or mental illness or persons who are economically or educationally disadvantaged, appropriate additional safeguards are included.

may be made available. The IRB has the authority to approve research, require modifications, or disapprove a research study. A researcher must receive some form of IRB approval before beginning to conduct research. Institutional review boards have the authority to suspend or terminate approval of research that is not conducted in accordance with IRB requirements or that has been associated with unexpected serious harm to subjects.

Institutional review boards also have mechanisms for reviewing research in an expedited manner where there is minimal risk to research subjects (Federal Code, 1983). An expedited review usually shortens the length of the review process. Keep in mind that although a researcher may determine that a project involves minimal risk, the IRB makes the final determination and the research may not be undertaken until then. A full list of research categories eligible for expedited review is available from any IRB office. It includes the following:

- Collection of hair and nail clippings in a nondisfiguring manner
- Collection of excreta and external secretions including sweat
- Recording of data on subjects 18 years or older, using noninvasive procedures routinely employed in clinical practice
- Voice recordings
- Study of existing data, documents, records, pathological specimens, or diagnostic data

An expedited review does not automatically exempt the researcher from obtaining informed consent.

The *Federal Register* is a publication that contains updated information about federal guidelines for research involving human subjects. Every researcher should consult an agency's research office to ensure that the application being prepared for IRB approval adheres to the most current requirements. Nurses who are critiquing published research should be conversant with current regulations to determine whether ethical standards have been met.

Special Legal and Ethical Considerations Related to Protecting Basic Human Rights

Researchers are advised to consult their agency's IRB for the most recent federal and state rules and guidelines when considering research involving the elderly, children, the mentally ill, prisoners, the deceased, the unborn, students, and persons with AIDS. In addition, researchers should consult the IRB before planning research that potentially involves an oversubscribed research population, such as organ transplantation patients, AIDS patients, or "captive" and convenient populations, such as prisoners. It should be emphasized that use of special populations does not preclude undertaking research; extra precautions must be taken, however, to protect their rights.

Davis (1981a) reminds us that a society can be judged by the way it treats its most vulnerable people—a point worth remembering in research that involves children and the elderly. In addition, Davis continues a cogent argument, "To ensure continuing progress in pediatric research and practice, experimentation is necessary. If the consent requirement is taken seriously to the point of excluding research in children, then children themselves will be the ultimate sufferers" (Davis, 1981b, p. 247).

Mitchell discussed the National Commission's concept of assent versus consent in regard to pediatric research. *Assent* contains three fundamental elements:
1. A basic understanding of what the child will be expected to do and what will be done to the child
2. A comprehension of the basic purpose of the research
3. An ability to express a preference regarding participation

In contrast to assent, *consent* requires a relatively advanced level of cognitive ability. Informed consent reflects competency standards requiring abstract appreciation and reasoning regarding the information provided. The issue of assent versus consent is an interesting one when one determines at what age children can make meaningful decisions about participating in research. In terms of the work by Piaget regarding cognitive ability, children at age 6 and older can participate in giving assent. Children at age 14 and older, although not legally authorized to give sole consent unless they are emancipated minors, can make such decisions as capably as adults (Mitchell, 1984).

Federal regulations require parental permission whenever a child is involved in research unless otherwise specified, for example, in cases of child abuse or mature minors at minimal risk (Broome & Stieglitz, 1992). If the research involves more than minimal risk and does not offer direct benefit to the individual child, both parents must give permission. When individuals reach maturity, usually at 18 years of age in cases of research, they may render their own consent. They may do so at a younger age if they have been legally declared emancipated minors. Questions regarding this should be addressed to the IRB and/or research administration office and not left to the discretion of the researcher to answer.

Dubler (1987), as an advocate for the vulnerable elderly who are of increasing dependence and declining cognitive ability, states that elders are precisely the class of persons who were historically and are potentially vulnerable to abuse and for whom the law must struggle to fashion specific protections. The issue of the legal competence of elders is often raised. There is no issue if the potential subject can supply legally effective informed consent. Competence is not a clear "black or white" situation. The complexity of the study may affect one's ability to consent to participate. For example, an elderly person may be able to consent to participate in a simple observation study but not in a clinical drug trial.

The issue of the necessity of requiring the elderly to provide consent often arises. Dubler (personal communication, 1993) refers to the research regulations that provide that requirements for some or all of the elements of informed consent may be waived for the following:
1. The research involves no more than minimal risk to the subjects.
2. The waiver or alteration will not adversely affect the rights and welfare of the subjects.
3. The research could not feasibly be carried out without the waiver or alteration.
4. Whenever appropriate, the subjects will be provided with additional pertinent information after participation.

No vulnerable population may be singled out for study because it is simply convenient. For example, prisoners may not be studied simply because they are an available and convenient group. Prisoners may be studied if the study pertains to them, that is, studies concerning the effects and processes of incarceration. Students are often a convenient group. They must not be singled out as research subjects because of convenience; the research questions must have some bearing on their status as students.

Researchers and patient caregivers involved in research with vulnerable people are well advised to seek advice from appropriate IRBs, clinicians, lawyers, ethicists, and others. In all cases, the burden should be on the investigator to show the IRB that it is appropriate to involve vulnerable subjects in research.

SCIENTIFIC MISCONDUCT AND FRAUD
Fraud

Periodically articles reporting unethical actions of researchers appear in the professional and lay literature. Data may have been falsified or fabricated or subjects may have been coerced to participate in a research study (Abdellah, 1990; Hawley

& Jeffers, 1992; Thomas, 1991). In a climate of "publish or perish" in academic and scientific settings and declining research dollars, there is increasing pressure on academics and scientists to produce significant research findings. Job security and professional recognition are coveted, essential, and often predicated on being a productive scientist and prolific writer. These pressures have been known to overpower some people, who then take shortcuts, fabricate data, and falsify findings to advance their positions.

The risks are many, including harming research subjects or basing clinical practice on false data. Nurses, as advocates of patient welfare and professional practice, should be aware that, albeit ideally rare, there are occasions when misconduct of the researcher is observed or suspected. In such cases, nurses are advised to contact the appropriate group, such as the IRB, to assure that this matter receives appropriate attention and review.

Misconduct

Of equal importance is the issue of basing practice on reports that appear in journals, where subsequent research and reports on those subjects change the scientific basis for practice. Journals may print corrections or further research in follow-up reports that are buried, obscure, or underreported. A physician, Lawrence K. Altman (1988), stated, "Such shortcomings are critically important because the thousands of journals that cover a range of specialties are the central reservoir of scientific knowledge. They are the standard references for crediting discoveries and determining treatments." It is incumbent on nurses as patient advocates and research consumers to keep up-to-date on scientific reports related to nursing practice and adjust practice as directed by ever-evolving research findings.

Unauthorized Research

At times, ad hoc or informal and unauthorized research does go on, including product testing. Although the testing may seem to be harmless, again it is not the purview of the investigator to make that determination. Nurses must carefully avoid being involved in unauthorized research for a number of reasons (Hanks, 1984b):

- These treatments or methods of care are usually not monitored as closely for untoward effects, hence exposing the client to unwarranted risk
- Clients' rights to informed consent in clinical trials are not protected
- The success or failure of these unrecorded trials contributes nothing to the organized scientific knowledge of the efficacy or complications of the treatment
- The lack of independent quality supervision allows deviations from the adopted experimental program that may eliminate the program's effectiveness.

Sometimes the nurse plays the dual role of researcher and caregiver. In that situation, the nurse must question whether there may be risks inherent in the research that do not exist in the care. Even when these risks are clearly identified—and they must be—the caregiver must be comfortable that the level of risk is acceptable and that the **benefits** outweigh the **risks.** Patients must feel comfortable in refusing to participate in the caregiver's research while continuing to require the nurse's care. It must be made clear to patients that they may refuse to participate or withdraw from the study at any time without consequence or compromise to their care or relationship to the institution. The nurse in this dual role must consider whether the research will incur additional expense for the patient, whether that is warranted, and whether the subject has been apprised of such expenses.

PRODUCT TESTING

Nurses are often approached by manufacturers to test products on patients. Moore (1984) points out that all nurses should be aware of the Food and Drug Administration guidelines and regulations for *testing of medical devices* before they initiate any form of clinical testing. Medical devices are classified under Section 513 in the Federal Food, Drug and Cosmetic Act according to the extent of control necessary to ensure safety and effectiveness of each device. Classes related to product testing are defined in Table 13-3 (p. 336).

It is important that nurses be aware of their own institution's policies for **product testing.** The class of the product will obviously make a difference to the institution's position. If a nurse suspects that, for example, a Class II device is being tested in an ad hoc or unauthorized manner and without patient consent, this should be discussed with a supervisor or other appropriate authorities.

LEGAL AND ETHICAL ASPECTS OF ANIMAL EXPERIMENTATION

The federal laws that have been written to protect **animal rights** in research emanate from an interesting history of attitudes toward animals and the value people place on them. Animal activists (e.g., the Animal Liberation Front) and antivivisectionist societies began to gain considerable public attention in the 1970s. Of interest, however, is the fact that the oldest piece of legislation controlling animal experimentation goes back to 1876 in the United Kingdom. With the increase in the use of animals in research after World War II, a number of states passed legislation called "pound seizure laws" that allowed and even mandated the release of unclaimed animals from pounds to laboratories. The first pound seizure law was enacted in 1949; not until 1972 was the first law of that type repealed. In 1966 in the United States, the first Laboratory Animal Welfare Act was passed. The act did not deal with what we consider today to be some of the most salient issues related to animal experimentation—for example, pain management—and amendments continued to be passed to address these concerns. The 1970 Act provided for the establishment of an institutional Animal Care and Use Committee (ACUC), one member of which must be a veterinarian. The United States Department of Agriculture

Table 13-3   Classes Related to Product Testing

	Examples
CLASS I: GENERAL CONTROLS	
Included in Class I are devices whose safety and effectiveness can be reasonably guaranteed by the general controls of the Good Manufacturing Practices Regulations. The Regulations part of the act ensures that manufacturers will follow specific guidelines for packaging, storing, and providing specific product instructions.	Ostomy supplies
CLASS II: PERFORMANCE STANDARDS	
General controls are insufficient in this case to ensure safety and efficacy of the product, and the manufacturer must provide this assurance in the form of information.	Cardiac pacemakers, sutures, surgical metallic mesh, and biopsy needles
CLASS III: PREMARKET APPROVAL	
This class includes devices whose safety and effectiveness are insufficiently ensured by general controls and for which performance standards are insufficient to ensure safety and effectiveness. These products are represented to be life-sustaining or life-supporting, are implanted into the body, or present a potential, unreasonable risk of illness or injury to the patient. Devices in this class are required to have approved applications for premarket approval. Extensive laboratory, animal, and human studies, which often require 2 to 3 years to complete, are required for Class III devices.	Heart valves, bone cements, contact lenses, and implantable devices left in the body for 30 days or longer

(USDA) oversees compliance with animal welfare acts and holds institutions' administration accountable for such compliance.

In 1985 President Reagan signed PL 99-108, which contains the "Improved Standards for the Laboratory Animals' Act." Provisions in the series of acts and amendments to acts pertaining to animal experimentation include, but are by no means limited to, the list that appears in the box on p. 337 (PHS Policy on Humane Care, 1985).

This section serves only as an introduction to the concept of legal/ethical issues related to animal experimentation. Principles of protection of animal rights in research have evolved over time. Animals, unlike humans, cannot give informed consent, but other conditions related to their welfare must not be ignored. Nurses who encounter the use of animals in research should be alert to their rights.

BASIC PROVISIONS OF ACTS PERTAINING TO ANIMAL EXPERIMENTATION

1. The transportation, care, and use of animals should be in accordance with the Animal Welfare Act and other applicable federal laws, guidelines, and policies.
2. Procedures involving animals should be designed and performed with consideration of their relevance to human or animal health, the advancement of knowledge, or the good of society.
3. The animals selected for a procedure should be of an appropriate species and quality and the minimum number required to obtain valid results. Methods such as mathematical models, computer simulation, and in vitro biological systems should be considered.
4. Proper use of animals, including the avoidance or minimization of discomfort, distress, and pain when consistent with sound scientific practices, is imperative. Unless the contrary is established, investigators should consider that procedures that cause pain or distress in human beings may cause pain or distress in other animals.
5. Procedures with animals that may cause more than temporary or slight pain or distress should be performed with appropriate sedation, analgesia, or anesthesia. Surgical or other painful procedures should not be performed on unanesthetized animals paralyzed by chemical agents.
6. Animals that would otherwise suffer severe or chronic pain or distress that cannot be relieved should be painlessly killed at the end of the procedure or, if appropriate, during the procedure.
7. The living conditions of animals should be appropriate for their species and contribute to their health and comfort. Normally the housing, feeding, and care of all animals used for biomedical purposes must be directed by a veterinarian or other scientist trained and experienced in the proper care, handling, and use of the species being maintained or studied. In any case, veterinary care shall be provided as indicated.
8. Investigators and other personnel shall be appropriately qualified and experienced for conducting procedures on living animals. Adequate arrangements shall be made for their in-service training, including the proper and humane care and use of laboratory animals.
9. Where exceptions are required in relation to the provisions of these principles, the decisions should not rest with the investigators directly concerned but should be made, with regard to principle 2, by an appropriate review group, such as an institutional animal research committee. Such exceptions should not be made solely for the purposes of teaching or demonstration.

CRITIQUING THE LEGAL AND ETHICAL ASPECTS OF A RESEARCH STUDY

Research articles and reports often do not contain detailed information regarding the degree to which or all the ways in which the investigator adhered to the legal-ethical principles presented in this chapter. Space considerations in articles pre-

CRITIQUING CRITERIA

1. Was the study approved by IRB or other agency committee members?
2. Is there evidence that informed consent was obtained from all subjects or their representatives? How was it obtained?
3. Were the subjects protected from physical or emotional harm?
4. Were the subjects or their representatives informed about the purpose and nature of the study?
5. Were the subjects or their representatives informed about any potential risks that might result from participation in the study?
6. Did the benefits of the study outweigh the risks?
7. Were subjects coerced or unduly influenced to participate in this study? Did they have the right to refuse to participate or withdraw without penalty? Were vulnerable subjects used?
8. Were appropriate steps taken to safeguard the privacy of subjects? How have data been kept anonymous and/or confidential?

clude extensive documentation of all legal and ethical aspects of a research study. Lack of written evidence regarding the protection of human rights does not imply that appropriate steps were not taken.

The critiquing criteria that appear in the box above provide guidelines for evaluating the legal-ethical aspects of a research report. Although research consumers reading a research report will not see all areas explicitly addressed in the research article, they should be aware of them and should determine that the researcher has addressed them before gaining IRB approval to conduct the study. A nurse who is asked to serve as a member of an IRB will find the critiquing criteria useful in evaluating the legal-ethical aspects of the research proposal.

Information about the legal-ethical considerations of a study is usually presented in the methods section of a research report. The subsection on the sample or data collection methods is the most likely place for this information. The author most often indicates in a few sentences that informed consent was obtained and that approval from an IRB or similar committee was granted. It is likely that a paper will not be accepted for publication without such a discussion. This also makes it almost impossible for unauthorized research to be published. Therefore when a research article provides evidence of having been approved by an external review committee, the reader can feel confident that the ethical issues raised by the study have been thoroughly reviewed and resolved.

To protect subject and institutional privacy, the locale of the study frequently is described in general terms in the sample subsection section of the report. For example, the article might state that data were collected at a 350-bed community hospital in the Northeast, without mentioning its name. Protection of subject privacy may be explicitly addressed by statements indicating that anonymity or confidentiality of data was maintained or that grouped data were used in the data analysis.

Determining whether participants were subjected to physical or emotional risk is often accomplished indirectly by evaluating the study's methods section. The reader evaluates the **risk-benefit ratio,** that is, the extent to which the benefits of the study are maximized and the risks are minimized such that subjects are protected from harm during the study.

For example, a study by Hickey, Owen, and Froman (1992), validating two measures of cardiac risk factor self-efficacy related to diet and exercise, compared subjects engaged in cardiac rehabilitation programs and members of running clubs with respect to accomplishment of diet and exercise goals as a measure of self-efficacy. The benefits to the participants were exercise and diet programs, in which they already were involved, that are presumed to decrease cardiac risk. Risk is minimized because subjects either were healthy runners or had received clearance to participate in a cardiac rehabilitation program. The subjects' time exercising is time they were spending anyway; the time spent completing the self-efficacy questionnaires could be minimized through organization and timely scheduling of research activities. Thus the evaluator could infer from a description of the method that the benefits were greater than the risks and subjects were protected from harm. The obligation to balance the risks and benefits of a study is the responsibility of the researcher. However, the research consumer reading a research report also should be confident that subjects have been protected from harm.

When considering the special needs of vulnerable subjects, research consumers should be sensitive to whether the special needs of groups, unable to act on their own behalf, have been addressed. For instance, has the right to self-determination been addressed by the informed consent protocol identified in the research report? For example, in a study by Meininger, Stashinko, and Hayman (1991) investigating the psychometric properties of the Mathews Youth Test for Health as a measure of type A behavior in school-age twin children, informed consent was obtained from the parents of the 6- to 11-year-old twins and the twins gave their assent before test administration.

When qualitative studies are reported, verbatim quotes from informants often are incorporated into the findings section of the article. In such cases the reader will evaluate how effectively the author protected the informant's identity, either by using a fictitious name or withholding information such as age, gender, occupation, or other potentially identifying data.

It should be apparent from the preceding sections that although the need for guidelines for the use of human and animal subjects in research is evident and the principles themselves are clear, there are many instances when the nurse must use best judgment both as a patient advocate and as a researcher when evaluating the ethical nature of a research project. In any research situation, the basic guiding principle of protecting the patient's human rights must always apply. When conflicts arise, the nurse must feel free to raise suitable questions with appropriate resources and personnel. In an institution these may include contacting the researcher first and then, if there is no resolution, the director of nursing research and the chairperson of the IRB. In cases where ethical considerations in a research article are in question, clarification from a colleague, agency, or IRB is indicated. The nurse should pursue his or her concerns until satisfied that the patient's rights and his or her rights as a professional nurse are protected.

KEY POINTS

- Ethical and legal considerations in research first received attention after World War II during the Nuremberg Trials, from which developed the Nuremberg Code. This became the standard for research guidelines protecting the human rights of research subjects.
- The National Research Act, passed in 1974, created the National Commission for the Protection of Human Subjects of Biomedical and Behavioral Research. The findings, contained in the *Belmont Report,* discuss three basic ethical principles (respect for persons, beneficence, and justice), which underlie the conduct of research involving human subjects. Federal regulations developed in response to the Commission's report provide guidelines for informed consent and institutional review board (IRB) protocols.
- The American Nurses Association's Commission on Nursing Research published *Human Rights Guidelines for Nursing in Clinical and Other Research* in 1975, for protection of human rights of research subjects. It is relevant to nurses as researchers, as well as caregivers. The ANA Code for Nurses is integral with the Research Guidelines.
- Protection of human rights includes:
  1. Right to self-determination
  2. Right to privacy and dignity
  3. Right to anonymity and confidentiality
  4. Right to fair treatment
  5. Right to protection from discomfort and harm
- Procedures for protecting basic human rights include gaining informed consent, which illustrates the ethical principle of respect, and obtaining institutional review board (IRB) approval, which illustrates the ethical principles of respect, beneficence, and justice.
- Special consideration should be given to studies involving vulnerable populations, such as children, the elderly, prisoners, and those who are mentally or physically disabled.
- Scientific fraud or misconduct represents unethical conduct and must be monitored as part of professional responsibility. Informal, ad hoc, or unauthorized research may expose patients to unwarranted risk and may not protect subject rights adequately.

- Nurses who are asked to be involved in product testing should be aware of Food and Drug Administration Guidelines and Regulations for Testing Medical Devices before becoming involved in product testing and, perhaps, violating guidelines for ethical research.
- Animal rights need to be protected, and regulations for animal research have evolved over time. Nurses who encounter the use of animals in research should be alert to their rights.
- Nurses as consumers of research must be knowledgeable about the legal-ethical components of a research study so they can evaluate whether appropriate protection of human or animal rights has been ensured by a researcher.

REFERENCES

Abdellah, F. (1990). Scientific misconduct: Myth or reality? *Journal of Professional Nursing,* 6, *1:* 61-63.

Altman, L. K. (1988, May 31). A flaw in the research process: Uncorrected errors in journals. Medical Science, *The New York Times.*

American Nurses' Association. (1975). *Guidelines for nurses in clinical and other research.* Kansas City, MO: Author.

American Nurses' Association. (1985). *Code for nurses with interpretive statements.* Kansas City, MO: Author.

Andrews, E.L. (1993, February 3). U.S. resumes granting patents on genetically altered animals. *New York Times,* C1.

Brink, P.J. (1992). Autonomy versus do no harm. *Western Journal of Nursing Research, 14* (3), 264-266.

Broome, M.E., and Stieglitz, K.A. (1992). The consent process and children. *Research in Nursing and Health, 15,* 147-152.

Burd, S. (1993). Scientists oppose diversity rule for clinical trials in NIH bill. *Chronicle of Higher Education,* April 7, 1993, A26.

Code of Federal Regulations, 45 CFR 46, Protection of Human Subjects, OPRR Reports, Revised March 8, 1983.

Cook, R. (1981). *Brain.* New York: Signet.

Creighton, H. (1977). Legal concerns of nursing research. *Nursing Research, 26* (4), 337-340.

Davis A. (1981a). Ethical issues in gerontological nursing research. *Geriatric Nursing, 2,* 267-272.

Davis, A. (1981b). Ethical issues in nursing research. *Western Journal of Nursing Research, 3* (2), 247-248.

Davis, A. (1990). Ethical similarities internationally. *Western Journal of Nursing Research, 12* (5), 685-688.

Department of Health and Human Services. (1981). Final regulations amending basic HHS policy for the protection of human research subjects. *Federal Regulations, 46, 16.*

Dubler, N.N. (1987). Legal judgements and informed consent in geriatric research. *Journal of the American Geriatric Society, 35,* 545-549.

Fowler, M.D.M. (1988). Ethical issues in nursing research: A call for an international code of ethics for nursing research. *Western Journal of Nursing Research, 3* (10), 352-355.

Hanks, G.E. (1984a). Implementing human research regulations: second biennial report on the adequacy and uniformity of federal rules and policies and of their implementation, for the study of ethical problems in medicine and biomedical and behavioral research, March 1983.

Hanks, G.E. (1984b). The dangers of ad hoc protocols. *Journal of Clinical Oncology, 2,* 1177-1178.

Hawley, D.J., and Jeffers, J.M. (1992). Scientific misconduct as a dilemma for nursing. *Image, 24* (1), 51-55.

Hershey, N., and Miller, R.D. (1976). *Human experimentation and the law.* Germantown, MD: Aspen.

Hickey, M.L., Owen, S.V., and Froman, R.D. (1992). Instrument development: cardiac diet and exercise self-efficacy. *Nursing Research, 41* (6), 347-351.

Katz, J. (1972). *Experimentation with human beings.* New York: Russell Sage Foundation.

Levine, R.J. (1979). Clarifying the concepts of research ethics. *Hastings Center Report, 93* (3), 21-26.

Levine, R.J. (1986). *Ethics and regulation of clinical research* (2nd ed.). Baltimore-Munich: Urban and Schwartzenberg.

Meininger, J.C., Stashinko, E.E., and Hayman, L.L. (1991). Type A behavior in children: psychometric properties of the Mathews youth test for health. *Nursing Research, 40* (4), 221-227.

Milgrim, S. (1963). Behavioral study of obedience. *Journal of Abnormal and Social Psychology, 67* (4), 371-377.

Mitchell, K. (1984). Protecting children's rights during research. *Pediatric Nursing, 10,* 9-10.

Moore, L. (1984). Conducting clinical trials. *Journal of Enterostomal Therapy, 11,* 229-232.

National Commission for the Protection of Human Subjects of Biomedical and Behavioral Research. (1978). *Belmont report: Ethical principles and guidelines for research involving human subjects* (DHEW Publication No. 05). Washington, DC: U.S. Government Printing Office. 78-0012.

Public Health Service Policy on Humane Care in Use of Lab Animals by Awardee Institution. (1985, June 25). *NIH Guidelines for Grants and Contracts, 14* (8).

Rempusheski, V.F. (1991). Elements, perceptions, and issues of informed consent. *Applied Nursing Research, 4* (4), 201-204.

Robb, I.H. (1900). *Nursing ethics: for hospital and private use.* Milwaukee, WI: G.N. Gaspar.

Rothman, D.J. (1982). Were Tuskegee and Willowbrook studies in nature? *Hastings Center Report, 12* (2), 5-7.

Thomas, S. (1991). Research fraud: when the pressure to publish manifests. *Tennessee Nurse, 54* (1), 17-18.

ADDITIONAL READINGS

Annas, G.J., and Healey J. (1974). The client rights advocate. *Journal of Nursing Administration, 4,* 25-31.

Applebaum, P.S., and Roth, L.H. (1982). Competency to consent to research. *Archives of General Psychiatry, 39,* 951-958.

Armiger, Sr.B. (1977). Ethics of nursing research: profiles, principles, perspective. *Nursing Research, 25* (5), 330-336.

Beecher, H.K. (1966a). Ethics and clinical research. *New England Journal of Medicine, 274,* 1354-1360.

Beecher, H.K. (1966b). Consent in clinical experimentation: myth and reality. *Journal of the American Medical Association, 195,* 34-35.

Davis, A.J. (1989). Clinical nurses' ethical decision making in situations of informed consent. *Advances in Nursing Science, 11,* 63-69.

Davis, A.J. (1988). The clinical nurses' role in informed consent. *Journal of Professional Nursing, 4,* 88-91.

Department of Health and Human Services. (1988, May). Policy on informing those tested about HIV sero status.

Goldberg, R.J. (1984). Disclosure of information to adult cancer clients: Issues and update. *Journal of Clinical Oncology, 2,* 948-955.

Levine, R.J. (1983). Research involving children: An interpretation of the new regulations. *IRB: A Review of Human Subjects Research, 5,* 1-5.

May, K.A. (1979). The nurse as researcher: Impediment to informed consent? *Nursing Outlook, 27,* 36-39.

Melnick, V.L., Dubler, N.N., Weisbard, A., and Butler, R.N. (1984). Clinical research in senile dementia of the Alzheimer type: Suggested guidelines addressing the ethical and legal issues. *Journal of the American Geriatrics Society, 32,* 531-536.

Orlans, F.B., Simmonds, R.C., and Dodds, W.J. (1987). Effective animal care use committees. A special issue of *Laboratory Animal Science.*

Robinson, G., and Merav, A. (1976). Informed consent: recall by clients tested postoperatively. *The Annals of Thoracic Surgery, 22,* 209-212.

Rothman, D. (1991). *Strangers at the bedside.* New York: Basic Books.

Rothman, D. (1987). Ethics and human experimentation: Henry Beecher revisited. *New England Journal of Medicine, 317,* 1195-1199.

Rowen, A.H. (1984). *Of mice, models and men: A critical evaluation of animal research.* Albany, NY: State University of New York Press.

CHAPTER 14

Data Collection Methods

MARGARET GREY

LEARNING OBJECTIVES

After reading this chapter the student should be able to do the following:

♦ Define the types of data collection methods used in nursing research.

♦ List the advantages and disadvantages of each of these methods.

♦ Critically evaluate the data collection methods used in published nursing research studies.

KEY TERMS

close-ended item	operational definition
concealment	operationalization
consistency	physiological measurement
content analysis	questionnaires
Delphi technique	reactivity
interrater reliability	records or available data
intervention	scale
interviews	scientific observation
Likert scales	social desirability
objective	systematic
open-ended item	

Nurses use all of their senses when collecting data from the patients for whom they provide care. Nurse researchers also have available many ways to collect information about their research subjects. The major difference between the data collected when performing patient care and the data collected for the purpose of research is that the data collection methods employed by researchers need to be objective and systematic. By *objective*, we mean that the data must not be influenced by anyone who collects the information; by *systematic*, we mean that the data must be collected in the same way by everyone who is involved in the collection procedure.

The methods that researchers use to collect information about subjects are the identifiable and repeatable operations that define the major variables being studied. Operationalization is the process of translating the concepts that are of interest to a researcher into observable and measurable phenomena. There may be a number of ways to collect the same information. For example, a researcher interested in measuring anxiety physiologically could do so by measuring sweat gland activity or by administering an anxiety scale, such as the State-Trait Anxiety Scale for Children (Speilberger, 1973). The researcher could also observe children to see whether they displayed anxious behavior. The method chosen by the researcher would depend on a number of decisions regarding the problem being studied, the nature of the subjects, and the relative costs and benefits of each method.

This chapter's purpose is to familiarize the student with the various ways that researchers collect information from and about subjects. The chapter provides nursing research consumers with the tools for evaluating the selection, utilization, and practicality of the various ways of collecting data.

MEASURING VARIABLES OF INTEREST

To a large extent the success of a study depends on the quality of the data collection methods chosen and employed. Researchers have many types of methods available for collecting information from subjects in research studies. Determining what measurement to use in a particular investigation may be the most difficult and time-consuming period in study design. In addition, because nursing research is still developing, researchers are beginning to have an array of quality instruments with adequate reliability and validity (see Chapters 10 and 15) from which to choose. This aspect of the research process demands painstaking efforts of the researcher. Thus the process of evaluating and selecting the available tools to measure variables of interest is of critical importance to the potential success of the study. In this section we discuss the selection of measures and the implementation of the data collection process.

You will find that researchers can use many different ways to collect information about phenomena of interest to nurses. We are interested in biological and physical indicators of health, such as blood pressure and heart rates, but nurses are also interested in complex psychosocial questions presented by patients. Psychosocial variables, such as anxiety, hope, social support, and self-concept, may be measured by several different techniques, such as observation of behavior or self-reports of feelings or attitudes by means of interviews or questionnaires. Researchers may also use data that have already been collected for another purpose, such as records, diaries, or other media, to study phenomena of interest.

As you can surmise, choosing the most appropriate method and instrument is difficult. The method must be appropriate to the problem, the hypothesis, the setting, and the population. For example, if a researcher is interested in studying the behavior of 3-year-old children in day-care, it probably would not be sensible to provide the children with some kind of paper-and-pencil test. Whereas the children might be able to draw on the paper, they would not be likely to answer written questions appropriately.

Selection of the data collection method begins during the literature review. In Chapter 5 one purpose of the review noted is to provide clues to instrumentation. As the literature review is conducted, the researcher begins to explore how previous investigators defined and operationalized variables similar to those of interest in the current study. The researcher uses this information to define conceptually the variables to be studied. Once a variable has been defined conceptually, the researcher returns to the literature to define the variable operationally. This **operational definition** translates the conceptual definition into behaviors or verbalizations that can be measured for the study. In this second literature review the researcher searches for measuring instruments that might be used as is or adapted for use in the study. If instruments are available, the researcher needs to obtain permission for their use from the author.

An example may illustrate the relationship of the conceptual and operational definitions. Stress research is popular with researchers from many disciplines, including nursing. Definitions of stressors may be psychological, social, or physiological. If a researcher is interested in studying stressors, the researcher needs first to define what he or she means by the concept of stressor. For example, Holmes and Rahe (1967) defined the stressful life event as any occurrence that required change or adaptation. This definition implies that it is the event that is stressful, not how the individual appraises the event. According to this conceptual definition, the researcher could use a Life Event Checklist (operational definition) to determine the degree of stress encountered by subjects in the study. If the researcher disagreed with this definition and supported the definition that events are stressful only when individuals appraise them as such (Lazarus & Folkman, 1984), another approach to measurement would be consistent with that view.

It is often the case that no suitable measuring device exists, so the researcher needs to decide whether the variable is important to the study and whether a new device should be constructed. This is often a problem in nursing research, because many variables of interest have not been studied. The construction of new instruments for data collection that have reasonable reliability and validity (see Chapter 15) is a most difficult task. Sometimes researchers decide not to study a variable if no suitable measuring device exists; at other times the researcher may decide to invest time and energy in tool development (Chapter 10). Either decision is acceptable depending on the goals of the study and the goals of the researcher.

Whether the researcher uses available methods or creates new ones, once the variables have been operationally defined in a manner consistent with the aims of the study, the population to be studied, and the setting, the researcher will determine how the data collection phase of the study will be implemented. This decision deals with how the instruments for data collection will be given to the subjects. Consistency is the most important issue in this phase.

Consistency means that the data are collected from each subject in the study in exactly the same way or as close to the same way as possible. Consistency can minimize the bias introduced when more than one person collects the data. Thus the researcher must consider ways to minimize subjects' anxiety and to maintain their motivation to complete the data collection process (Given, Keilman, Collins, & Given, 1990), and data collectors must be carefully trained and supervised (Collins, Given, Given, & King, 1988). To ensure consistency in data collection, researchers must rehearse data collectors in the methods to be used in the study so that each person collects the information in the same way. Information about how to observe and collect data often is included in a kind of "cookbook" for the research project. A researcher may spend several months training research assistants to collect data systematically and reliably. If data collectors are used, the reader should expect to see some comment about their training and the consistency with which they collected the data for the study. For example, in the study by Stewart Fahs and Kinney (1991; Appendix A), the procedure by which the consistency of measurement was assured is clearly presented. Nurses watched a videotape, participated in a live teaching session, and held training sessions. Further, because ratings were done by the investigator and three research assistants, interrater reliability for the measurement of bruising was obtained. The index of agreement in this study was a Pearson correlation of 0.94 to 0.99, demonstrating high levels of agreement among the observers. **Interrater reliability** (see Chapter 15) is the consistency of observations between two or more observers; it often is expressed as a percentage of agreement among raters or observers or a coefficient of agreement that considers the element of chance (coefficient Kappa).

DATA COLLECTION METHODS

In general, data collection methods can be divided into the following five types: physiological, observational, interviews, questionnaires, and records or available data. Each of these methods has a specific purpose, as well as certain pros and cons inherent in its use. We discuss each type of data collection method and then compare its respective uses and problems.

Physiological or Biological Measurement

In everyday practice, nurses collect physiological data about patients, such as their temperature, pulse rate, and blood pressure. Such data frequently are useful to nurse researchers as well, as in the study by Stewart Fahs and Kinney (1991), reprinted in Appendix A. The purpose of the study was to evaluate three subcutaneous injection sites for low-dose heparin therapy. To study this problem, it was important for the researchers to measure bruising similarly in all of the subjects. Refer to the section "Measures." Note how the authors describe the measurement of the bruising, as well as the interrater reliability coefficient obtained by comparing the various observers. In addition, these researchers collected data about patients' activated partial thromboplastin time (aPTT) because this physiological measure demonstrated that the heparin administered at the various sites was effective.

The study by Stewart Fahs and Kinney is an excellent example of the use of a particular type of data collection method—physiological. **Physiological measurement** and biological measurement involve the use of specialized equipment to determine physical and biological status of subjects. Frequently such measures also require specialized training. Such measures can be physical, such as weight or temperature; chemical, such as blood glucose level; microbiological, as with cultures; or anatomical, as in radiological examinations. What separates these measurements from others used in research is that they require the use of special equipment to make the observation. We can say, "This subject feels warm," but to determine how warm the subject is requires the use of a sensitive instrument, a thermometer.

Heidenreich and Giuffre (1990) did a study to determine whether the axillary site was a valid site for the measurement of temperature in the postoperative patient. They used four different measures of temperature in 18 patients. Thus they were able to discern which of the four measures most accurately reflected the core temperature. The study required careful standardization of the procedures so that the instruments were all used in the same way.

Physiological or biological measurement is particularly suited to the study of several types of nursing problems. The aforementioned example is typical of studies dealing with ways to improve the performance of certain nursing actions, such as measuring and recording of patients' physiological data. Physiological measures may be important criteria for determining the effectiveness of certain nursing actions. An experimental study by Gift et al. (1992) tested the effectiveness of a taped relaxation message in reducing dyspnea and anxiety in patients with chronic obstructive pulmonary disease. The authors used a combination of measures, including a portable skin temperature monitor and a peak flow meter to determine airway obstruction. They found that the taped relaxation message was effective in reducing airway obstruction, as well as feelings of anxiety and dyspnea.

This study (Gift et al., 1992) illustrates a type of research that is a priority for the National Institute for Nursing Research: studies of the interface between biology and behavior (termed *biobehavioral interface*). The study by Grey, Cameron, & Thurber (1991; Appendix B) also illustrates this type of work, since the authors were interested not only in describing the psychological adaptation of children with diabetes, but also in relating that adaptation to the physiological measurement of metabolic control of the diabetes.

The advantages of using physiological data collection methods include their objectivity, precision, and sensitivity. Such methods are generally quite objective, because unless there is a technical malfunction, two readings of the same instrument taken at the same time by two different nurses are likely to yield the same result. Because such instruments are intended to measure the variable being studied, they offer the advantage of being precise and sensitive enough to pick up subtle variations in the phenomenon of interest. It is also unlikely that a subject in a study can deliberately distort physiological information.

Physiological measurements are not without inherent disadvantages, however. Some instruments, if they are not available through a hospital, may be quite expensive to obtain. In addition, such instruments often require specialized knowledge and training to be used accurately. Another problem with such measurements is that just by using them, the variable of interest may be changed. Although some researchers think of these instruments as being nonintrusive, the presence of some types of devices might change the measurement. For example, the presence of a heart rate monitoring device might make some patients anxious and increase their heart rate. In addition, nearly all types of measuring devices are affected in some way by the environment. Even a simple thermometer can be affected by the subject drinking something hot immediately before the temperature is taken. Thus it is important to consider whether the researcher controlled such environmental variables in the study. Finally, there may not be a physiological way to measure the variable of interest. Occasionally researchers try to force a physiological parameter into a study in an effort to increase the precision of measurement. However, if the device does not really measure the phenomenon of interest, the validity of its use is suspect.

Observational Methods

Sometimes nurse researchers are interested in determining how subjects behave under certain conditions. For example, the researcher might be interested in how children respond to painful situations. We might ask children how painful an experience was, but they may not be able to answer the question, may not be able to quantify the amount of pain, or may distort their responses to please the researcher. Therefore sometimes observing the subject may give a more accurate picture of the behavior in question than asking the subject.

Although observing the environment is a normal part of living, **scientific observation** places a great deal of emphasis on the objective and systematic nature of the operation. The researcher is not merely looking at what is happening, but rather is watching with a trained eye for certain specific events. To be scientific, observations must fulfill the following four conditions:

1. The observations undertaken are consistent with the study's specific objectives.
2. There is a standardized and systematic plan for the observation and the recording of data.
3. All of the observations are checked and controlled.
4. The observations are related to scientific concepts and theories.

Observation is particularly suitable as a data collection method in complex research situations that are best viewed as total entities and that are difficult to measure in parts, such as studies dealing with the nursing process, parent-child interactions, or group processes. In addition, observational methods can be the best way to operationalize some variables of interest in nursing research studies, particularly individual characteristics and conditions, such as traits and symptoms, verbal and nonverbal communication behaviors, activities and skill attainment, and environmental characteristics.

A study of the effect of a strategy to promote night sleep in hospitalized 3- to 8-year old children was conducted by White, Williams, Alexander, Powell-Cope, and Conlon (1990). Asking young children about their sleep behaviors is not likely to be reliable or valid, so the researchers used a number of observational tools to describe children's sleep onset latency and distress. The Sleep Onset Latency Behavior Catalog is a list of 54 behaviors in eight conceptual categories (distress, self-soothing, communication, pleasure, neutral, sleep, active, and inactive) of child subjects and others in the child's environment. The catalog is used to encode data by using a computer-based recording system, the Senders Signals and Receivers System. The researchers note that observers were trained in the use of the system and the behavioral catalog. Training tapes were used to practice encoding behaviors. Average interrater reliability was 79%. In the study the researchers demonstrated that a recording of a parent telling a story significantly reduced the length of time it took children to fall asleep compared with stories recorded by strangers and no story groups.

Observational methods can be distinguished also by the role of the observer. This role is determined by the amount of interaction between the observer and those being observed. Each of the following four basic types of observational roles is distinguishable by the amount of **concealment** or **intervention** implemented by the observer:

1. Concealment without intervention
2. Concealment with intervention
3. No concealment without intervention
4. No concealment with intervention

These methods are illustrated in Fig. 14-1, and examples are given later.

Concealment

		Yes	No
Intervention	Yes	Researcher hidden Some intervention	Researcher open Some intervention
	No	Researcher hidden No intervention	Researcher open No intervention

Fig. 14-1   Types of observational roles in research.

Concealment refers to whether the subjects know that they are being observed, and **intervention** deals with whether the observer provokes actions from those who are being observed. The study described previously (White et al., 1990) is an excellent example of no concealment with intervention. The researchers were not concealed in their observations, but they did intervene with the children. Suppose the researcher believed that by being open to the subjects, the subjects' behavior would change. For example, if these researchers wanted to replicate their studies with older children who might be more suggestive in response to the presence of a known investigator, the researchers might employ concealment with intervention. When a researcher is concerned that the subjects' behavior will change as a result of being observed, the type of observation most commonly employed is that of concealment without intervention. In this case the researcher watches the subjects without their knowledge of the observation, but he or she does not provoke them into action. Often such concealed observations use hidden television cameras, audiotapes, or one-way mirrors. Concealment without intervention often is used in observational studies of children. You may be familiar with rooms with one-way mirrors, where a researcher can observe the behavior of the occupants of the room without being observed by them. Such studies allow for the observation of children's natural behavior and often are used in developmental research. No concealment without intervention also is commonly used for observational studies. In this case, the researcher obtains informed consent from the subject to be observed and then simply observes his or her behavior.

Observing subjects without their knowledge may violate assumptions of informed consent, and therefore researchers face ethical problems with this type of approach. However, sometimes there is no other way to collect such data and the data collected are unlikely to have negative consequences for the subject; therefore the disadvantages of the study are outweighed by the advantages. Further, the problem often is handled by informing subjects after the observation and allowing them opportunity to refuse to have their data included in the study and to discuss any question they might have. This process is called *debriefing*.

When the observer is neither concealed nor intervening, the ethical question is not a problem. Here the observer makes no attempt to change the subjects' behavior and informs them that they are to be observed. Because the observer is present, this type of observation allows a greater depth of material to be studied than if the observer is separated from the subjects by an artificial barrier, such as a one-way mirror. Participant observation is a commonly used observational technique where the researcher functions as a part of a social group to study the group in question. The problem with this type of observation is **reactivity**, the Hawthorne effect, or the distortion created when the subjects change behavior because they are being observed (see Chapter 8).

In the study by White et al. (1990), the researchers used unconcealed observation, because the children and parents had given full consent for participation in the study. They also performed an intervention—the use of recorded stories by parents or a stranger or the presence of a parent—so the method was no concealment with intervention. No concealment with intervention is employed when the researcher is observing the effects of some intervention introduced for scientific purposes. Because the subjects know that they are participating in a research study, there are few problems with ethical concerns, but reactivity is a problem with this type of study. Gill, Behnke, Conlon, McNeely, and Anderson (1988) studied the effect of nonnutritive sucking on behavioral state of preterm infants. Because infants cannot report their behavior, they must be observed. The researchers were not hidden from the infants, so the observation was not covert, but they did intervene by providing some infants with pacifiers (nonnutritive sucking). By using the Anderson Behavioral State Scale, a structured tool for observing infant behavior, the researchers found that nonnutritive sucking was an effective modulator of behavioral state.

Concealed observation with intervention involves staging a situation and observing the behaviors that are evoked in the subjects as a result of the intervention. Because the subjects are unaware of their participation in a research study, this type of observation has fallen into disfavor and rarely is used in nursing research.

Observations may be structured or unstructured. Unstructured observational methods, such as those suggested by West, Bondy, and Hutchinson (1991) for working with the elderly, are not characterized by a total absence of structure but usually involve collecting descriptive information about the topic of interest. In participant observation the observer keeps field notes that record the activities, as well as the observer's interpretations of these activities. Field notes usually are not restricted to any particular type of action or behavior; rather, they intend to paint a picture of a social situation in a more general sense. Another type of unstructured observation is the use of anecdotes. Anecdotes are not necessarily funny but usually focus on the behaviors of interest and frequently add to the richness of research reports by illustrating a particular point.

On the other hand, structured observations, such as the Sleep Onset Latency Behavior Catalog and the Anderson Behavioral State Scale, involve specifying in advance what behaviors or events are to be observed and preparing forms for record keeping, such as categorization systems, checklists, and rating scales. Whichever system is employed, the observer watches the subject and then marks on the recording form what was seen. In any case, the observations must be similar among the observers (see earlier discussion and Chapter 15 for an explanation of interrater reliability). Thus it is important that observers be trained to be consistent in their observations and ratings of behavior.

Scientific observation has several advantages as a data collection method, the main one being that observation may be the only way for the researcher to study the variable of interest. For example, what people say they do often is not what they really do. Therefore if the study is designed to obtain substantive findings about human behavior, observation may be the only way to ensure the validity of the findings. In addition, no other data collection method can match the depth and variety of information that can be collected when using these techniques. Such techniques also are quite flexible in that they may be used in both experimental and nonexperimental designs and in laboratory and field studies.

As with all data collection methods, observation also has its disadvantages. We mention the problems of reactivity and ethical concerns when we discuss the concealment and intervention dimensions. In addition, data obtained by observational techniques are vulnerable to the bias of the observer. Emotions, prejudices, and values all can influence the way that behaviors and events are observed. In general, the more the observer needs to make inferences and judgments about what is being observed, the more likely it is that distortions will occur. Thus in judging the adequacy of observational methods, it is important to consider how observational tools were constructed and how observers were trained and evaluated.

Interviews and Questionnaires

Subjects in a research study often have information that is important to the study and that can be obtained only by asking the subject. Such questions may be asked orally by a researcher in person or over the telephone in an interview, or they may be asked in the form of a paper-and-pencil test. Both interviews and questionnaires have the purpose of asking subjects to report data for themselves, but each has unique advantages and disadvantages as well. **Interviews** are a method of data collection where a data collector questions a subject verbally. Interviews may be face-to-face or performed over the telephone, and they may consist of open-ended or close-ended questions. On the other hand, **questionnaires** are paper-and-pencil instruments designed to gather data from individuals about knowledge, attitudes, beliefs, and feelings.

Survey research relies almost entirely on questioning subjects with either interviews or questionnaires, but these methods of data collection also can be used in other types of research. No matter what type of study is conducted, the purpose of questioning subjects is to seek information. This information may be of either direct interest, such as the subject's age, or indirect interest, such as when the researcher uses a combination of items to estimate to what degree the respondent has some trait or characteristic. An intelligence test is an example of how an individual item is combined with several others to develop an overall scale of intelligence. When items of indirect interest are combined to obtain an overall score, the measurement tool is called a *scale*.

The investigator determines the content of an interview or questionnaire from the literature review (see Chapter 5). When evaluating these methods, the reader should consider the content of the schedule, the individual items, and the order of the items. The basic standard for evaluating the individual items in an interview or questionnaire is that the item must be clearly written so that the intent of the question and the nature of the information sought are clear to the respondent. The only way to know whether the questions are understandable to the target respondents is to pilot test them in a similar population. Items also must ask only one question, be free of suggestion, and use correct grammar. Items also may be **open-ended items** or **close-ended items.** *Open-ended* items are used when the researcher wants the subjects to respond in their own words or when the researcher does not know all of the possible alternative responses. *Close-ended* items are used when there is a fixed number of alternative responses. Many scales use a fixed response format called a Likert scale.

Likert scales are lists of statements on which respondents indicate, for example, whether they "strongly agree," "agree," "disagree," or "strongly disagree." Sometimes more fine distinctions are given or there may be a neutral category. The use of the neutral category, however, sometimes creates problems because it often is the most frequent response and this response is difficult to interpret. Fixed-response items also can be used for questions requiring a "yes" or "no" response or when there are categories, such as with income. Structured, fixed-response items are best used when the question has a fixed number of responses and the respondent is to choose the one closest to the right one. Fixed-response items have the advantage of simplifying the respondent's task and the researcher's analysis, but they may miss some important information about the subject. Unstructured response formats allow such information to be included but require a special technique to analyze the responses. This technique is called **content analysis** and is a method for the objective, systematic, and quantitative description of communications and documentary evidence.

The box on p. 355 shows a few items from a survey of pediatric nurse practitioners (Grey & Flint, 1989). The first items are taken from a list of similar items, and they are both closed and of a Likert-type format. Note that respondents are asked to choose how strongly they agree with each item. In using these questions in the survey, we are forcing the respondent to choose from only these answers because we think that these will be the only responses. The only possible alternative response is to skip the item and leave it blank. On the other hand, sometimes we have no idea or we have only a limited idea of what the respondent will say, or we want the answer in the respondent's own words, as with the second set of items. Here, the respondent may also leave the item blank but we are not forcing the subject to make a particular response.

Interviews and questionnaires commonly are used in nursing research. Both are strong approaches to gathering information for research, because they approach the task directly. In addition, both have the ability to obtain certain kinds of information, such as the subjects' attitudes and beliefs, that would be difficult to obtain without asking the subject directly. All methods that involve verbal reports, however, share a problem with accuracy. There is often no way to know whether what we are

EXAMPLES OF CLOSE-ENDED AND OPEN-ENDED QUESTIONS

CLOSE-ENDED (LIKERT-TYPE SCALE)

A. How satisfied are you with your current position?
1. Very satisfied
2. Moderately satisfied
3. Undecided
4. Moderately dissatisfied
5. Very dissatisfied

B. To what extent do the following factors contribute to your current level of positive satisfaction?

	Not at all	Very little	Somewhat	Moderate amount	A great deal
1. % of time in patient care	1	2	3	4	5
2. Types of patients	1	2	3	4	5
3. % of time in educational activity	1	2	3	4	5
4. % of time in administration	1	2	3	4	5

CLOSE-ENDED

A. On an average, how many clients do you see in one day?
1. 1 to 3
2. 4 to 6
3. 7 to 9
4. 10 to 12
5. 13 to 15
6. 16 to 18
7. 18 to 20
8. More than 20

B. How would you characterize your practice?
1. Too slow
2. Slow
3. About right
4. Busy
5. Too busy

OPEN-ENDED

A. Are there incentives that National Association of Pediatric Nurse Associates and Practitioners ought to provide for members that are currently not being done?

_____

_____

_____

_____

told is indeed true. For example, people are known to respond to questions in a way that makes a favorable impression. This response style is known as **social desirability**. Because there is no way to tell whether the respondent is telling the truth or responding in a socially desirable way, the researcher usually is forced to assume that the respondent is telling the truth.

Questionnaires and interviews also have some specific purposes, advantages, and disadvantages. Questionnaires and paper-and-pencil tests are most useful when there is a finite set of questions to be asked and the researcher can be assured of the clarity and specificity of the items. Questionnaires are desirable tools when the purpose is to collect information. If questionnaires are too long, they are not likely to be completed. Face-to-face techniques or interviews are best used when the researcher may need to clarify the task for the respondent or is interested in obtaining more personal information from the respondent. Telephone interviews allow the researcher to reach more respondents than face-to-face interviews, and they allow for more clarity than questionnaires.

Grey et al. (1991; Appendix B) used a combination of interview and questionnaires to study the influence of age, coping behavior, and self-care on psychological, social, and physiological adaptation in children and adolescents with diabetes. One of the measures of social adaptation is the Child and Adolescent Adjustment Profile, which is a parent interview measuring the social role performance of children and adolescents in the areas of productivity, peer relations, dependency, hostility, and withdrawal. Obtaining a more complete evaluation of the adaptation of the children, however, required that the children also report on their own feelings. This was accomplished by using the Self-Perception Profile for Children, which is a questionnaire dealing with children's feelings of competence in several areas. Thus the researchers were able to report both the children's and their parents' accounts of the child's overall adaptation. This use of multiple measures gives a more complete picture than the use of just one measure.

Researchers face difficult choices when determining whether to use interviews or questionnaires. The final decision is often based on what instruments are available and their relative costs and benefits.

Both face-to-face and telephone interviews offer some advantages over questionnaires. All things being equal, interviews are better than questionnaires because the response rate is almost always higher and this helps to eliminate bias in the sample (see Chapter 15). Respondents seem to be less likely to hang up the telephone or to close the door in an interviewer's face than to throw away a questionnaire. Another advantage of the interview is that some people, such as children, the blind, and the illiterate, could not fill out a questionnaire but they could participate in an interview. With an interview, the data collector knows who is giving the answers. When questionnaires are mailed, for example, anyone in the household could be the person who supplies the answers.

Interviews also allow for some safeguards to be built into the interview situation. Interviewers can clarify misunderstood questions and observe the level of the respondent's understanding and cooperativeness. In addition, the researcher has strict control over the order of the questions. With questionnaires, the respondent can answer questions in any order. Sometimes changing the order of the questions can change the response.

Finally, interviews allow for richer and more complex data to be collected. This is particularly so when open-ended responses are sought. Even when close-ended response items are used, interviews can probe to understand why a respondent answered in a particular way.

Questionnaires also have certain advantages. They are much less expensive to administer than interviews, because interviews may require the hiring and training of interviewers. Thus if a researcher has a fixed amount of time and money, a larger and more diverse sample can be obtained with questionnaires. Questionnaires also allow for complete anonymity, which may be important if the study deals with sensitive issues. Finally, the fact that no interviewer is present assures the researcher and the reader that there will be no interviewer bias. Interviewer bias occurs when the interviewer unwittingly leads the respondent to answer in a certain way. This problem is especially pronounced in studies that use unstructured interview formats. A subtle nod of the head, for example, could lead a respondent to change an answer to correspond with what the researcher wants to hear.

Records or Available Data

All of the data collection methods discussed thus far concern the ways that nurse researchers gather new data to study phenomena of interest. Not all studies, though, require a researcher to acquire new information. Sometimes existing information can be examined in a new way to study a problem. The use of records and available data sometimes is considered to be primarily the province of historical research, but hospital records, care plans, and existing data sources, such as the census, are frequently used for collecting information. What sets these studies apart from a literature review is that these available data are examined in a new way, are not merely summarized, and answer specific research questions. **Records or available data,** then, are forms of information that are collected from existing materials, such as hospital records, historical documents, or videotapes, and are used to answer research questions in a new manner.

The use of available data has certain advantages. Because the data collection step of the research process often is the most difficult and time-consuming, the use of available records often allows for a significant savings of time. If the records have been kept in a similar manner over time, as with the National Health and Examination Surveys, analysis of these records allows for the examination of trends over time. The time series study in Chapter 9 (Jones, Robertson, & Pieper, 1992) is an example of this type of study. In addition, the use of available data decreases problems of reactivity and response set bias. The researcher also does not have to ask individuals to participate in the study.

On the other hand, institutions are sometimes reluctant to allow researchers to have access to their records. If the records are kept so that an individual cannot be identified, this is usually not a problem. However, the Privacy Act, a federal law, protects the rights of individuals who may be identified in records. Another problem that affects the quality of available data is that the researcher has access only to those records that have survived. If the records available are not representative of all of the possible records, the researcher may have a problem with bias. Often there is no way to tell whether the records have been saved in a biased manner, and the researcher has to make an intelligent guess as to their accuracy. For example, a researcher might be interested in studying socioeconomic factors associated with the suicide rate. These data are frequently underreported because of the stigma attached to suicide, and so the records would be biased.

Another problem is related to the authenticity of the records. The distinction of primary and secondary sources is as relevant here as it was in discussing the literature review (see Chapter 5). A book, for example, may have been ghostwritten but credit accorded to the known author. It may be difficult for the researcher to ferret out these types of subtle biases.

Nonetheless, records and available data constitute a rich source of data for study. Aber and Hawkins (1992) provide an interesting example of the use of available data in studying the image of nurses in advertisements. In this study the researchers were interested in determining whether nurses were portrayed in advertising as professionals or as physician helpers. They examined 313 different advertisements in medical and nursing journals by using a standardized content analysis. They found that nurses were portrayed as sex objects, ornaments, and physicians' handmaidens.

CONSTRUCTION OF NEW INSTRUMENTS

As already mentioned in this chapter and Chapter 10, researchers sometimes cannot locate an instrument or method with acceptable reliability and validity to measure the variable of interest. This often is the case when testing a part of a nursing theory or when evaluating the effect of a clinical intervention. A recent example is provided by the work of Melnyk (1990), who was interested in the reasons that individuals seek or do not seek health care. One such construct is that of perceived barriers to care. She undertook a study to operationalize the concept of barriers by identifying potential barriers with a special procedure called a **Delphi procedure.** Then the items were tested for reliability and classified using factor analysis (see Chapter 17). Finally, this classification led to the development of a scale that was tested.

Tool development is complex and time-consuming. It consists of the following steps:
* Define the construct to be measured
* Formulate the items
* Assess the items for content validity
* Develop instructions for respondents and users
* Pretest and pilot test the items
* Estimate reliability and validity

To define the construct to be measured requires that the researcher develop an expertise in the construct. This requires an extensive review of the literature and of all tests and measurements that deal with related constructs. The researcher will use all of this information to synthesize the available knowledge so that the construct can be defined (see Chapters 5 and 10).

Once defined, the individual items measuring the construct can be developed. The researcher will develop many more items than are needed to address each aspect of the construct or subconstruct. The items are evaluated by a panel of experts in the field so that the researcher is assured that the items measure what they are intended to measure (content validity; see Chapter 15). Eventually the number of items will be decreased, because some items will not work as they were intended and they will be dropped. In this phase the researcher needs to ensure consistency among the items, as well as consistency in testing and scoring procedures.

Finally, the researcher administers the test to a group of people who are similar to those who will be studied in the larger investigation. The purpose of this analysis to determine the quality of the instrument as a whole (reliability and validity), as well as the ability of each item to discriminate individual respondents (variance in item response). The researcher also may administer a related instrument to see if the new instrument is sufficiently different from the older one.

It is important that researchers who invest significant amounts of time in tool development publish those results. This type of research serves not only to introduce other researchers to the tool but ultimately to enhance the field, because our ability to conduct meaningful research is limited only by our ability to measure important phenomena.

CRITIQUING DATA COLLECTION METHODS

Evaluating the adequacy of data collection methods from written research reports is often problematic for new nursing research consumers. This is because the tool itself is not available for inspection and the reader may not feel comfortable about judging the adequacy of the method without seeing it. However, a number of questions can be asked as you read to judge the method chosen by the researcher. These questions are listed in the box on pp. 360-361.

All studies should have clearly identified data collection methods. The conceptual and operational definitions of each important variable should be present in the report. Sometimes it is useful for the researcher to explain why a particular method was chosen. For example, if the study dealt with young children, the researcher may explain that a questionnaire was deemed to be an unreasonable task, so an interview was chosen.

Once you have identified the method chosen to measure each variable of interest, you should decide if the method used was the best way to measure the variable. If a questionnaire was used, for example, you might wonder why the decision was made not to use an interview. In addition, consider whether the method was appropriate to the clinical situation. Does it make sense to interview patients in the recovery room, for example?

Once you have decided whether all relevant variables are operationalized appropriately, you can begin to determine how well the method was carried out. For studies using physiological measurement, it is important to determine whether the

CRITIQUING CRITERIA

1. Are all of the data collection instruments clearly identified and described?
2. Is the rationale for their selection given?
3. Is the method used appropriate to the problem being studied?
4. Is the method used appropriate to the clinical situation?
5. Are the data collection procedures similar for all subjects?

PHYSIOLOGICAL MEASUREMENT

1. Is the instrument used appropriate to the research problem and not forced to fit it?
2. Is a rationale given for why a particular instrument was selected?
3. Is there a provision for evaluating the accuracy of the instrument and those who use it?

OBSERVATIONAL METHODS

1. Who did the observing?
2. Were the observers trained to minimize any bias?
3. Was there an observational guide?
4. Were the observers required to make inferences about what they saw?
5. Is there any reason to believe that the presence of the observers affected the behavior of the subjects?
6. Were the observations performed using the principles of informed consent?

INTERVIEWS

1. Is the interview schedule described adequately enough to know whether it covers the subject?
2. Is there clear indication that the subjects understood the task and the questions?
3. Who were the interviewers, and how were they trained?
4. Is there evidence of any interviewer bias?

QUESTIONNAIRES

1. Is the questionnaire described well enough to know whether it covers the subject?
2. Is there evidence that subjects were able to perform the task?
3. Is there clear indication that the subjects understood the questionnaire?
4. Are the majority of the items appropriately close- or open-ended?

CRITIQUING CRITERIA—cont'd

AVAILABLE DATA AND RECORDS

1. Are the records that were used appropriate to the problem being studied?
2. Are the data examined in such a way as to provide new information and not summarize the records?
3. Has the author addressed questions of internal and external criticism?
4. Is there any indication of selection bias in the available records?

instrument was appropriate to the problem and not forced to fit it. The rationale for selecting a particular instrument should be given. For example, it may be important to know that the study was conducted under the auspices of a manufacturing firm that provided the measuring instrument. In addition, provision should be made to evaluate the accuracy of the instrument and those who use it.

Several considerations are important when reading studies that use observational methods. Who were the observers, and how were they trained? Is there any reason to believe that different observers saw events or behaviors differently? Remember that the more inferences the observers are required to make, the more likely there will be problems with biased observations. Also consider the problem of reactivity; in any observational situation, the possibility exists that the mere presence of the observer could change the behavior in question. What is important here is not that reactivity could occur, but rather how much reactivity could affect the data. Finally, consider whether the observational procedure was ethical. The reader needs to consider whether subjects were informed that they were being observed, whether any intervention was performed, and whether subjects had agreed to be observed.

Interviews and questionnaires should be clearly described to allow the reader to decide whether the variables were adequately operationalized. Sometimes the researcher will reference the original report about the tool, and the reader may wish to read this study before deciding if the method was appropriate for the present study. The respondents' task should be clear. Thus provision should be made for the subjects to understand both their overall responsibilities and the individual items. Who were the interviewers in the interview situation? Does the researcher explain how they were trained to decrease any interviewer bias?

Available data are subject to internal and external criticism. Internal criticism deals with the evaluation of the worth of the records. Internal criticism primarily refers to the accuracy of the data (see Chapter 11). The researcher should present evidence that the records are genuine. External criticism is concerned with the authenticity of the records. Are the records really written by the first author? Finally, the reader should be aware of the problems with selective survival. The researcher may not have an unbiased sample of all of the possible records in the problem area, and this may have a profound effect on the validity of the results.

Finally, the reader should consider the data collection procedure. Is any assurance provided that all of the subjects received the same information? In addition, it is important to try to determine whether all of the information was collected in the same way for all of the subjects in the study.

Once you have decided that the data collection method used was appropriate to the problem and the procedures were appropriate to the population studied, the reliability and validity of the instruments themselves need to be considered. These characteristics are discussed in the next chapter.

KEY POINTS

- Data collection methods are described as being both objective and systematic. The data collection methods of a study provide the operational definitions of the relevant variables.
- Types of data collection methods include physiological, observational, interviews, questionnaires, and available data or records. Each method has advantages and disadvantages.
- Physiological measurements are those methods that use technical instruments to collect data about patients' physical, chemical, microbiological, or anatomical status. Such instruments are particularly suited to the study of the effectiveness of nursing care and the ways to improve the provision of nursing care. Physiological measurements are objective, precise, and sensitive. However, they may be very expensive and they may distort the variable of interest.
- Observational methods frequently are used in nursing research when the variables of interest deal with events or behaviors. Scientific observation requires preplanning, systematic recording, controlling the observations, and relationship to scientific theory. This method is best suited to research problems that are difficult to view as a part of a whole. Observers may be passive or active and concealed or obvious. Observational methods have several advantages, the most important one being the flexibility of the method to measure many types of situations. In addition, observation allows for a great depth and breadth of information to be collected, depending on the problem being studied. Observation has several disadvantages, too. Reactivity, or the distortion of data as a result of the observer's presence, is a common problem in nonconcealed observations. If the observer is concealed, however, there are ethical considerations. Finally, observations may be biased by the person who is doing the observing.
- Interviews and questionnaires are the most commonly used data collection methods in nursing research. Both have the purpose of asking subjects to report data for themselves. Items on questionnaire and interview schedules may be of direct or indirect interest and can be combined into scales. Scales provide an estimate of the degree to which the respondent possesses some trait or characteristic. Either

open-ended or close-ended questions may be used when asking subjects questions. The form of the question should be clear to the respondent, free of suggestion, and grammatically correct.

- Questionnaires, or paper-and-pencil tests, are particularly useful when there are a finite number of questions to be asked and the researcher is sure that the questions are clear and specific. Questionnaires also are much less costly in time and money to administer to a large number of subjects, particularly if the subjects are geographically widespread. Another advantage of questionnaires over interviews is that questionnaires have the potential to be completely anonymous. In addition, there is no possibility of interviewer bias.

- Interviews are best used when a large response rate and an unbiased sample are important, because the refusal rate for interviews is much less than that for questionnaires. Interviews also allow for some portions of the population who would be precluded by the use of a questionnaire, such as children and the illiterate, to participate in the study. An interviewer can clarify the questions and maintain the order of the questions for all participants.

- Records and available data also are an important source for research data. The use of available data may save the researcher considerable time and money when conducting a study. This data collection method reduces problems with both reactivity and ethical concerns. However, records and available data are subject to problems of availability, authenticity, and accuracy.

- A critical evaluation of data collection methods should emphasize the appropriateness, objectivity, and consistency of the method employed.

REFERENCES

Aber, C.S.M., & Hawkins, J.W. (1992). Portrayal of nurses in advertisements in medical and nursing journals. *Image: Journal of Nursing Scholarship, 24,* 289-293.

Collins, C., Given, B., Given, C.W., & King, S. (1988). Interviewer training and supervision. *Nursing Research, 37,* 122-124.

Gift, A.G., Moore, T., & Soeken, K. (1992). Relaxation to reduce dyspnea and anxiety in COPD patients. *Nursing Research, 41,* 242-245.

Gill, N.E., Behnke, M., Conlon, M., McNeely, J.B., & Anderson, G.C. (1988). Effect of nonnutritive sucking on behavioral state in preterm infants before feeding. *Nursing Research, 37,* 147-150.

Given, B.A., Keilman, L.J., Collins, C., & Given, C.W. (1990). Strategies to minimize attrition in longitudinal studies. *Nursing Research, 39* (3), 184-186.

Grey, M., & Flint, S. (1989). 1988 NAPNAP membership survey: Characteristics of member's practice. *Journal of Pediatric Health Care, 3,* 336-341.

Grey, M., Cameron, M.E., & Thurber, F.W. (1991). Coping and adaptation in children with diabetes. *Nursing Research, 40,* 144-148.

Heidenreich, T., & Giuffre, M. (1990). Postoperative temperature measurement. *Nursing Research, 39* (3), 153-155.

Holmes, T.H., & Rahe, R.H. (1967). The social readjustment rating scale. *Journal of Psychosomatic Research, 11,* 213-218.

Lazarus, R.S., & Folkman, S. (1984). Coping and adaptation. In W.D. Gentry (Ed.), *The handbook of behavioral medicine* (pp. 22-325). New York: Guildford.

Melnyk, K.A.M. (1990). Barriers to care: Operationalizing the variable. *Nursing Research, 39,* 108-112.

Seaman, C.C.H., & Verhonick, P.J. (1982). *Research methods for undergraduate students in nursing.* Norwalk, CT: Appleton-Century-Crofts.

Speilberger, C.D. (1973). *Manual for the state-trait anxiety inventory for children.* Palo Alto, CA: Consulting Psychologists.

Stewart Fahs, P.S., & Kinney, M.R. (1991). The abdomen, thigh, and arm as sites for subcutaneous sodium heparin injections. *Nursing Research, 40* (4), 204-207.

West, M., Bondy, E., & Hutchinson, S. (1991). Interviewing institutionalized elders: Threats to validity. *Image: Journal of Nursing Scholarship, 23,* 171-176.

White, M.A., Williams, P.D., Alexander, D.J., Powell-Cope, G.M., & Conlon, M. (1990). Sleep onset latency and distress in hospitalized children. *Nursing Research, 39* (3), 134-139.

ADDITIONAL READINGS

Butz, A.M., & Alexander, C. (1991). Use of health diaries with children. *Nursing Research, 40,* 59-61.

DeKeyser, F.G., & Puch, L.C., (1990). Assessment of the reliability and validity of biochemical measures. *Nursing Research, 39,* 314-317.

Gold, D.R., Weiss, S.T., Tager, I.B., Segal, M.R., & Speizer, F.E. (1989). Comparison of questionnaire and diary methods in acute childhood respiratory illness surveillance. *American review of respiratory diseases, 139,* 847-849.

Hutchinson, S., & Wilson, H.S. (1992). Validity threats in scheduled semistructured research interviews. *Nursing Research, 41,* 117-119.

Jones, E.J., & Kay, M. (1992). Instrumentation in cross-cultural research. *Nursing Research, 41,* 186-188.

Morse, J.M. (1991). Approaches to qualitative-quantitative methodological triangulation. *Nursing Research, 40,* 120-123.

Nield, M., & Kim, M.J. (1991). The reliability of magnitude estimation for dyspnea measurement. *Nursing Research, 40,* 17-19.

Sandelowski, M. (1991). Telling stories: Narrative approaches in qualitative research. *Image: Journal of Nursing Scholarship, 23,* 161-165.

Strickland, O.L., & Waltz, C.F. (1988). *Measurement of nursing outcomes: measuring client outcomes* (Vol. 1). New York: Springer.

Waltz, C.F., & Strickland, O.L. (1988). *Measurement of nursing outcomes: measuring client outcomes* (Vol. 2). New York: Springer.

GERI LoBIONDO-WOOD
JUDITH HABER

LEARNING OBJECTIVES

After reading this chapter the student should be able to do the following:

♦ Discuss how measurement error can affect the outcomes of a research study.
♦ Discuss the purposes of reliability and validity.
♦ Define reliability.
♦ Discuss the concepts of stability, equivalence, and homogeneity as they relate to reliability.
♦ Compare and contrast the estimates of reliability.
♦ Define validity.
♦ Compare and contrast content, criterion-related, and construct validity.
♦ Identify the criteria for critiquing the reliability and validity of measurement tools.
♦ Use the critiquing criteria to evaluate the reliability and validity of measurement tools.

KEY TERMS

chance error	interrater reliability
concurrent validity	item-total correlation
construct validity	Kuder-Richardson coefficient
content validity	parallel or alternate form
convergent validity	predictive validity
criterion-related validity	reliability
Cronbach alpha	split-half reliability
divergent validity	stability
equivalence	systematic error
error variance	test
homogeneity	test-retest reliability
hypothesis testing validity	validity
internal consistency	

Measurement of nursing phenomena is a major concern of nursing researchers. Unless measurement tools validly and reliably reflect the concepts of the theory being tested, conclusions drawn from the empirical phase of the study will be invalid and will not advance the development of nursing theory. Issues of reliability and validity are of central concern to the researcher, as well as the critiquer of research. From either perspective the measurement tools that are used in a research study must be evaluated in terms of the extent to which reliability and validity have been established. Many new constructs are relevant to nursing theory, and a growing number of established measurement instruments are available to researchers. However, investigators frequently face the challenge of developing new instruments and, as part of that process, establishing the reliability and validity of those tools.

In other contexts investigators use tools that have been developed by researchers in nursing or other disciplines. They must evaluate the tools they select to be certain that they are valid and reliable measures—that they accurately operationalize the constructs being tested.

The critiquer of research, when reading research studies and reports, must assess the reliability and validity of the instruments used in the study to determine the soundness of these selections in relation to the constructs under investigation. The appropriateness of the tools and the extent to which reliability and validity are demonstrated have a profound influence on the findings and the internal and external validity of the study. Invalid measures produce invalid estimates of the relation-

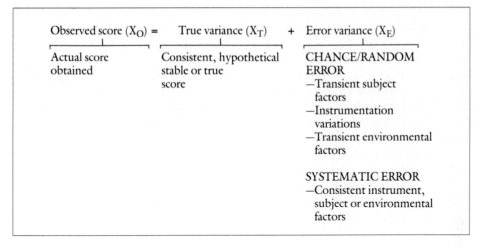

Observed score (X_O) =   True variance (X_T)   +   Error variance (X_E)

| Actual score obtained | Consistent, hypothetical stable or true score | CHANCE/RANDOM ERROR
—Transient subject factors
—Instrumentation variations
—Transient environmental factors

SYSTEMATIC ERROR
—Consistent instrument, subject or environmental factors |

Fig. 15-1   Components of observed scores.

ships between variables, thus affecting internal validity. The use of invalid measures produces inaccurate generalizations to the populations being studied, thus affecting external validity and the ability to apply or not apply research findings in clinical practice. As such, the assessment of reliability and validity is an extremely important task for the research critiquer.

Regardless of whether a new or already developed measurement tool is used in a research study, evidence of reliability and validity is of crucial importance to the research investigator and evaluator.

The purpose of this chapter is to examine the major types of reliability and validity and demonstrate the applicability of these concepts to the development, selection, and evaluation of measurement tools in nursing research.

RELIABILITY, VALIDITY, AND MEASUREMENT ERROR

Researchers may be concerned about whether the scores that were obtained for a sample of subjects were consistent, true measures of the behaviors and thus an accurate reflection of the differences between individuals. The extent of variability in test scores that is attributable to error rather than a true measure of the behaviors would be the **error variance.**

An observed test score that is derived from a set of items actually consists of the true score plus error (Fig. 15-1). The error may be either *chance error,* or *random error,* or it may be what is known as *systematic error.* Validity is concerned with systematic error, whereas reliability is concerned with random error (Waltz, Strickland, and Lenz, 1991). Chance or random errors are errors that are difficult to control, such as a respondent's anxiety level at the time of testing. **Random** errors are unsystematic in nature. Random errors are a result of a transient state in the subject, in the context of the study, or in the administration of the instrument (Jennings & Rogers, 1989). For example, perceptions or behaviors that occur at a specific point in time, such as anxiety, are known as a state or transient characteristic and are often beyond the awareness and control of the examiner. Another example of random error is in a study that measures blood pressure. Random error could occur by misplacement of the cuff, not waiting for a specific time period before taking the blood pressure, and random placement of the arm in relationship to the heart while measuring blood pressure.

Systematic or constant error is measurement error that is attributable to relatively stable characteristics of the study population that may bias their behavior and/or cause incorrect instrument calibration. Such error has a systematic biasing influence on the subjects' responses and thereby influences the validity of the instruments. For instance, level of education, socioeconomic status, social desirability, response set, or other characteristics may influence the validity of the instrument by altering measurement of the "true" responses in a systematic way.

For example, a subject who wants to please the investigator may constantly answer items in a socially desirable way, thus making the estimate of validity inaccurate. Systematic error occurs also when an instrument is improperly calibrated. Consider a scale that consistently weighs a person 2 pounds less than the actual body weight. The scale could be quite reliable (that is, capable of reproducing the precise measurement), but the result is consistently invalid.

VALIDITY

Validity refers to whether a measurement instrument accurately measures what it is supposed to measure. When an instrument is valid, it truly reflects the concept it is supposed to measure.

A valid instrument that is supposed to measure anxiety does so; it does not measure some other construct, such as stress. A reliable measure can consistently rank participants on a given construct, such as anxiety, but a valid measure correctly measures the construct of interest. A measure can be reliable but not valid. Let us say that a researcher wanted to measure anxiety in patients by measuring their body temperatures. The researcher could obtain highly accurate, consistent, and precise temperature recordings, but such a measure could not be a valid indicator of anxiety. Thus the high reliability of an instrument is not necessarily congruent with evidence of validity. However, a valid instrument is reliable. An instrument cannot validly measure the attribute of interest if it is erratic, inconsistent, and inaccurate.

There are three major kinds of validity that vary according to the kind of information provided and the purpose of the investigator. They are *content validity, criterion-related validity,* and *construct validity.* A critiquer of research articles will want to evaluate whether sufficient evidence of validity is present and whether the type of validity is appropriate to the design of the study and instruments used in the study.

Content Validity

Content validity represents the universe of content, or the domain of a given construct. The universe of content provides the framework and basis for formulating the items that will adequately represent the content. When an investigator is developing a tool and issues of content validity arise, the concern is whether the measurement tool and the items it contains are representative of the content domain the researcher intends to measure. The researcher begins by defining the concept and identifying the dimensions that are the components of the concept. Those items that reflect the concept and its dimensions are formulated.

When the researcher has completed this task, the items are submitted to a panel of judges who are considered to be experts about this concept. Researchers typically request that the judges indicate their agreement with the scope of the items and the extent to which the items reflect the concept under consideration (Berk, 1990).

Hickey, Owen, and Froman (1992) developed two tools to measure diet and exercise self-efficacy, reflected by two common and modifiable cardiac risk factors—inactivity and improper diet. On the basis of a review of the literature from which conceptual definitions and items were derived, the researchers submitted 30 items that reflected cardiac diet self-efficacy (CDSEI) and 30 items that reflected cardiac exercise self-efficacy (CESEI) to a multidisciplinary panel of 10 experts in cardiac rehabilitation and self-efficacy. The experts were asked to indicate how well each item fit within its subdimension: that is, diet or exercise, on a 5-point scale (1 = very poor fit; 5 = excellent fit). Experts' ratings were tallied, and items were retained if they received a mean score of at least 3 on their fit. Nineteen items remained on the CDSEI and 18 items on the CESEI.

A subtype of content validity is face validity. *Face validity* is a rudimentary type of validity that verifies basically that the instrument gives the appearance of measuring the concept. It is an intuitive type of validity in which colleagues or subjects are asked to read the instrument and evaluate the content in terms of whether it appears to reflect the concept the researcher intends to measure. This procedure may be useful in the tool development process in relation to determining readability and clarity of content. However, it should in no way be considered a satisfactory alternative to other types of validity.

Criterion-Related Validity

Criterion-related validity indicates to what degree the subject's performance on the measurement tool and the subject's actual behavior are related. The criterion is usually the second measure, which assesses the same concept under study.

Two forms of criterion-related validity are concurrent and predictive. Concurrent validity refers to the degree of correlation of two measures of the same concept administered at the same time. A high correlation coefficient indicates agreement between the two measures. Predictive validity refers to the degree of correlation between the measure of the concept and some future measure of the same concept. Because of the passage of time, the correlation coefficients are likely to be lower for predictive validity studies.

Abraham, Neundorfer, and Currie (1992) assessed concurrent validity of the Geriatric Depression Scale (GDS) by correlating scores on the GDS with those from the Zung Self-Rating Depression Scale and the Hamilton Rating Scale for Depression, two well-established tools for the assessment of depression in adults. Significant positive correlations between the Geriatric Depression Scale and the Zung Self-Rating Depression Scale ($r = .84$) and the Hamilton Rating Scale for Depression ($r = .83$) provided support for concurrent validity of the GDS.

Hickey et al. (1992) assessed predictive validity of the CDSEI and CESEI. Scores on the CDSEI and CESEI on entry into a cardiac rehabilitation program (CRP) were correlated with subsequent scores related to diet and exercise goal attainment. Significant positive correlations were found between initial diet and exercise self-efficacy levels of the 101 CRP participants and their subsequent diet ($r = .62; p < .0001$) and exercise ($r = .53; p < .0001$) goal attainment.

Construct Validity

Construct validity is based on the extent to which a test measures a theoretical construct or trait. It attempts to validate a body of theory underlying the measurement and testing of the hypothesized relationships. Empirical testing confirms or fails to confirm the relationships that would be predicted among concepts and, as such, provides greater or lesser support for the construct validity of the instruments measuring those concepts. The establishment of construct validity is a complex process, often involving several studies and several approaches. The hypothesis testing, factor analytic, convergent and divergent, and contrasted-groups approaches are discussed.

Hypothesis-Testing Approach

When the **hypothesis-testing** approach is employed, the investigator uses the theory or concept underlying the measurement instrument's design to develop hypotheses regarding the behavior of individuals with varying scores on the measure, to gather data to test the hypotheses, and to make inferences, on the basis of the findings, concerning whether the rationale underlying the instrument's construction is adequate to explain the findings.

For example, Haber (1990) used a hypothesis-testing approach to establish the construct validity of the Level of Differentiation of Self Scale (LDSS), a tool that theoretically was derived from the cornerstone concept of the Bowen Theory (1978) differentiation of self. As illustrated in Table 15-1, Haber derived five hypotheses that represented propositions related to differentiation of self, stress, anxiety, and adult dysfunction. Statistically significant findings provided support for the hypotheses and, as such, for the theoretical basis and conceptual accuracy of the LDSS.

Table 15-1   Construct Validity Estimation by Hypothesis Testing Strategy: The LDSS

Hypotheses	Findings	
	F ratio	Pearson r
1. Differentiation of self and negative impact ratings of stressful life events will have an additive effect on adult dysfunction.	21.31* 6.44†	
2. There will be a negative relationship between differentiation of self and trait anxiety.		−0.52*
3. There will be a negative relationship between differentiation of self and state anxiety.		−0.43*
4. There will be a negative relationship between differentiation of self and adult dysfunction.		−0.53*
5. Negative impact ratings of stressful life events will have a greater impact than positive impact ratings on adult dysfunction.	58.74* 1.50	

From The Haber Level of Differentiation of Self Scale by J.E. Haber. In C. Waltz and O. Strickland (Eds.), 1990, *The measurement of educational and clinical outcomes*, vol. 4, New York: Springer.
*$p < 0.001$.
†$p < 0.01$.

Convergent and Divergent Approaches

Two strategies for assessing construct validity include convergent and divergent approaches.

Convergent validity refers to a search for other measures of the construct. When two or more tools that theoretically measure the same construct are identified, they are both administered to the same subjects. A correlational analysis is performed. If the measures are positively correlated, convergent validity is said to be supported. In the development of the Health Related Hardiness Scale (HRHS), Pollack and Duffy (1990) established convergent validity by correlating the HRHS with Kobasa's Hardiness Scale. The statistically significant but moderate positive correlation of .54 between the two scales supported the idea that the HRHS was measuring hardiness.

Divergent validity searches for instruments that measure the opposite of the construct. It refers to the ability to differentiate the construct from others that may be similar. If the divergent measure is negatively related to other measures, validity for the measure is strengthened. In the development of the Miller Hope Scale (MHS) (1988), divergent validity was established by correlating the MHS with the Hopelessness Scale. A negative correlation, $r = −0.54$, between the MHS and Hopelessness Scale was obtained, thereby lending support to the divergent validity of the MHS.

A specific method of assessing convergent and divergent validity is the *multi-*

trait-multimethod approach. Similar to the approach described, this method, proposed by Campbell and Fiske (1959), also involves examining the relationship between indicators that should measure the same construct and between those that should measure different constructs. However, a variety of measurement strategies are used. For example, anxiety could be measured by:
• Administering the State-Trait Anxiety Inventory
• Recording blood pressure readings
• Asking the subject about anxious feelings
• Observing the subject's behavior
The results of one of these measures should then be correlated with results of each of the others in a multitrait-multimethod matrix (Waltz, Strickland, & Lenz, 1991). A study designed to develop, validate, and norm a measure of dimensions of interpersonal relationships including social support, reciprocity, and conflict by Tilden, Nelson, and May (1990) used the multitrait-multimethod approach to validity assessment. The two traits of social support and conflict of the Interpersonal Relationship Inventory (IPRI) were each measured with two different methods—a subject self-report tool and an investigator observation visual analog rating. Reciprocity was not included because of its high correlation with social support.

The use of multiple measures of a concept decreases systematic error. A variety of data collection methods, such as self-report, observation, interview, and collection of physiological data, will also diminish the effect of systematic error.

Contrasted-Groups Approach

When the *contrasted-groups* approach (sometimes called the *known-groups* approach) to the development of construct validity is used, the researcher identifies two groups of individuals who are suspected to score extremely high or low in the characteristic being measured by the instrument. The instrument is administered to both the high- and low-scoring group, and the differences in scores obtained are examined. If the instrument is sensitive to individual differences in the trait being measured, the *mean performance* of these two groups should differ significantly and evidence of construct validity would be supported. A *t* test or analysis of variance is used to statistically test the difference between the two groups. In the study by Hickey et al. (1992) on diet and exercise self-efficacy, the contrasted-groups approach was established by studying the differences in mean CDSEI and CESEI scores between cardiac rehabilitation participants and marathon runners. As predicted, the marathon runner sample reported significantly higher diet and exercise self-efficacy scores than did cardiac rehabilitation participants. Table 15-2 illustrates the mean scores of both groups, as well as the *t* scores that signify the differences between the sample groups.

Factor Analytic Approach

A final approach to assessing construct validity is *factor analysis.* This is a procedure that gives the researcher information about the extent to which a set of items measures the same underlying construct or dimension of a construct. Factor analysis assesses the degree to which the individual items on a scale truly cluster together

Table 15-2   *T*-Test Results of CDSEI and CESEI Scores Between Cardiac Rehabilitation Participants and Marathon Runners

CDSEI	*n*	*M*	*SD*	*SE*	*T*
Runners	54	4.44	.57	.08	
					4.58†
Cardiac sample	370	4.00	.63	.03	
CESEI	*n*	*M*	*SD*	*SE*	*T*
Runners	54	4.40	.58	.08	
					2.89*
Cardiac sample	370	4.11	.63	.03	

From M.L. Hickey, S.V. Owen, and R.D. Froman, 1992, *Nursing Research, 41:* 6, 347-351.
*p = .004.
*p = .0001.

around one or more dimensions. Items designed to measure the same dimension should load on the same factor; those designed to measure differing dimensions should load on different factors (Nunnally, 1978; Anastasi, 1988). This analysis will indicate also whether the items in the instrument reflect a single construct or several constructs.

A factor analysis was carried out by Haber (1990) during the establishment of construct validity of the LDSS. The original scale consisted of a 32-item, two-subscale instrument. Findings from three factor analytic studies indicated that 24 of the 32 items loaded on factor I, only 6 loaded on factor II, and 2 did not load significantly on either factor. As a result of these and other findings, a decision was made to revise the LDSS as a 24-item unidimensional scale that measures one rather than two aspects of the concept of differentiation of self.

RELIABILITY

Reliable people are people whose behavior can be relied on to be consistent and predictable. **Reliability** of a research instrument likewise is defined as the extent to which the instrument yields the same results on repeated measures. Reliability is then concerned with consistency, accuracy, precision, stability, equivalence, and homogeneity. Concurrent with the questions of validity or after they are answered, the researcher and the critiquer of research ask the question of how reliable is the instrument? A reliable measure is one that can produce the same results if the behavior is measured again by the same scale. Reliability then refers to the proportion of accuracy to inaccuracy in measurement. In other words, if we use the same or comparable instruments on more than one occasion to measure a set of behaviors that ordinarily remain relatively constant, we would expect similar results if the tools are reliable. The three main attributes of a reliable scale are *stability, homogeneity,* and *equivalence.* The stability of an instrument refers to the instrument's ability to produce the same results with repeated testing. The homogeneity of an instrument means that all the items in a tool measure the same concept or characteristic. An instrument is said to exhibit equivalence if the tool produces the same results when equivalent or parallel instruments or procedures are used. Each of these attributes and the means to estimate them will be discussed. Before these are discussed an understanding of how to interpret reliability is essential.

Reliability Coefficient Interpretation

Because all the attributes of reliability are concerned with the degree of consistency between scores that are obtained at two or more independent times of testing, they often are expressed in terms of a correlation coefficient. The reliability coefficient ranges from 0 to 1. The reliability coefficient expresses the relationship between the error variance, true variance, and the observed score. A zero correlation indicates that there is no relationship. When the error variance in a measurement instrument is low, the reliability coefficient will be closer to 1. The closer to 1 the coefficient is, the more reliable the tool. For example, a reliability coefficient of a tool is reported to be 0.89. This tells the reader that the error variance is small and the tool has little measurement error. On the other hand, if the reliability coefficient of a measure is reported to be 0.49, the error variance is high and the tool has a problem with measurement error. For a tool to be considered reliable, a level of 0.70 or higher is considered to be an acceptable level of reliability. The interpretation of the reliability coefficient depends on the proposed purpose of the measure. There are five major tests of reliability that can be used to calculate a reliability coefficient. The test(s) used depends on the nature of the tool. They are known as test-retest, parallel or alternate form, item-total correlation, split-half, Kuder-Richardson (KR-20), Cronbach's alpha, and interrater reliability. These tests are discussed as they relate to the attributes of stability, equivalence, and homogeneity (see box on p. 375). There is no best means to assess reliability in relationship to stability, homogeneity, and equivalence. The critiquer of research should be aware that the method of reliability that the researcher uses should be consistent with the investigator's aim.

Stability

An instrument is thought to be stable or to exhibit **stability** when the same results are obtained on repeated administration of the instrument. Researchers are concerned with the stability of an instrument when they want the instrument to be able to measure the concept consistently over a period of time. Measurement over time is important when an instrument is used in a longitudinal study and therefore will be used on several occasions. Stability is also a consideration when the researcher is conducting an intervention study that is designed to effect an alteration in a specific variable. In this case the instrument is administered once and again later after the alteration or change intervention has been completed. The tests that are used to estimate stability are *test-retest* and *parallel* or *alternate form*.

MEASURES USED TO TEST RELIABILITY

STABILITY
Test-retest reliability
Parallel or alternate form

HOMOGENEITY
Item-total correlation
Split-half reliability
Kuder-Richardson coefficient
Cronbach's alpha

EQUIVALENCE
Parallel or alternate form
Interrater reliability

Test-Retest Reliability

Test-retest reliability is the administration of the same instrument to the same subjects under similar conditions on two or more occasions. Scores on the repeated testing are compared. This comparison is expressed by a correlation coefficient, usually a Pearson *r* (see Chapter 16). The interval between repeated administrations varies and depends on the phenomenon being measured. For example, if the variable that the test measures is related to the developmental stages in children, the interval between tests should be short. The amount of time over which the variable was measured should also be recorded in the report. An example of an instrument that was tested for test-retest reliability is the Work Impediment Scale (WAS) (Gulick, 1991), which was designed to rate situations that impede or enhance work capabilities of persons with multiple sclerosis (MS). Test-retest correlation coefficients for WAS subscales (mobility, hand function, cognitive, general body state, pain, environmental barrier, heavy labor) obtained at 1 and 3 weeks for 51 MS subjects were .91, .88, .83, .76, .88, .77, and .81, respectively. The magnitude of these correlations supports the idea that the WAS has the attribute of stability.

Parallel or Alternate Form

Parallel or alternate form reliability is applicable and can be tested only if two comparable forms of the same instrument exist. It is like test-retest reliability in that the same individuals are tested within a specific interval, but it differs because a different form of the same test is given to the subjects on the second testing. Parallel forms or tests contain the same types of items that are based on the same domain or concept, but the wording of the items is different. The development of parallel forms is desired if the instrument is intended to measure a variable for which a researcher believes that "test-wiseness" will be a problem. For example, there are two alternate forms of the Partner Relationship Inventory (Hoskins, 1988) that may be used in a repeated-measures design. An item on one scale ("I am able to tell my partner how I feel") is consistent with the paired item on the second form ("My partner tries to understand my feelings").

Another example of a parallel test is the Multidimensional Health Locus of Control Scale (Wallston, Wallston, & DeVellis, 1978), which was designed to measure three dimensions or sources of reinforcement for health-related behaviors. This scale has parallel forms for studies that incorporate a repeated-measures design. Examples of parallel items are "If I get sick, it is my own behavior that determines how soon I get well." This item compares with "If I get sick, I have the power to make myself well again." As can be seen, the two items, although worded differently, reflect the same idea. Practically speaking, it is difficult to develop alternate forms of an instrument when one considers the many issues of reliability and validity of an instrument. If alternate forms of a test exist, they should be highly correlated if the measures are to be considered reliable.

Homogeneity

Another attribute of an instrument related to reliability is the **internal consistency** or homogeneity with which the items within the scale reflect or measure the same concept. This means that the items within the scale correlate or are complementary to each other. This also means that a scale is unidimensional. A unidimensional scale is one that measures one concept. For example, a scale that is designed to measure anxiety should not be designed to measure depression as well. There are scales, such as the Interpersonal Relationship Inventory (Tilden et al., 1990), that do contain two or more concepts or dimensions within them. If that is the case, the researcher should identify this for the reader and should also have tested separately each concept within the scale. The internal consistency of items allows the investigator to tally the items and obtain a total score for the concept. The total score is then used in the analysis of data. Homogeneity can be assessed by using one of four methods: *item-total correlations, split-half reliability, Kuder-Richardson (KR-20) coefficient,* or *Cronbach's alpha.*

Item to Total Correlations

Item to total correlations measure the relationship between each of the items and the total scale. When item to total correlations are calculated, a correlation for each item on the scale is generated (Table 15-3). Items that do not achieve a high correlation may be deleted from the instrument. Usually in a research study, not all the item to total correlations are reported unless the study is a report of a methodological study. Typically the lowest and highest correlations are reported. An example of an item to total correlation report is "Item-total correlations . . . were computed for the 51 item HRHS. A minimum total criterion item-total correlation level of .25 was set for inclusion in the scale. Ten items failed to meet this criterion level and were dropped. Of the remaining 41, all but 5 items had item-total corre-

Table 15-3   Examples of Item to Total Correlations from Computer-Generated Data

Item	Item to total correlation
1	0.5096
2	0.4455
3	0.4479
4	0.4369
5	0.4139
6	0.4016

lations above .30. An examination of the correlation matrix showed no redundant items. Correlations ranged from ± .01 to .51" (Pollack & Duffy, 1990).

The investigators eliminate items that have too low a correlation, whereas they examine others to ensure that they are high enough to be measuring the same concept without being redundant. If item to total correlations are found to be too high, they are considered to be redundant and therefore not complementary to each other (Anastasi, 1988). This is unlike the other errors of reliability in which a higher correlation is generally a better correlation.

Split-Half Reliability

Split-half reliability involves dividing a scale into two halves and making a comparison. The halves may be odd-numbered and even-numbered items or a simple division of the first from the second half, or items may be randomly selected as to the halves that will be analyzed opposite one another. The split-half provides a measure of consistency in terms of sampling the content. The two halves of the test or the contents in both halves are assumed to be comparable, and a reliability coefficient is calculated. If the scores for the two halves are approximately equal, the test may be considered reliable. A formula called the Spearman-Brown formula is one method used to calculate the reliability coefficient. In a study investigating the appraisal of pain and coping in cancer patients, Arathuzik (1991) obtained a split-half reliability rating of .85 from a pilot test of the Pain Experience Inventory with 30 patients with metastatic breast cancer who were experiencing pain.

Kuder-Richardson (KR-20) Coefficient

The **Kuder-Richardson** (KR-20) coefficient is the estimate of homogeneity used for instruments that have a dichotomous response format. A dichotomous response format is one in which the question asks for a yes/no or a true/false response. The technique yields a correlation that is based on the consistency of responses to all the items of a single form of a test that is administered one time. Strauss and Sawin (1990) developed the Krantz Health Opinion Survey (KHOS), which is designed to measure one's preferences for information and control over one's health care. Because the response format for the KHOS and the Information and Behavior Control subscales is binary (yes/no), the KR 20 was used to deter-

	Definitely yes	Yes	Uncertain	No	Definitely no
I am uncertain about being pregnant	5	4	3	2	1
The baby seems to know when I feel tense or anxious	5	4	3	2	1

Fig. 15-2 Examples of a Likert scale. (From LoBiondo-Wood, G., O'Rourke Vito, K., & Brage, D. [1990, July]. *The prenatal maternal attachment scale: A methodological study.* Paper presented at the NAACOG's Research Conference Meeting, Denver, CO.)

mine the internal consistency of the items. Kuder-Richardson-20 reliability coefficient for KHOS subscales ranged from .68 to .78, indicating a moderate level of internal consistency reliability.

Cronbach's Alpha

The fourth and most commonly used test of internal consistency is **Cronbach's alpha.** Many tools used to measure psychosocial variables and attitudes have a Likert scale response format. A Likert scale format asks the subject to respond to a question on a scale of varying degrees of intensity between two extremes. The two extremes are anchored by responses such as "strongly agree" to "strongly disagree" or "most like me" to "least like me." The points between the two extremes may range from 1 to 5 or 1 to 7. Subjects are asked to circle the response closest to how they feel. Fig. 15-2 provides examples of items from a tool that uses a Likert scale format. Cronbach's alpha compares each item in the scale simultaneously with each other. Examples of reported Cronbach's alpha are in the box on p. 379.

Equivalence

Equivalence is either the consistency or agreement among observers using the same measurement tool or the consistency or agreement among alternate forms of a tool. An instrument is thought to demonstrate equivalence when two or more observers have a high percentage of agreement of an observed behavior or when alternate forms of a test yield a high correlation. There are two methods to test equivalence: *interrater reliability* and *alternate or parallel form.*

Interrater Reliability

Some measurement instruments are not self-administered questionnaires but are direct measurements of observed behavior. Instruments that depend on direct observation of a behavior that is to be systematically recorded need to be tested for **interrater reliability.** To accomplish interrater reliability, two or more individuals should make an observation or one observer observe the behavior on several occa-

---

EXAMPLES OF REPORTED CRONBACH'S ALPHA

Perlow, M. (1992, p. 206): "The Perlow Self Esteem Survey (PSES) had a Cronbach's alpha of .86. The alpha value is quite high, indicating that . . . the PSES has demonstrated internal consistency."

Miller, J.F., and Powers, M.J. (1988, p. 8): "Cronbach's alpha on the Miller Hope Scale using 522 respondents was .93."

Wheeler, K. (1990, p. 194): Cronbach's alpha (N = 81) was found to be .94 for the entire 33-item Perception of Empathy Inventory (PEI).

LoBiondo-Wood, G., O'Rourke Vito, K., Brage, D. (1990): "Cronbach's alpha for the 29 items relevant to all stages of pregnancy (N = 650) was .89."

---

sions. The observers should be trained or oriented to the definition of the behavior to be observed. In the method of direct observation of behavior, the consistency or reliability of the observations between observers is extremely important. In the instance of interrater reliability, the reliability or consistency of the observer is tested rather than the reliability of the instrument. Interrater reliability is expressed as a percentage of agreement between scorers or as a correlation coefficient between the scores assigned to the observed behaviors.

In the development of the Braden Scale for Predicting Pressure Sore Risk, the researchers conducted three studies to determine interrater reliability (Bergstrom, Braden, Laguzza, & Holman, 1987). The three studies used different levels of nursing personnel to rate the items of pressure sore risk. The report of the interrater reliability assessment in the first study is as follows:

> Subjects were rated by both the Registered Nurse (RN) and Graduate Student (GS) for a period of 1 to 7 weeks. Scores on admission ranged from 11 to 15; on discharge, from 11 to 22. There were a total of 86 pairs of RN and GS observations. Pearson product moment correlation between observers was r = .99, p <.001. The percent agreement, a more conservative measure of reliability than a correlation (Goodwin & Prescott, 1981), was 88%. In no case was the total score by the two raters more than 1 point different. (p. 207)

The researchers further describe the other two studies they conducted to establish interrater reliability. In the other two studies they use both percentage agreement and correlation coefficients. On the basis of these three studies and others noted by the researchers in the article, they established that the Braden Scale is a highly reliable instrument when used by registered nurses, primary nurses, and graduate nurses to measure pressure sore risk. But they note that the interrater reliability between licensed practical nurses and nursing assistants was not highly correlated. The researchers review the reasons for this and conclude that the tool should most appropriately be used by caregivers who are registered nurses.

CRITIQUING CRITERIA

1. Was an appropriate method used to test the reliability of the tool?
2. Is the reliability of the tool adequate?
3. Was an appropriate method(s) used to test the validity of the instrument?
4. Is the validity of the measurement tool adequate?
5. If the sample from the developmental stage of the tool was different from the current sample, were the reliability and validity recalculated to determine if the tool is still adequate?
6. Have the strengths and weaknesses of the reliability and validity of each instrument been presented?
7. Are strengths and weaknesses of instrument reliability and validity appropriately addressed in the discussion, limitations, or recommendations sections of the report?

Another example of interrater reliability is given in the study conducted by Stewart Fahs and Kinney (1991), who studied the differential effect of three injection sites for low-dose heparin therapy in relation to thromboplastin time and bruising. The bruises measured in this study were soft tissue injuries resulting from the trauma of subcutaneous injections of heparin. Over a 4-month period, 105 injection sites were used to calculate interrater reliability with respect to occurrence and size of bruises. Ratings were done by the principal investigator and three research assistants. The Pearson correlation coefficients ranged from $r = .94$ to $.99$, indicating a high degree of interrater reliability.

Parallel or Alternate Form

Parallel or alternate form was described under the heading Stability. Use of parallel forms is then a measure of stability and equivalence. The procedures for assessing equivalence using parallel forms are the same.

CRITIQUING RELIABILITY AND VALIDITY

Reliability and validity are two crucial aspects in the critical appraisal of a measurement instrument. Criteria for critiquing reliability and validity are presented in the box above. The reviewer evaluates an instrument's level of reliability and validity and the manner in which they were established. In a research report the reliability and validity for each measure should be presented. If these data have not been presented at all, the reviewer must seriously question the merit and use of the tool and the study's results.

In an article about the proliferation of unreliable and invalid questionnaires, Rempusheski (1990) stresses that when psychometric principles in general, but including those related to reliability and validity, are violated, the product, that is the instrument used, impacts on the profession, the organization, and the individuals within the organization. It is the ethical responsibility of the critiquer to question the reliability and validity of instruments used in research studies and to examine the findings in light of the quality of the instruments used and the data presented. The following discussion highlights key areas related to reliability and validity that should be evident to the critiquer in a research article.

Appropriate reliability tests should have been performed by the developer of the measurement tool and should then have been included by the current user in the research report. If the initial standardization sample and the current sample have different characteristics, the reader would expect (1) that a pilot study for the present sample would have been conducted to determine if the reliability was maintained or (2) that a reliability estimate was calculated on the current sample. For example, if the standardization sample for a tool that measures "satisfaction in an intimate heterosexual relationship" comprises undergraduate college students and if an investigator plans to use the tool with married couples, it would be advisable to establish the reliability of the tool with the latter group.

The investigator determines which type of reliability procedures are used in the study, depending on the nature of the measurement tool and how it will be used. For example, if the instrument is to be administered twice, the critiquer might determine that test-retest reliability should have been used to establish the stability of the tool. If an alternate form has been developed for use in a repeated-measures design, evidence of alternate form reliability should be presented to determine the equivalence of the parallel forms. If the degree of internal consistency among the items is relevant, an appropriate test of internal consistency should be presented. In some instances more than one type of reliability will be presented, but the evaluator should determine whether all are appropriate. For example, the Kuder-Richardson formula implies that there is a single right or wrong answer, making it inappropriate to use with scales that provide a format of three or more possible responses. In such cases another formula is applied, such as Cronbach's coefficient alpha formula. Another important consideration is the acceptable level of reliability, which varies according to the type of test. Coefficients of reliability of 0.70 or higher are desirable. The validity of an instrument is limited by its reliability; that is, less confidence can be placed in scores from tests with low reliability coefficients.

Satisfactory evidence of validity is probably the most difficult item for the reviewer to ascertain. It is this aspect of measurement that is most likely to fall short of meeting the required criteria. Validity studies are time-consuming, as well as complex, and sometimes researchers will settle for presenting minimal validity data. Therefore the critiquer should closely examine the item content of a tool when evaluating its strengths and weaknesses and try to find conclusive evidence of content validity. However, in the body of a research article it is most unusual to have more than a few sample items available for review. Because that is the case, the critiquer should determine whether the appropriate assessment of content validity was used to meet the researcher's goal. Such procedures provide the reviewer with assurance that the tool is psychometrically sound and that the content of the items is consistent with the conceptual framework and construct definitions. Construct and criterion-related validity are some of the more precise statistical tests of whether the tool measures what it is supposed to measure. Ideally an instrument should provide evidence of content validity, as well as criterion-related or construct validity, before a reviewer invests a high level of confidence in the tool.

The reader would also expect to see the strengths and weaknesses of instrument reliability and validity presented in the discussion, limitations, and/or recommendations section of a research article. In this context the reliability and validity might be discussed in relation to other tools devised to measure the same variable. The relationship of the findings to strengths and weaknesses in instrument reliability and validity would be another important discussion point. Finally, recommendations for improving future studies in relation to instrument reliability and validity should be proposed (Rempusheski, 1990). For example, in the discussion section of a study investigating pain and coping in cancer patients, Arathuzik (1991) appropriately reports the weaknesses in reliability and validity of the Pain Inventory and Pain Coping tools developed for this study. She indicates that the tools had been tested only for content validity and reliability and only with a small pilot sample. She further highlights weaknesses in reliability, that is, marginally acceptable internal consistency reliability coefficients for the Pain Coping Tool (.71) and low item-total correlations of some of its subscale items (>.20), signifying a question of their relatedness to the total scale. In addition, Cronbach's alpha for the Meaning-Harm subscale of the Pain Inventory was only .59, even though the alpha for the overall scale was acceptable at .84. Although Arathuzik does indicate that further research is needed to determine the validity of both instruments and strengthen their reliability, she does not discuss the effect of the just-cited weaknesses in relation to the hypotheses and the findings of the study.

As you can see, the area of reliability and validity is complex. These aspects of research reports can be evaluated to varying degrees. The research consumer should not feel inhibited by the complexity of this topic but may use the guidelines presented in this chapter to systematically assess the reliability and validity aspects of a research study. Collegial dialogue also is an approach to evaluating the merits and shortcomings of an existing, as well as a newly developed, instrument that is reported in the nursing literature. Such an exchange promotes the understanding of methodologies and techniques of reliability and validity, stimulates the acquisition of a basic knowledge of psychometrics, and encourages the exploration of alternative methods of observation, and the use of reliable and valid tools in clinical practice.

KEY POINTS

• Reliability and validity are crucial aspects of conducting and critiquing research.
  • Validity refers to whether an instrument measures what it is purported to measure, and it is a crucial aspect of evaluating a tool. Three types of validity

are content validity, criterion-related validity, and construct validity. The choice of a validation method is important and is made by the researcher on the basis of the characteristics of the measurement device in question and its utilization.

- Reliability refers to the accuracy/inaccuracy ratio in a measurement device. The major tests of reliability are the following: test-retest, parallel or alternate form, split-half, item-total correlation, Kuder-Richardson, Cronbach's alpha, and interrater reliability. Again, the selection of a method for establishing reliability will depend on the characteristics of the tool, the testing method that is used for collecting data from the standardization sample, and the kinds of data that are obtained.

REFERENCES

Abraham, I.L., Neundorfer, M.M., & Currie, L.J. (1992). Effects of group interventions on cognition and depression in nursing home residents, *Nursing Research, 41:* (4), 196-202.

Anastasi, A. (1988). *Psychological testing.* (6th ed.). New York: Macmillan.

Arathuzik, M.D. (1991). The appraisal of pain and coping in cancer patients. *Western Journal of Nursing Research. 13:* (6), 714-731.

Bergstrom, N., Braden, B.J., Laguzza, A., & Holman, V. (1987). The Braden scale for predicting pressure sore risk, *Nursing Research, 36,* 205-210.

Berk, R.A. (1990). Importance of expert judgment in content-related validity evidence. *Western Journal of Nursing, 12* (5), 659-671.

Bowen, M. (1978). On the differentiation of self. In M. Bowen (Ed.), *Family therapy in clinical practice* (pp. 467-528). New York: Jason Aronson.

Campbell, D., & Fiske, D. (1959). Convergent and discriminant validation by the matrix. *Psychological Bulletin, 53,* 273-302.

Gulick, E.E. (1991). Reliability and validity of the work assessment scale for persons with multiple sclerosis. *Nursing Research, 40,* (2), 107-112.

Haber, J.E. (1990). The Haber Level of Differentiation of Self Scale. In O. Strickland & C. Waltz (Eds.) *The measurement of educational and clinical outcomes* (Vol. 4). New York: Springer.

Hickey, M.I., Owen, S.V., & Froman, R.D. (1992). Instrument development: Cardiac diet and exercise self-efficacy. *Nursing Research, 41* (6), 347-351.

Hoskins, C.N. (1988). *The Partner Relationship Inventory.* Palo Alto, CA: Consulting Psychologists Press.

Jennings, B.M., & Rogers, S. (1989). Managing measurement error. *Nursing Research, 38,* 186-187.

LoBiondo-Wood, G., O'Rourke Vito K., & Brage, D. (1990). *The prenatal maternal attachment scale: a methodological study.* Paper presented at the NAACOG Research Conference Meeting, Denver, CO.

Miller, J.F., & Powers, M.J. (1988). Development of an instrument to measure hope. *Nursing Research, 37,* 6-10.

Nunnally, J.C. (1978). *Psychometric theory.* New York: McGraw-Hill.

Perlow, M. (1992). Validity and reliability of the PSES. *Western Journal of Nursing Research, 14* (2), 201-210.

Pollack, S.E. & Duffy, M.E. (1990). The health-related hardiness scale: Development and psychometric analysis, *Nursing Research, 39* (4), 218-222.

Rempusheski, V.F. (1990). The proliferation of unreliable and invalid questionnaires. *Applied Nursing Research, 3* (4), 174-176.

Stewart Fahs, P.S., & Kinney, M.R. (1991). The abdomen, thigh, and arm as sites for subcutaneous sodium heparin injections. *Nursing Research, 40* (4), 204-207.

Strauss, S.S., & Sawin, K.J. (1990). The Krantz health opinion survey: A measurement model. In O. Strickland & C. Waltz (Eds.), *The measurement of educational and clinical outcomes* (Vol. 4, pp. 229-249). New York: Springer.

Tilden, V.P., Nelson, C.A., & May, B.A. (1990). The IPR inventory: Development and psychometric characteristics. *Nursing Research, 39* (6), 337-343.

Wallston, K.S., Wallston, B.S., & DeVellis, B.S. (1978). Development of the multidimensional health locus of control (MHLC) scales. *Health Education Monographs, 6,* 160-170.

Waltz, C., Strickland, O., & Lenz, E. (1991). *Measurement in nursing research* (3rd ed.). Philadelphia: F.A. Davis.

Wheeler, K. (1990). Perception of empathy inventory. In O. Strickland & C. Waltz (Eds.), *The measurement of educational and clinical outcomes* (Vol. 4, pp. 181-198). New York: Springer.

ADDITIONAL READINGS

Berk, R.A. (1990). Importance of expert judgement in content-related validity evidence. *Western Journal of Nursing Research, 12* (5), 659-671.

Grubba, C.J., Popovich, B., & Jirovec, M.M. (1990). Reliability and validity of the Popovich scale in home health care assessments. *Applied Nursing Research, 3* (4), 161-163.

Laschinger, H.K.S. (1992). Intraclass correlations as estimates of interrater reliability in nursing research. *Western Journal of Nursing Research, 14* (2), 246-251.

Reineck, C. (1991). Nursing research instruments: Pathway to resources. *Applied Nursing*

Thomas, S.D., Hathaway, D.K., & Arheart, K.L. (1992). Face validity. *Western Journal of Nursing Research, 14* (1), 109-112.

Weinert, C., & Tilden, V.P. (1990). Measures of social support: Assessment of validity. *Nursing Research, 39* (4), 212-216.

CHAPTER
16

Descriptive Data Analysis

ANN BELLO

LEARNING OBJECTIVES

After reading this chapter the student should be able to do the following:

♦ Define descriptive statistics.
♦ State the purposes of descriptive statistics.
♦ Identify the levels of measurement in a research study.
♦ Describe a frequency distribution.
♦ List measures of central tendency and their use.
♦ List measures of variability and their use.
♦ Critically analyze the descriptive statistics used in published research studies.

KEY TERMS

descriptive statistics	modality
frequency distribution	mode
interval measurement	nominal measurement
kurtosis	normal curve
levels of measurement	ordinal measurement
mean	percentile
measurement	range
measures of central tendency	ratio measurement
measures of variability	semiquartile range
median	standard deviation
modal percentage	Z score

After carefully collecting data, the researcher is faced with the task of organizing the individual pieces of information so that the meaning is clear. It would be neither practical nor helpful to the reader to list individually each piece of data collected. The researcher must choose methods of organizing the raw data based both on the kind of data collected and on the hypothesis that was tested.

Statistical procedures are used to give organization and meaning to data. Procedures that allow researchers to describe and summarize data are known as **descriptive statistics**. Procedures that allow researchers to estimate how reliably they can make predictions and generalize findings based on the data are known as *inferential statistics* (see Chapter 17). Descriptive statistical techniques reduce data to manageable proportions by summarizing them, and they also describe various characteristics of the data under study. Descriptive techniques include measures of central tendency, such as mode, median, and mean; measures of variability, such as modal percentage, range, and standard deviation; and some correlation techniques, such as scatter plots. The research consumer does not need a detailed knowledge of how to calculate these statistics but does need an understanding of their meaning, use, and limitations.

Measures of central tendency describe the average member of the sample, whereas **measures of variability** describe how much dispersion is in the sample. If a researcher reported that the average age of one nursing class was 22 years, with the youngest member 18 and the oldest 25, and that in another nursing class students had an average age of 22 years, but the youngest member was 17 and the oldest 45, the reader would form a very different picture of the two classes. In both cases the average member of the sample was the same, but in the second class there was much greater variation or dispersion in the age of the members of the class.

Descriptive statistics may be presented in several ways in a research report. The data may be reported in words in the text of the report or summarized in tables or graphs. Whatever the method of presentation, the report should give the reader a clear and orderly picture of the research results.

This chapter and the next are designed to provide the reader of nursing research with an understanding of statistical procedures. This chapter focuses on the understanding and evaluation of descriptive statistical procedures, and the next chapter discusses inferential statistical procedures. To evaluate the appropriateness of the statistical procedures used in a study, the research consumer should have an understanding of the **levels of measurement** that are appropriate to each statistical technique.

LEVELS OF MEASUREMENT

Measurement is the assignment of numbers to objects or events according to rules (Kerlinger, 1986). Every event that is assigned a specific number must be similar to every other event assigned that number; for example, male subjects may be assigned the number 1 and female subjects the number 2. The measurement level is determined by the nature of the object or event being measured. Levels of measurement in ascending order are nominal, ordinal, interval, and ratio. The levels of measurement are the determining factors of the type of statistics to be used in analyzing data.

The higher the level of measurement, the greater the flexibility the researcher has in choosing statistical procedures. Every attempt should be made to the use the highest level of measurement possible so that the maximum amount of information will be obtained from the data (see Table 16-1).

Nominal Measurement

Nominal measurement is used to classify objects or events into categories. The categories are mutually exclusive; the object or event either has the characteristic or does not have it. The numbers assigned to each category are nothing more than labels; such numbers do not indicate more or less of a characteristic. Examples of nominal level measurement can be used to categorize a sample on such information as gender, hair color, marital state, or religious affiliation. In Stewart Fahs and Kinney's (1991) study of injection sites for subcutaneous sodium heparin, there are several examples of nominal level measurement, including the presence or absence of bruises at each site, gender of subject, and subject's medical diagnosis (see Appendix A). The nominal level of measurement allows the least amount of mathematical manipulation. Most commonly the *frequency* of each event is counted, as well as the *percent of the total* each category represents. In Table 16-1 of their study, Stewart Fahs and Kinney summarize the bruise count by injection site for each injection (see Appendix A).

Table 16-1   Summary Table

Measurement	Description	Measures of central tendency	Measures of variability
Nominal	Classification	Mode	Modal percentage, range, frequency distribution
Ordinal	Relative rankings	Mode, median	Range, percentile, semiquartile range, frequency distribution
Interval	Rank ordering with equal intervals	Mode, median, mean	Range, percentile, semiquartile range, standard deviation
Ratio	Rank ordering with equal intervals and absolute zero	Mode, median, mean	All

Ordinal Measurement

Ordinal measurement is used to show relative rankings of objects or events. The numbers assigned to each category can be compared, and a member of a higher category can be said to have more of an attribute that one in a lower category. The intervals between numbers on the scale are not necessarily equal nor is zero an absolute zero. For example, ordinal measurement is used to formulate class rankings where one student can be ranked higher or lower than another. However, the difference in actual grade point average between students may differ widely. Grey, Cameron, and Thurber's (1991; Appendix B) study of coping and adaptation in children with diabetes measured sexual maturation with an ordinal level scale, the Tanner scale. The Tanner scale assesses the development of secondary sex characteristics on a 5-point scale. A low number reflects less development of the secondary sex characteristics, but it is not possible to say a score of 5 represents 5 times more sexual development than a score of 1.

Ordinal level data are limited in the amount of mathematical manipulation possible. In addition to what is possible with nominal data, *medians, percentiles*, and *rank order coefficients of correlation* can be calculated.

Interval Measurement

Interval measurement shows rankings of events or objects on a scale with equal intervals between the numbers. The zero point remains arbitrary. For example, interval measurements are used in measuring temperatures on the Fahrenheit scale. The distances between degrees are equal, but the zero point is arbitrary. Stewart Fahs and Kinney (1991) used the activated partial thromboplastin time (aPTT), a coagulation test, to measure the effectiveness of the low-dose heparin. The results are reported in seconds, but the zero point is related to the control used and is not absolute.

In many areas in the social sciences, including nursing, there is much controversy over the classification of the level of measurement of intelligence, aptitude, and personality tests, with some regarding these measurements as ordinal and others as interval. The research consumer needs to be aware of this controversy and to look at each study individually in terms of how the data are analyzed (Kerlinger, 1986). Interval level data allow more manipulation of data, including the addition and subtraction of numbers and the *calculation of means*. This additional manipulation is why many want to argue for the higher classification level. The Child and Adolescent Adjustment Profile and the Self-Perception Profile for Children are used as interval measures by Grey et al. (1991) in their study of coping and adaptation in diabetic children.

Ratio Measurement

Ratio measurement shows rankings of events or objects on scales with equal intervals and absolute zeros. The number represents the actual amount of the property the object possesses. This is the highest level of measurement, but it is usually achieved only in the physical sciences. Examples of ratio level data are height, weight, pulse, and blood pressure. Stewart Fahs and Kinney's (1991) study (see Appendix A) used ratio measurement in reporting the diameter of the bruises on the skin after injection of heparin.

All mathematical procedures can be performed on data from ratio scales. Therefore the use of any statistical procedure is possible as long as it is appropriate to the design of the study (see Chapter 17).

FREQUENCY DISTRIBUTION

One of the most basic ways of organizing data is in a **frequency distribution.** In a *frequency distribution* the number of times each event occurs is counted or the data are grouped and the frequency of each group is reported. An instructor reporting the results of an examination could report the number of students receiving each grade or could group the grades and report the number in each group. Table 16-2 shows the results of an examination given to a class of 51 students. The results of the examination are reported in several ways. The columns on the left give the raw data *tally* and the *frequency* for each grade, whereas the columns on the right give the grouped-data tally and grouped frequencies. Grey et al. (1991), in their study of children with diabetes, rather than reporting the results for each child, place the children in Tanner groups and report the results for each group (see Appendix B).

When data are grouped, it is necessary to define the size of the group or the *interval width* so that no score will fall into two groups. The grouping of the data in Table 16-2 prevents overlap; each score falls into only one group. If the grouping had been 70 to 80 and 80 to 90, scores of 80 would have fallen into two categories.

Table 16-2   Frequency Distribution

Individual			Group		
Score	Tally	Frequency	Score	Tally	Frequency
90	|	1	>89	|	1
88	|	1			
86	|	1	80-89	Ⱶ Ⱶ Ⱶ	15
84	Ⱶ |	6			
82	||	2	70-79	Ⱶ Ⱶ Ⱶ	23
80	Ⱶ	5		Ⱶ |||	
78	Ⱶ	5			
76	|	1	60-69	Ⱶ Ⱶ	10
74	Ⱶ ||	7			
72	Ⱶ ||||	9	<59	||	2
70	|	1			
68	|||	3			
66	||	2			
64	||||	4			
62	|	1			
60		0			
58	|	1			
56		0			
54	|	1			
52		0			
50		0			
TOTAL		51			51

Mean, 73.1; standard deviation, +12.1; median, 74; mode, 72; range, 36 (54-90).

The grouping should allow for a precise presentation of the data without serious loss of information. Very large interval widths lead to loss of data information and may obscure patterns in the data. If the test scores in Table 16-2 had been grouped as 40 to 69 and 70 to 99, the pattern of the scores would have been obscured.

Information about frequency distributions may be presented in the form of a table, such as Table 16-2, or in graphic form. Fig. 16-1 illustrates the most common graphic forms: the histogram and the frequency polygon. The two graphic methods are similar in that both plot scores or percentages of occurrence against frequency. The greater the number of points plotted, the smoother the resulting graph. The shape of the resulting graph allows for observations that will further describe the data.

MEASURES OF CENTRAL TENDENCY

Measures of central tendency answer questions such as "What does the average nurse think?" and "What is the average temperature of patients on a unit?" They yield a single number that describes the middle of the group. They summarize the

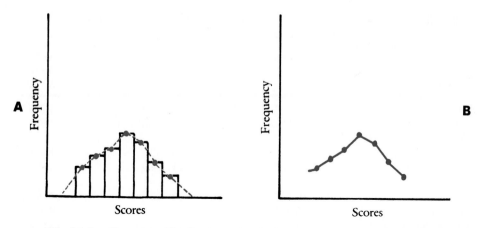

Fig. 16-1 Frequency distributions. **A,** Histogram and **B,** frequency polygon.

members of a sample. Therefore they are known as *summary statistics* and are sample-specific. Because they are sample-specific, they change with each sample. Grey et al. (1991; Appendix B), in their study of coping and adaptation in children with diabetes, list the means and standard deviations for each of the variables by Tanner groupings (Table 16-3). These scores represent the average of each variable and the amount of variation in each group on each variable. For example, Tanner group 1 had an average state anxiety score of 28.8 with a variation of ±4.2. This means that 68% of the Tanner group 1 scored between 24.6 and 33 on the measure of state anxiety.

Summary statistics also may be reported in narrative form as illustrated by the following excerpt from Conn's (1991) study of self-care actions taken by older adults for flu and colds:

> Interviews were conducted with 118 women and 42 men. Fifty-five percent of the subjects lived in a family setting and 45% lived alone. Subjects' ages ranged from 65 to 94 years *(M = 77.2, SD = 7.7).* The average household income was $16,950 per year (range $2,887 to $80,000). Two subjects were Asian and the remainder were white. Subjects reported none to 6 chronic illnesses (M = 1.6, SD = 1.4) and none to 11 prescription medications (M = 3.2, SD = 1.6). Eighteen subjects (11%) rated their health as excellent, 81 (51%) as good, 49 (31%) as fair, and 12 (7%) as poor. Forty-nine subjects (31%) reported their health state interfered a great deal with activities, 61 (38%) reported a little interference by health state, and 50 (31%) reported their health state did not interfere with activities.

The characteristics of a sample in a study are described in terms of summary statistics. The mean test score reported in Table 16-2 is an example of such a statistic. If a different group of students was given the same test, it is likely that the mean would be different.

The term *average* is a nonspecific, general term. In statistics there are three measures of central tendency: the *mode*, the *median*, and the *mean*. Depending on

Table 16-3   Illustration of Data Reporting: Differences in Adaptation and Coping by Stages of Sexual Maturation

Variable	Tanner 1 M(SD) (N = 34)	Tanner 2-4 M(SD) (N = 39)	Tanner 5 M(SD) (N = 25)
State anxiety	28.8 (4.2)	30.8(4.4)	33.7(5.7)
Depression	6.1(5.8)	6.2(5.6)	9.7(7.7)
CAAP			
Peer relations	14.4(2.1)	13.4(2.7)	11.9(3.4)
Dependency	9.4(2.2)	11.5(2.1)	10.8(2.5)
SPPC			
School	19.6(4.4)	17.7(3.4)	15.9(4.2)
Behavior	20.5(2.6)	18.6(3.5)	18.3(3.1)
Hemoglobin A_1	9.8(2.9)	11.2(3.8)	13.9(4.4)
A-COPE			
Avoid problems	17.6(1.9)	18.0(2.6)	19.0(2.4)
Vent feeling	16.5(2.7)	13.4(3.4)	13.9(3.1)
Relaxation	8.8(2.5)	9.8(2.4)	10.8(2.4)
CHIP			
Fam. integration	40.7(7.3)	41.3(7.6)	35.5(7.9)
SCQ	40.0(6.5)	41.9(6.3)	43.1(5.9)
LEC	8.1(6.4)	8.5(4.4)	7.7(3.9)

From *"Coping and Adaptation in Children with Diabetes"* by M. Grey, M.E. Cameron, and F.W. Thurber, 1991, *Nursing Research, 40,* p. 3.
M, Mean; *SD,* standard deviation; *N,* number.

the distribution, these measures may not all give the same answer to the question, "What is the average?" Each measure of central tendency has a specific use and is most appropriate to specific kinds of measurement and types of distributions.

Mode

The **mode** is the most frequent score or result, and it can be obtained by inspection of the frequency distribution table or graph. A distribution can have more than one mode. The number of modes contained in a distribution is called the **modality** of the distribution. Figs. 16-2, *A* and *E,* and 16-3 show unimodal or one-peak distributions. Fig. 16-2, *B,* shows a bimodal or two-peaked distribution. Multimodal distributions having two or more peaks are shown in Fig. 16-2, *B* and *D.* Table 16-4 (on p. 395) illustrates how the change in a few scores can change the modality of a distribution from unimodal to bimodal.

The mode is most appropriately used with nominal data but can be used with all levels of measurement (see Table 16-1). It cannot be used for any subsequent calculations, and it is unstable; that is, the mode can fluctuate widely from sample to sample from the same population. A change in just one score in Table 16-2 would change the mode from 72.

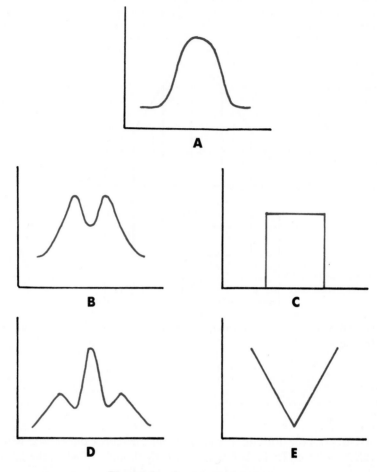

Fig. 16-2   Symmetrical shapes.

Median

The **median** is the middle score or the score where 50% of the scores are above it and 50% of the scores are below it. The median is not sensitive to extremes in high and low scores. In the series of scores in Table 16-2 the twenty-sixth score will always be the median regardless of how high the highest or low the lowest score. It is best used when the data are skewed (see The Normal Distribution in this chapter) and the researcher is interested in the "typical" score. For example, if age is a variable and there is a wide range with extreme scores that may affect the mean, it would be appropriate to also report the median. The median is easy to find by either inspection or calculation and can be used with ordinal or higher data (see Table 16-1).

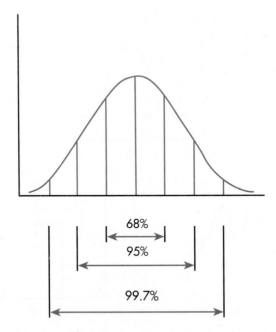

Fig. 16-3 The normal distribution (mesokurtosis) and associated standard deviations.

Mean

The **mean** is the arithmetic average of all the scores and is used with interval or ratio data (see Table 16-1). It is what is usually thought of when the term *average* is used in general conversation and is the most widely used measure of central tendency. Most tests of significance use the mean (see Chapter 17). The mean is affected by every score but is more stable than the median or mode, and of the three measures of central tendency, it is the most constant or least affected by chance. The larger the sample size, the less affected the mean will be by a single extreme score. The mean is generally considered the single best point for summarizing data. In Table 16-4 the mean is the least affected by the change in the distribution from unimodal to bimodal.

When one compares the measures of central tendency, the mean is the most stable and the median the most typical of these statistics. If the distribution is symmetrical and unimodal, the mean, median, and mode will coincide. If the distribution is skewed, the mean will be pulled in the direction of the long tail of the distribution. With a skewed distribution, all three statistics should be reported. For example, national income in the United States is skewed. The mean wage differs from the median wage, because the large salaries are so much greater than the low salaries.

Table 16-4   Measures of Central Tendency

Score	Frequency	Measure
35	卌	
36	卌 |||	Mode
37	||||	Median, mean
38	卌	
39	卌	
40	卌		
35	卌	
36	卌 |||	Mode
37	|||	Mean
38	||||	Median
39	卌 |||	Mode
40	卌	

THE NORMAL DISTRIBUTION

The concept of the normal distribution is a theoretical one, based on the observation that data from repeated measures of interval or ratio level group themselves about a midpoint in a distribution in a manner that closely approximates the **normal curve** illustrated in Fig. 16-3. In addition, if the means of a large number of samples of the same interval or ratio data are calculated and plotted on a graph, that curve also approximates the normal curve. This tendency of the means to approximate the normal curve is termed the *sampling distribution of the means.* The mean of the sampling distribution of the means is the mean of the population (see Chapter 17).

The normal curve is one that is symmetrical about the mean and is unimodal. The mean, median, and mode are equal. An additional characteristic of the normal curve is that a fixed percentage of the scores falls within a given distance of the mean. As shown in Fig. 16-3, about 68% of the scores or means will fall within ±1 standard deviation (SD) of the mean; 95% within ±2 SD of the mean; and 99.7% within ±3 SD of the mean.

Skewness

Not all samples of data approximate the normal curve. Some samples are *nonsymmetrical* and have the peak off center. If one tail is longer than the other, the distribution is described in terms of *skew.* In a positive skew the bulk of the data are at the low end of the range and there is a longer tail pointing to the right or the positive end of the graph. Worldwide individual income has a positive skew, with most individuals in the low-to-moderate range and very few in the upper range. The mean in a positive skew is to the right of the median. In a negative skew the bulk of

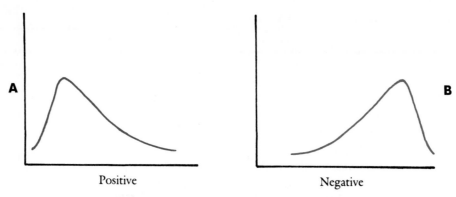

Fig. 16-4   **A,** Positive and **B,** negative skews.

the data are in the high range and there is a longer tail pointing to the left or the negative end of the graph. Age at death in the United States has a negative skew, since most deaths occur at older ages. In a negative skew the mean is to the left of the median. Fig. 16-4 illustrates positive and negative skew. In each diagram the peak is off center and one tail is longer.

Symmetry

When the two halves of a distribution are folded over and they can be superimposed on each other, the distribution is said to be *symmetrical*. In other words, the two halves of the distribution are mirror images of each other. The overall shape of the distribution does not affect symmetry. Although the shapes in Fig. 16-2 are different, they are all symmetrical; however, only Fig. 16-2, *A,* approximates the normal curve.

Symmetry and modality are independent. Look at Figs. 16-2, *A,* and 16-3. These are all unimodal, but Fig. 16-4 is skewed, whereas Fig. 16-2, *A,* is symmetrical.

Kurtosis

Kurtosis is related to the peakness or flatness of a distribution. The peakness or flatness of a distribution is related to the spread of the data. The farther the data are spread out on a scale, the flatter the peak. The distribution that peaks sharply is called *leptokurtic,* whereas a broad, flat distribution is *platykurtic.* Fig. 16-5 illustrates kurtosis. Neither the leptokurtic nor the platykurtic distributions approximate the normal curve or mesokurtic distribution.

INTERPRETING MEASURES OF VARIABILITY

Variability or dispersion is concerned with the spread of data. Samples with the same mean could differ in both distribution (kurtosis) and skew. Variability mea-

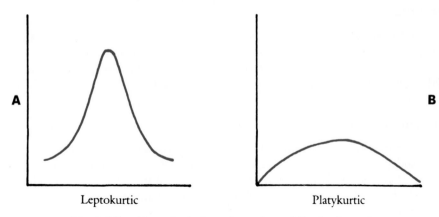

Leptokurtic   Platykurtic

Fig. 16-5   Kurtosis. **A,** Leptokurtosis, and **B,** platykurtosis.

sures answer the questions "Is the sample homogeneous or heterogeneous?" and "Is the sample similar or different?" If a researcher measures oral temperatures in two samples, one sample drawn from a healthy population and one sample from a hospitalized population, it is possible that the two samples will have the same mean. However, it is likely that there will be a wider range of temperatures in the hospitalized sample than in the healthy sample. Measures of variability are used to describe these differences in the dispersion of data.

As with measures of central tendency, the various measures of variability are appropriate to specific kinds of measurement and types of distributions.

Modal percentage is used with nominal data and is the percentage of cases in the mode. A high modal percentage is indicative of decreased variability.

Range

The **range** is the simplest but most unstable measure of variability. Range is the difference between the highest and lowest scores. A change in either of these two scores would change the range. The range should always be reported with other measures of variability. The range in Table 16-2 is 36, but this could easily change with an increase or decrease in the high score of 90 or the low score of 54.

Semiquartile Range

The **semiquartile range** (semiinterquartile range) indicates the range of the middle 50% of the scores. It is more stable than the range, since it is less likely to be changed by a single extreme score. It lies between the upper and lower quartiles, the upper quartile being the point below which 75% of the scores fall and the lower quartile being the point below which 25% of the scores fall. The middle 50% of the scores in Table 16-2 lies between 68 and 78, and the semiquartile range is 10.

Percentile

A **percentile** represents the percentage of cases a given score exceeds. The median is the 50% percentile, and in Table 16-2 it is a score of 74. A score in the 90th percentile is exceeded by only 10% of the scores. The zero percentile and the 100th percentile are usually dropped (McNemar, 1969).

Standard Deviation

The **standard deviation** (SD) is the most frequently used measure of variability, and it is based on the concept of the normal curve (see Fig. 16-3). It is a measure of average deviation of the scores from the mean and as such should always be reported with the mean. It takes all scores into account and can be used to interpret individual scores.

Because the mean (X) and standard deviation (SD) for the examination in Table 16-2 was 73.1 ± 12.1, a student should know that 68% of the grades were between 85.1 and 61. If the student received a grade of 88, he would know he did better than most of the class, whereas a grade of 58 would indicate he did not do as well as most of the class. Table 16-3, from the study by Grey et al. (1991), reports the mean and standard deviation of each of the study variables by Tanner group. As illustrated in this table, the mean depression score for the Tanner 5 group was 9.7 and the standard deviation was 7.7. This means that 68% of the Tanner 5 group depression scores would be expected to fall between 2.0 and 17.4. This table allows the reader to inspect the data and get a feel for the variation the data contain.

The standard deviation is used in the calculation of many inferential statistics (see Chapter 17). One limitation of the standard deviation is that it is expressed in terms of the units used in the measurement and cannot be used to compare means that have different units. If researchers were interested in the relationship between height measured in inches and weight measured in pounds, it would be necessary for them to convert the height and weight measurements to standard units or Z scores.

Z Scores

The **Z score** is used to compare measurements in standard units. Each of the scores is converted to a Z score, and then the Z scores are used to examine the relative distance of the scores from the mean. A Z score of +1.5 means that the observation is 1.5 SD above the mean, whereas a score of −2 means that the observation is 2 SD below the mean. By using Z scores, a researcher can compare results from scales that use different units, such as height and weight.

Many measures of variability exist. The modal frequency is the easiest to calculate, but the standard deviation is the most useful. The standard deviation and the semiquartile range always exist and are unique for each sample. The standard deviation is the most stable statistic. Transformation of scores to Z scores allows comparison between scores that have different measurement units.

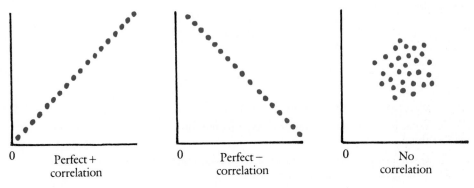

| 0 | Perfect + | 0 | Perfect − | 0 | No |
| | correlation | | correlation | | correlation |

Fig. 16-6   Scatter plots.

CORRELATION

Correlations are used to answer the question "To what extent are the variables related?" Correlations are used most commonly with ordinal or higher level data. Most correlations are discussed in Chapter 17, but here we will briefly mention scatter plots, which are visual representations of the strength and magnitude of the relationship between two variables. The strength of the correlation is demonstrated by how closely the data points approximate a straight line. In a positive correlation, the higher the score on one variable, the higher the score on the other. Temperature and pulse are positively correlated; that is, a rise in temperature generally is associated with a rise in the pulse rate. In a negative correlation, the higher the score on one measure, the lower the score on the other measure. A decrease in blood volume is generally associated with a rise in the pulse rate. Fig. 16-6 illustrates a perfect positive correlation, a perfect negative correlation, and no correlation. In most research, correlation results lie between these extremes.

CRITIQUING DESCRIPTIVE STATISTICS

Many students who have not had a course in statistics feel that they cannot critique descriptive statistics. However, the student should be able to critically analyze the use of statistics even if the student does not understand the derivation of the numbers presented. What is most important in critiquing this aspect of a research study is that the procedures for summarizing the data make sense in light of the purpose of the study. The criteria for critiquing descriptive statistics are presented in the box on p. 400.

Before the reader can decide whether the statistics employed make sense, it is important to return to the beginning of the paper and determine the purpose of the study. Although all studies use descriptive statistics to summarize the data obtained, many studies go on to use identical statistics to test specific hypotheses (see Chapter 17). If a study is an exploratory one, it is possible that only descriptive statistics will be presented, since their purpose is to describe the characteristics of a population.

CRITIQUING CRITERIA

1. Were appropriate descriptive statistics used?
2. What level of measurement is used to measure each of the major variables?
3. Is the sample size large enough to prevent one extreme score from affecting the summary statistics used?
4. What descriptive statistics are reported?
5. Were these descriptive statistics appropriate to the level of measurement for each variable?
6. Are there summary statistics for each major variable?
7. Is there enough information present to judge the results?
8. Are the results clearly and completely stated?
9. If tables and graphs are used, do they agree with the text and extend it or do they merely repeat it?

Just as the hypotheses should flow from the problem and purpose of a study, so should the hypotheses suggest the type of analysis that will follow. The hypotheses should indicate the major variables that the reader can expect to have presented in summary form. Each of the variables in the hypotheses should be followed in the results section with appropriate descriptive information.

After studying the hypotheses, the reader should proceed to the methods section. Using the operational definition provided, the reader identifies the level of measurement employed to measure each of the variables that were listed in the hypotheses. From this information the reader should be able to determine the measures of central tendency and variability that should be employed to summarize the data. For example, you would not expect to see a mean used as a summary statistic for the normal variable of gender. In all likelihood, gender would be reported as a frequency distribution. The reader should expect that the means and standard deviations will be provided for measurements performed at the interval level. The sample size is another aspect of the methods section that is important when evaluating the researcher's use of descriptive statistics. The larger the sample, the less chance that one outlying score will affect the summary statistics.

Only after these aspects of the study have been examined should the reader begin to consider the results presented by the researcher. Each important variable should have an appropriate measure of central tendency and variability presented. If tables or graphs are used, they should agree with the information presented in the text. The tables and the charts should be clearly and completely labeled. If the researcher presents grouped frequency data, the groups should be logical and mutually exclusive. The size of the interval in grouped data should not obscure the pattern of the data nor should it create an artificial pattern. Each table and chart should be referred to in the text, but each should add to the text—not merely repeat it. Each table or graph should have an obvious connection to the study being reported. For example, one table may describe the sample and another may present data relevant to the hypotheses being studied. Table 16-4 illustrates a clearly presented table; each group is mutually exclusive, and the data in the table agree with the data in the text.

The results should be written so that they are understandable to the intended audience. The audience for nursing research is the average practicing nurse. Thus the descriptive information presented should be clear enough that the reader can determine the usefulness of the study in the individual practice situation.

Descriptive statistics cannot be critiqued apart from the study as a whole. Each part of the research paper must make sense in relation to the entire paper. Therefore the reader should evaluate each portion of the paper in relation to what has preceded it. As such, the evaluation of the descriptive statistics must precede the evaluation of the inferential statistics.

The following is a partial critique of Stewart Fahs and Kinney's (1991) study of the abdomen, thigh, and arm as sites for subcutaneous sodium heparin injections; only one option is chosen at each step:

Purpose of study:	To determine the occurrence of bruising at selected injection sites
Hypothesis:	Null hypothesis (no difference in occurrence of bruising at selected sites)
Dependent variable:	Occurrence of bruising
Conceptual definition:	A bruise is a discolored, purpuric lesion
Operational definition:	Bruise or no bruise
Level of measurement:	Nominal (bruise or no bruise)

	Expected	*Reported*
Summary statistics:	Number of bruises at each site	In Table 1—bruise count by site
Measure of variability:	Percentage of injections resulting in bruise	In text—percentage of sites bruised

Sample size:	105 individuals with repeated injections
Conclusion:	Reported statistics are appropriate for the problem, hypothesis, and level of measurement; sample size is large enough to prevent one score from having a large effect on the mean

KEY POINTS

- Descriptive statistics are a means of describing and organizing data gathered in research.
- The four levels of measurement are nominal, ordinal, interval, and ratio. Each has appropriate descriptive techniques associated with it.
- Measures of central tendency describe the average member of a sample. The mode

is the most frequent score, the median is the middle score, and the mean is the arithmetic average of the scores. The mean in the most stable and useful of the measures of central tendency, and with the standard deviation it forms the basis for many of the inferential statistics described in Chapter 17.

- The frequency distribution presents data in tabular or graphic form and allows for the calculation or observations of characteristics of the distribution of the data, including skewness, symmetry, modality, and kurtosis.
  - In nonsymmetrical distributions the degree and direction of the pull of the peak off center are described in terms of skew.
  - In speaking of modality the number of peaks is described as unimodal, bimodal, or multimodal.
  - The relative spread of the data is described by kurtosis.
  - Each characteristic of the frequency distribution is independent.
- Measures of variability reflect the spread of the data.
  - The modal percentage is the percent of the cases in the mode.
  - The ranges reflect differences between high and low scores.
  - The standard deviation is the most stable and useful measure of variability. It is derived from the concept of the normal curve. In the normal curve, sample scores and the means of large numbers of samples group themselves around the midpoint in the distribution, with a fixed percentage of the scores falling within given distances of the mean. This tendency of means to approximate the normal curve is called the sampling distributions of the means. A Z score is the standard deviation converted to standard units.
- The scatter plot shows a measure of correlation.
- When critiquing published research reports, special emphasis should be given to the relationship of levels of measurement and appropriate descriptive techniques.

REFERENCES

Conn, V. (1991). Self-care actions taken by older adults for influenza and colds. *Nursing Research, 40*(3), 176-181.

Grey, M., Cameron, M.E., & Thurber, F.W. (1991). Coping and adaptation in children with diabetes. *Nursing Research, 40*(4), 144-149.

Kerlinger, F.N. (1986). *Foundations of behavioral research.* (2nd ed). New York: Holt, Reinhart & Winston.

Stewart Fahs, P.S., & Kinney, M. R. (1991). The abdomen, thigh, and arm as sites for subcutaneous sodium heparin injections. *Nursing Research, 40*(4), 204-207.

ADDITIONAL READINGS

Bluman, A.G. (1992). *Elementary statistics,* Dubuque, IA: Wm. C. Brown.

Knapp, T.R. (1993). Treating ordinal scales as ordinal scales. *Nursing Research, 42*(3), 184-186.

Moore, D.S. (1991). *Statistics: Concepts and controversies.* New York: W.H. Freeman.

Triola, M.F. (1989). *Elementary Statistics* (4th ed.). Redwood City, CA: Benjamin Cummings.

Waltz, C.F., & Bausell, R.B. (1981). *Nursing research: Design, statistics and computer analysis.* Philadelphia: F.A. Davis.

Waltz, C.F., Strickland, O.L., & Lenz, E.R. (1991). *Measurement in nursing research* (2nd ed.). Philadelphia: F.A. Davis.

Weimer R.C. (1987). *Applied Elementary Statistics.* Monterey, CA: Brooks/Cole.

CHAPTER 17

Inferential Data Analysis

MARGARET GREY

LEARNING OBJECTIVES

After reading this chapter the student should be able to do the following:

* Identify the purpose of inferential statistics.
* Distinguish between a parameter and a statistic.
* Explain the concept of probability as it applies to the analysis of sample data.
* Distinguish between type I and type II error and its effect on a study's outcome.
* Distinguish between parametric and nonparametric tests.
* List the commonly used statistical tests and their purposes.
* Critically analyze the statistics used in published research studies.

KEY TERMS

analysis of covariance (ANCOVA)	null hypothesis
	parameter
analysis of variance (ANOVA)	parametric statistics
chi-square (χ^2)	path analysis
correlation	Pearson correlation
degrees of freedom	coefficient, or Pearson r
Fisher's exact probability test	probability
inferential statistic	sampling error
level of significance (alpha level)	scientific hypothesis
	standard error of the mean
multiple analysis of variance (MANOVA)	t statistic
	type I error
multiple regression	type II error
nonparametric statistic	

Inferential statistics are used to analyze the data collected in a research study. The reader of research studies needs to understand the purpose and application of statistics. Although it may be useful also to understand how statistical procedures are conducted, such knowledge is not critical to understanding published research findings. The purpose of this chapter is to demonstrate how researchers use inferential statistics to make conclusions about larger groups (the population of interest) from sample data. Basic concepts and terminology are presented in the sections that follow so that the reader can begin to make sense of the statistics used in research papers. Those readers who desire a more advanced discussion should refer to the Additional Readings section at the end of this chapter.

DESCRIPTIVE AND INFERENTIAL STATISTICS

In the previous chapter we discuss *descriptive statistics,* the statistics that are used when the researcher needs to summarize the data. In this chapter we turn our attention to the use of inferential statistics. *Inferential statistics* combine mathematical processes and logic that allows researchers to test hypotheses about a population using data obtained from probability samples. Statistical inference is generally used for two purposes: to estimate the probability that statistics found in the sample accurately reflect the population parameter and to test hypotheses about a population.

In the first purpose a *parameter* is a characteristic of a population, whereas a *statistic* is a characteristic of a sample. We use statistics to estimate population parameters. Suppose we randomly sample 100 people with chronic lung disease and use an interval scale to study their knowledge of the disease. If the mean score for these subjects is 65, the mean represents the *sample statistic*. If we were able to study every subject with chronic lung disease, we also could calculate an average knowledge score and that score would be the *parameter for the population*. As you know, a researcher rarely is able to study an entire population, so inferential statistics allow the researcher to make statements about the larger population from studying the sample.

The example given alludes to two important qualifications of how a study must be conducted so that inferential statistics may be used. First, it was stated that the sample was randomly selected (see Chapter 15). Because you already are familiar with the advantages of probability sampling, it should be clear that if we wish to make statements about a population from a sample, that sample must be representative. All procedures for inferential statistics are based on the assumption that the sample was drawn with a known probability. Second, it was stated that the scale had to reach the interval level of measurement. This is because the mathematical operations involved in doing inferential statistics require this level of measurement.

HYPOTHESIS TESTING

The second and most commonly used purpose of inferential statistics is hypothesis testing. Statistical hypothesis testing allows researchers to make objective decisions about the outcome of their study. The use of statistical hypothesis testing allows researchers to answer such questions as "How much of this effect is a result of chance?" or "How strongly are these two variables associated with each other?"

The procedures used when making inferences are based on principles of negative inference. In other words, if a researcher studied the effect of a new educational program for patients with chronic lung disease, the researcher would actually have two hypotheses—the **scientific hypothesis** and the **null hypothesis** (see Chapter 7). The research or *scientific* hypothesis is that which the researcher believes will be the outcome of the study. In our example the scientific hypothesis would be that the educational intervention would have a marked impact on the outcome in the experimental group beyond that in the control group. The *null hypothesis*, which is the hypothesis that actually can be tested by statistical methods, would state that there is *no* difference between the groups. Inferential statistics use the null hypothesis for testing the validity of a scientific hypothesis in sample data. The null hypothesis states that there is no actual relationship between the variables and that any observed relationship or difference is merely a function of chance fluctuations in sampling.

The concept of the null hypothesis is often confusing. An example may help to clarify this concept. The study by Grey, Cameron, and Thurber (1991; Appendix B) provides a good example. The authors were interested in determining whether age was an important influence on psychological, social, and physiological adaptation of children with diabetes. The *scientific* hypothesis was that adolescents would have poorer adaptation than younger children. This hypothesis was based on clinical knowledge and previous findings in the literature. On the basis of this hypothesis, the authors then determined whether the scores on the scales used differed among preadolescents, middle adolescents, and later adolescents by using inferential statistics. The researchers used the *null hypothesis*—that there were no differences between the groups of children—to test this scientific hypothesis. The authors found that the preadolescent children were less depressed, were less anxious, coped in more positive ways, had fewer adjustment problems, and had better metabolic control than the older children. In other words, the investigators found that the differences in the scores among the groups were large enough that they were unlikely to be caused by chance, and the null hypothesis was *rejected*.

Note that the researcher would *reject* the null hypothesis. All statistical hypothesis testing is a process of disproof or rejection. It is impossible to prove that a scientific hypothesis is true, but it is possible to demonstrate that the null hypothesis has a high probability of being incorrect. To reject the null hypothesis, then, is considered to show support for the scientific hypothesis and is the desired outcome of most studies that use inferential statistics (see Chapter 7).

PROBABILITY

The researcher can never prove the scientific hypothesis but can show support for it by rejecting the null hypothesis; that is, show that the null hypothesis has a high probability of being incorrect. We have now introduced the theory underlying all of the procedures discussed in this chapter—probability theory. **Probability** is a concept that we talk about all the time, such as the chance of rain today, but we have a difficult time defining it. The *probability* of an event is the event's long-run relative frequency in repeated trials under similar conditions. In order words, the statistician does not think of the probability of obtaining a single result from a single study but rather of the chances of obtaining the same result from an idealized study that can be carried out many times under identical conditions. It is the notion of repeated trials that allows researchers to use probability to test hypotheses.

Statistical probability is based on the concept of **sampling error.** Remember that the use of inferential statistics is based on random sampling. However, even when samples are randomly selected, there is always the possibility of some errors in sampling. Therefore the characteristics of any given sample may be different from those of the entire population. Suppose a group of researchers has at their disposal a large group of patients with decubitus ulcers and they wish to study the average length of time for ulcers to heal with the usual nursing care. If the researchers studied the entire population, they might obtain an average healing time of 50 days, with a standard deviation of 10 days. Now suppose that the researchers did not have the money necessary to study all of the patients but wished instead to do several consecutive studies of these patients. For this study they first draw a sample of 25 patients, calculate the mean and standard deviation, and replace the subjects in the population before drawing the next sample. The researchers repeat this process

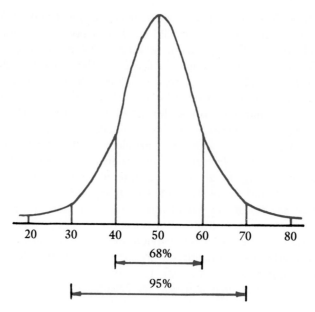

Fig. 17-1   Sampling distribution of the means.

many times so that they might end up with 50 different means. If the researchers then placed the means in a frequency distribution, it might appear as in Fig. 17-1. This frequency distribution is a sampling distribution of the means. It illustrates that the researchers might find that one sample's mean might be 50.5, the next 47.5, the next 62.5, and so on. The tendency for statistics to fluctuate from one sample to another is known as *sampling error.*

Sampling distributions are theoretical. In practice, researchers do not routinely draw consecutive samples from the same population; usually they compute statistics and make inferences based on one sample. However, the knowledge of the properties of the sampling distribution—*if* these repeated samples are hypothetically obtained—permits the researcher to draw a conclusion based on one sample. This is possible because the sampling distribution of the means has certain known properties.

The sampling distribution of the means followed a normal curve, and the mean of the sampling distribution will be the mean of the population. As is discussed in the previous chapter, the fact that the sampling distribution of the means is normal tells us several other important things. When scores are normally distributed, we know that 68% of the cases will fall between +1 SD and −1 SD or that the probability is 68 out of 100 that any one randomly drawn sample mean will lie within the range of values between ±1 SD. In the example given, if we drew only one sample, we would have a 68% chance of finding a sample mean that fell between 40 and 60. The standard deviation of a theoretical distribution of sample means is called the **standard error of the mean.** The word *error* is used because the various means that make up the distribution contain some error in their estimates of the population mean. The error is considered to be standard because it implies the magnitude of the average error, just as a standard deviation implies the average variation from one mean. The smaller the standard error, the less variable are the sample means and the more accurate are those means as estimates of the population value.

Although researchers rarely construct sampling distributions, standard error can be estimated because it bears a systematic relationship to the sample standard deviation and the size of the sample. This tells us that increasing the size of the sample will increase the accuracy of our estimates of population parameters. It should make intuitive sense that to increase the size of a sample will decrease the likelihood that one outlying score will dramatically affect the sample mean (see Chapter 16). The other reason that the sampling distribution is so important is that there are sampling distributions for all statistics. Researchers consult these distributions when making determinations about rejecting the null hypothesis.

TYPE I AND TYPE II ERRORS

The researcher's decision to accept or reject the null hypothesis is based on a consideration of how probable it is that the observed differences are a result of chance alone. Because data on the entire population are not available, the researcher can never flatly assert that the null hypothesis is or is not true. Thus statistical inference is always based on incomplete information about a population and it is possible for errors to occur when making this decision. There are two types of error in statistical inference: **type I error** and **type II error.**

Let us return to the example of the study by Grey and colleagues (1991; Appendix B) of preadolescents and adolescents with diabetes. Remember that the null hypothesis of the study was that there would be no differences in adjustment between preadolescents and adolescents. Approximately 30 children were in each of three groups: preadolescent, middle adolescent, and postpubertal. The authors found that there were significant differences in adaptation between the groups of children. If the differences that were found were truly a function of chance (e.g., because this group of children was unusual in some way) and if the number studied was too small, a type I error would occur. *Type I error* is the researchers' rejection of the null hypothesis when it is actually true. If on the other hand, the researchers had found that the three age-groups did not differ but they had studied only a few children, a type II error might occur. A *type II error* is the researchers' acceptance of a null hypothesis that is actually false. The relationship of the two types of error is shown in Fig. 17-2. In a practice discipline, type I errors are usually considered more serious. This is because if a researcher declares that differences exist where none is present, the potential exists for patient care to be affected adversely.

Level of Significance

The researcher does not know when an error in statistical decision making has occurred. It is possible to know only that the null hypothesis is indeed true or

	REALITY	
Conclusion of test of significance	Null hypothesis is true	Null hypotheses is not true
Not statistically significant	Correct conclusion	Type II error
Statistically significant	Type I error	Correct conclusion

Fig. 17-2   Outcome of statistical decision making.

false if data from the total population are available. However, the researcher can control the risk of making type I errors by setting the **level of significance** before the study begins. The importance of setting the level of significance before the study is conducted is explained in detail by Slakter, Wu, and Suzuki-Slakter (1991). The *level of significance* is the probability of making a type I error, or the probability of rejecting a true null hypothesis. The minimum level of significance acceptable for nursing research is 0.05. If the researcher sets *alpha*, or the level of significance, at 0.05, the researcher is willing to accept the fact that if the study were done 100 times, the decision to reject the null hypothesis would be wrong 5 times out of those 100 trials. If as is sometimes done, the researcher wants to have a smaller risk of rejecting a true null hypothesis, the level of significance may be set at 0.01. In this case the researcher is willing to be wrong only once in 100 trials. The decision as to how strictly the alpha level should be set depends on how important it is to not make an error. For example, if the results of a study are to be used to determine whether a great deal of money should be spent in an area of nursing care, the researcher may decide that the accuracy of the results is so important that an alpha level of 0.01 is chosen. In most studies, however, alpha is set at 0.05.

Perhaps you are thinking that researchers should always use the lowest alpha level possible, because it makes sense that researchers would like to keep the risk of both types of errors at a minimum. Unfortunately, decreasing the risk of making a type I error increases the risk of making a type II error. What this means is that the stricter the researcher is in preventing the rejection of a true null hypothesis, the more likely is the possibility that a false null hypothesis will be accepted. Therefore the researcher always has to accept more of a risk of one type of error when setting the alpha level.

Practical Versus Statistical Significance

The reader should realize that there is a difference between statistical significance and practical significance. When a researcher tests a hypothesis and finds that it is statistically significant, this means that the finding is unlikely to have happened by chance. In other words, if the level of significance has been set at 0.05, the odds are 19 to 1 that the conclusion the researcher makes on the basis of the statistical test performed on sample data is correct. The researcher would reach the wrong conclusion only 5 times in 100. In other words, the researcher would obtain this result by chance alone only 5 times in 100.

Suppose a researcher is interested in the effect of loud rock music on the behavior of laboratory mice. The researcher could design an experiment to study this question and find that loud music makes the mice act strangely. A statistical test suggests that this finding is not the result of chance. However, such a finding may or may not have practical significance, even though the finding has statistical significance. Although some would argue that this study might have relevance to understanding the behavior of teenagers, some would argue also that the study has no practical value. Thus the findings of a study may have statistical significance, but they may have no practical value or significance. Although researchers should consider the practicality of a problem in the early stages of a research project (see Chapters 4 and 7), a distinction between the statistical and practical significance of the findings should also be made when discussing the results of a study. Some people believe that if findings are not statistically significant, they have no practical value. Consider the study by Stewart Fahs and Kinney (1991; Appendix A), who studied three injection sites for low-dose heparin therapy. In this study the scientific hypothesis was also the null hypothesis and the researchers indeed confirmed the null hypothesis. These findings have practical importance because they reject common practice on the basis of scientific findings.

TESTS OF STATISTICAL SIGNIFICANCE

Tests of significance may be *parametric* or *nonparametric*. Most of the studies in nursing research literature use parametric tests, which have the following three attributes: (1) they involve the estimation of at least one parameter; (2) they require measurement on at least an interval scale; and (3) they involve certain assumptions about the variables being studied. These assumptions usually include that the variable is normally distributed in the overall population. In contrast to parametric tests, nonparametric tests of significance are not based on the estimation of population parameters, so they involve less restrictive assumptions about the underlying distribution. Nonparametric tests usually are applied when the variables have been measured on a nominal or ordinal scale.

There has been some debate about the relative merits of the two types of statistical tests. The moderate position taken by most researchers and statisticians is that nonparametric statistics are best used when the data cannot be assumed to be at the interval level of measurement or when the sample is small and the normality of the underlying distribution cannot be inferred. However, if these assumptions can be made, most researchers prefer to use **parametric statistics** because they are more powerful and more flexible than **nonparametric statistics.**

There are many different statistical tests of significance that researchers use to test hypotheses. The procedure and the rationale for their use are similar from test to test. Once the researcher has chosen a significance level and collected the data,

Table 17-1   Tests of Differences Between Means

Level of measurement	One group	Two groups		More than two groups
		Related	Independent	
NONPARAMETRIC				
Nominal	Chi-square	Chi-square Fisher exact probability	Chi-square	Chi-square
Ordinal	Kolmogorov-Smirnov	Sign test Wilcoxon matched pairs Signed rank	Chi-square Median test Mann-Whitney U	Chi-square
PARAMETRIC				
Interval or ratio	Correlated *t* ANOVA (repeated measures)	Correlated *t*	Independent *t* ANOVA	ANOVA ANCOVA MANCOVA

the data are used to compute the appropriate test statistic. For each test there is a related theoretical distribution that shows the probable and improbable values for that statistic. On the basis of the statistical result and the values in the distribution, the researcher either accepts or rejects the null hypothesis and then reports both the statistical result and its probability. Thus a researcher may perform a statistical test called a *t* test, obtain a value of 8.98, and report that it is statistically significant at the $p < 0.05$ level. This means that the researcher had 5 chances out of 100 to be wrong in concluding that this result could not have been obtained by chance. In addition, the likelihood of finding a statistic that is high enough to be statistically significant is increased as the sample size increases. This likelihood is indicated by the degrees of freedom that are often reported with the statistic and the probability value. Degrees of freedom is usually abbreviated as *df.*

Tables 17-1 and 17-2 show the most commonly used inferential statistics. The test that is used depends on the level of the measurement of the variables in question and the type of hypothesis being studied. Basically these statistics test two types of hypotheses: (1) that there is a difference between groups (Table 17-1); or (2) that there is a relationship between two or more variables (Table 17-2).

Tests of Difference

Suppose a researcher has done an experimental study using an after-only design (see Chapter 9). What the researcher hopes to determine is that the two randomly assigned groups are different after the introduction of the experimental treatment. If the measurements taken are at the interval level, the researcher would use

Table 17-2   Tests of Association

Level of measurement	Two variables	More than two variables
NONPARAMETRIC		
Nominal	Phi coefficient	Contingency coefficient
	Point-biserial	
Ordinal	Kendall's tau	Discriminant function analysis
	Spearman rho	
PARAMETRIC		
Interval or ratio	Pearson r	Multiple regression
		Path analysis
		Canonical correlation

the t test to analyze the data. If the t statistic was found to be high enough as to be unlikely to have occurred by chance, the researcher would reject the null hypothesis and conclude that the two groups were indeed more different than would have been expected on the basis of chance alone. In other words, the researcher would conclude that the experimental treatment had the desired effect. A study by Gardner (1991) illustrates the use of the t statistic. The author was interested in comparing primary and team nursing in several areas, and she used the t statistic to determine that there were significant differences in quality of patient care measures between primary and team nursing.

Parametric Tests

The t **statistic** is commonly used in nursing research. This statistic tests whether two group means are different. Thus, this statistic is used when the researcher has two groups, and the question is whether the mean scores on some measure are more different than would be expected by chance. To use this test the variables must have been measured at the interval or ratio level, and the two groups must be independent. By *independent* we mean that nothing in one group helps to determine who is in the other group. If the groups are related, as when samples are matched (see Chapter 12), and the researcher also wants to determine differences between the two groups, a paired or correlated t test would be used.

The t statistic illustrates one of the major purposes of research in nursing—to demonstrate that there are differences among groups. Groups may be naturally occurring collections, such as age-groups, or they may be experimentally created. The type of test that is used for any particular study depends primarily on whether the researcher is examining differences in one, two, or more groups and whether the data to be analyzed are nominal, ordinal, or interval.

Sometimes a researcher has more than two groups, as in the study in Appendix B (Grey et al., 1991). In Table 1 of the study (Appendix B), the researchers report data about differences among the children at different developmental stages. Because there were three groups and the data are at the interval level, the researchers used the statistic known as the **analysis of variance (ANOVA)**. Analysis of variance, like the t statistic, tests whether group means differ, but rather than testing each pair of means separately, ANOVA considers the variation among all groups. In other studies the researchers are interested in differences that occur before and after something occurs. This is the case in the study by Stewart Fahs and Kinney (1991; Appendix A). In Table 3 the authors present the results of their analysis of differences among the injection groups before and after injections. The appropriate statistic is the repeated measures analysis of variance, because this statistic takes into account the fact that multiple measures affect the potential range of scores.

In other cases, particularly in experimental work, the researchers use t tests or ANOVA to determine whether random assignment to groups was effective in creating groups that are equivalent before introduction of the experimental treatment. In this case the researcher wants to show that there is no difference among the groups. In a study by O'Sullivan and Jacobson (1992) of the effects of a special treatment program for teen mothers, the authors report, "There were no statistically significant differences between the experimental group, the control group, and the refusals in maternal age, length of prenatal care, whether or not the adolescent had a previous pregnancy, and complications of the mother or infant at delivery" (pp. 211-212). Suppose, however, that these groups had differed on length of prenatal care. For the researchers to conclude that their experimental program was effective, they would need to control statistically for length of prenatal care. This is done by using the technique of **analysis of covariance (ANCOVA)**. ANCOVA also measures differences among group means, and it uses a statistical technique to equate the groups under study on an important variable. Another expansion of the notion of analysis of variance is **multiple analysis of variance (MANOVA)**, which is used also to determine differences in group means, but it used when there is more than one dependent variable.

Nonparametric Tests

In the example from O'Sullivan and Jacobson (1992), we noted that the researchers tested whether the subjects in the experimental or treatment group were similar in the number of complications of pregnancy. The number of complications of pregnancy is not interval level data, so the researchers could not test this difference with any of the tests discussed thus far. When data are at the nominal level and the researcher wants to determine whether groups are different, the researcher uses another very commonly used statistic, the **chi-square** (χ^2). Chi-square is a nonparametric statistic that is used to determine whether the frequency in each category is different from what would be expected by chance. As with the t test and ANOVA, if the calculated chi-square is high enough, the researcher would conclude that the frequencies found would not be expected on the basis of chance alone and the null hypothesis would be rejected. Although this test is quite robust and can be used in many different situations, it cannot be used to compare frequencies when samples are small and expected frequencies are less than 6 in each cell. In these instances the **Fisher's exact probability test** is used. An example of the use of chi-square to determine differences among groups can be found in Aber and Hawkins (1992). They studied the content of nursing journals to determine whether the images of nurses reflect the roles they play in health care. Because their data were frequencies, they used the chi-square statistic to compare different types of nursing portrayals.

When the data are ranks, or at the ordinal level, researchers have several other nonparametric tests at their disposal. These include the Kolmogorov-Smirnov test, the sign test, the Wilcoxon matched pairs test, and the signed rank test for related groups, and the median test and the Mann-Whitney U test for independent groups. Explanation of these tests is beyond the scope of this chapter; those readers who desire further information are referred to the Additional Readings section at the end of the chapter.

A randomized clinical trial by Naylor (1990) of the effects of a comprehensive discharge planning protocol implemented by a gerontological nurse specialist illustrates the use of several of these statistical tests. The researcher was interested in comparing the new method of discharge planning with usual discharge planning. Although the patients were randomly assigned to experimental and treatment groups, it was important to determine whether the random assignment procedure succeeded in creating equivalent groups, especially because the sample was small. For data measured at the nominal level, such as gender and race, the chi-square statistic was used. For data measured at the interval level, such as age, the *t*-test was used. Finally, to test the effect of the intervention, either ANOVA or chi-square was used, depending on the level of measurement.

Tests of Relationships

Researchers often are interested in exploring the relationship between two or more variables. Such studies use statistics that determine the **correlation,** or the degree of association, between two or more variables. Tests of the relationships between variables are sometimes considered to be descriptive statistics when they are used to describe the magnitude and direction of a relationship of two variables in a sample and the researcher does not wish to make statements about the larger population. Such statistics can also be inferential when they are used to test hypotheses about the correlations that exist in the target population.

Null hypothesis tests of the relationships between variables assume that there is no relationship between the variables. Thus when a researcher rejects this type of null hypothesis, the conclusion is that the variables are in fact related. Suppose a researcher is interested in the relationship between the age of patients and the length of time it takes them to recover from surgery. As with other statistics discussed, the researcher would design a study to collect the appropriate data and then analyze the data using measures of association. In the example, age and length of time until recovery can be considered to be interval level measurements. The researcher would use a test called the **Pearson correlation coefficient,** or **Pearson** *r*, or the Pearson product moment correlation coefficient. Once the Pearson *r* is calculated, the researcher consults the distribution for this test to determine whether the value obtained is likely to have occurred by chance. Again the research reports both the value of the correlation and its probability of occurring by chance.

The interpretation of correlation coefficients often is difficult for students who are learning statistics. Correlation coefficients can range in value from $+1.0$ to -1.0 and also can be zero. A zero coefficient means that there is no relationship between the variables. A perfect positive correlation is indicated by a $+1.0$ coefficient, and a perfect negative correlation by a -1.0 coefficient. We can illustrate the meaning of these coefficients by using the example from the previous paragraph. If there was no relationship between the age of the patient and the time he or she required to recover from surgery, the researcher would find a correlation of zero. However, if the correlation were $+1.0$, this would mean that the older the patient, the longer it took him or her to recover. A negative coefficient would imply that the younger the patient, the longer it would take him or her to recover. Of course, relationships are rarely perfect. The magnitude of the relationship is indicated by how close the correlation comes to the absolute value of 1. Thus a correlation of -0.76 is just as strong as a correlation of $+0.76$, but the direction of the relationship is opposite. In addition, a correlation of 0.76 is stronger than a correlation of 0.32. When a researcher tests hypotheses about the relationships between two variables, the test considers whether the magnitude of the correlation is large enough not to have occurred by chance. This is the meaning of the probability value or the p value reported with correlation coefficients. As with other statistical tests of significance, the larger the sample, the greater the likelihood of finding a significant correlation. Therefore researchers also report the degrees of freedom associated with the test performed.

Refer again to the paper by Grey, Cameron, and Thurber (1991; Appendix B) on the influence of age, coping behavior, and self-care on psychological, social, and physiological adaptation in preadolescents and adolescents with diabetes. Table 2 (in Appendix B) in that paper (reprinted on p. 529) contains the correlation coefficients that describe the relationships among all of the pairs of variables. For example, the correlation coefficient for age and time since diagnosis was 0.32, suggesting that as children get older they are more likely to have had diabetes longer. This reflects a moderate correlation, and it indicates that approximately 10.4% (0.32×0.32) of the variability in time since diagnosis is explained by age.

Nominal and ordinal data also can be tested for relationships by nonparametric statistics. When two variables being tested have only two levels (such as gender: male/female; yes/no), the phi coefficient can be used to express relationships. When the researcher is interested in the relationship between a nominal variable and an interval variable, the point-biserial correlation is used. Spearman rho is used to determine the degree of association between two sets of ranks, as is Kendall's tau. All of these correlation coefficients may range in value from $+1.0$ to -1.0. These tests are shown in Table 17-2. Naylor (1990) used the phi coefficient to determine the relationship of type of discharge planning and length of time since discharge.

Nursing problems rarely are so simple that they can be explained by only two variables. When researchers are interested in studying complex relationships among more than two variables, they use techniques other than those we have discussed thus far.

When researchers are interested in understanding more about a problem than just the relationship between two variables, they often use a technique called mul-

tiple regression, which measures the relationship between one interval level dependent variable and several independent variables. Multiple regression is the expansion of correlation to include more than two variables, and it is used when the researcher wants to determine what variables contribute to the explanation of the dependent variable and to what degree. For example, a researcher may be interested in determining what factors help women decide to breast-feed their infants. A number of variables, such as the mother's age, previous experience with breast-feeding, number of other children, and knowledge of the advantages of breast feeding, might be measured and then analyzed to see whether they, separately and together, predict the length of breast-feeding. Such a study would require the use of multiple regression. The results of a study such as this might help nurses to know that a younger mother with only one other child might be more likely to benefit from a teaching program about breast-feeding than an older mother with several other children.

The reader of research reports often will see multiple regression techniques described as forward solution, backward solution, or stepwise solution. These are techniques that are used in multiple regression to find the smallest group of variables that will account for the greatest proportion of variance in the dependent variable. In the *forward solution* the independent variable with the highest correlation with the dependent variables is entered first, and the next variable is the one that will increase the explained variance the most. In the *backward solution* all variables are entered into the solution and each variable is deleted to see whether the explained variance drops significantly. The stepwise solution is a combination of the two approaches. In general, all of the approaches give similar, although not identical, results (Munro, Visintainer, & Page, 1986).

Suppose the individual who was researching breast-feeding was interested in not just breast-feeding but also maternal satisfaction. *Canonical correlation* is used when there is more than one dependent variable. If the data are nominal or ordinal, the contingency coefficient or discriminant function analyses are used. These last tests are beyond the scope of this text; further information can be found in the Additional Readings section.

Refer again to the study by Grey et al. (1991; Appendix B). They were interested in furthering the understanding of the stress-adaptation model of coping with chronic illness. To do so, they needed to go beyond the analysis of relationships between two variables. Table 3 shows the results of this analysis. The column titled "Beta" reflects the amount of relationship between the variables when the other variables are included. The R^2 listed at the bottom of the table shows the amount of variability in the dependent variable that is accounted for by the independent variables. For example, for adjustment, the total variance explained is 34%. The remaining columns in the table report the statistical test results used to determine the relative importance of each of the variables in the regression. This table is a commonly used and accepted way to show results of a multiple regression analysis.

Advanced Statistics

Sometimes researchers are interested in even more complex problems. For example, DeMaio-Esteves (1990) used the transactional cognitive theory of psychological stress and coping to study the effects of daily stress, introspectiveness, and coping efforts on perceived health status. On the basis of the theory, the author postulated that daily stress would affect perceived health status both directly and through the mediating variables of introspectiveness and coping efforts. To test this mediating effect requires a type of advanced statistics called **path analysis.** In path analysis the researcher hypothesizes how variables are related and in what order and then tests how strong those relationships or paths are.

This notion of testing specific relationships in a specific order can be extended further to test hypothesized variables that are made up of several measures. A technique called *LISREL* tests path models made up of variables that are not actually measured. For example, a researcher might study the concept of self-esteem and use three different measures to determine subjects' levels of self-esteem. The researcher would test how carefully these three measures actually measure self-esteem by testing a measurement model using LISREL. Because many of the variables of interest to nursing are not easily defined and measured and because we are ultimately interested in causal models, LISREL is becoming more commonly used in nursing studies; for examples, see Braden (1990) and Mishel, Padilla, Grant, and Sorenson (1991). In both examples the researchers were testing theories about complex problems and the LISREL technique allowed them the opportunity to study complex interactions among variables simultaneously.

Another advanced technique often used in nursing research is factor analysis. Factor analysis helps us to understand concepts more fully and contributes to our ability to measure concepts reliably and validly (see Chapter 15). *Factor analysis* takes a large number of variables and groups them into a smaller number of factors. It is used to reduce a set of data so that it may be easily described and used. In addition, factor analysis is used for instrument development and theory development. In instrument development, factor analysis is used to group individual items on a scale into meaningful factors or subscales. Gulick (1991), for example, was interested in testing the reliability and validity of the Work Assessment Scale for persons with multiple sclerosis. Factor analysis was used to determine whether the scale actually measured the concepts that they intended the instrument to measure.

Many other statistical techniques are available to nurse researchers. Consult any of the statistics sources listed in the Additional Readings section if further information is desired or if a test not discussed is included in a study of interest to you.

CRITIQUING INFERENTIAL STATISTICAL RESULTS

Many students find that critiquing inferential statistics is difficult or even impossible if they have not taken a course in statistics. Although there is some merit to this feeling, there are aspects of the statistical analysis that should be possible to critique without the benefit of years of statistics course work. Important questions to consider when critiquing the use of inferential statistics are listed in the box on p. 419.

The first place to begin critiquing the statistical analysis of a research report is with the hypothesis. The hypothesis should indicate to you what type of statistics will be used. If the hypothesis indicates that a relationship will be found, you should expect to find indexes of correlation. If the study is experimental or quasiexperimental, the hypothesis would indicate that the author is looking for differences between the groups studied, and you would expect to find statistical tests of differences between means.

Then as you read the methods section of the paper, consider what level of measurement the author has used to measure the important variables. If the level of measurement is interval or ratio, the statistics most likely will be parametric statistics. On the other hand, if the variables are measured at the nominal or ordinal level, the statistics used should be nonparametric. Also consider the size of the sample, and remember that samples have to be large enough to permit the assumption of normality. If the sample is quite small, for example, 5 to 10 subjects, the researcher may have violated the assumptions necessary for inferential statistics to be used. Thus the important question is whether the researcher has provided enough justification to use the statistics presented.

Finally, consider the results as they are presented. There should be enough data presented for each hypothesis studied to determine whether the researcher actually examined each hypothesis. The tables should accurately reflect the procedure performed and be in harmony with the text. For example, the text should not indicate that a test reached statistical significance, while the tables indicate that the probability value of the test was above 0.05. If the researcher has used analyses that are not discussed in this text, you may want to refer to a statistics text to decide whether the analysis was appropriate to the hypothesis and the level of measurement.

There are two other aspects of the data analysis section that the reader should critique. The paper should not read as if it were a statistical textbook. The results of the study in the text of the paper should be clear enough to the average reader so that the reader can determine what was done and what the results were. In addition, the author should attempt to make a distinction between practical and statistical significance. Some results may be statistically significant, but their practical importance may be doubtful. If this is so, the author should note it. Alternatively, you may find yourself reading a research report that is elegantly presented, but you come away with a "so what?" feeling. Such a feeling may indicate that the practical significance of the study and its findings have not been adequately explained in the report.

Note that the critical analysis of a research paper's statistical analysis is not done in a vacuum. It is possible to judge the adequacy of the analysis only in relationship to the other important aspects of the paper: the problem, the hypotheses, the design, the data collection methods, and the sample. Without consideration of these aspects of the research process, the statistics themselves have very little meaning. Statistics can lie; thus it is most important that the researcher use the appropriate statistic for the problem. For example, a researcher may sometimes use a nonparametric statistic when it appears that a parametric statistic is appropriate. Because parametric statistics are more powerful than nonparametric, the result of the parametric analysis may not have been what the researcher expected. However, the nonparametric result might be in the expected direction, so the researcher reports only that result.

Example of the Use and Critique of Inferential Statistics

Earlier in this chapter reference was made to a study of injection sites for subcutaneous heparin injections (Stewart Fahs & Kinney, 1991; Appendix A). The purpose of the study was to evaluate three subcutaneous injection sites for low-dose heparin therapy. This statement of purpose implies that the authors were interested in looking at differences among groups. Therefore the reader should expect that the analysis will consist of statistical tests that examine differences between means, such as ANOVA or the t-test.

The major variables, prothrombin time and bruise size, were measured using standard methods at the interval or ratio level so that parametric tests could be used. There were 101 subjects randomly assigned to three groups—an adequate sample. The researchers used ANOVAs to determine that the three groups had equivalent bleeding times before the heparin injections.

The hypotheses were tested using ANOVA. This test is appropriate to the problem, since the researcher was interested in differences among the injection sites. Results for each of the hypotheses are presented, and they suggest that there is no difference in efficacy of heparin injections among the three injection sites. Tables agree with the text, and the results are understandable to the reader. The discussion points out limitations to the study. Clear implications for practice are found, and they support the practical significance of the study. The statistical level of significance was set at 0.05 and is consistent throughout the paper. Therefore the researchers' statistics were appropriate to the study's purpose, method, sample, and levels of measurement.

KEY POINTS

- Inferential statistics are a tool to test hypotheses about populations from sample data.
- Because the sampling distribution of the means follows a normal curve, researchers are able to estimate the probability that a certain sample will have the same properties as the total population of interest. Sampling distributions provide the basis for all inferential statistics.
- Inferential statistics allow researchers to estimate population parameters and to test hypotheses. The use of these statistics allows researchers to make objective decisions about the outcome of the study. Such decisions are based on the rejection or acceptance of the null hypothesis, which states there is no relationship between the variables.
- If the null hypothesis is accepted, this result indicates that the findings are likely to have occurred by chance. If the null hypothesis is rejected, the researcher accepts the scientific hypothesis of a relationship being present between the variables and that this relationship is unlikely to have been found by chance.
- Statistical hypothesis testing is subject to two types of error: type I and type II.
  - Type I error occurs when the researcher rejects a null hypothesis that is actually true.
  - Type II error occurs when the researcher accepts a null hypothesis that is actually false.
  - The researcher controls the risk of making a type I error by setting the alpha level, or level of significance. Unfortunately, reducing the risk of a type I error by reducing the level of significance increases the risk of making a type II error.
- The results of statistical tests are reported to be significant or nonsignificant. Statistically significant results are those whose probability of occurring is less than 0.05 or 0.01, depending on the level of significance set by the researcher.
- Commonly used parametric and nonparametric statistical tests include those that test for differences between means, such as the t test and ANOVA, and those that test for differences in proportions, such as the chi-square test.
- Tests that examine data for the presence of relationships include the Pearson r, the sign test, the Wilcoxon matched-pairs, signed ranks test, and multiple regression.

- Advanced statistical procedures include path analysis, LISREL, and factor analysis.
- The most important aspect of critiquing statistical analyses is the relationship of the statistics employed to the problem, design, and method used in the study. Clues to the appropriate statistical test to be used by the researcher should stem from the researcher's hypotheses. The reader also should determine if all of the hypotheses have been presented in the paper.

REFERENCES

Aber, C.S. & Hawkins, J.W. (1992). Portrayal of nurses in advertisements in medical and nursing journals. *Image: Journal of Nursing Scholarship, 24,* 289-293.

Braden, C.J. (1990). A test of the self-help model: Learned response to the chronic illness experience. *Nursing Research, 39,* 42-46.

DeMaio-Esteves, M. (1990). Mediators of daily stress and perceived health status in adolescent girls. *Nursing Research, 39,* 360-364.

Gardner, K. (1991). A summary of findings of a five-year comparison study of primary and team nursing. *Nursing Research, 40,* 113-117.

Grey, M., Cameron, M.E., & Thurber, F.W. (1991). Coping and adaptation in children with diabetes. *Nursing Research, 40,* 144-148.

Gulick, E.E. (1991). Reliability and validity of the Work Assessment Scale for persons with Multiple Sclerosis. *Nursing Research, 40,* 107-112.

Mishel, M.H., Padilla, G., Grant, M., & Sorenson, D.S. (1991). Uncertainty in illness theory: A replication of the mediating effects of mastery and coping. *Nursing Research, 40,* 236-240.

Munro, B.H., Visintainer, M.A., & Page, E.B. (1986). *Statistical methods for health care research.* Philadelphia: J.B. Lippincott.

Naylor, M.D. (1990). Comprehensive discharge planning for hospitalized elderly: A pilot study. *Nursing Research, 39,* 156-161.

O'Sullivan, A.L., & Jacobson, B.S. (1992). A randomized trial of a health care program for first-time adolescent mothers and their infants. *Nursing Research, 41,* 210-215.

Slakter, M.J., Wu, Y.W.B., & Suzuki-Slakter, N.S. (1991). *, **, and ***: Statistical nonsense at the .00000 level. *Nursing Research, 40,* 248-249.

Stewart Fahs, P.S., & Kinney, M.R. (1991). The abdomen, thigh, and arm as sites for subcutaneous sodium heparin injections. *Nursing Research, 40,* 204-207.

ADDITIONAL READINGS

Asher, A.B. (1976). *Causal modeling.* Beverly Hills, CA: Sage.

Blaloch, H.M. (1972). *Causal inferences in nonexperimental research.* New York: W.W. Norton.

Ferketich, S., & Muller, M. (1990). Factor analysis revisited. *Nursing Research, 39,* 59-62.

Jacobson, B.S., Tulman, L., & Lowery, B.J. (1991). Three sides of the same coin: The analysis of paired data from dyads. *Nursing Research, 40,* 359-363.

Joreskog, K.G., & Sorbom, D. (1979). *Advances in factor analysis and structural equation models.* Cambridge, MA: Clark Abt.

Kerlinger, F.N., & Pedhazur, E.J. (1986). *Foundations of behavioral research* (2nd ed.). New York: Holt, Rinehart, & Winston.

Knapp, T.R. (1990). Treating ordinal scales as interval scales: An attempt to resolve the controversy. *Nursing Research, 39,* 121-125.

Pedhazur, E.J. (1982). *Multiple regression in behavioral research* (2nd ed.). New York: Holt, Rinehart & Winston.

Wikoff, R.L., & Miller, P. (1991). Canonical analysis in nursing research. *Nursing Research, 40,* 367-370.

Wu, Y.W.B., & Slakter, M.J. (1990). Increasing the precision of data analysis: planned comparisons versus omnibus tests. *Nursing Research, 39,* 251-253.

Youngblut, J.M., Loveland-Cherry, C.J., & Horan, M. (1990). Data management issues in longitudinal research. *Nursing Research, 39,* 188-189.

LEARNING OBJECTIVES

After reading this chapter the student should be able to do the following:

♦ Discuss the difference between the results sections of a study and the discussion of the results.

♦ Identify the format of the results section.

♦ Determine if both statistically supported and statistically nonsupported findings are discussed.

♦ Determine whether the results are objectively reported.

♦ Describe how tables and figures are used in a research report.

♦ List the criteria of a meaningful table.

♦ Identify the format and components of the discussion of the results.

♦ Determine the purpose of the discussion section.

♦ Discuss the importance of interpreting both supported and nonsupported hypotheses.

♦ Discuss the importance of including generalizations and limitations of a study in the report.

♦ Determine the purpose of including recommendations in the study report.

KEY TERMS

finding   limitation
generalizability   recommendation

The ultimate goals of nursing research are to develop nursing theory and knowledge, to substantiate and improve nursing practice, thereby widening the scientific basis of the nursing profession. Nursing research serves not only nurses but also those individuals, families, and groups with whom nurses interact in a multitude of health care settings. From the viewpoint of the research consumer, the analysis of the results, interpretations, and generalizations that a researcher generates from a study becomes a highly important piece of the research project. The final sections of a research report are generally entitled *results* and *discussion,* and it is here that the researcher puts the final pieces of the jigsaw puzzle together to view the total picture with a critical eye. This process is analogous to *evaluation,* the last step in the nursing process. The reader of a research report may view these last sections as an easier step for the investigator, but it is here that a most critical and creative process comes into use. It is in these final sections of the report, after the statistical procedures have been applied, that the researcher will interrelate the statistical or numerical findings to the theoretical framework, literature, methods, hypotheses, and problem statements.

The final sections of published research reports generally are titled *results* and *discussion,* but other topics, such as limitations of findings, implications for future research, and nursing practice, recommendations, and conclusions may be separately addressed or subsumed within these sections. The presentational format of these areas is a function of the author's and the journal's stylistic considerations. The function of these final sections is then to interrelate all aspects of the research process and to discuss, interpret, and identify the limitations and generalizations relevant to the investigation and thereby further nursing research. The goal of this chapter is to introduce the student to the purpose and content of the final sections of a research investigation where data are presented, interpreted, discussed, and generalized. An understanding of what an investigator presents in these sections will assist the research consumer to critically analyze an investigator's findings.

FINDINGS

The findings of a study are the results, conclusions, interpretations, recommendations, generalizations, implications for future research, and nursing practice, and will be addressed by separating the presentation into two major areas. These two areas are the results and the discussion of the results. The results section will

Table 18-1   Examples of Reported Statistical Results

Statistical test	Examples of reported results
Mean	$M = 118.28$
Standard deviation	SD = 62.5
Pearson correlation	$r = -0.39$, p < .01
Analysis of variance	F = 3.59, df = 2, 48, p < .05
t test	$t = 2.65$, p < .01
Chi-square	$\chi^2 = 2.52$, df = 1, p < .05

focus on the results or statistical findings of the study, and the discussion of the results section will focus on the remaining topics. For both sections the rule applies, as it does to all other sections of a report, that the content needs to be presented clearly, concisely, and logically.

Results

The results section of a research report is considered to be the data-bound section of the report. It is here that the researcher presents the quantitative data or numbers generated by the descriptive and inferential statistical tests. The results of the data analysis set the stage for the interpretations or discussion section that follows the results. The results section should then reflect the problem and hypothesis tested. The information from each hypothesis should be sequentially presented. The tests used to analyze the data should be mentioned. If the exact test that was used is not explicitly stated, then the values obtained should be noted. This is done by providing the numerical values of the statistics and stating the specific correlation and probability level, or t value (see Chapters 16 and 17). Examples of these can be found in Table 18-1. These numbers and their signs should not frighten the novice. These numbers are important, but there is much more to the research process than the numbers. They are one piece of the whole. Chapters 16 and 17 conceptually present the meanings of the numbers found in studies for the novice consumer. Whether the consumer only superficially understands statistics or has an in-depth knowledge of statistics, it should be obvious to the reader that the results are clearly stated, and the presence or lack of statistically significant results should be noted. The Additional Readings list at the end of this chapter also provides further detail for those interested in the application of statistics.

The researcher is bound to present the data for all of the hypotheses posed, such as whether the hypotheses were accepted, rejected, supported, or not supported. If the data supported the hypotheses, it may be assumed that the hypotheses were proved, but this is not true. It does not necessarily mean that the hypotheses were proved; it means only that the hypotheses were supported and that the results suggest that the relationships as posed in the hypotheses, which were derived from the theoretical framework, were probably logical. The beginning research consumer may think that if a researcher's results were not supported statistically or only partially supported, the study is irrelevant or possibly should not have been published, but this also is not true. If the data are not supported, the critiquer should not expect the researcher to bury the work in a file. It is as important for a critiquer of research to review and understand nonsupported studies as it is for the researcher. Information obtained from nonsupported studies often can be as useful as data obtained from supported studies. Nonsupported studies can be used to suggest limitations of particular aspects of a study's design and procedures. Data from nonsupported studies may suggest that current modes of practice or current theory in an area may not be supported by research and therefore need to be reexamined and researched further. Data then assist a profession to generate new knowledge, as well as prevent stagnation of knowledge.

Generally it has been noted that an investigator will interpret the results in a separate section of the report. At times the reader may find that the results section contains the results and the researcher's interpretations, which generally fall into the discussion section. Integrating the results with the discussion in a report becomes the decision of the author. Integration of both sections may be used when a study contains several segments that may be viewed as fairly separate subproblems of a major overall problem.

An example of this type of integration is found in a study by Ventura, Young, Feldman, Pastore, Pikula, and Yates (1985). In this study the investigators' purpose was to provide cost-related data from an intervention study in the care of patients with peripheral vascular disease (PVD). The study looked at various aspects of cost and hospitalization, such as vascular-related costs and outpatient usage. Instead of two sections titled *results* and *discussion*, the investigators integrated both of these areas and discussed these areas as subproblems of the overall problem. The encompassing title that addressed results and discussion in this study was labeled *Hospitalization* and *Costs*. Subproblems or related areas tested and discussed were titled as follows: costs—PVD; costs—vascular related; costs—nonvascular; costs—combined total; outpatient hospital usage and time allocation; and costs for intervention. The investigators thus made use of conceptually discrete portions that flowed back to the overall problem. If integration is done in this manner, it should be consistent; that is, if one hypothesis or question is integrated, all should be. The presentation should not take on a haphazard use of integration. In the Ventura study a consistent approach was used. Overall the reader will generally find the data results in a separate section from the interpretation or discussion of the results.

The investigator also should demonstrate objectivity in the presentation of the results. A quote like: "A paired t test revealed a significant difference between these means, $t = 2.73$; $p < 0.05$. Given the size of the sample, the power of the statistical test to prevent a type II error was examined. Although 0.80 is the recommended standard, the power level was approximately 0.77" (Cole, 1993, p. 109) is the appropriate means to express results. The investigator would be accused of lacking objectivity if he had stated the results in the following manner: "A paired t test showed surprisingly that there was a significant difference between the means." Opinions or reactionary statements to the data in the results section therefore are

EXAMPLES OF RESULTS SECTION

QUANTITATIVE STUDIES

Pearson correlations for the total sample indicated that family stress and parental coping were not significantly related to family adaptation. A significant negative correlation was found between social support and family adaptation for the total sample ($p < .05$). (LoBiondo-Wood, Bernier-Henn, Williams; 1992, p. 263).

Differences in time 1, time 2, and time 3 family functioning for mothers and fathers and child development between employment status were examined with two-sample t tests. . . . Two significant differences were obtained. At time 1 and time 3, employed mothers report higher FFS (Family Functioning Scores) than unemployed mothers, t (58) = 2.05, p = 0.05; and t (36.45) = 2.13, p = 0.04; respectively (Youngblut, Loveland-Cherry, & Horan, 1993, p. 37).

To determine whether the sociodemographic characteristics of the women influenced the presence of selected risk factors, the variables of age, education, parity, and marital status were recoded in a binary format. This analysis revealed significant differences. Significantly more nonwhite subjects had inadequate prenatal care (χ^2 = 7.685, p = 0.006) and practiced pica (χ = 3.56, p = 0.005). (Fogel, 1993, p. 37).

QUALITATIVE STUDIES

Deliberation (regarding breast cancer treatment) occurs while the decision maker seeks and evaluates the alternatives and gathers information required to make a choice. Subjects thought about the alternatives, talked with friends and family, and sorted out their feelings about the choices confronting them (Pierce, 1993, p. 25). (The researcher details the meaning of this and provides examples of subjects' responses).

Preparers (patients adapting to cancer treatment) described a process leading to their decision to use specific strategies to prepare for treatment. The preparers first confronted the horror of diagnosis: "I was devastated (by the diagnosis)," "I got panicky. I mean at that point I thought I was dying"; "I went into a cold sweat"; "I was too scared and overwhelmed to deal with it" (Lev, 1992, p. 600). (The researcher provides further examples of the concept and a conceptual map of the subjects' strategies.)

inappropriate. The box above provides examples of objectively stated results from both quantitative and qualitative studies. It is the investigator's responsibility to respond objectively to the results. This is accomplished in the section titled Discussion of Results. The investigator then uses the discussion of the results section to respond to and interpret the results, with a careful reflection on all aspects of the study that preceded the results.

The reader of a research report should keep in mind that the data presented are considerably reduced. A great deal more data or numbers are generated in a study, but only the critical numbers of each test need to be presented in a report. An

Table 18-2   Mean Surface Area (mm^2) and Standard Deviation by Injection and Site at Hour of Measurement Postinjection

	Injection 1 72 hours ($n = 101$)		Injection 2 60 hours ($n = 101$)		Injection 3 48 hours ($n = 97$)	
	M	SD	M	SD	M	SD
Abdomen	85.71	(295.57)	88.42	(368.94)	19.17	(44.94)
Thigh	95.15	(286.71)	200.20	(616.94)	118.69	(263.70)
Arm	219.39	(498.59)	151.69	(383.87)	176.07	(299.56)

From "The Abdomen, Thigh, and Arm as Sites for Subcutaneous Sodium Heparin Injections" by P.S. Stewart Fahs and M.R. Kinney, 1991, *Nursing Research, 40,* 204-207.

example of summarized descriptive data is seen when only the means and standard deviations of age, education, income, and years married are presented rather than all of the subject information listed. Including all of the data in a published report would be too cumbersome. Individual data may be presented when a case study design is used. The condensation of data is done both in the written text and through the use of tables and figures. The use of tables and figures can facilitate the presentation of large amounts of data generated by the study.

In the study by Stewart Fahs and Kinney (1991; Appendix A), the researchers developed tables to present the results visually. Table 18-2 provides the descriptive results (means and standard deviation) by injection and site at the hour of measurement postinjection, and Table 18-3 provides the results of testing for differences in bruise surface area of injection sites measured at 72, 60, and 48 hours, regardless of injection site, using the repeated measure analysis of variance (ANOVA) test. These tables allow the researchers to provide a more thorough explanation and discussion of the results. The results section then can be viewed as a summation section. Both the results of the descriptive and inferential statistics are presented for each hypothesis posed. No data should be omitted that would preclude the critiquer from gaining a full picture of the results. If tables and figures are used, they need to be concise. Although the text is the major mode of communicating the results, the tables and figures serve a supplementary but independent role. The role of tables and figures is to report results with some detail that the investigator does not enter into the text. This does not mean that tables and figures should not be mentioned in the text. The amount of detail that the author uses in the text to describe the specific tabled data varies with the needs of the researcher. If the text includes everything that is found in the table, the table should not appear. A good table is one that meets the following criteria:

1. Supplements and economizes the text
2. Has precise titles and headings
3. Does not repeat the text

An example of a table that meets these criteria can be found in the study by Grey, Cameron, and Thurber (1991; Appendix B). The research team wanted to report the correlations among the model's variables and the demographic variables.

Table 18-3   Repeated Measure ANOVA

Variable	SS	df	MS	F-ratio	F-value
SURFACE AREA **(72 Hours)**					
Between subjects	386656.5	02	193382.3	1.37	.26
Within subjects	13870580.9	98	141536.5		
SURFACE AREA **(60 Hours)**					
Between subjects	207055.5	02	103527.7	.47	.63
Within subjects	21532142.8	98	219715.7		
SURFACE AREA **(48 Hours)**					
Between subjects	404498.0	02	202249.0	3.69	.03
Within subjects	5038643.5	95	141536.5		

From "The Abdomen, Thigh, and Arm as Sites for Subcutaneous Sodium Heparin Injections" by P.S. Stewart Fahs and M.R. Kinney, 1991, *Nursing Research, 40,* 204-207.

Because of the number of variables, it is much clearer for the reader to have a table that easily and clearly summarizes the results as this table does. To describe each one of these in the text of the article would not have economized space and would have been difficult to visualize. The table developed by the researchers (Table 18-4) allows the readers not only to visualize the variables quickly but to assess the results.

The research consumer will find a well-written results section is systematic, logical, concise, and drawn from all of the analyzed data. All that is written in the results section should be geared to letting the data reflect the testing of the problems and hypotheses. The length of this section therefore depends on the scope and breadth of the analysis.

Discussion of the Results

In the final section of the report the investigator interpretively discusses the results of the study. It is in this section that a skilled researcher makes the data come alive. The researcher gives the numbers in quantitative studies or the concepts in qualitative studies meaning and interpretation. The reviewer may ask where the investigator extracted the meaning that is applied in this section. If the researcher does the job properly, you will find a return to the beginning of the study. The researcher returns to the earlier points in the study where a problem statement was identified and independent and dependent variables were related on the basis of a sound theoretical framework and literature review. It is in this section that the researcher discusses both the supported and nonsupported data. In this final section the limitations or weaknesses of a study are discussed in light of the design and the sample or

Table 18-4   Variable Correlation Matrix $N = 103$

Variable	Age	Time	STAIC	CDI	LEC	SCQ	CHIP	COPE	CAAP	SPPC	M (SD)
Time since dx (Time)	.32										5.3(3.9)
State Anxiety (STAIC)	.40	.07									29.2(4.7)
Depression (CDI)	.15	−.10	.62								6.2(5.9)
Stressors (LEC)	−.01	.14	−.03	.14							8.2(5.2)
Self-Care (SCQ)	.06	−.17	−.11	−.07	.14						41.8(6.7)
Parent Coping (CHIP)	−.05	−.15	.14	−.25	−.29	.13					88.5(19.5)
Child Coping (COPE)	−.30	.06	.38	−.37	.19	.27	.20				171.0(25.9)
Adjustment (CAAP)	−.17	−.05	−.27	−.32	−.15	.12	.06	.10			67.4(14.1)
Self-Worth (SPPC)	−.15	.01	−.43	−.68	.11	.06	.07	.15	.38		19.8(3.4)
Hemoglobin A$_1$ (HgbA$_1$)	.43	.23	.34	.23	.12	.08	.04	.28	−.09	−.27	1.1(3.9)

From "Coping and Adaptation in Children with Diabetes" by M. Grey, M.E. Cameron, and F.W. Thurber, 1991, *Nursing Research, 40,* 144-149.

data collection procedures. When the data are supported with a statistical significance, the discussion and interpretation are seen as a relatively easy task. The critiquer should find a discussion of how the theoretical framework was supported. In addition, the reviewer should also see the investigator's attempt to look at the data for additional or previously unrealized relationships.

Even if the data are supported, the reviewer should not believe it to be the final word. Downs (1984) cautions that the researcher critiquer should not be overwhelmed by small p values, since they are not indicative of research breakthroughs. To the critiquer of a research study this means that statistical significance in a research study does not always mean that the results of a study are clinically significant. As the body of nursing research grows, so does the profession's ability to critically analyze beyond the tests of significance and assess a research study's applicability to practice. Chapter 3 reviews methods to think about and analyze the usefulness of research findings. Also, within the nursing literature, discussion about clinical significance is emerging (Becker, 1993; LeFort, 1993; Mercer, 1984; Polit & Sherman, 1990; Slakter, Wu, & Suzuki-Slakter, 1991). As indicated throughout this text, many important pieces in the research puzzle need to fit together for a study to be evaluated as a well-done project. Therefore researchers and reviewers should accept statistical significance with prudence. Statistically significant findings are not the sole means of establishing the study's merit. Other aspects, such as theory, sample, instrumentation, and methods, also should be considered.

When the results are not statistically supported, the researcher also returns to the theoretical framework and analyzes the earlier thinking process. Results of non-supported hypotheses do not require the investigator to go on a fault-finding tour of each piece of the project. Such a course can then become an overdone process. All research has weaknesses. This analysis is an attempt to identify the weaknesses and to suggest what the possible problem or problems were in the study. At times the theoretical thinking is correct, but the researcher finds problems or limitations that could be attributed to the tools (see Chapters 14 and 15), the sampling methods (see Chapter 12), the design (see Chapters 8 through 11), or the analysis (see Chapters 16 and 17). Therefore when results are not supported, the investigator attempts to go on a *fact*-finding tour rather than a *fault*-finding one. The purpose of the discussion then is not to show humility or one's technical competence but rather to enable the reviewer to judge the validity of the interpretations drawn from the data and the general worth of the study (Kerlinger, 1986).

It is in the discussion section of the report that the researcher ties together all the loose ends of the study. It is from this point that reviewers of research can begin to think about clinical relevance, the need for replication, or the germination of a new idea for a prospective research study. Finally, the reviewer of a research project should find this section either in separate sections or subsumed within the discussion section, and it should include **generalizability** and recommendations for future research, as well as a summary or a conclusion.

Generalizations (generalizability) are inferences that the data are representative of similar phenomena in a population beyond the study's sample. Reviewers of research are cautioned not to generalize beyond the population on which a study is based. Beware of research studies that may overgeneralize. Generalizations that draw conclusions and make inferences within a particular situation and at a particular time are appropriate. An example of such a generalization is drawn from a study conducted by Baillie, Norbeck, and Barnes (1988) that was designed to examine the effects of stress and social support and their interaction with psychological well-being in family caregivers of impaired elderly. The researchers, when discussing the sample in light of the results, appropriately noted.

> The ability to generalize the findings is limited by the nonrandom, predominately middle-class nature of the sample. Although the measure of perceived stress and social support had high internal consistency reliability, further work with more developed measures is needed to validate these findings. Because social support was strongly related to the psychological well-being of these caregivers, additional research is needed to explore factors that contribute to satisfaction with social support. (p. 450)

This type of statement is important for reviewers of research. It helps to guide thinking in terms of a study's clinical relevance, and it also suggests areas for further research (see Chapter 3). One study does not provide all of the answers, nor should it. It has been said that a good study is one that raises more questions than it answers. So the research consumer should not view an investigator's review of limi-

EXAMPLES OF RESEARCH RECOMMENDATIONS AND PRACTICE IMPLICATIONS

RESEARCH RECOMMENDATIONS

"Further research is needed not only on patients' perceptions of bruises, but also on any discomfort they experience, whether physiologic or psychologic. The possible fear patients may have of injections in the abdomen, compared to the extremities, and the convenience to patients and nurses of using alternative sites should be studied" (Stewart Fahs & Kinney, 1991, p. 207).

"Although the study has a number of limitations, including nonprobability sampling and lack of an actual measurement of patients' activities after surgery (a major concern being the possible social desirability bias in patient reportings), the study findings suggest implications for further research and practice" (Rice, Mullin, & Jarosz, 1992, p. 258).

PRACTICE IMPLICATIONS

"The results of this investigation, combined with findings from these previous studies, do not support published recommendations on the length of time to postpone oral temperature measurement after ingestion of cold liquids. The recommended 5 min is too brief for accurate measurement regardless of the time of day. The 30-min recommendation will provide accurate results but this long time span is an inefficient use of time, especially if it delays treatment" (Cole, 1993, p. 110).

"Pain ratings by children and nurses were found to be significantly different, supporting previous literature. This finding should influence practice by encouraging health care providers to consider assessing a child's pain from more than just their own perception, which is likely to be different from the child's perception" (Schneider & LoBiondo-Wood, 1992, p. 161).

tations, generalizations, and implications of the findings for practice as lack of research skill. These final steps of evaluation are critical links to the refinement of practice and the generation of future research. Evaluation of research, like evaluation of the nursing process, is not the last link in the chain but a connection between findings that may serve to improve nursing theory and nursing practice.

The final area that the investigator integrates into the discussion section is the recommendations. The *recommendations* are the investigator's suggestions for the study's application to practice, theory, and further research. This requires the investigator to reflect on the question "What contribution to nursing does this study make?" For examples of recommendations for future research and implications for nursing practice, see the box above. This evaluation places the study into the realm of what is known and what needs to be known before being utilized. Fawcett (1982) noted, "It is through future exploration of the dissemination and utilization of research in nursing practice that the science of nursing will become an entity with

=== **CRITIQUING CRITERIA** ===

1. Are all of the results of each hypothesis presented?
2. Is the information regarding the results concisely and sequentially presented?
3. Are the tests that were used to analyze the data presented?
4. Are the results presented objectively?
5. If tables or figures are used, do they meet the following standards:
   a. They supplement and economize the text.
   b. They have precise titles and headings.
   c. They are not repetitious of the text.
6. Are the results interpreted in light of the hypotheses and theoretical framework and all of the other sections that preceded the results?
7. If the data are supported, does the investigator provide a discussion of how the theoretical framework was supported?
8. If the data are not supported, does the investigator attempt to identify the weaknesses and suggest what the possible problems were in the study?
9. Does the investigator discuss the study's clinical relevance?
10. Are any generalizations made?
11. Are the generalizations within the scope of the findings or beyond the findings?
12. Are any recommendations for future research stated or implied?

which to be reckoned." This thought is critical and has been reaffirmed by many nurse researchers in the past decade, such as Hinshaw (1988), Gortner (1990), Gennaro and Vessey (1991), Brink (1992), and Stetler (in press).

CRITIQUING THE RESULTS AND DISCUSSION

Criteria for critiquing the results and the discussion of the results sections are found in the box above.

The results and the discussion of the results are the researcher's opportunity to examine the logic of the hypothesis(es) posed, the theoretical framework, the methods, and the analysis. This final section requires as much logic, conciseness, and specificity as was employed in the preceding steps of the research process. The consumer should be able to identify statements of the type of analysis that was used and whether the data statistically supported the hypothesis(es). These statements should be straightforward and not reflect bias (see Table 18-2). Auxiliary data or serendipitous findings also may be presented. If such auxiliary findings are presented, they should be as dispassionately presented as were the hypothesis data. The statistical tests used also should be noted. The numerical value of the obtained data also should be presented (see Table 18-1). The presentation of the tests, the numerical values found, and the statements of support or nonsupport should be clear, concise, and systematically reported. For illustrative purposes that facilitate readability the researchers should present extensive findings in tables.

The discussion section should interpret the data, the gaps, the limitations of the study, and the conclusions, as well as give recommendations for further research. Drawing these aspects into the study should give the consumer a sense of the relationship of the findings to the theoretical framework. Statements reflecting the underlying theory are necessary, whether or not the hypotheses were supported.

If the findings were not supported, the consumer should, as the researcher did, attempt to identify, without fault-finding, possible methodological problems. Finally, a concise presentation of the study's generalizability and the implications of the findings for practice and research should be evident. The last presentation can help the research consumer to begin to rethink clinical practice, provoke discussion in clinical settings (see Chapters 19 and 20), and find similar studies that may support or refute the phenomena being studied to more fully understand the problem.

KEY POINTS

- The analysis of the findings is the final step of a research investigation. It is in this section that the consumer will find the results printed in a straightforward manner.
- All results should be reported whether or not they support the hypothesis. Tables and figures may be used to illustrate and condense data for presentation.
- Once the results are reported, the researcher interprets the results. In this presentation, usually titled Discussion, the consumer should be able to identify the key topics being discussed. The key topics, which include an interpretation of the results, are the limitations, generalizations, implications, and recommendations for future research.
- The section on interpretation of the results is where the researcher draws together the theoretical framework and makes interpretations based on the findings and theory. Both statistically supported and nonsupported results should be interpreted. If the results are not supported, the researcher should discuss the results reflecting on the theory, as well as possible problems with the methods, procedures, design, and analysis.
- The researcher should present limitations or weaknesses of the study. This presentation is important, because it affects the study's generalizability. The generalizations or inferences about similar findings in other samples also are presented in light of the findings.
- The research consumer should be alert for sweeping claims or overgeneralizations

that a researcher may state. An overextension of the data can alert one to possible researcher bias.

The recommendations provide the consumer with suggestions regarding the study's application to practice, theory, and future research. These recommendations furnish the critiquer with a final perspective of the researcher on the utility of the investigation.

REFERENCES

Baillie, V., Norbeck, J.S., & Barnes, L.E. (1988). Stress, social support, and psychological distress of family caregivers of the elderly. *Nursing Research, 37*:217-222.

Becker, P.T. (1993). A lingering identity crisis. *Research In Nursing and Health, 16,* 87-88.

Brink, P. (1992). Nursing care makes a difference [Editorial]. *Western Journal of Nursing Research, 14,* 416-417.

Cole, F. (1993). Temporal variation in the effects of iced water on oral temperature. *Research In Nursing And Health, 16,* 107-112.

Downs, F.S. (1984). *A sourcebook of nursing research* (3rd ed.). Philadelphia: F.A. Davis.

Fawcett, J. (1982). Utilization of nursing research findings. *Image, 14,* 57-59.

Fogel, C.I. (1993). Pregnant inmates: Risk factors and pregnancy outcomes. *Journal of Obstetric, Gynecologic, and Neonatal Nursing, 22,* 33-40.

Gennaro, S., & Vessey, J. (1991). Making practice perfect. *Nursing Research, 40,* 529.

Gortner, S. (1990). Nursing values and science: Toward a science philosophy. *Image, 22,* 101-105.

Grey, M., Cameron, M.E., & Thurber, F.W. (1991). Coping and adaptation in children with diabetes. *Nursing Research, 40,* 144-149.

Hinshaw, A.S. (1988). Using research to shape health policy. *Nursing Outlook, 36,* 21-24.

Kerlinger, F.N. (1986). *Foundations of behavioral research* (2nd ed.). New York: Holt, Rinehart & Winston.

LeFort, S.M. (1993). The statistical versus clinical significance debate. *Image, 25,* 57-62.

Lev, E.L. (1992). Patients' strategies for adapting to cancer treatment. *Western Journal of Nursing Research, 14,* 595-611.

LoBiondo-Wood, G., Bernier-Henn, M., & Williams, L. (1992). Impact of the child's liver transplant on the family: Maternal perspective. *Pediatric Nursing, 18,* 461-466.

Mercer, R.T. (1984). Nursing research: The bridge to excellence in practice. *Image, 16,* 47-51.

Pierce, P.F. (1993). Deciding on breast cancer treatment: A description of decision behavior. *Nursing Research, 42,* 22-27.

Polit, D.F., & Sherman, R.E. (1990). Statistical power in nursing research. *Nursing Research, 39,* 365-369.

Rice, V.H., Mullin, M.H., & Jarosz, P. (1992). Preadmission self-instruction effects on postadmission and postoperative indicators in CABG patients: Partial replication and extension. *Research In Nursing and Health, 15,* 253-259.

Schneider, E.M., & LoBiondo-Wood, G. (1992). Perceptions of procedural pain: Parents, nurses, and children. *Children's Health Care, 21,* 157-162.

Slakter, M.J., Wu, Y.W.B., & Suzuki-Slakter, N.S. (1991). *, **, and ***: Statistical nonsense at the .00000 level. *Nursing Research, 40,* 248-249.

Stetler, C.B. (in press). Refinement of the Stetler/Marram model for application and research findings to practice. *Nursing Outlook.*

Stewart Fahs, P.S., & Kinney, M.R. (1991). The abdomen, thigh, and arm as sites for subcutaneous sodium heparin injections. *Nursing Research, 40,* 204-207.

Ventura, M.R., Young, D.E., Feldman, M.J., Pastore, P., Pikula, S., and Yates, M.A. (1985). Cost savings as an indicator of successful nursing intervention. *Nursing Research, 34,* 50-53.

Youngblut, J.M., Loveland-Cherry, C.J., & Horan, M. (1993). Maternal employment, family functioning and preterm infant development at 9 and 12 months. *Research In Nursing & Health, 16,* 33-44.

ADDITIONAL READINGS

Abraham, I.L., Nadzam, D.M., & Fitzpatrick, J.J. (1989). *Statistics and quantitative methods in nursing.* Philadelphia: W.B. Saunders.

Knapp, R.G. (1985). *Basic statistics for nurses* (2nd ed.). New York: John Wiley & Sons.

Pedhazer, E.J. (1986). *Multiple regression in behavioral research,* (2nd ed.). New York: Holt, Rinehart, & Winston.

Voliker, B.J. (1984). *Multivariate statistics for nursing research.* New York: Grune & Stratton.

Waltz, C. & Bausell, R.B. (1991). *Nursing research: Design, statistics, and computer analysis.* Philadelphia: F.A. Davis.

CRITIQUE AND APPLICATION

Using Research in Practice

MARA M. BAUN

Critical care nursing provides an opportunity for exciting challenges in patient care but at the same time requires a high level of technical competence of the caregiver. Patients in intensive care units (ICUs) are at critical stages in their illnesses, so interventions that might be considered relatively routine for most patients can be accompanied by quite deleterious consequences. Neither are all critically ill patients alike. Thus critical care nurses need to make accurate assessments based on research data and protocols in "tailoring" care for each individual patient.

One frequently performed procedure for intubated and mechanically ventilated patients is endotracheal suctioning (ETS). Although most critical care texts suggest that each patient may respond differently to the procedure, in practice nurses often suction patients according to a unit protocol or the method they were taught, giving little regard to whether that prescribed protocol is "right" for a given patient. For some patients who have essentially normal lungs (e.g., liver transplantation patients), routine ETS procedures usually suffice. As long as the basic requirements of hyperoxygenation are met, these patients do not have any deleterious consequences of ETS and frequently are extubated within a few hours after surgery, as soon as they are fully awake.

Patients in acute respiratory failure, on the other hand, respond entirely differently to each aspect of the ETS procedure. Because these patients may already be somewhat desaturated, they may have little margin of tolerance for the decrease in oxygen that accompanies ETS. Usually they are also being maintained on positive end expiratory pressure (PEEP) on the ventilator to keep their airways open. Thus techniques such as hyperinflation before and after ETS may augment the positive pressure already present in the thorax. This reduces the venous return to the heart and thereby decreases cardiac output, further compromising their already compromised cardiovascular systems. Our laboratory research (Baun, Rudy, Stone, & Turner, in press) as well as that of others (Stone, Vorst, Lanham, & Zahn, 1989) has demonstrated quite convincingly that both decreased and increased arterial pressure can result from these hyperinflations. Patients receiving PEEP, particularly those with increased pulmonary vascular resistance, are particularly susceptible. Thus careful assessment based on research protocols must be implemented so that during suctioning the same key dependent variables used in the research are assessed for the individual patient.

On the basis of the individual's response to the interventions used, the procedure can then be modified. For example, a patient whose arterial pressure increases markedly during an ETS procedure that includes hyperinflation with an anesthesia bag might be suctioned through a modified endotracheal tube adapter while receiving tidal volume breaths from the ventilator rather than receiving lung hyperinflations from the anesthesia bag. Familiarity with the research on ETS would assist the critical care nurse in identifying the key variables to be monitored and in implementing the therapeutic alternatives available. The result would be less deleterious side effects to the patient and maintenance of patency of the patient's airway.

As you can see, research is an integral part of practice, not just an exercise to be mastered to complete one's education. It can assist the nurse in providing the best possible care for patients and have a significant impact on the care of many patients through establishing research-based protocols.

REFERENCES

Baun, M.M., Rudy, E., Stone, K.S., & Turner, B. Differences between open and closed systems of endotracheal suctioning with and without positive end expiratory pressure in an oleic acid–injured model of acute respiratory failure (in press). *American Journal of Critical Care.*

Stone, K.S., Vorst, E.C., Lanham, B., & Zahn, S. (1989). Effects of lung hyperinflation on mean arterial pressure and postsuctioning hypoxemia. *Heart & Lung, 18*(4), 377-385.

CHAPTER 19

Evaluating Quantitative Research Studies

JUDITH A. HEERMANN
BETTY CRAFT

LEARNING OBJECTIVES

After reading this chapter the student should be able to do the following:

- Identify the influence of stylistic considerations on the presentation of a research report.
- Identify the purpose of the critiquing process.
- Describe the criteria of each step of the critiquing process.
- Evaluate the strengths and weaknesses of a research report.
- Discuss the implications of the findings of a research report for nursing practice.
- Construct a critique of a research report.

	KEY TERMS	
replication	scientific merit	
research base		

To determine the merit of a research report, each component of a research study is examined. Criteria designed to assist the consumer in judging the relative value of a research report are found in previous chapters. An abbreviated set of questions (see Table 19-1, pp. 443-446) summarizing the more detailed criteria is used in this chapter as the framework for two sample research critiques. These critiques are included to exemplify the process of evaluating reported research for potential application to practice and thus extending the **research base** for nursing. For clarification, readers are encouraged to refer to the earlier chapters for the detailed presentation of the critiquing criteria and explanations of the research process. The criteria and examples in this chapter apply to quantitative studies.

STYLISTIC CONSIDERATIONS

Before beginning to critique research studies, the evaluator should realize several important aspects related to the world of publishing. First, different journals have different publication goals and target specific professional markets. For example, *Nursing Research* is a journal that publishes articles on the conduct or results of research in nursing. *The Journal of Obstetric, Gynecologic, and Neonatal Nursing* also publishes research articles but, in addition, includes articles related to the knowledge, experience, trends, and policies in obstetrical, gynecological, and neonatal nursing. The emphasis in this latter journal is broader in that it contains clinical and theoretical as well as research articles. Consequently the style and content of the manuscript varies according to the type of journal to which it is being submitted.

Second, the author of a research article prepares the manuscript using both personal judgment and specific guidelines. *Personal judgment* refers to the researcher's expertise developed in the course of designing, executing, and analyzing the study. As a result of this expertise, the researcher is in the position to judge which content is most important to communicate to the profession. The decision is a function of the following:

• The level of study: experimental or nonexperimental
• The focus of the study: basic or clinical
• The audience to which the results will be most appropriately communicated

Table 19-1   Major Content Sections of a Research Report and Related
Critiquing Guidelines

Section	Questions to guide evaluation
Problem statement and purpose (see Chapter 7)	1. What is the problem and/or purpose of the research study? Is it appropriately stated? 2. Does the problem or purpose statement express a relationship between two or more variables, e.g., between an independent and a dependent variable? If so, what is/are the relationship(s)? Are they testable? 3. Does the problem statement and/or purpose specify the nature of the population being studied? What is it? 4. What significance of the problem has been identified, if any, by the investigator?
Review of literature and theoretical framework (see Chapters 5 and 6)	1. What concepts are included in the review? Of particular importance, note those concepts that are the independent and dependent variables and how they are conceptually defined. 2. Does the literature review make explicit the relationships among the variables or place the variables within a theoretical/conceptual framework? What are the relationships? 3. What gaps or conflicts in knowledge about the problem are identified? How does this study intend to fill those gaps or resolve those conflicts? 4. Are the references cited by the author mostly primary or mostly secondary sources? Give an example of each. 5. What are the operational definitions of the independent and dependent variables? Do they reflect the conceptual definitions?
Hypotheses or research questions(s) (see Chapter 7)	1. What hypothesis(es) or research questions are stated in the study? Are they appropriately stated? 2. If research questions are stated, are they used in addition to hypotheses or to guide an exploratory study? 3. What are the independent and dependent variables in the statement of each hypothesis/research question? 4. If hypotheses are stated, is the form of the statement statistical (null) or research? 5. What is the direction of the relationship in each hypothesis, if indicated? 6. Are the hypotheses testable?
Sample (see Chapter 12)	1. How was the sample selected? 2. What type of sampling method is used in the study? Is it appropriate to the design? 3. To what population may the findings be generalized? What are the limitations in generalizability?

Continued.

Table 19-1   Major Content Sections of a Research Report and Related Critiquing Guidelines—cont'd

Section	Questions to guide evaluation
	4. Does the sample reflect the population as identified in the problem or purpose statement?
	5. Is the sample size appropriate? How is it substantiated?
Research design (see Chapters 8 to 10)	1. What type of design is used in the study?
	2. What is the rationale for the design classification?
	3. Does the design seem to flow from the proposed problem statement, theoretical framework, literature review, and hypothesis?
Internal validity (see Chapter 8)	1. Discuss each of the threats to the internal validity of the study.
	2. Does the design have controls at an acceptable level for the threats to internal validity?
External validity (see Chapter 8)	1. What are the limits to generalizability in terms of external validity.
Research approach (see Chapters 13, 14 and 15)	
Methods (see Chapter 14)	1. What type(s) of data collection method(s) is/are used in the study?
	2. Are the data collection procedures similar for all subjects?
Legal-Ethical Issues (see Chapter 13)	1. How have the rights of subjects been protected?
	2. What indications are given that informed consent of the subjects has been ensured?
Instruments (see Chapter 14)	1. Physiological measurement
	a. Is a rationale given for why a particular instrument/method was selected? If so, what is it?
	b. What provision is made for maintaining the accuracy of the instrument and its use, if any?
	2. Observational methods
	a. Who did the observing?
	b. How were the observers trained to minimize bias?
	c. Was there an observational guide?
	d. Were the observers required to make inferences about what they saw?
	e. Is there any reason to believe that the presence of the observers affected the behavior of the subjects?
	3. Interviews
	a. Who were the interviewers? How were they trained to minimize bias?
	b. Is there evidence of any interviewer bias? If so, what is it?

Table 19-1   Major Content Sections of a Research Report and Related Critiquing Guidelines—cont'd

Section	Questions to guide evaluation
	4. Questionnaires a. What is the type and/or format of the questionnaire (e.g., Likert, open-ended)? 5. Available data and records a. Are the records that were used appropriate to the problem being studied? b. Are these data being used to describe the sample or for hypothesis testing?
Reliability and validity (see Chapter 15)	1. What type of reliability is reported for each instrument? 2. What level of reliability is reported? Is it acceptable? 3. What type of validity is reported for each instrument? 4. Does the validity of each instrument seem adequate? Why?
Analysis of data (see Chapters 16 and 17)	1. What level of measurement is used to measure each of the major variables? 2. What descriptive or inferential statistics are reported? 3. Were these descriptive or inferential statistics appropriate to the level of measurement for each variable? 4. Are the inferential statistics used appropriate to the intent of the hypothesis(es)? 5. Does the author report the level of significance set for the study? If so, what is it? 6. If tables or figures are used, do they meet the following standards? a. They supplement and economize the text. b. They have precise titles and headings. c. They are not repetitious of the text.
Conclusions, implications, and recommendations (see Chapter 18)	1. If hypothesis(es) testing was done, was/were the hypothesis(es) supported or not supported? 2. Are the results interpreted in the context of the problem/purpose, hypothesis, and theoretical framework/literature reviewed? 3. What does the investigator identify as possible limitations and/or problems in the study related to the design, methods, and sample? 4. What relevance for nursing practice does the investigator identify, if any? 5. What generalizations are made? 6. Are the generalizations within the scope of the findings or beyond the findings? 7. What recommendations for future research are stated or implied?

Continued.

Table 19-1 Major Content Sections of a Research Report and Related Critiquing Guidelines—cont'd

Section	Questions to guide evaluation
Application and utilization for nursing practice (see Chapter 3)	1. Does the study appear valid? That is, do its strengths outweigh its weaknesses?
	2. Are there other studies with similar findings?
	3. What risks/benefits are involved for patients if the research findings would be used in practice?
	4. Is direct application of the research findings feasible in terms of time, effort, money, and legal/ethical risks?
	5. How and under what circumstances are the findings applicable to nursing practice?
	6. Should these results be applied to nursing practice?
	7. Would it be possible to replicate this study in another clinical practice setting?

Guidelines are provided by each journal for preparing research manuscripts for publication. The following major headings are essential sections in the research report:

- Introduction
- Methodology
- Results
- Discussion

Depending on stylistic considerations related to authors' preferences and the publishing journal's requirements, specific content is included in each section of the research report. Stylistic variations as factors influencing the presentation of the research study are distinct from the focus of evaluating the reported research for scientific merit. Constructive evaluation is based on objective, unbiased, and impartial appraisal of the study's strengths and limitations. This is a step that precedes consideration of the relative worth of the findings for clinical application to nursing practice. Such judgments are the hallmark of promoting a sound theory base for quality nursing practice.

Critique of Research Study: Sample No. 1

The study "Preadmission Self-Instruction Effects on Postadmission and Postoperative Indicators in CABG Patients: Partial Replication and Extension" by Virginia Hill Rice, PhD, RN, FAAN; Marlene H. Mullin, MSN, RN; and Patricia Jarosz, MSN, RN, published in *Research in Nursing & Health* (1992), is critiqued. The article is presented in its entirety and is followed by the critique on p. 456.

Preadmission Self-Instruction Effects on Postadmission and Postoperative Indicators in CABG Patients: Partial Replication and Extension*

Virginia Hill Rice, Marlene H. Mullin, and Patricia Jarosz

Fifty adult coronary artery bypass graft surgery patients were randomly assigned to preadmission self-instruction or posthospital admission instruction of therapeutic exercises (e.g., coughing). Self-instructed subjects reported higher positive mood scores, performed correctly significantly more exercise behaviors, and required less teaching time following hospital admission. Postoperatively, no group differences were found on mood states, physical activity, analgesic use, or length of hospital stay. Both groups, however, tended to use less pain medication than that reported by other researchers and experience shorter hospital stays than that assigned under the Diagnostic Related Groups prescription. © John Wiley & Sons, Inc.

The purpose of this study was to compare the effects of two approaches to teaching postoperative therapeutic exercise (preadmission self-instruction and postadmission instruction by a nurse) on postadmission mood state, exercise per-

formance, and teaching time, and on postoperative recovery. This study was, in part, a replication and extension of an earlier study (Rice & Johnson, 1984). Although CABG surgery contributes to an overall improvement in the quality of life for many individuals with coronary artery disease, the surgery itself can be a significant stressor with a potential for resulting anxiety, pain, postoperative complication, and extended hospital stay (Christopherson & Pfeiffer, 1980; King, 1985; King, Norsen, Robertson, & Hicks, 1987; King & Parrinello, 1988; Lepczyk, Raleigh, & Rowley, 1990; Rakoczy, 1977; Wallwork & Caine, 1985).

A stress-coping theoretical framework (Lazarus & Folkman, 1984) was adopted for the present study to conceptualize the use of exercise behaviors as a form of direct action coping and indicators of postoperative recovery as elements of somatic health. Lazarus and Folkman suggest that individuals confronted by a stressful situation such as surgery will evaluate its implications for their well-being (primary appraisal), weigh their resources for coping with it (secondary appraisal), may change their original perception based on new information (reappraisal), and select a coping strategy appropriate to the nature of the stressor and their resources for dealing with it.

In this framework, coping is viewed as a dynamic process that directs how a

*© 1992 John Wiley & Sons, Inc. Reprinted from *Research in Nursing & Health*, 1992, 15, 253–259. Used with permission.
Virginia Hill Rice, PhD, RN, FAAN is an associate professor of adult health in the Wayne State University College of Nursing, Detroit, MI and a fellow of the American Academy of Nursing. Marlene H. Mullin, MSN, RN is a cardiovascular clinical nurse specialist at Sinai Hospital, Detroit, MI. Patricia Jarosz, MSN, RN was a part-time clinical instructor at Wayne State University College of Nursing and a doctoral student at the University of Michigan, Ann Arbor, MI.
The study was funded by the American Heart Association of Michigan.
This article was received on January 14, 1991, was revised, and accepted for publication on February 5, 1992.

person will deal with a situation, what the concerns are, and what the emotional response will be. Coping strategies are those efforts (e.g., direct actions, indirect actions, intrapsychic responses, and information seeking) that one makes to manage demands that tax or exceed one's resources. Lazarus and Folkman (1984) suggest that individuals use a combination of these coping strategies when confronted by a threat such as surgery. They note that "the prime importance of appraisal and coping processes is that they affect adaptational outcomes" (p. 181) which include social functioning, life satisfaction or morale, and somatic health.

One way to facilitate coping with stressors such as surgery is through the use of psychoeducational interventions that include health related information, psychosocial support, and teaching of self-care skills (e.g., coughing and deep breathing). Using meta-analysis, a number of researchers have reported positive effects for such interventions in reducing negative emotional responses, pain, and discomfort, and in facilitating recovery (e.g., Devine & Cook, 1983, 1986; Hathaway, 1986; Mumford, Schlesinger & Glass, 1982). Researchers (Miller & Shada, 1978; Parrinello, 1984) studying cardiac patients have reported that these patients value preoperative instruction of postoperative therapeutic exercises among other types of perioperative information because it allows them an opportunity to participate in their own recovery.

With today's shortened length of hospital stay, the time available for nurses to instruct patients in exercise behaviors while they are in the hospital is limited. Lipetz, Bussigel, Bannerman, and Risley (1990), in their study of 'barriers' to patient education, reported

that 81% of the nurses in their sample believed patients were not in the hospital long enough to be given adequate information and/or instructions. To allow patients the time needed to learn and to practice new behaviors it seems reasonable to provide them with information/instructions prior to their hospital admission, and there is evidence to suggest that this is a viable alternative to initiating patient teaching following hospital admission.

Levesque, Grenier, Kirouac, and Reidy (1984) and Lepczyk, Raleigh, and Rowley (1990) asked individuals to come to the hospital for information and/or instructions prior to their actual admission for scheduled surgery. Study findings showed lowered anxiety scores for instructed patients in the first study and greater knowledge gain for patients taught preadmission in the second. Although having individuals come to the hospital for information/instructions on an outpatient basis may save time and money for the hospital, it is probably costly for patients who have to come for the teaching. A more cost-effective and less labor intensive approach would be to send written materials to the patient at home for self-instruction and learning prior to hospital admission.

Self-instruction or self-directed learning affords the individual an opportunity to learn, practice, and master new behaviors in a familiar environment at his/her own rate (Hill & Smith, 1985). Learning time for developing new skills can vary for individuals and practice is often necessary for gaining control of motor behaviors (Redman, 1984). Having the exercise information at home prior to hospital admission theoretically gives the individual both the time and opportunity needed to learn them.

Support for this notion is provided by

Christopherson and Pfeiffer (1980) who examined knowledge gain, anxiety, and length of stay in cardiac surgery patients who had been given perioperative information and instructions following their cardiac catheterization but prior to their later readmission for cardiac surgery. They found that subjects who did not choose to read the preadmission information had lower information scores and were, on the average, two days longer in the intensive care unit and in the hospital compared to those who did read the material. No differences were found as a function of the length of time preadmission that patients had the information (1 to 2 days vs. 3 to 35 days) and no differences were found on reported anxiety. Although patients completed a knowledge questionnaire, there was no actual performance evaluation of the coughing, deep breathing, and other exercises described in the information booklets.

Rice and Johnson (1984) found that patients sent an exercise booklet with specific directions and feedback cues could perform significantly more of the targeted behaviors than those sent nonspecific directions for doing the exercises, or no preadmission instructions. Both self-instructed groups required significantly less teaching time following hospital admission than subjects with no preadmission information, although these groups did not differ from one another. Not examined in this study or the others above, however, was the impact, if any, of preadmission teaching on subjects' overall positive and negative mood states and on postoperative recovery. Thus, the present study is intended to fill this gap and is, in part, a replication and extension of the earlier study in a different patient population. "Replication, especially conceptual replication,

seems especially important when the underlying motivation for research is the application of the results to the clinical practice of nursing" (Johnson, Fuller, Endress, & Rice, 1978, p. 111). If the original findings can be replicated with different subjects, differing situational factors, and minor variations in procedure, then far greater confidence can be placed in these results than would be the case for an exact replication.

Based on the literature cited and theoretical considerations of Lazarus and Folkman (1984), it was hypothesized that CABG patients sent preadmission self-instructions would on hospital admission: (1) have more positive and less negative moods, (2) perform correctly more of the exercise behaviors, and (3) require less teaching time than those instructed postadmission. It also was hypothesized that preadmission instructed patients would postoperatively: (4) report higher positive and lower negative mood scores, (5) have higher physical activity scores, (6) use fewer analgesics, and (7) experience shorter hospital stays. In this study, performance of self-taught or nurse-taught exercise behaviors was viewed as direct actions taken by the patient to facilitate his/her own recovery. The postoperative variables of positive mood state, physical activity, use of analgesics, and length of hospital stay were all viewed as indicators of somatic health.

METHOD
Subjects

A convenient sample of 55 adults scheduled for first time elective CABG surgery without cardiac catheterization, who had not had other major surgery within the previous year, and who were not health professionals met the study criteria and were randomly assigned to one of the two instruction conditions. Five persons, two assigned to the preadmission and three to the postadmission group, refused to participate; no specific reasons were given for the refusals. Based on a formulation of 80% power, a medium critical effect size of 0.4 for each of the dependent variables, and a significance level of .05 for one-tailed *t* tests of means, a sample size of 48 was deemed sufficient to test the study hypotheses (Kraemer & Thiemann, 1987). There were 21 men and 4 women in the preadmission group; 2 subjects were black. In the postadmission group there were 20 men and 5 women; 1 subject was black. The majority (85%) of the subjects in both groups reported moderate incomes and were proprietors of small businesses, skilled workers, operatives, and service workers. No differences between the groups were found for age, education, cardiopulmo-

nary bypass pump time, aortic clamp time, or length of time in the Intensive Care Unit postoperatively (see Table 1).

Intervention

Subjects assigned to the preadmission group were sent a self-instructional exercise booklet entitled *Exercises for a Speedy Recovery* 6 to 10 days prior to their scheduled admission for surgery. The booklet, initially developed for an earlier study (Rice & Johnson, 1984), provided step-by-step instructions for performing coughing, deep breathing, leg movement, and ambulation exercises followed by feedback cues to help persons determine if they were doing them correctly. Content for the booklet was derived from the literature (e.g., Lindeman & Van Aernam, 1971) and it was pretested for readability and understandability. In addition, it was evaluated for

Table 1   Demographic and Perioperative Indicators for Preadmission and Postadmission Teaching Groups

Indicators	Preadmission teaching (*n* = 25)		Postadmission teaching (*n* = 25)		
	M	*SD*	*M*	*SD*	*t*
Age (Years)	60.4	8.3	60.0	7.4	.17
Education (Years)	11.5	2.2	12.3	3.1	1.04
Cardiopulmonary pump time (Min)	84.6	32.9	86.6	30.6	.23
Aortic clamp time (Min)	54.6	22.3	52.9	18.5	.28
Intensive care unit time (Hr)	44.1	6.7	45.6	14.2	.48

Note. All *t* values were nonsignificant.

content validity by three Recovery Room nurse clinicians. The booklet also was used to teach patients in the postadmission instruction group.

Measures

Mood was assessed using the Mood Adjective Checklist (MACL) which consists of 24 adjectives describing three positive (well-being, relaxed, and happy) and three negative (helplessness, anxiety, and anger) feeling states; there are four adjectives to describe each emotion (Radloff & Helmreich, 1968). Subjects were asked to indicate on a 4-point scale, ranging from *not at all* to *very much,* how well each adjective described their feelings "right then." Scores for the positive and negative moods were summed separately, yielding a range of 12 to 48 units for each subscale. In this study alpha coefficients were .84 for the positive moods, and .78 for the negative moods; the positive and negative mood subscale scores were negatively correlated ($r = -.40$, $p = <.010$) with one another. Although other researchers (e.g., Johnson et al., 1978; Padilla et al., 1979) have used the Mood Adjective Checklist, reliability and validity values were not reported. Padilla et al. (1979) did find a six-factor structure for the measure.

Preoperative performance was assessed using an Exercise Checklist which listed the 34 exercise behaviors found in the *Exercises for a Speedy Recovery* intervention booklet. The booklet and Exercise Checklist were developed in an earlier study (Rice & Johnson, 1984) and content and face validity established by a panel of three medical-surgical clinical specialists who judged the behaviors on the Exercise Checklist as reflective of those described in the booklet. Nurses observed whether or not subjects performed the component behaviors of coughing, deep breathing, leg exercises, turning in bed, and ambulation and then checked their presence or absence on the Checklist. One point was given for each component behavior performed; possible scores ranged from 0 to 34. The amount of time it took for patients to perform all 34 behaviors correctly was recorded as teaching time and ranged from 6 to 51 min. Initially, interrater reliability was determined between the investigator and three surgical nurse data collectors for the number of behaviors performed and for the amount of time it took for patients to perform the behaviors in a small group ($N = 5$) of subjects. Percentages of agreement were 88% and 92%, respectively.

Postoperative mood states were obtained using the Mood Adjective Checklist described earlier. Physical activity was determined by asking patients on the fifth postoperative day how many times they had gotten out of bed in the previous 24 hr. Each time patients reported getting out of bed was given a score of one; scores ranged from 2 to 30. Construct validity for this measure was assessed by asking patients to indicate elsewhere on the Postoperative Questionnaire the number of times that they had walked to the chair, to the bathroom, and in the hall; summing these scores and then comparing them with those on the first measure. Correlational analysis revealed a coefficient of .89 between the two measures.

Analgesic use was determined by averaging patients' daily doses of pain medications for each of the first three postoperative days; medications were grouped into those given by injection (e.g., meperidine) and those taken by mouth (e.g., acetaminophen). Length of stay was the number of days that the patient was in the hospital for CABG surgery.

Procedure

Subjects assigned to the preadmission instruction group and who agreed to participate were sent the exercise booklet. Following hospital admission, a nurse who was not aware of the patient's group assignment visited all patients, obtained an informed consent, and asked patients to provide mood and demographic data. Patients then were asked to demonstrate how they would cough, deep breathe, do leg exercises, get out of bed, and walk after their surgery. The nurse noted when patients began the exercises and the presence or absence of the 34 behaviors on the Exercise Checklist. If a behavior was missed or performed incorrectly, the nurse instructed the patient until all behaviors were done correctly without cues or assistance. The finish time was noted. Another nurse visited subjects on the fifth postoperative day and obtained information on mood states, physical activity, and analgesic use.

RESULTS

The means, standard deviations, and t values for the postadmission variables are shown in Table 2. Analysis revealed that individuals sent the preadmission instructions reported more positive moods, performed more of the exercise behaviors, and required less teaching time following hospital admission.

The means, standard deviations, and t values for the postoperative variables are in Table 3. Postoperatively, the study groups did not differ from each other on mood scores. However, both groups reported higher positive mood scores postoperatively than on hospital admission, paired $t(25) = 4.98$ and 6.65 respective, both $p = <.01$. In addition, groups did not differ on reported physical activity or in their use of analgesics. Initial examination of length of stay data revealed unequal variance for the pread-

Table 2   Comparison of Postadmission Moods, Exercise Behaviors and Teaching Time by Intervention Group

Indicators	Preadmission teaching (n = 25)		Postadmission teaching (n = 25)		
	M	SD	M	SD	t
Mood					
Positive	27.6	4.7	24.7	5.5	1.99*
Negative	22.4	6.7	21.8	5.2	.72
Exercise behaviors					
(Range 0-34)	16.9	11.0	6.0	5.5	4.43**
Teaching time					
(Mins)	10.2	4.7	14.2	8.8	2.05*

*$p = <.05$. **$p = <.0001$.

mission ($M = 8.9$, $SD = 2.22$) and postadmission ($M = 11.0$, $SD = 7.0$) groups, with one patient in the latter group being hospitalized for 40 days with a stroke. When this outlier was excluded from the analysis, no differences were found between the two groups on length of stay.

DISCUSSION

The purpose of this study was to replicate, in part, major findings of an earlier study (Rice & Johnson, 1984) with a sample of CABG patients and to extend that work by examining postoperative recovery variables. Similar postadmission results were found in the current study; CABG patients sent the same self-instructional booklet performed more exercise behaviors and required less teaching time to achieve evident mastery of the exercises on hospital admission than patients not sent preadmission instructions. Findings show that preadmission self-instructed patients in the current study correctly performed, on average, 16.9 of the exercise behaviors as compared to patients in the earlier study who did 13.2. The higher degree of physiological threat posed by the nature of the surgery (i.e., coronary artery bypass graft surgery versus cholecystectomy) may have been a motivating factor for why patients in the current study learned more of the exercise behaviors. The amount of teaching time required by preadmission self-instructed subjects in the current study was similar to preadmission self-instructed patients in the earlier study, 10.2 min as compared to 9.6 min. The savings in teach-

Table 3   Comparison of Postoperative Moods, Physical Activity, Analgesic Use and Length of Hospital Stay by Intervention Group

Indicators	Preadmission teaching (n = 25)		Postadmission teaching (n = 25)		
	M	SD	M	SD	t
Moods					
Positive	31.8	5.3	31.3	5.9	.32
Negative	24.7	7.8	22.6	8.6	1.12
Physical activity	9.7	7.0	7.4	5.5	1.22
Injection analgesics					
Day 1	3.4	1.8	3.5	1.9	.29
Day 2	2.1	1.3	2.0	1.0	.41
Day 3	0.9	1.1	1.4	1.7	1.21
Oral analgesics					
Day 1	0.1	0.6	0.0	0.0	.44
Day 2	0.8	0.9	0.7	0.6	.46
Day 3	1.5	1.5	1.5	1.8	.17
Length of hospital stay[a]	8.9	2.2	9.8	3.7	1.04

Note. All *t* values were nonsignificant.

[a]$n = 24$ subjects in the postadmission group.

ing time was about 4 min in the current study and 3 min in the earlier study. Whether these average time "savings" are clinically or economically meaningful needs to be explored further. Part of the answer may lie in why patients took the time to learn the exercises at all.

One reason why patients may have taken the time to learn the exercises was to help themselves cope with the upcoming threatening event of surgery. This was evidenced by the more positive mood scores reported by preadmission instructed patients in the current study. This finding supports Lazarus and Folkman's (1984) position that direct action is one means by which individuals cope with new and/or threatening events and that effective coping results in more positive emotions. Preadmission information may have allowed for a more positive appraisal of the threat in terms of its implications for well being. Although the exercise booklet did not provide patients with information about the surgery itself, it did suggest behaviors that would be expected of them postoperatively and what actions they could take to effect their own recovery. This finding is consistent with other research (e.g., King, 1985; Miller & Shada, 1978; Parrinello, 1984) in which information has been identified as an important need for surgical patients. Future research should include measures of perceived threat appraisal to more closely examine the proposed link between meeting informational needs and reducing threat. Additional research also will be needed to examine what additional benefits patients experience by getting preadmission information.

Although preadmission instructed patients reported higher positive moods on hospital admission, they did not differ from the postadmission instructed patients on negative moods; both groups had moderately negative mood states. Considering the seriousness of cardiac surgery and the risks often associated with it, it is probably not realistic to expect exercise information alone to reduce negative feelings associated with such an event. The effects of preadmission information which deals with the other aspects of the upcoming hospital experience (e.g., the impact of the diagnosis itself) should be examined. Different types of information may be needed to facilitate coping with the many aspects of the perioperative experience (Barsevick & Johnson, 1990; Johnson, Christman, & Stitt, 1985; King, 1985; Levesque et al., 1984).

Recovery variables indicated that patients in both groups reported significantly higher positive mood scores on the fifth day postsurgery than they had on hospital admission although they did not differ from one another. This increase in postoperative well-being has been reported in other studies with surgical patients (e.g., Devine & Cook, 1986; Levesque et al., 1984) as well as cardiac patients (King, 1985) and is probably related to a general sense of relief that the threat of surgery is over and recovery is in progress. Additional findings of this research do not allow for inferences regarding a differential impact of preadmission self-instruction on other aspects of postoperative recovery. No differences were found between the study groups on postoperative physical activity, use of analgesics, or length of hospital stay. Patients in this study, however, were given less pain medication than that reported in another study with CABG patients (King et al., 1987). Perhaps knowing how to do the postoperative exercises correctly resulted in less pain and a reduced need for analgesics. Although the length of stay was similar for both study groups, the overall mean of 9.4 days was less than that expected under the Diagnostic Related Group prescription (i.e., 11.2 days) for CABG without cardiac catheterization (DRG 107) based on prospective payment from Medicare (Office of Federal Register, 1990). This finding is consistent with other studies (e.g., Christopherson & Pfeiffer, 1980) in which patient teaching has been shown to be a factor in shortened hospital stay.

The value of preadmission teaching of therapeutic exercises may be translated into lower costs associated with shortened lengths of hospital stay, particularly if nursing does not have the time nor opportunity to teach all patients following hospital admission for surgery. If presurgical patients can learn the exercise behaviors at home on their own, this will reduce the amount of time that is needed by nursing to teach the patient following hospital admission. Although the study has a number of limitations, including nonprobability sampling and lack of an actual measurement of patients' activities after surgery (a major concern being the possible social desirability bias in patient reportings), the study findings suggest implications for further research and practice.

Sending information to patients at home before their diagnostic and/or surgical experience, particularly information on behaviors that are to be learned, is an important and unique opportunity for nursing to provide more comprehensive care. Such information should not eliminate the need for postadmission teaching, but would allow nursing to use the valuable time following hospital ad-mission more effectively to review/reinforce materials that have been sent to the patient's home or to provide other types of information and/or support.

REFERENCES

Barsevick, A., & Johnson, J. (1990). Preference for information and involvement, information seeking, and emotional responses of women undergoing colposcopy. *Research in Nursing & Health, 13,* 1-7.

Christopherson, B., & Pfeiffer, C. (1980). Varying the time of information to alter preoperative anxiety and postoperative recovery in cardiac surgery patients. *Heart & Lung, 9,* 854-861.

Devine, E., & Cook, T. (1983). A meta-analytic analysis of the effects of psycho-educational interventions on length of postsurgical hospital stay. *Nursing Research, 32,* 267-274.

Devine, E., & Cook, T. (1986). Clinical and cost-saving effects of psychoeducational interventions with surgical patients: A meta-analysis. *Research in Nursing & Health, 9,* 89-105.

Hathaway, D. (1986). Effect of preoperative instructions on postoperative outcomes: A meta-analysis. *Nursing Research, 35,* 269-275.

Hill, L., & Smith, N. (1985). *Self-care nursing: Promotion of health* (2nd ed.). Norwalk, CT: Appleton & Lange.

Johnson, J., Christman, N., & Stitt, C. (1985). Personal control interventions: Short- and long-term effects in surgical patients. *Research in Nursing & Health, 8,* 131-145.

Johnson, J., Fuller, S., Endress, P., & Rice, V.H. (1978). Altering patients' responses to surgery: An extension and replication. *Research in Nursing & Health, 1,* 111-121.

King, K. (1985). Measurement of coping strategies, concerns, and emotional responses in patients undergoing coronary artery bypass grafting. *Heart & Lung, 14,* 579-586.

King, K., Norsen, L., Robertson, R., &

Hicks, G. (1987). Patient management of pain medication after cardiac surgery. *Nursing Research, 36,* 145-150.

King, K., & Parrinello, K. (1988). Patient perceptions of recovery from coronary artery bypass grafting after discharge from the hospital. *Heart & Lung, 17,* 708-715.

Kraemer, H., & Thiemann, S. (1987). *How many subjects?* Beverly Hills, CA: Sage.

Lazarus, R., & Folkman, S. (1984). *Stress, appraisal, & coping.* New York: Springer.

Lepczyk, M., Raleigh, E., & Rowley, C. (1990). Timing of preoperative patient teaching. *Journal of Advanced Nursing, 15,* 300-306.

Levesque, L., Grenier, R., Kirouac, S., & Reidy, M. (1984). Evaluation of a presurgical group program given at two different times. *Research in Nursing & Health, 7,* 227-236.

Lindeman, C., & Van Aernam, B. (1971). Nursing intervention with the presurgical patient: The effect of structured and unstructured preoperative teaching. *Nursing Research, 20,* 319-332.

Lipetz, M., Bussigel, M., Bannerman, J., & Risley, B. (1990). What is wrong with patient education programs? *Nursing Outlook, 36,* 184-189.

Miller, P., & Shada, E. (1978). Preoperative information and recovery of open-heart surgery patients. *Heart & Lung, 7,* 486-493.

Mumford, E., Schlesinger, H., & Glass, G. (1982). The effects of psychological intervention on recovery from surgery and heart attacks: An analysis of the literature. *American Journal of Public Health, 72,* 141-150.

Office of Federal Register. (1990, Tuesday, September 4). *National archives and record administration* (Vol. 55, No. 171). Washington DC: U.S. Government Printing Office.

Padilla, G., Grant, M., Wong, H., Hansen, B., Hanson, R., Bergstrom, N., & Kubo, W. (1979). Subjective distresses of nasogastric tube feeding. *Journal of Parenteral and Enteral Nutrition, 3,* 53-57.

Parrinello, K. (1984). Patients' evaluations of a teaching booklet for arterial bypass surgery. *Patient Education and Counseling, 5,* 183-188.

Radloff, R., & Helmreich, R. (1968). *Groups under stress.* New York: Appleton-Century-Crofts.

Rakoczy, M. (1977). The thoughts and feelings of patients in the waiting period prior to cardiac surgery. *Heart & Lung, 6,* 280-287.

Redman, B. (1984). *The process of patient education.* (5th ed.). St. Louis: Mosby.

Rice, V.H., & Johnson, J. (1984). Preadmission self-instruction booklets, postadmission exercise performance, and teaching time. *Nursing Research, 33,* 147-151.

Wallwork, J., & Caine, N. (1985). A comparison of the quality of life of cardiac transplant patients and coronary artery bypass graft patients before and after surgery. *Quality of Life and Cardiovascular Care, 2,* 317-331.

INTRODUCTION TO CRITIQUE NO. 1

The article "Preadmission Self-Instruction Effects on Postadmission and Postoperative Indicators in CABG Patients: Partial Replication and Extension" by Rice, Mullin, and Jarosz (1992) is critically examined in terms of its quality and the potential usefulness of the findings for application to nursing practice.

Problem and Purpose

The authors state the purpose of this **replication** study was "to compare the effects of two approaches to teaching postoperative therapeutic exercise (preadmission self-instruction and postadmission instruction by a nurse) on postadmission mood state, exercise performance, and teaching time and on postoperative recovery" (p. 253). In this purpose statement, the two teaching approaches are the independent variable affecting the dependent variables of postadmission mood state, exercise performance and teaching time and of postoperative recovery. Although not included in the purpose statement, the population is later specified as CABG patients. Thus the research problem is embedded in the purpose statement.

Rice et al. (1992) identify the significance of the problem when they note that although CABG surgery contributes to improved quality of life in patients with coronary artery disease, the surgery itself may be a significant stressor with potential negative consequences, such as "anxiety, pain, postoperative complication, and extended hospital stay" (p. 253). Psychoeducational interventions are identified as a way to facilitate coping with the stressors associated with surgery.

Review of Literature and Definitions

Concepts discussed in the literature review are coping strategies, psychoeducational interventions, time (timing) of instruction, self-directed learning, and adaptational outcomes. The theoretical framework adopted for this study is Lazarus and Folkman's stress-coping model. Exercise behaviors are viewed as an example of direct action coping to be developed through the use of psychoeducational intervention (teaching postoperative therapeutic exercise) to improve somatic health, an indicator of adaptational outcome. Somatic health was conceptualized as comprising moods, postoperative physical activity, analgesic use, and length of hospital stay. Timing and self-directed learning are discussed as parameters of the psychoeducational intervention believed to be important to the outcome. Thus all key concepts are defined.

Knowledge gaps identified are the lack of performance evaluation of exercise and evaluation of the subjects' overall mood states and postoperative recovery after preadmission teaching. The authors propose replicating and extending previous research to a different population and incorporating the measurement of exercise performance and mood states.

An appropriate theoretical base is derived almost entirely from primary sources. The reference to Rice and Johnson (cited by Rice et al., 1992, p. 253) is an example of a primary source, since it is identified as the study undergoing **replication** and extension. The reference selected to illustrate the use of a secondary source (p. 254) is a textbook by Redman that describes the process of patient education and is used to support the premise that learning time varies and that practice is often needed.

The independent variable of psychoeducational instruction was operationalized as the use of the self-instructional booklet "Exercises for a Speedy Recovery" for both preadmission and postadmission groups. The booklet was mailed 6 to 10 days before admission for surgery to those subjects in the preadmission group and used to guide the postadmission instruction for the other group.

The dependent variables of mood, performance of exercise behaviors, and teaching time are measured preoperatively, whereas mood, physical activity, analgesic use, and hospital stay are measured postoperatively. Preoperative and postoperative mood states are operationalized by the Mood Adjective Checklist (MACL); performance of exercise behavior is measured through use of the Exercise Checklist listing 34 behaviors from the Exercises for Speedy Recovery booklet; teaching time is identified as the amount of time patients took to perform all 34 of the behaviors. Physical activity is operationalized by asking the patients on the fifth postoperative day to report the number of times they got out of bed in the previous 24 hours. "Analgesic use was determined by averaging patients' daily dose of pain medications for each of the first three postoperative days; medications were grouped into those given by injection (e.g., meperidine) and those taken by mouth (e.g., acetaminophen). Length of stay was the number of days that the patient was in the hospital for CABG surgery" (p. 256).

Hypotheses and/or Research Questions

Hypotheses rather than research questions are used appropriately in this study. The hypotheses are "that CABG patients sent preadmission self-instructions would on hospital admission: (1) have more positive and less negative moods, (2) perform correctly more of the exercise behaviors, and (3) require less teaching time than those instructed postadmission" and "it also was hypothesized that preadmission instructed patients would postoperatively: (4) report higher positive and lower negative mood scores, (5) have higher physical activity scores, (6) use fewer analgesics, and (7) experience shorter hospital stays" (pp. 254-255). The independent variable is type of instruction (preadmission self-instruction or postadmission instruction). The dependent variables are preoperative and postoperative moods, exercise behaviors, teaching time, physical activity scores, analgesic use, and length of hospital stay. The hypotheses, stated in research form, are appropriately directional, since they predict that the patients in the preadmission self-instruction group will have *more* positive and *less* negative moods preoperatively and postoperatively, will be able to perform *more* exercise behaviors correctly with *less* teaching time, will have *higher* physical activity scores, will use *fewer* analgesics, and will have *shorter* hospital stays.

Sample

The convenience sample was recruited from those "adults scheduled for first-time elective CABG surgery without cardiac catheterization, who had not had other major surgery within the previous year, and who were not health professionals" (p. 255). The use of a nonprobability sample limits generalization to the sample itself. The sample selected for inclusion in the research project matches the population proposed after the purpose statement when CABG surgery is identified as a potentially significant stressor. The 50 subjects who agreed to participate exceeded the sample size of 48 reported as sufficient to test the study hypotheses. There is no indication as to how the sample size was decided.

Research Design

Consistent with the experimental design used by the authors, the independent variable is manipulated by mailing the "Exercises for a Speedy Recovery" booklet before admission to the subjects in the experimental group and including a control group of subjects receiving instruction after admission. Subjects are randomly assigned to one of the two instructional groups. The logic underlying the research design is discerned by examining the purpose statement, which proposes investigating the effect of two approaches to teaching postoperative therapeutic exercise: the theoretical framework (as presented in the literature review), which supports the efficacy of enhancing patient coping through the use of a psychoeducational intervention designed to enhance adaptational outcome; and the hypotheses, which predict enhanced postoperative performance in the experimental group.

Internal Validity

Examination of threats to internal validity reveals no indication of difficulty associated with history or maturation with this adult population over a brief time span. Selection bias is controlled for by specific selection criteria used to identify subjects who are randomly assigned to groups. In addition, the groups do not differ on selected demographic and perioperative indicators. Although two subjects assigned to the preadmission group and three to the postadmission group refused to participate, the examination of groups for similarity described previously negates the threat of mortality. A potential threat caused by instrumentation, acknowledged by the authors, is associated with possible social desirability resulting from reliance on patient report of postoperative activity. Although the Mood Adjective Checklist is administered both preoperatively and postoperatively, the threat of testing (internal validity) seems minimal. The research design adequately controls for threats to internal validity.

External Validity

Generalizability of findings is limited by the use of a nonprobability sampling technique. The findings may be generalized only to the sample.

Research Approach

Methods

Data collection methods include questionnaires, observation, and use of available records. Data collection procedures are consistent and systematic for both the experimental and control groups and occur at the time of admission and 5 days postoperatively. Rice et al. (1992) report obtaining informed consent on admission.

Instruments

Preoperative performance is based on three surgical nurses' observations of subjects. Training of the observers is implied in the report of established interrater reliability with the investigator. The observational guide used is the Exercise Checklist. The observers are required to determine whether the subject performed each of the 34 behaviors on the Exercise Checklist and the amount of time it took to achieve correct performance. The only apparent effect on subject performance is the intended increase in behaviors performed correctly after instruction.

One questionnaire used is the Mood Adjective Checklist, which requires subjects to rate each of 24 adjectives on a 4-point Likert scale ranging from *not at all* to *very much*. The Postoperative Questionnaire is used to collect patients' self-report of physical activity in two places on the questionnaire. Although the formats of these questions are not specified, the data are reported as a summing of specified activities occurring while out of bed and comparing with the total times reportedly out of bed.

It appears that analgesic use and length of hospital stay are determined appropriately from chart review. These data are used for hypotheses testing.

Reliability and Validity

The Mood Adjective Scale is reported to have internal consistency with alpha coefficients of .84 for positive moods and .78 for negative moods in this study; these are above the acceptable limit of .70. Interrater reliability of 88% is reported for the rating of exercise performance and 92% for determination of time necessary for patients to perform the exercise behaviors, which are also within acceptable limits. No reliability information is reported for the Postoperative Questionnaire or for the measures of analgesic use and length of hospital stay.

Construct validity is adequately supported for the Mood Adjective Checklist; divergent validity is indicated through the negative correlation of the positive and negative mood subscales and with a previously established six-factor structure. It is assumed that the factor analysis supports the presence of three positive and three negative feeling states, and the negative correlation between the positive and negative subscale scores supports that the scales measure different feeling states.

The content and face validity for the Exercise Checklist in relation to the intervention booklet are established by three recovery room nurses; this number seems adequate. Pretesting of the booklet for readability and understanding (face validity) was conducted.

Construct validity is reported for the measure of physical activity from the Postoperative Questionnaire through a correlation of .89 between two measures. This measure seems an appropriate and accurate indicator of physical activity.

Validity of analgesic use and length of stay is not reported.

Analysis of Data

The Mood Adjective Checklist is an interval level of measurement derived by summing the ratings of the 12 adjectives for each of the positive and negative subscales, resulting in a score ranging from 12 to 48. Both preoperative performance measures are ratios: a score for the number of behaviors performed on admission and the number of minutes teaching time required to perform all 34 behaviors correctly. Postoperative measures of the number of times out of bed, daily doses of pain medications, and number of days hospitalized postoperatively are all ratio level measures.

Rice et al. (1992) report results of data analyses using descriptive and inferential statistics. Descriptive statistics reported are frequencies, percentages, means, and standard deviations for sample description, and means and standard deviations for summarizing measures of postadmission and postoperative dependent variables. Results of the analysis using inferential statistics are reported. The *t* test establishes comparability of the groups by testing for differences in age, education, cardiopulmonary pump time, aortic clamp time, and intensive care unit time of patients, as well as for differences between the two groups' postadmission moods, exercise behaviors, and teaching time, and their postoperative moods, physical activity, injection analgesics, oral analgesics, and length of hospital stay.

The statistics reported are appropriate for use with interval or ratio data. The use of inferential statistics to test differences in the specified variables postadmission and postoperatively in the experimental and control groups is appropriate to testing the hypotheses that the patients receiving preadmission instruction will have more positive mood states, perform more exercise behaviors correctly, require less teaching time, have higher activity scores, use fewer analgesics, and have shorter hospital stays. The level of significance set for the study is not specified but assumed to be .05.

Three tables are used to present detailed information. These tables are precisely titled and headed, and they supplement the content on data analyses presented in the narrative. Unnecessary repetition is avoided.

Conclusions, Implications, Recommendations

The hypotheses predict differences between CABG patients sent preadmission self-instructions and CABG patients instructed postadmission. On postadmission, the hypotheses that CABG patients sent preadmission self-instruction would have more positive moods, perform more exercise behaviors correctly, and require less teaching time are supported. The prediction that these patients would have less negative moods is not supported. Postoperatively, the hypotheses that preadmission-instructed patients would report higher positive and lower negative mood scores, have higher physical activity scores, use fewer analgesics, and experience shorter hospital stays are not supported.

The authors appropriately interpret the findings in relation to the study's purpose: that of comparing the effects of two approaches to teaching postoperative therapeutic exercise to the application of the Lazarus stress and coping framework and to previous research. Rice et al. (1992) identify the study's limitations as non-probability sampling and reliance on patients' self-report of activities after surgery rather than on direct measurement.

The researchers identify clinical relevance of preadmission teaching of therapeutic exercise as potentially lowering costs through shorter hospitalization and shortening teaching time postadmission. The authors are appropriately cautious in not making any generalizations beyond the potential clinical relevance and further indicate that the study's findings do not allow for any inferences regarding the impact of preadmission self-instruction on aspects of postoperative recovery.

The authors do identify a number of areas for further research. These include determination of clinical or economic importance of time saved through use of preoperative self-instruction, determination of additional benefits gained by patients' receiving preadmission information, closer examination of the proposed link between meeting needs for information and reduced threat through measures of perceived threat appraisal, and examination of different types of information related to the perioperative experience that would facilitate coping.

Application to Nursing Practice

The research conducted seems valid. The study is conceptualized from an existing theoretical framework and contributes to the accumulation of nursing knowledge by building upon previous research. The methodological design provides a precise test of the hypotheses. The weaknesses identified are limited to the use of nonprobability sampling and the threat of instrumentation produced by reliance on patients' self-report of postoperative physical activities.

The present research provides a partial replication of previous research by Rice and Johnson. Postadmission results are similar in the two studies. Patients provided preadmission self-instruction perform more exercise behaviors and require less teaching time than patients instructed postadmission.

For patients who would be taught postoperative exercises on admission, no apparent risks are identified in the use of the preoperative self-instructional exercise booklet. The potential benefit to the patient is enhanced postoperative recovery.

The authors' identification of potential time, effort, and monetary savings associated with the use of preoperative self-instruction seems realistic. The balance of potential benefits without apparent risks for patients supports feasibility of application. According to the Stetler model for research utilization, the presence of two studies with similar findings suggests readiness for translation/application to nursing practice (see Chapter 3). Replication of the research with other populations and settings is possible and advisable.

Critique of a Research Study: Sample No. 2

The study "Relocation Appraisal, Functional Independence, Morale, and Health of Nursing Home Residents" by Kathleen A. Gass, PhD, RN; Gail Gausted, MSN, RN; Marilyn T. Oberst EdD, RN; and Susan Hughes, MS, RN, published in *Issues in Mental Health Nursing* (1992), is critiqued. The article is presented first and is followed by the critique on p. 474.

Relocation Appraisal, Functional Independence, Morale, and Health of Nursing Home Residents*

Kathleen A. Gass, PhD, RN
Rutgers, The State University, College of Nursing, Newark, New Jersey

Gail Gaustad, MSN, RN
Meriter Hospital, Madison, Wisconsin

Marilyn T. Oberst, EdD, RN

Susan Hughes, MS, RN
School of Nursing, University of Wisconsin, Madison, Wisconsin

Relocation to a nursing home can be stressful and may result in mental and physical illness. Appraisal, or the meaning assigned to relocation, can influence relocation outcome. This study examined the relationships between appraisal of relocation and 30 nursing home residents' psychological and physical health, morale, functional independence, and demographic and situational factors, including age, gender, income, education, prior residence, participation in the decision to relocate, and preparation for the move. Positive, benign, and challenge appraisals were related to higher morale and functional independence. Threat appraisal was related to poorer psychological health and lower morale. Harm-loss appraisal was associated with lower morale and lower functional independence. Preparation for the move was related to higher positive appraisal, higher morale, functional independence, and lower harm-loss scores. Implications include the need to assess people's appraisal of relocation so as to plan strategies that prevent relocation stress.

People 65 years and older are the largest growing sector of the population in the United States today. Increased longevity has resulted in an increase in demand and need for health care services, including nursing home placement. Experts estimate that more than 20% of Americans over 65 will spend some time in a nursing home and these people are often functionally dependent and frail (Freudenheim, 1987). Relocation from one residence to another can be a stressful event for older adults that may precipitate illness or death (Pruncho & Resch, 1988; Thomasma et al., 1990; Young, 1990). Lieberman (1961) observed a rise in the mortality rate of nursing home applicants within 1 year of admission. Older adults who experienced a radical environmental change became more pessimistic about their health than those who experienced a moderate or no environmental change (Bourestom & Pastalan, 1975). Although the direction of causality for failing health was not established, Spasoff et al. (1978) found that new residents' functional health declined during 4 weeks following relocation and this decline persisted at one year. Nirenberg (1983) observed more withdrawn, passive behaviors, including a decrease in interactive behaviors, talking, food consumption, grooming, cleaning activities, and vigor from subjects with lower functioning following relocation, while higher functioning subjects were found to be more active and outgoing. Other researchers have found relocation to have minimal or no effects on health

---

*Issues in Mental Health Nursing, 13:239-253, 1992. Copyright © 1992 by Hemisphere Publishing Corporation. Reprinted with permission.

outcomes (Borup et al., 1980; Pablo, 1977), including very little effect on life satisfaction, morale, and behavioral patterns (Raasoch et al., 1977).

Research has been focused on the identification of factors that influence relocation outcome (Burnette, 1986). Environmental preparation for the move (Amenta et al., 1984; Haddad, 1981; Pablo, 1977; Wolanin, 1978; Zweig & Csank, 1975), participation in selecting the residence, and choices while living in the nursing home (Kapp, 1991; Pohl & Fuller, 1980; Poplawski, 1983; Schulz & Brenner, 1977) have been identified as conditions that relate to a positive relocation outcome, as well as high morale and better functional status (Pino et al., 1978). Positive attitude about the move, younger age, female gender, good health, high life satisfaction, frequent contacts with friends and kin, having not lived in a neighborhood for a long time, improved environment, and higher economic and social status are reported to be predictors of a positive relocation outcome (Borup et al., 1980; Blenker, 1967; Hasselkus, 1978; Kasl, 1972; Kowalski, 1981; Mirotznik & Ruskin, 1984; Pablo, 1977; Stein et al., 1985). Some investigators have found opposite findings or no differences in the effects of some of these factors on relocation outcome, such as Kowalski (1978) who found that females had a higher mortality rate than males and that age was not related to mortality following relocation.

One factor that likely influences relocation outcome is the appraisal or meaning assigned to relocation by the older person. Interestingly, few attempts have been made to assess appraisal in stressful situations (Folkman & Lazarus, 1980; Gass, 1987; Gass & Chang, 1989;

Oberst et al., 1989). While the importance of a positive attitude or realistic perception about the move has been reported in the literature (Stein et al., 1985; Rosswurm, 1983), no studies were found that have focused on a systematic examination of the meaning of relocation to older persons and how meaning is related to some relocation predictors and health outcome. The way in which the individual appraises the situation may be a more meaningful predictor of risk for morbidity or mortality following relocation than other variables mentioned previously, because appraisal guides coping responses (Lazarus & Folkman, 1984).

The purposes of this study were to examine relationships between appraisal of relocation and nursing home residents' (1) functional independence, (2) perceived physical and psychological health, (3) morale, and (4) demographic and situational factors, including age, gender, economic status, educational level, type of prior residence, and extent of participation in the decision to relocate. Three hypotheses were tested: (1) Relocated older adults who appraise relocation to the nursing home more positively will have higher functional independence, higher self-ratings of psychological and physical health status, and higher morale than relocated older adults who appraise relocation less positively; (2) There are differences in appraisal of relocation for recently relocated older adults who have had different types of prior residence, different participation in the decision-making process to relocate to a nursing home, and different gender; (3) There is a relationship between older adults' appraisal of relocation and their age, economic status, and educational level.

METHODOLOGY
Sample

A convenience sample of 30 recently relocated older adult nursing home residents from nine long-term care facilities in the midwest was studied. The criteria for inclusion in the study were English-speaking people: aged 60 or older; admitted to the nursing home one year ago or less with no prior history of nursing home admission; able to correctly identify themselves by first or last name and place of residence; with no history of moderate to severe cognitive or psychiatric impairment; able to see and hear. Subjects ranged in age from 68 to 96 years ($\bar{x}$ age = 83.8), with the majority being female (76.7%, n = 23) and widowed (76.7%). The mean years in last residence prior to nursing home admission was 18.31 years (SD = 17.37). Eighty percent (n = 24) of all the residents expected to stay within the nursing home indefinitely. Characteristics of the sample and characteristics of the relocation situation are presented in Tables 1 and 2, respectively.

Theoretical Framework

The theoretical framework that guided this study was Lazarus and Folkman's (1984) stress-appraisal-coping framework, which postulates that potentially stressful situations such as relocation are repeatedly evaluated in terms of their significance or meaning to the individual's

Table 1   Characteristics of the Sample

Variable and categories	Number reporting	(%)
Educational level		
Less than ninth grade	9	30.0
9 to 12 years	7	23.3
High school with additional education	13	43.4
Missing	1	3.3
Economic status		
Less than $10,000 per year	18	60.0
$10,000 to $25,000 per year	9	30.0
$25,000 to $50,000 per year	3	10.0
Major health problems		
Mobility problems	21	70.0
Sensory losses	5	16.7
Diabetes	2	6.7
Chronic obstructive pulmonary disease	1	3.3
Missing	1	3.3
Type of prior residence		
Living independently in the community in own home or apartment	20	66.7
Senior housing facility	10	33.3

Table 2   Characteristics of the Relocation Situation

Variable and categories	Number reporting	(%)
Reasons for relocation		
Inability to live independently	12	40.0
Illness or injury	10	33.3
Need for medical care or physician's order	6	20.0
Request of children	2	6.7
Decision period prior to admission to the nursing home		
Less than 1 week	19	63.2
1 to 4 weeks	5	16.7
Greater than 1 month to 6 months	2	6.7
Greater than 6 months	2	6.7
Missing	2	6.7
Degree of participation in the decision to relocate		
No participation	11	36.7
Agreed with family, friends, and/or health care providers on the need for nursing home care	7	23.3
Made the decision independently	6	20.0
Selected the nursing home for relocation	5	16.7
Missing	1	3.3
Type of preparation received prior to relocation to the nursing home		
No preparation	14	46.6
Talked with a resident who lived in a nursing home	6	20.0
Received verbal information from family, friends, and/or health providers	5	16.7
Received reading materials	2	6.7
Visited the nursing home prior to relocation	2	6.7
Missing	1	3.3

well-being, and that this evaluation guides coping responses. Primary appraisal, which focuses on meaning, helps the person to identify whether the situation is stressful, while secondary appraisal determines what can be done about it. There are three kinds of primary appraisal: irrelevant, benign-positive, and stressful. An irrelevant appraisal results when an event has no implications for the individual's well-being. Relocation has not been perceived as an irrelevant event. When a favorable or definitely positive outcome is anticipated, the situation is viewed as benign or positive, respectively. A situation is appraised as stressful when it is appraised as: a harm or loss in which the damage is already done; a threat or the potential for harm or losses; or a challenge, which is a difficult situation with an opportunity for mastery or gain (Folkman & Lazarus, 1980). While a challenge appraisal is stressful, it is a positive and higher level response than appraisal of a situation as a threat or harmful loss. Thus positive, benign, and challenge appraisal types are favorable or positive responses while harm-loss and threat appraisal types are negative responses. The processes of primary and secondary appraisal are repetitive, allowing for reappraisal of the situation. Primary and secondary appraisal reoccur until the stressor is neutralized or adaptation results.

Procedure

The data collection procedure involved the Directors of Nursing of nine long-term care facilities who were mailed a letter that described the study and sought their assistance in identifying residents who fit the selection criteria for participation. A follow-up telephone call was made to the Directors of Nursing to schedule an appointment to discuss the study. The Director of Nursing or a designated staff member met with the residents and assessed their interest in participating in the study. Residents who decided to participate met with a nurse researcher who explained the study in detail and obtained informed consent. During a 45- to 60-min interview, residents completed the Relocation Appraisal Scale, Self Ratings of Physical and Psychosocial health, and the Background Information Questionnaire. The Katz Index was completed by a nursing assistant who cared for the resident, and the Behavior Morale Scale (BMS) was completed by both a nursing assistant and one researcher who were familiar with the resident. The average of the nursing assistant's and researcher's BMS scores was used in the analysis.

Instruments

The Relocation Appraisal Scale (RAS) is a newly developed 79-item self-report instrument designed to measure the meaning of nursing home relocation in terms of the degree of five appraisal dimensions: (1) harm/loss (17 items), (2) threat (18 items), (3) challenge (17 items), (4) benign (13 items), and (5) positive (14 items). The items were generated to address broadly defined areas that were suggested in the research and clinical literature to be affected by relocation. These areas include responsibilities, life-style, physical health, emotional health, personal loss/growth, relationships, independence, control, goals, finances, self-esteem, mobility, self-care, and personal privacy. Content validity of the questionnaire was established through input from relocated older adults, health care providers involved in the care of people relocated to a nursing home, and people knowledgeable about the stress-appraisal-coping framework that guided the development of the instrument. The internal consistency reliabilities of the RAS for this initial study were threat, $\alpha = .88$; harm/loss, $\alpha = .84$; challenge, $\alpha = .89$; benign, $\alpha = .54$; and positive, $\alpha = .90$. Construct validity for the RAS was not established in this study. Construct validity of the RAS will be assessed in future studies by examining relationships among types of relocation appraisal and ways of coping, psychological health, and physical health within the context of Lazarus and Folkman's (1984) theoretical framework. A five-point Likert response format is used, with choices ranging from 1 (very untrue) to 5 (very true). Higher scores on each of the five appraisal subscales represent greater amounts of that appraisal dimension. Examples of items are shown in Table 3.

Self-Ratings of Physical and Psychological Health were measured by using Cantril ladders, which are equal-interval 10-point scales ranging from 1 to 10, 1 representing poor physical or psychological health and 10 representing per-

Table 3   Relocation Appraisal Scale: Examples of Items

Subscales

Threat

 I worry that friends and/or family might withdraw from me.
 I fear I might lose control over my life.
 I worry that I'll have to give up a lot of things in the future.

Harm/loss

 I've had real financial losses as a result of this move.
 My relationships with family and friends have suffered a lot.
 I feel a sense of loss at the things I've had to give up.

Challenge

 This move really challenges me to find new ways of maintaining my own independence.
 It's going to be hard to meet all of my responsibilities, but I feel confident that I can do so.
 It's hard to keep feeling good emotionally, but I feel I can meet this challenge.

Benign

 This move to this nursing home does not affect my life-style.
 My responsibilities will continue to be what they were before moving to the nursing home.
 This move isn't especially stressful for me.

Positive

 My physical health has improved since I came to the nursing home.
 I feel better about myself since the move.
 It has been easier to care for myself since moving here.

fect physical or psychological health (Palmore & Luikart, 1972). The respondent was asked to rate his or her physical and psychological health on the scales. An adapted version of the Cantril ladder has been used with elderly subjects (Engle & Graney, 1985-1986) with a reported test/retest reliability of .57 (Palmore & Luikart, 1972).

The Katz Index of Independence in Activities of Daily Living was used to measure the independence of subjects in their performance of six hierarchically related functions: (1) bathing, (2) dressing, (3) toileting, (4) transferring, (5) continence, and (6) feeding. The observer used the six-item observational rating scale and identified one of the three degrees of independent-dependent behavior for each of the six functions.

The observer rated subjects' activities of daily living status as they existed during a 2-week period preceding the evaluation, using the guidelines on the scoring sheet for the instrument. Interrater reliability coefficients for the Katz Index are .95 and .98 (Kane & Kane, 1981).

The Behavior Morale Scale (BMS), developed by MacElveen (1977), consists of a set of observable behaviors indicative of morale. The rater observed verbal and nonverbal behavior of subjects for a brief period, and then rated them on each of 17 items on the BMS using a five-point scale. Items focus on posture, body attitude, motor movements, facial expression, speech and verbalizations, and general attitude. A high BMS score indicates high morale. Cronbach coefficient alpha reliability for the BMS in the present study was .94 (researcher's observations) and .91 (nursing assistant's observations).

A Background Information Questionnaire was developed to obtain demographic data and information on situational factors reported to influence relocation outcome. Questions focused on age, gender, economic status, educational level, prior living circumstance, participation in the decision to relocate, length of decision period before relocation, and preparation for the move. All instruments were pretested for clarity, time, and ease of administration.

The time between relocation of the resident to the nursing home and the interview was less than 1 month (6.7%), 1 to 3 months (23.3%), 4 to 6 months (36.7%), 7 to 9 months (6.7%), and 10 to 12 months (26.6%). Pearson Product-Moment correlations and t-tests were used to test the hypotheses.

RESULTS

The first hypothesis was partially supported (see Table 4). Significant negative relationships were found between the challenge, benign, and positive subscales of the RAS and the Katz Index. That is, older adults who appraised relocation as a challenge or a benign or positive experience had higher functional independence. A positive relationship was found between the harm-loss appraisal subscale and the Katz Index scores: Those who appraised relocation as a harm-loss had lower functional independence. Threat appraisal was not significantly related to functional independence. A significant negative relationship was found between threat appraisal and psychological health. Appraisal was not significantly related to self-rating of physical health. Psychological and physical health rating mean scores were 6.90 (SD = 2.60) and 5.50 (SD = 2.37), respectively. More positive relocation appraisals (positive, benign, and challenge) were significantly related to higher morale in residents, while negative appraisals (threat and harm-loss) were related to lower morale.

The second hypothesis was not supported. There were no differences in scores on any of the appraisal subscales when the group was analyzed by type of prior residence, involvement in the relocation decision, or gender.

The third hypothesis was partially supported. Educational level was negatively related to challenge ($r = -.31$, $p < .05$) and positive ($r = -.33$, $p < .05$) appraisals of relocation. No significant relationships were found between types of relocation appraisal and age or economic status.

Other situational variables were

Table 4   Pearson Product-Moment Correlations Between Relocation Appraisal Subscales and the Katz Index, Self Ratings of Health, and Behavior Morale Scores

Relocation appraisal subscales	Katz index	Psychological health rating	Physical health rating	Behavior morale scale
Threat	.13	−.40*	−.21	−.42*
Harm/loss	.32*	−.20	−.41	−.44*
Challenge	−.32*	.23	.07	.33*
Benign	−.35*	.11	.16	.56**
Positive	−.40*	.15	−.02	.40*

*$p < .05$; **$p < .001$.

found to be related to some of the appraisal subscales, functional independence, and morale. Length of the decision period before relocation was negatively correlated with challenge scores ($r = -.39$, $p < .05$) and positively correlated with harm-loss scores ($r = .46$, $p < .01$). Preparation for the move was positively correlated with positive appraisal scores ($r = .36$, $p < .05$) and Behavior Morale scores ($r = .35$, $p < .05$), and negatively correlated with harm-loss scores ($r = -.33$, $p < .05$) and Katz scores ($r = -.40$, $p < .05$).

DISCUSSION

People moving to a nursing home are seldom asked how they view the move. Findings suggest that appraisal or the meaning of relocation is an important factor that is related to residents' functional independence, rating of psychological health, and morale. The higher the challenge, positive, and benign appraisals of relocation, the greater the person's functional independence. However, the higher the harm/loss appraisal, the lower the person's functional independence. Findings are in agreement with other studies, which have found more negative relocation outcomes among residents with impaired or limited physical functioning (Killian, 1970; Pino et al., 1978). Threat appraisal was not significantly related to functional ability. A threat appraisal is future-oriented and is concerned with harms and losses that have not yet taken place but are anticipated. This nonsignificant finding may be explained by the relocation event having already occurred and many subjects' expressions of limited future orientation within their current environment. As threat appraisal of relocation

increased, older adults rated their psychological health more poorly. Lack of significant findings on the rating of physical health may be a reflection of small sample size and the difficulty expressed by many subjects in differentiating aging effects on physical health from the effects of relocation appraisal on physical health.

The results of this study indicated that the positive types of appraisal (i.e., challenge, positive, and benign appraisals) were associated with high morale. Conversely, negative relocation appraisals of harm/loss and threat were correlated with low morale. Since morale is a fluctuating state rather than a trait or unchanging attribute, many situational determinants, such as the meaning of the move, may affect morale and also be open to intervention. Learning how to reappraise the move to a nursing home more positively may in turn improve morale of residents.

No significant differences were found between people who had lived in the community and those who resided in a senior congregate housing facility prior to admission. This may be related to the similarity of the living environments in the community dwelling and senior housing facilities. Findings are in agreement with Borup (1982), who found that degree of environmental change did not affect relocation outcome.

Surprisingly, the results indicated no significant differences in appraisal of relocation between those who participated in the decision-making process to move and those who did not. The findings of this study conflict with prior research findings that suggest that voluntary participation in the move is an important factor in positive relocation outcome (Carp, 1977; Lawton & Yaffe, 1970).

Voluntary participation allows for greater perceived controllability or predictability, thereby contributing to less harmful effects on the person (Schulz & Brenner, 1977). Lack of significant differences may be a reflection of the quality of participation. Eighteen of the subjects reported participation in the decision-making process, with 63.3% reporting a decision period of less than 1 week prior to admission. This brief decision period was most often due to hospitalization prior to admission. The quality of participation in the decision to relocate may have been influenced by a stressful event, namely, hospitalization, and the actual degree of controllability and preparation may have been limited. The time period available to decide about relocating to a nursing home and preparation for the move may be more critical variables affecting relocation appraisal than participation in the decision to relocate. Findings suggested that the shorter the decision period regarding relocation, the higher the challenge and the lower the harm-loss appraisals by residents. Preparation for relocation was related to higher positive and lower harm-loss appraisals as well as higher functional independence and morale.

Age and economic status were not significantly related to relocation appraisal and there were no gender differences in appraisal. The small sample of males may have influenced these results. Unexpectedly, the challenge and positive appraisals were negatively related to educational level. The higher the educational level of the residents, the lower their challenge and positive appraisals of relocation. Further research is needed to explain these findings. It may be that older adults with more education have more knowledge about relocation, and thus perceive it as less of a challenge, or they have had to give up more conveniences that they had when living independently in the community, which makes them perceive relocation less positively.

LIMITATIONS AND RECOMMENDATIONS FOR FUTURE RESEARCH

Several limitations of the study may have influenced the findings. A small convenience sample was studied, composed primarily of healthy females. Subjects had resided in the nursing home 1 year or less, making it difficult to ascertain whether relocation appraisals were the result of the relocation event itself, or a function of living within institutional settings with different staff, health services, and social activity characteristics. Recommendations for future research are: to study a larger random sample to facilitate more generalizability of findings, and to design a longitudinal study to assess relocation appraisal prior to the event of relocation and several times during 1 year following relocation in order to investigate changes in relocation appraisal over time and how changes influence functioning, morale, and health ratings of residents. Further reliability testing of the Relocation Appraisal Scale is warranted using a larger, more heterogeneous population of nursing home residents. The Relocation Appraisal subscales, with the exception of the benign subscale, have good reliability. Three items on the benign subscale had less than .1 corrected item correlation. These items included "This move doesn't affect my financial security"; "This move doesn't affect my relationships with others"; and "This move hasn't affected my ability to stay mobile or move about on my own." Improved reliability on the benign subscale may result with the revision or exclusion of these troublesome items and inclusion of additional favorable items in future testing of the instrument.

IMPLICATIONS

Findings from this study have implications for nursing for the delivery of quality mental health care to nursing home residents. However, caution is warranted when considering these implications since the RAS is in the early stages of development and further testing and evaluation is needed. Policies that address assessment of appraisal of relocation for nursing home residents needed to be developed and implemented. Assessment of the meaning of relocation to older persons can be accomplished by using questionnaires such as the Relocation Appraisal Scale as a part of a preadmission or admission screening. Assessment can provide knowledge of types of relocation appraisal and can help identify older adults at risk for negative relocation appraisal, which may result in mental health problems or poor morale. Problem areas such as a person's financial worries, concern over carrying out responsibilities, and unwelcome life-style changes can be pinpointed. If preadmission screening reveals that an older person has a negative perception of the relocation experience, nurses can teach and assist these older adults to mobilize effective coping strategies and resources to enhance successful relocation. Appraisal of relocation may change over time, which suggests that there may be a need to reassess periodically how residents view their relocation to their new home rather than to rely on the initial evaluation.

Preparation should be an integral part of relocation plans for all elderly people and their families and should focus on the positive aspects of the new home. Residents with negative appraisals of relocation may learn how to reappraise the relocation situation more positively through preparation and counseling that might include a discussion of positive and negative meanings about the move, concerns and needs identified on screening, and choices available to them in their new home such as preferred floor, possessions, room, and roommate. Preparation should also include a discussion of: written information related to admission criteria, financial requirements, activities, programs, and visitation schedules; medical and nursing care available in the nursing home; and tours or slide shows of the facility. Opportunities for questions and answers about the new home need to be provided. For some older people, the nurse may need to provide emotional and social support prior to, during, and after relocation. This can be effectively accomplished through a staff-resident buddy system where the nurse buddy visits the resident daily and assists him or her to view the move as a resource rather than a negative experience. The nurse buddy imparts an optimistic and favorable attitude toward relocating and provides opportunities for meaningful involvement. Preparation and counseling can help make the relocation process more predictable and enhance feelings of control that will influence positive feelings about moving to the nursing home and may reduce mental health problems. Findings suggest that type of appraisal of relocation is related to nursing home residents' psychological health, morale, and functional independence. Nurses need to assess the older person's appraisal of the relocation event so as to effectively plan and implement strategies that promote successful relocation and manage or prevent relocation stress.

REFERENCES

Amenta, M., Weiner, A., & Amenta, D. (1984). Successful relocation. *Geriatric Nursing, 11,* 356-360.

Blenker, M. (1967). Environment change and the aging individual. *The Gerontologist, 7,* 101-105.

Borup, J.H. (1982). The effects of varying degrees of inter-institutional environmental change on long-term care patients. *The Gerontologist, 22,* 409-417.

Borup, J.H., Gallego, D.T., & Hefferman, P. (1980). Relocation: its effect on health functioning and mortality. *The Gerontologist, 20,* 468-479.

Bourestom, N.C., & Pastalan, L. (1975). *Final report, forced relocation: setting, staff and patient effects.* University of Michigan, Ann Arbor: Institute of Gerontology.

Burnette, K. (1986). Relocation and the elderly: changing perspectives. *Journal of Gerontological Nursing, 12,* 6-11.

Carp, F.M. (1977). The impact of environmental settings on the lives of older people. *The Gerontologist, 7,* 106-108.

Engle, V.E., & Graney, M.J. (1985-86). Self-assessed and functional health of older women. *International Journal of Aging and Human Development, 22,* 301-313.

Folkman, S., & Lazarus, R.S. (1980). An analysis of coping in a middle-aged community sample. *Journal of Health and Social Behavior, 21,* 219-239.

Freudenheim, M. (1987). Officials warn of gaps in insurance for the aged. *New York Times,* Jan. 16.

Gass, K.A. (1987). The health of conjugally bereaved older widows: the role of appraisal, coping and resources. *Research in Nursing and Health, 10,* 39-47.

Gass, K.A., & Chang, A.S. (1989). Appraisals of bereavement, coping, resources, and psychosocial health dysfunction in widows and widowers. *Nursing Research, 38,* 31-36.

Haddad, L. (1981). Intra-institutional relocation: measured impact upon geriatric patients. *Journal of the American Geriatrics Society, 29,* 86-88.

Hasselkus, B.R. (1978). Relocation stress and the elderly. *The American Journal of Occupational Therapy, 32,* 631-636.

Kane, R.A., & Kane, R.L. (1981). *Assessing the elderly: a practical guide to measurement.* Lexington, MA: Lexington Books, DC Heath.

Kapp, M.B. (1991). Health care decision making by the elderly: I get by with a little help from my family. *The Gerontologist, 31,* 619-623.

Kasl, S.V. (1972). Physical and mental effects of involuntary relocation and institutionalization on the elderly: a review. *American Journal of Public Health,* March, 377-383.

Killian, E.C. (1970). Effects of geriatric transfer on mortality rates. *Social Work, 15,* 19-26.

Kowalski, N.C. (1978). Fire at a home for the aged: a study of short term mortality following dislocation of elderly residents. *Journal of Gerontology, 33,* 601-602.

Kowalski, N.C. (1981). Institutional relocation: current programs and applied approaches. *The Gerontologist, 21,* 512-519.

Lawton, M.P., & Yaffe, S. (1970). Mortality and morbidity and voluntary change of residence by older people. *Journal of the American Geriatrics Society, 18,* 823-831.

Lazarus, R.S., & Folkman, S. (1984). *Stress, appraisal and coping.* New York: Springer.

Lieberman, M.A. (1961). Relationship of mortality rates to entrance to a home for the aged. *Geriatrics, 16,* 515-519.

MacElveen, P.M. (1977). An observational measure of patient morale: the behavior-morale scale. In M. Batey (Ed.), *Communicating nursing research: nursing research in the bicentennial year* (Vol. 9). Boulder, CO: Western Interstate Commission for Higher Education.

Mirotznik, J., & Ruskin, A.P. (1984). Inter-institutional relocation and its effects on health. *The Gerontologist, 24,* 286-291.

Nirenberg, T.D. (1983). Relocation of institutional elderly. *Journal of Consulting and Clinical Psychology, 51,* 693-701.

Oberst, M.T., Thomas, S.E., Gass, K.A., & Ward, S.E. (1989). Caregiving demands and appraisal of stress among family caregivers. *Cancer Nursing, 12,* 209-215.

Pablo, R.Y. (1977). Intra-institutional relocation: its impact on long-term care patients. *The Gerontologist, 17,* 426-435.

Palmore, E., & Luikart, C. (1972). Health and social factors related to life satisfaction. *Journal of Health and Social Behavior, 13,* 68-80.

Pino, C.J., Rosica, L.M., & Carter, T.J. (1978). The differential effects of relocation on nursing home patients. *The Gerontologist, 18,* 167-172.

Pohl, J.M., & Fuller, S.S. (1980). Perceived choice, social interaction, and dimensions of morale of residents in a home for the aged. *Research in Nursing and Health, 3,* 147-157.

Poplawski, B. (1983). The stress of relocation. *Nursing Homes, 11,* 33-34.

Pruncho, R.A., & Resch, N. (1988). Institutional relocation: mortality effects. *The Gerontologist, 28,* 311-317.

Raasoch, J., Willmuth, R., Thomson, L., & Hyde, R. (1977). Intra-hospital transfer: effects on chronically ill psychogeriatric patients. *Journal of the American Geriatric Society, 25,* 281-284.

Rosswurm, M.A. (1983). Relocation and the elderly. *Journal of Gerontological Nursing, 9,* 632-637.

Schulz, R., & Brenner, G. (1977). Relocation of the aged: a review and theoretical analysis. *Journal of Gerontology, 32,* 323-333.

Spasoff, R., Kraus, A., Beattie, E., Holden, D., Lawson, J., Rodenburg, M., & Woodcock, G. (1978). A longitudinal study of elderly residents of long-stay institutions. *The Gerontologist, 18,* 281-292.

Stein, S., Linn, M.W., & Stein, E.M. (1985). Patients' anticipation of stress in nursing home care. *The Gerontologist, 25,* 88-94.

Thomasma, M., Yeaworth, R.C., & McCabe, B.W. (1990). Moving day: relocation and anxiety in institutionalized elderly. *Journal of Gerontological Nursing, 16,* 18-25.

Wolanin, M. (1978). Relocation of the elderly. *Journal of Gerontological Nursing, 4,* 47-50.

Young, H. (1990). The transition of relocation to a nursing home. *Holistic Nursing Practice, 4,* 74-83.

Zweig, J.P., & Csank, J.Z. (1975). Effects of relocation on chronically ill geriatric patients of a medical unit: mortality rates. *Journal of the American Geriatric Society, 23,* 132-136.

INTRODUCTION TO CRITIQUE NO. 2

This critique examines the research reported by Gass, Gaustad, Oberst, and Hughes (1992) that "examined the relationships between appraisal of relocation and 30 nursing home residents' psychological and physical health, morale, functional independence, and demographic and situational factors" (p. 239). The purpose of this critique is to determine the quality of the research on the basis of the information provided in the report as well as its potential usefulness for nursing practice.

Problem and Purpose

The identified purposes are "to examine relationships between appraisal of relocation and nursing home residents' (1) functional independence, (2) perceived physical and psychological health, (3) morale, and (4) demographic and situational factors, including age, gender, economic status, educational level, type of prior residence, and extent of participation in the decision to relocate" (p. 241). The variables examined in this study include whether nursing home residents' appraisal of relocation is related to their perceived physical and psychological health, morale, and demographic and situational factors. The population specified is nursing home residents.

The authors appropriately identify the significance of the problem of relocation through their discussion of the increasing number of people over 65 in the United States, which has produced a greater need for health care, including nursing home placement. The potential impact of relocation on health with the possibility of illness and death support further study.

Review of Literature and Definitions

Consistent with the study's purpose, literature review includes the following concepts: older persons experiencing relocation, health in institutionalized elders, factors associated with relocation outcome, and appraisal of meaning assigned to relocation. Appraisal of relocation is identified as one factor likely to influence relocation outcome and is seen as significant "because appraisal guides coping responses" (p. 241). Appraisal of relocation is conceptually defined as "the meaning assigned to relocation by the older person" (p. 241). The relationship of these variables is based on Lazarus and Folkman's theory of stress-appraisal-coping.

The authors identify a gap in the literature as the lack of studies systematically examining the meaning of relocation, and its relationship of relocation predictors and health outcomes.

The majority of the sources cited by these authors are primary. The reference by Spasoff et al., in which the authors report their research, constitutes a primary source (cited in Gass et al., 1992). The article by Kasl (cited in Gass et al., 1992) appears to be a review of literature and therefore is an example of a secondary source.

Adequate measurement or operationalization of the variables is accomplished as follows: the subjects' appraisal of their relocation by use of the Relocation Appraisal Scale, their health status by use of Self-Ratings of Physical and Psychological Health, subjects' functional independence by observers' use of the Katz Index of Independence of Daily Living, and subjects' morale through use of the Behavior Morale Scale. Economic status, education, prior residence, length of decision period before relocation, and subjects' participation in the decision to relocate are measured via the Background Information Questionnaire.

Hypotheses and/or Research Questions

No research questions are used, but three hypotheses consistent with the review of the literature are stated in research form. They are the following:

1. Relocated older adults who appraise relocation to the nursing home more positively will have higher functional independence, higher self-ratings of psychological

and physical health status, and higher morale than relocated older adults who appraise relocation less positively.

    2. There are differences in appraisal of relocation for recently relocated older adults who have had different types of prior residence, different participation in the decision-making process to relocate to a nursing home, and different gender.

    3. There is a relationship between older adults' appraisal of relocation and their age, economic status, and educational level. (p. 241)

The first hypothesis is directional, indicating that the subjects who have more positive appraisal of their relocation will have higher functional independence, self-ratings of health status, and morale. Hypotheses numbers 2 and 3 are nondirectional, indicating differences and relationships but no direction. This is compatible with the review of the literature.

In the first hypothesis the independent variable is the appraisal of relocation, and the dependent variables are functional independence, self-ratings of psychological and physical health status, and morale. In the second hypothesis, types of prior residence, participation in the decision-making process to relocate to a nursing home, and gender are the variables identified as varying with the differences in appraisal of relocation. The third hypothesis predicts relationships among age, economic status, educational level, and older adults' appraisal of relocation.

Sample

The sample was selected by contacting nine directors of nursing in long-term care facilities who identified older adult nursing home residents who met the inclusion criteria. The directors of nursing or their designated staff identified those residents interested in participating. Then a nurse researcher met with interested residents, explained the study, and those who consented to participate were included in the study. This results in a nonprobability convenience sample and necessitates caution in generalizing beyond the sample. The sample is congruent with the purpose that designates the population as nursing home residents. The sample size is small, considering the number of variables being studied. However, the size may be considered adequate for the early stage of studying the identified problem and piloting the newly developed Relocation Appraisal Scale.

Research Design

Gass et al. (1992) use a nonexperimental design, specifically a correlational design. Correlational designs are nonexperimental, since there is no manipulation of an independent variable. This type of design permits the determination of whether two or more variables are related, as well as the direction and strength of the relationships. The design is consistent with the purposes of examining relationships between appraisal of relocation and the variables extrapolated from the literature review. The relationships of the variables are described by the stress and coping theoretical framework and expressed in the three stated hypotheses.

Internal Validity

Although the threats to internal validity are most clearly applicable to experimental research designs, attention to the relationships among the identified variables and rival interpretations that might potentially compromise the study is necessary for correlational designs as well. Possible threats of history, maturation, and mortality are not identified for this study. Testing is not a problem, since measures are taken only one time. Selection bias is noted as the major threat to internal validity because of the use of a small convenience sample. The lack of random selection negates control for such variables as differences in subjects' life experiences and differences in length of time since relocation. Potential threats associated with instrumentation occur in the use of multiple nursing assistants who provided care to the subjects to rate subjects' activity-of-daily-living status during a preceding 2-week period, as well as the averaging of a nursing assistant's and a researcher's score on the Behavior Morale Scale. Training of the nursing assistants in use of the observational instruments and interrater reliability checks are not reported. Confidence in the results is limited by these potential threats to internal validity.

External Validity

Generalizibility is limited to the sample because of the effect of sample selection.

Research Approach

Methods

Questionnaires and observations are used to collect data. Data collection procedures are described as the same for all subjects: the residents completed the questionnaires during an interview. The details of timing and management of the completion of the Katz Index and Behavior Morale Scale are not reported. It is evident that ethical standards are met; Gass et al. (1992) report that informed consent is obtained by a nurse researcher during the interview.

Instruments

Observations by nursing assistants are recorded by using the Katz Index of Independence in Activities of Daily Living. Both a nursing assistant and a nurse researcher complete the Behavior Morale Scale, which is based on brief periods of observations of verbal and nonverbal behaviors of the subjects. Both guides require the raters to make judgments about observed behaviors to rate subjects' functional independence and morale. The fact that the training of the observers is not described limits the ability to evaluate the consistency of the raters in the data collection process.

Three questionnaires are used. The Relocation Appraisal Scale is a 79-item instrument measuring five dimensions of appraisal and uses a Likert response format with responses ranging from 1 to 5 (very untrue to very true). The Self-Ratings of Physical and Psychological Health questionnaire used Cantril ladders, which are described as equal-interval 10-point scales ranging from 1 (poor health) to 10 (perfect health). However, the format of the Background Information Questionnaire is not described.

Reliability and Validity

Acceptable levels of internal consistency reliabilities reported from this study for the Relocation Appraisal Scale are .88 for threat, .84 for harm/loss, .89 for challenge, .54 for benign, and .90 for positive appraisal. The Self-Ratings of Physical and Psychological Health have a reported test/retest reliability of .57 indicating stability. No reliability is reported for the Background Information Questionnaire. Kane and Kane's "interrater reliability coefficients for the Katz Index" of .95 and .98 are cited by Gass et al. (1992, p. 246). Cronbach coefficient alphas indicating homogeneity for the Behavior Morale Scale are reported as .94 for the researcher's observations and .91 for the nursing assistant's observations in the study by Gass et al. (1992). The alpha of .54 for the benign appraisal subscale and the test/retest reliability of .57 for the self-rating scale are less than the desired .70 level. The other reported reliabilities are at acceptable levels.

Content validity for the Relocation Appraisal Scale is "established through input from relocated older adults, health care providers involved in the care of people relocated to a nursing home, and people knowledgeable about the stress-appraisal-coping framework that guided the development of the instrument" (Gass et al., 1992, p. 244). No information on the validity of the other instruments is provided. With so little information, the validity of the instruments must be questioned and the ability to generalize must be questioned.

Analysis of Data

Relocation appraisal subscale scores result from summing ratings of contributing items and as such are considered interval levels of measurement. Functional independence, measured by the Katz Index, is treated as interval by Gass et al. (1992) in the analysis, although the description lacks details necessary to ascertain the level of measurement. Self-ratings of psychological and physical health status use 10-point equal interval scales, treated as interval level. Determination of morale is based on a score derived from summing 17 items rated on a 5-point scale, an interval level of measurement. Types of prior residence, participation in the decision-making process, and gender appear to be used as the grouping variable for analyses using t tests and are considered a nominal level of measurement. Age is ratio level of measurement. Economic and educational level appear to have been treated as interval levels of measurement.

Descriptive statistics reported include range, frequency, mean, percentage, and standard deviation. The inferential statistic used was the Pearson product moment correlation. The descriptive statistics used are appropriate, as are the inferential statistical procedures, assuming interval levels of measurement. Pearson correlations test for the relationships specified in hypotheses one and three and t tests examine differences as predicted in hypothesis two. Gass et al. (1992) appear to be using .05 or less as the alpha level for significance, although this is not specifically stated.

Four tables are used to present detailed information. The tables are clearly titled and headed and supplement the content on data analyses presented in the narrative, thus preventing unnecessary repetition. Educational level, economic status, decision period before admission to the nursing home, and type of preparation received before relocation are reported as categorical data in tables 1 and 2, raising the question of whether more detailed information was collected on the Background Information Questionnaire, allowing its use as interval level for the Pearson Product-Moment correlations in the hypotheses testing.

Conclusions, Implications, Recommendations

The results of the hypotheses testing are mixed. Hypotheses one and three are partially supported. The second hypothesis is not supported. Gass et al. (1992) interpret the results within the stress-appraisal-coping framework and compare and contrast findings with previous research.

The two major limitations appropriately identified by the authors are (1) the size and makeup of the sample (primarily healthy women) and (2) the range of time of up to 1 year after relocation. These are identified as factors possibly clouding the interpretation of the findings in understanding relocation appraisals.

Possible clinical implications from the study are considered. Gass et al. (1992) appropriately identify the need for caution but also provide detailed suggestions for use of relocation appraisal by nurses in enhancing the coping of older adults and their families to "promote successful relocation and manage or prevent relocation stress" (p. 251). They note that the "findings suggest that type of appraisal of relocation is related to nursing home residents' psychological health, morale, and functional independence" (p. 251). This generalization is tentative (as indicated by the word *suggest*) but nicely reflects the complexity of the problem being studied and the preliminary findings about the problem appropriately.

Recommendations for future research include use of a larger sample that is randomly selected, use of a longitudinal design assessing relocation before the move and several times during the following year, and additional reliability testing of the Relocation Appraisal Scale.

Application to Nursing Practice

The study has merit, given the stage of the research program. The strengths include identification of a problem for which Gass et al. (1992) establish significance and frame conceptually within a theoretical model. A tool is developed for the major variable of concern with established content validity. The researchers address the limitations such as those associated with sample size and the need to establish reliability and validity of the Relocation Appraisal Scale. Additional limitations identified include lack of information on validity for several other instruments, as well as information on training of observers, use of multiple observers, and averaging of observers' scores.

The central variable of concern in this research—relocation appraisal—has not been examined in previous research. This omission is identified by the investigators in supporting the importance of studying the identified problem. Prior research findings related to selected variables in this study are reviewed and compared with present findings.

No risks are apparent in the incorporation of an assessment of relocation appraisal in planning relocation of elderly patients to nursing home settings. Benefits proposed by Gass et al. (1992) are management and prevention of relocation stress. Although there appear to be potential benefits without identified risks in assessing relocation appraisal, clinical application cannot be justified on the basis of the results of this study. The findings are not yet ready for direct application to practice. According to the Stetler model for research utilization, replication of the study is feasible and necessary (see Chapter 3).

REFERENCES

Gass, K.A., Gaustad, G., Oberst, M.T., & Hughes, S. (1992). Relocation appraisal, functional independence, morale, and health of nursing home residents. *Issues in Mental Health Nursing, 13,* 239-253.

Rice, V.H., Mullin, M.H., & Jarosz, P. (1992). Preadmission self-instruction effects on post-admission and postoperative indicators in CABG patients: Partial replication and extension. *Research in Nursing and Health, 15,* 253-259.

Stetler, C.M. (in press). Refinement of the Stetler/Marram model for application of research findings to practice. *Nursing Outlook.*

ADDITIONAL READINGS

American Psychological Association. (1983). *Publication manual of the American Psychological Association* (3rd ed.). Washington, DC: Author.

Funk, S.G., Tornquist, E.M., & Champagne, M.T. (1989). A model for improving the dissemination of nursing research. *Western Journal of Nursing Research, 11,* 361-367.

Kerlinger, F.N. (1986). *Foundations of behavioral research* (3rd ed.). New York: Holt, Rinehart, & Winston.

Larson, E. (1989). Using the CURN project to teach research utilization in a baccalaureate program. *Western Journal of Nursing Research, 11,* 593-599.

Stetler, C.B. (1985). Research utilization: Defining the concept. *Image: The Journal of Nursing Scholarship, 17,* 40-44.

Stetler, C.B., & Marram, G. (1976). Evaluating research for applicability in practice. *Nursing Outlook, 24,* 559-563.

CHAPTER 20

Evaluating the Qualitative Research Report

HELEN J. STREUBERT

LEARNING OBJECTIVES

After reading this chapter the student should be able to do the following:

- Identify the influence of stylistic considerations on the presentation of a qualitative research report.
- Identify the criteria for critiquing a qualitative research report.
- Evaluate the strengths and weaknesses of a qualitative research report.
- Describe the applicability of the findings of a qualitative research report.
- Construct a critique of a qualitative research report.

KEY TERMS

auditability   fittingness
credibility

Nursing research is focused on the generation of new knowledge. The information discovered through rigorous research methods assists nurses in the development, implementation, and evaluation of nursing interventions. For most of the early history of nursing research, nurse researchers have directed their endeavors toward objective, empirical research. The use of empiricism has contributed significantly to nursing. The compatibility of this approach with the phenomena of interest to nursing has been limited at times because of the focus on objectivity. Qualitative research is another means of generating nursing knowledge that provides opportunity for studying phenomena that are not able to be made objective. Because qualitative researchers are making important contributions to nursing, nurses should know how to evaluate qualitative research reports. In this chapter the reader is offered the criteria used to evaluate qualitative research studies. In addition, a published research report is presented to demonstrate the application of the criteria.

STYLISTIC CONSIDERATIONS

The presentation of a qualitative research report is different from that of a quantitative research report. In a qualitative research report, the reader will not find hypotheses, dependent and independent variables, large or randomized samples, statistical analyses, conceptual frameworks, or scaled instruments. Because the intent of the research is to describe or explain phenomena or culture, the report is generally written in a way that allows the researcher to convey the richness of the research. This is different from a quantitative research report. The goal of an empirical research report is to convey in an abbreviated manner the most critical aspects of the research findings. Numerical data that make up the findings section of a quantitative research article are reportable in abbreviated format. In contrast, the critique usually will include direct quotes from the participants that highlight themes. An example of this type of reporting can be found in Beck's (1992) study of postpartum depression. In describing the feeling of depression, the research participant described "going to the gates of hell and back. It was terrifying. I felt there was absolutely no way out of it. I was very suicidal. I loved my baby but I thought if this is the quality of life that I was going to have, there's no way. No way anybody can endure the kind of pain I was going through." (p. 168)

The ability of the qualitative researcher to convey the richness of the data and to do so within the publication guidelines of particular nursing journals is a challenge. In the past 5 to 6 years, more journals have recognized the importance of publishing qualitative research studies. Qualitative research studies are published most frequently in the following journals: *Image, Western Journal of Nursing Research, Advances in Nursing Science, Qualitative Health Research, Research in Nursing and Health,* and *Nursing Science Quarterly.*

Guidelines for the publication of research reports generally are listed in nursing publications. Criteria for publication of research based on the type of research method that is chosen—that is, quantitative versus qualitative—are not stated. The primary goal of all journal editors is to provide articles that are informative and interesting to their readers. To meet this goal, regardless of the type of research report, the editors prefer to publish articles that have scientific merit, present new knowledge, and will interest their readers. The challenge for the qualitative researcher, like the quantitative researcher, is to demonstrate the significance of the work and its scientific merit within the page limitations imposed by the journal of interest. The qualitative researcher also must be aware of the traditional evaluation of research within the context of empirical research and therefore the challenge of the necessity of presenting the richness of data but also imparting the scientific merit of the work in a concise report. In Table 20-1, pp. 484-485, the reader is provided with general criteria to be used in evaluating the scientific merit and significance of qualitative research. You are directed to Chapter 11 for additional information on the specifics of qualitative research design.

APPLICATION OF QUALITATIVE RESEARCH FINDINGS IN PRACTICE

The purpose of qualitative research is to describe or explain a phenomenon or culture. Because the goal is not to predict or control, the findings of qualitative research are used differently from findings of quantitative research. For example, the results of qualitative research are not generalizable to larger groups. The individual who plans to use the findings of qualitative research has the responsibility of validating whether the findings accurately reflect the phenomenon in another setting. For instance, Hutchinson (1986), in describing the process chemically dependent nurses experience as part of their addiction, articulated a theory regarding chemical dependence in nurses. The theory she described was *grounded* in human experience. If her theory accurately reflects the process chemically dependent nurses experience, her ideas are applicable to chemically dependent nurses. Nurses who wish to apply her findings must validate through their own practice whether the process is applicable to those nurses with whom they work. Validation of her findings through empirical research adds further support to the results and subsequently adds to the chain of nursing research knowledge.

Similar to the findings of qualitative studies of particular processes or experiences, the findings from qualitative studies of culture also must be viewed within a context. In other words, the descriptions of culture documented through ethnographic study are specific to the culture studied. In the case of ethnographic research, the information collected on cultural norms, values, and mores can be applied only to

Table 20-1   CRITIQUING GUIDELINES FOR QUALITATIVE RESEARCH

Section	Questions to guide evaluation
Statement of the phenomenon of interest	1. Is the phenomenon of interest clearly identified? 2. Has the researcher identified why the phenomenon requires a qualitative design for study? 3. Are the philosophical underpinnings of the research described?
Purpose	1. Is the purpose of conducting the research made explicit? 2. Does the researcher describe the projected significance of the work to nursing?
Method	1. Is the method used to collect data compatible with the purpose of the research? 2. Is the method adequate to address the phenomenon of interest? 3. If a particular approach is used to guide the inquiry, does the researcher complete the study according to the processes described?
Sampling	1. Does the researcher describe the selection of participants? Is purposive sampling used? 2. Are the informants who were chosen appropriate to inform the research?
Data collection	1. Is data collection focused on human experience? 2. Does the researcher describe data collection strategies (i.e., interview, observation, field notes)? 3. Is protection of human subjects addressed? 4. Is saturation of the data described? 5. Are the procedures for collecting data made explicit?
Data analysis	1. Does the researcher describe the strategies used to analyze the data? 2. Has the researcher remained true to the data? 3. Does the reader understand the procedures used to analyze the data? 4. Does the researcher address the credibility, auditability, and fittingness of the data?
Credibility	a. Do the participants recognize the experience as their own?
Auditability	a. Can the reader follow the thinking of the researcher?

Table 20-1   CRITIQUING GUIDELINES FOR QUALITATIVE RESEARCH—cont'd

Section	Questions to guide evaluation
	b. Does the researcher document the research process?
Fittingness	a. Are the findings applicable outside the study situation?
	b. Are the results meaningful to individuals not involved in the research?
	5. Is the strategy used for analysis compatible with the purpose of the study?
Findings	1. Are the findings presented within a context?
	2. Is the reader able to apprehend the essence of the experience from the report of the findings?
	3. Are the researcher's conceptualizations true to the data?
	4. Does the researcher place the report in the context of what is already known about the phenomenon?
Conclusions, implications, and recommendations	1. Do the conclusions, implications, and recommendations give the reader a context

the group studied. A nurse who is interested in the cultural values of senior citizens living in an apartment complex in New York could not use the results generated from a study of this group and apply it to senior citizens living in a nursing home in Louisiana. The findings of all qualitative research studies are context-bound.

Nurses who wish to use the findings of qualitative research in their practice must validate either through their own observations or through interaction with groups similar to the study participants whether the findings accurately reflect their experience.

Another use of qualitative research findings is to initiate examination of important concepts in nursing practice. For example, in a study conducted by Miller, Haber, and Byrne (1992), the researchers used phenomenology to examine the concept of caring. The focus of the study was on patient and nurse perceptions of caring in acute care settings. This study adds to the existing body of knowledge on the concept of caring and offers the reader direction on the focus for future research related to this concept.

Finally, qualitative research can be used to discover information about a phenomenon of interest that can lead to development of research instruments. When qualitative methods are used to direct the development of a structured research instrument, it is usually part of a larger empirical research project. Instruments developed from qualitative research are useful to practicing nurses because they are grounded in the reality of human experience with a particular phenomenon.

Critique of a Qualitative Research Study

The following study, "The Lived Experience of Postpartum Depression: A Phenomenological Study," by Cheryl Tatano Beck, D.N.Sc., C.N.M., R.N., published in *Nursing Research* (1992), is critiqued. The article is presented in its entirety and followed by the critique.

The Lived Experience of Postpartum Depression: A Phenomenological Study

Cheryl Tatano Beck

The purpose of this phenomenological study was to describe the essential structure of the lived experience of postpartum depression. Seven mothers who had suffered from postpartum depression were interviewed regarding their subjective experiences. Data were analyzed using Colaizzi's (1978) method of phenomenology. Forty-five significant statements were extracted and clustered into 11 themes. These results were integrated into the essential structure of postpartum depression. Postpartum depression was a living nightmare filled with uncontrollable anxiety attacks, consuming guilt, and obsessive thinking. Mothers contemplated not only harming themselves but also their infants. The mothers were enveloped in loneliness and the quality of their lives was further compromised by a lack of emotions and all previous interests. Fear that their lives would never return to normal was all encompassing.

Within days of the birth of her daughter, a young woman describes her terrifying bout with depression: "I was transformed from a competent lawyer into a new mother crippled with doubt, confusion, and unshakable sadness. Too terrified to hold my baby, I cried even more than she did. My nightmarish postpartum depression lasted for months" (Balk, 1990, p. 38). In the United States the reported incidence of postpartum depression has ranged from 10% (Saks et al., 1985) to 26% (Atkinson & Rickel, 1984). Postpartum depression not only may have devastating effects on mothers, as evidenced by the above quote, but also may have adverse consequences on young children's general behavioral and developmental functioning (Fleming, Ruble, Flett, & Shaul, 1988; Whiffen & Gotlib, 1989).

For clarification purposes, postpartum depression needs to be differentiated from maternity blues and postpartum psychosis. Postpartum depression is similar to a minor or major depressive episode as defined by the Research Diagnostic Criteria (Spitzer, Endicott, & Robins, 1978). The clinical signs and symptoms of postpartum depression are comparable to nonpostpartum depression such as feelings of inadequacy, anxiety, despair, lack of energy, loss of interest in sexual activities, and compulsive thoughts. The content of the mother's depressive thoughts, however, are concentrated on her sense of inability to love or to love adequately and on their ambivalence towards the infant (Chalmers & Chalmers, 1986). Maternity blues

Reprinted from *Nursing Research*, 1992, 41(3). © American Journal of Nursing Company. Used with permission.

is a common transitory phenomenon of mood changes that begins within the first few days after delivery and lasts from one day through the first 10 days postpartum or longer. Postpartum psychosis, on the other hand, is a severe illness that occurs in only one or two per 1,000 deliveries (Kendell, 1984). The clinical features of postpartum psychosis include delusions, hallucinations, incoherence or loosening of associations, and grossly disorganized or catatonic behavior (Gjerdingen, Froberg, & Wilson, 1986). The delusional content may reflect themes of childbirth.

Through quantitative research the signs and symptoms of postpartum depression have been identified and categorized. These studies have relied heavily on the use of questionnaires to assess postpartum depression. What has not been researched, however, is the lived experience of postpartum depression. A lived experience is how a person immediately experiences the world prereflectively (Husserl, 1970). This deeper understanding of the nature or meaning of postpartum depression can offer insights that will assist in understanding the world of women who experience postpartum depression. To understand how women experience postpartum depression prereflectively, without classifying or categorizing it into signs and symptoms, a phenomenological approach was used. The purpose of this study was to describe postpartum depression as it is experienced in everyday life and to answer the research question: What is the essential structure of the lived experience of postpartum depression?

Tilden, Nelson, and May (1990) suggested the use of qualitative research to enhance the content validity of quantitative instruments. Since researchers have placed heavy emphasis on quantitative scales to measure postpartum depression, data from this phenomenological study were used not only to describe the essential structure of postpartum depression but also to assess the content validity of some of these measurement scales.

Method
Sample

A purposive sample of seven mothers participated in the study. All the mothers had attended a local postpartum depression support group which the researcher had helped to facilitate over the past year. The support group met twice a month. Attendance at each support group meeting varied from two to 10. The ages of the seven mothers who participated in the study ranged from 22 to 38. Three of the women had college degrees, four had high school diplomas. Four mothers were primiparas, three were multiparas. Four mothers had vaginal deliveries, and the remaining three had cesarean deliveries. Postpartum depression developed in five of the mothers within the first three weeks after delivery. The other two women did not begin to experience postpartum depression until 6 months and 7 months after birth. Six of the seven women had been or still were under the care of a psychiatrist. All six had been diagnosed by their psychiatrists as having postpartum depression. Three women had been hospitalized and two had undergone shock treatments for postpartum depression. Only one mother had not been under a psychiatrist's care. She had depended solely on the support group for help. At the time of the interviews the range in the length of time since delivery for these mothers was 3 months to 2½ years.

Research Design

Phenomenology is both a philosophical movement and a research method in which the main objective is to examine and describe phenomena as they are consciously experienced. It is without theories about causes and as free as possible from unexamined preconceptions and presuppositions (Spiegelberg, 1975). A basic philosophical assumption of phenomenology is that one can know what one experiences only by attending to perceptions and meanings that awaken conscious awareness (Husserl, 1962). Subject and object are united in being in the world.

To achieve the goal of the phenomenological method, the discovery of the meaning of human experiences, researchers must reawaken their own presuppositions and make them appear by abstaining from them for a moment (Merleau-Ponty, 1956). This process, called bracketing, involves peeling away the layers of interpretation so the phenomena can be seen as they are, not as they are reflected through preconceptions. Bracketing does not eliminate perspective. It brings the experience into clearer focus. As the layers of meaning that give persons interpreted experiences are laid aside, what is left is the perceived world prior to interpretation and explanation (Oiler, 1986).

Procedure

After the research proposal received approval from the university's Human Subjects Review Committee, women who were attending a postpartum depression support group in the southeastern United States were approached to participate in the study. Once the informed consent sheet was signed by the mother, she was asked to respond verbally to the following statement:

"Please describe a situation in which you experienced postpartum depression. Share all the thoughts, perceptions, and feelings you can recall until you have no more to say about the situation."

Prior to each interview the researcher attempted to bracket her experiential knowledge in order to capture the empirical reality outside herself (Swanson-Kauffman & Schonwald, 1988) and to portray accurately the reality described by the mothers who participated in the study.

Mothers were interviewed privately, either in their own homes or after a support group meeting in the psychiatric facility where the group met. All the mothers' interviews were tape recorded and then transcribed. The same researcher conducted all of the interviews. In order to ensure a full, accurate description of the phenomenon under study, data collection continued until repetition of data occurred without any new themes.

Data Analysis

Each transcript of the mother's oral descriptions of a postpartum depression experience was analyzed using Colaizzi's (1978) phenomenological methodology. Colaizzi's six procedural steps are as follows:

1. All the subjects' oral or written descriptions are read in order to obtain a feel for them.
2. From each transcript significant statements and phrases that directly pertain to postpartum depression are extracted.
3. Meanings are formulated from these significant statements and phrases.
4. The formulated meanings are organized into clusters of themes.
5. The results of the data analysis so far

are integrated into an exhaustive description of postpartum depression.

6. To achieve final validation, the researcher returns to the participants with the exhaustive description. Any new relevant data that are obtained from the participants are incorporated into the fundamental structure of the experience.

Credibility, Auditability, and Fittingness

Efforts to limit potential bias included identification of the researcher's perspective and bracketing it prior to data collection and analysis. To help ensure the credibility of the data, three of the seven mothers who participated in the study reviewed the exhausting description of postpartum depression to validate that it accurately captured the essence of their lived experience. This "member check" has been suggested by Guba and Lincoln (1985) as a validity check. Numerous quotes from the mothers' oral descriptions of postpartum depression were included in the results of the study to provide thick, rich slices of data. Also, tapes of each mother's oral descriptions were transcribed verbatim. Intersubjective agreement between the researcher and an independent judge, a master's-prepared nurse with experience in phenomenological analysis, was achieved at each phase of data analysis. Upon discussion with this independent judge, two of the original theme clusters were combined into one cluster.

The auditability of the study was enhanced by adding Hycner's (1985) suggestion of listing for each theme cluster its subsumed formulated meanings and their original numeration. This step clarified the transition of formulated meanings to theme clusters. Fittingness of the study was increased by seeking out participants from a postpartum depression support group who not only had experienced the phenomenon under study but also were able to articulate their experiences.

Results

Forty-five significant statements regarding a postpartum depression experience were extracted from the transcripts. Examples of the significant statements and their corresponding formulated meanings are given in Table 1. After these formulated meanings were identified, they were organized into 11 clusters of themes. Table 2 contains an example of the decision trail used for two of the cluster themes. The original number of the significant statements from which the formulated meaning was derived is listed in parentheses in this table. Eleven theme clusters emerged from the data.

Theme 1

Mothers were enveloped in unbearable loneliness due to discomfort with others and a belief that no one else understood what they were experiencing.

Feelings of loneliness prevailed because mothers felt that no one really understood the nightmare they were going through. Mothers would attempt to explain what they were experiencing to their husbands, other family members, and friends, but most attempts were unsuccessful. Typically the mothers were told to "just snap out of it. You have a husband who loves you and a beautiful healthy baby. What more do you want!" Because mothers' pleas for understanding often fell on deaf ears, they began to isolate themselves, since they no longer felt comfortable around others. Only one woman reported that someone understood the nightmare she was living

Table 1   Selected Examples of Significant Statements of Postpartum Depression and Corresponding Formulated Meanings

Significant Statements	Formulated Meanings
1. I was very suicidal because there was no way anyone could endure the kind of pain I was going through.	1. Suicidal thoughts prevailed as her quality of life became intolerable.
2. You want to be okay and you try, but the fogginess and fatigue would set in.	2. Attempts to overcome the depression were hindered by the fogginess and fatigue.
3. I was like a baby because I had to be taken care of and couldn't be left alone.	3. She perceived she had regressed to an infancy state where she was incapable of taking care of herself.
4. I would think, not that I would hurt my baby, but what if I didn't intervene to help him or to give him something.	4. She was horrified by her thoughts of not intervening to help her baby if he needed her.
5. I would lie awake at night having a lot of obsessive thinking.	5. She was haunted by obsessive thoughts while trying to fall asleep.

Table 2   Examples of Two Theme Clusters with Their Subsumed Formulated Meanings

The mother envisioned herself as a robot stripped of all feelings, just going through the motions.
   a. She would just go through the mechanics when caring for her baby. (1)
   b. Feelings of emptiness prevailed. (6)
   c. She was unable to feel any emotions. (9)
   d. She felt like a robot who just went through the motions. (15)
   e. Sheer exhaustion left the mother with nothing to give herself or her baby. (37)

Shrouded in fogginess the mother's ability to concentrate diminished.
   f. She felt as if she was drifting in a fog with her mind filled with cobwebs. (3)
   g. Attempts to overcome the depression were hindered by the fogginess and fatigue. (8).
   h. Loss of both concentration and sometimes motor skills occurred. (23)
   i. She experienced being in a totally different dimension. (38).

Note: Numbers in parentheses indicate the original numbers of significant statements from which meanings were derived.

through. The person was her own mother, who had experienced the disorder after the birth of one of her children. However, it was not diagnosed as postpartum depression at the time.

Theme 2

Contemplating death provided a glimmer of hope to the end of their living nightmare.

While mothers were immersed in postpartum depression, the thought of leaving this world was enticing. One mother stated that she had never been that low in her whole life, where she thought death was the way to go. Suffering in their aloneness, women felt trapped, as though there was no way out of this living hell. One mother summed it up as:

going to the gates of hell and back. It was terrifying. I felt there was absolutely no way out of it. I was very suicidal. I loved my baby but I thought if this is the quality of life that I was going to have, there's no way. No way anybody can endure the kind of pain I was going through.

Theme 3

Obsessive thoughts of being a bad mother and of questioning what was happening to them consumed the mothers' waking hours.

During the day, mothers' minds were constantly filled with obsessive thinking such as, "What's wrong with me? Am I going crazy? Why can't I enjoy being with my baby? Will I ever be normal again?" Their obsessive thinking also centered on their perceptions of themselves as being horrible mothers and failures. Mothers suffering with postpartum depression believed that when others looked at them they were thinking what terrible mothers they were. Due to their obsessive thinking, at the end of the day mothers were physically and mentally exhausted. They longed for escape from these obsessive thoughts, though sleep was not possible on many nights because their minds were still racing with repetitive thoughts.

Theme 4

Haunted by the fear that any normalcy in their lives was irretrievable, the mothers grieved for their loss of self.

The women were frightened that their lives would never be normal again and that their happiness was gone forever. One mother put it succinctly when she revealed that:

My big fear was that I wasn't going to get better and even if I got better that I wasn't

going to be the same person I was before the experience; that I never would quite get over it.

The women mourned their loss of self, the way they used to be prior to postpartum depression. They felt as if their lives would never be right again. They believed there was no turning back, and this terrified them.

Theme 5

Life was empty of all previous interests and goals.

To further worsen matters during postpartum depression, mothers could not find solace in any of their usual interests or hobbies because they no longer were important to them. No enjoyment was derived from anything that once brought them pleasure, such as reading or bowling. Their previous interests could not provide even a temporary diversion for these mothers from their "living nightmare."

Women had no desire to even be with their husbands, or to have sex. As one mother expressed:

My husband and I would have sex. It just hurt. I wanted nothing to do with it. I just wanted him to leave me alone and not touch me.

Theme 6

The women carried a suffocating burden of fear and guilt over pondering harming their infants.

None of the women who participated in this study ever attempted to harm their babies. However, at times some of the mothers did contemplate harming them. Mothers were horrified that they could harbor such thoughts and were consumed with guilt. Once women began to contemplate hurting their infants, they were terrified that at some point they would actually carry out these thoughts. One mother stated:

Many times I would be on the verge of throwing my son at my husband. I felt such tremendous guilt that I just wanted to hurt myself.

Mothers also bore the burden of guilt over not giving their babies the love they felt the babies needed. The women feared that psychologically they were harming their infants. As one mother noted:

I always worried about my son. I knew I couldn't take care of him but I was always asking my mom to hold him and love him for me. I didn't want him to suffer. The guilt made it even worse and the fact I couldn't love him normally made it even worse.

Theme 7

Shrouded in fogginess, the mothers were unable to concentrate.

During postpartum depression mothers repeatedly reported their inability to concentrate. Mothers described it as "the fogginess would set in." When this happened, their minds seemed to be filled with cobwebs and their concentration level decreased. Women, for example, who had been avid readers prior to postpartum depression stopped reading because they had to reread each page at least three or four times due to their inability to concentrate. Another mother said:

If I went grocery shopping, it was like I was in a fog. I would do it but it would take me four hours to unload the bags and put them away. It was as if I just wasn't efficient at anything. Everything was a big, big deal to do.

Theme 8

Mothers envisioned themselves as robots stripped of all positive feelings, just going through the motions.

Feelings of emptiness prevailed during postpartum depression. Mothers described themselves as unable to feel any emotions other than anxiety, fear, and sadness. Mothers went through the motions of caring for their infants but felt no joy or love while doing these activities. For example, while feeding or bathing their babies, mothers described themselves as robots finishing their tasks without any emotion. Mothers said:

It was like a withdrawal of emotions. I didn't feel real. I felt as if I was acting. I went through the motions of my life without any of the joy.

I'd be having guests or family over for dinner and laughing and talking. All of a sudden it was like my personality was pulled right out of me and I'd just be quiet and look around. I'd start acting again.

Theme 9

Uncontrollable anxiety attacks led to a feeling of being on the edge of insanity.

During postpartum depression the sadness mothers constantly experienced was periodically shattered without warning by terrifying, uncontrollable anxiety attacks. The onset of these attacks was sudden and unexpected. Mothers thought they were literally losing their minds. Tingling hands, sweating, palpitations, and chest pain were some of the symptoms mothers experienced during an anxiety attack. Out of fear that they were dying, some women went to emergency rooms just to make certain they were not having a heart attack. An anxiety attack was described vividly by one woman as follows:

It's terrible. It's like the worst thing you can imagine. Think of how you would feel if your husband or child had been hit by a car and killed. Well, it would be as bad as what I felt during an anxiety attack.

Theme 10

Loss of control of mothers' emotions was alarming and difficult to accept.

Loss of control permeated all aspects of the mothers' lives. Women were frightened because they no longer were in control of their emotions or thoughts. For instance, even though obsessive thinking was driving some women to the brink of insanity, mothers had no control over their thoughts. They could not stop them. Mothers found this loss of control extremely difficult to accept. Even though the women desperately wanted to get out of their pain, they had no control over postpartum depression. One mother captured this theme by saying that:

I had no control and that was the scary thing. I felt trapped. I felt like there was absolutely no way out of this hell. These horrible feelings weren't going to leave no matter how hard I tried.

Theme 11

Besieged with insecurities the mothers needed to be mothered themselves.

During postpartum depression women were extremely insecure. They felt fragile, weak, and vulnerable. To these women the responsibility of motherhood was overwhelming. If they could not control even their own thoughts and feelings, how could they depend on themselves to care for another human being so tiny and helpless? The following quote

from one of the women in this study poignantly illustrates this theme:

It just snapped in me and there was no going back. Even though all of a sudden everybody rushed in to help, it didn't make any difference. I was like an infant. I had to be with my mother all the time. I needed help with the baby. The responsibility seemed absolutely enormous.

These 11 theme clusters comprised the fundamental structure of postpartum depression. Incorporated in this fundamental structure are two additional points, self-hatred and hypochondriasis, that one mother requested be included to more fully reflect her experience.

Discussion

Prior to this phenomenological study, research on postpartum depression had been based on quantitative designs. This quantitative research relied heavily on questionnaires to collect data. Do the responses elicited by these questionnaires adequately assess the lived experience of postpartum depression? The Beck Depression Inventory (BDI; Beck, Ward, & Mendelson, 1961), a generalized depression scale, has frequently been used to measure behavioral manifestations of postpartum depression. Cognitive distortion has been hypothesized by Beck (1972) as the core deficit in depression. His tool consists of 21 categories of symptoms and attitudes towards depression. Beck et al. (1961) stated that these items do not reflect any theory regarding the etiology or underlying psychological processes in depression. When the 21 symptoms in the Beck Depression Inventory are compared with the 11 theme clusters of this phenomenological study, only three of the 11 theme clusters can be found in the BDI: contemplating death, loss of interests, and guilt. The BDI does address, however, both of the additional symptoms one mother suggested be included in the exhaustive description, self-hatred and hypochondriasis. Anxiety, which was a major component of the lived experience of postpartum depression revealed by all the mothers in the study, is not included in the BDI. Other cluster themes such as obsessive thoughts, loss of control, and thoughts of hurting the baby also were not included in this tool. As evidenced by the findings of this study, a generalized depression scale such as the BDI does not measure all of the specifics of postpartum depression, nor should it be expected to. Nurse researchers need to seriously consider whether to use a generalized depression scale in future studies on postpartum depression.

Even one of the newest instruments designed specifically to detect postpartum depression, the Edinburgh Postnatal Depression Scale (Cox, Holden, & Sagovsky, 1987) does not include most of the cluster themes of postpartum depression that emerged in this study. Only thoughts of harming oneself, anxiety, and fear are assessed by the Edinburgh Postnatal Depression Scale.

Even though a woman does not need to exhibit every symptom of postpartum depression to be diagnosed as experiencing this disorder, quantitative instruments should include the gamut of possible behavioral manifestations from which a mother can rate her symptomatology. The fundamental structure of postpartum depression developed from this phenomenological study can be a starting point for methodological research focused on developing a quantitative instrument to measure postpartum depression specifically.   **NR**

REFERENCES

Atkinson, A., & Rickel, A. (1984). Postpartum depression in primiparous parents. *Journal of Abnormal Psychology, 93,* 115-119.

Balk, L. (1990, November). I couldn't cope with motherhood. *Working Mother,* 38-43.

Beck, A. (1972). *Depression: Causes and treatment.* Philadelphia: University of Pennsylvania Press.

Beck, A., Ward, C., & Mendelson, M. (1961). An inventory of measuring depression. *Archives of General Psychiatry, 4,* 561-571.

Chalmers, B., & Chalmers, B. (1986). Postpartum depression: A revised perspective. *Journal of Psychosomatic Obstetrics and Gynecology, 5,* 93-105.

Colaizzi, P. (1978). Psychological research as the phenomenologist views it. In R. Valle & M. King (Eds.), *Existential phenomenological alternative for psychology* (pp. 48-71). New York: Oxford University Press.

Cox, J., Holden, J., & Sagovsky, R. (1987). Detection of postnatal depression: Development of the 10-item Edinburgh Postnatal Depression Scale. *British Journal of Psychiatry, 150,* 782-786.

Fleming, A., Ruble, D., Flett, G., & Shaul, D. (1988). Postpartum adjustment in first time mothers: Relations between mood, maternal attitudes and mother-infant interactions. *Developmental Psychology, 24,* 71-81.

Gjerdingen, D., Froberg, D., & Wilson, D. (1986). Postpartum mental and physical problems. *Postgraduate Medicine, 80,* 133-145.

Guba, E., & Lincoln, Y. (1985). *Naturalistic inquiry.* Beverly Hills, CA: Sage Publications.

Husserl, E. (1962). *Ideas; General introduc-*

tion to pure phenomenology. New York: Macmillan.

HUSSERL, E. (1970). *The crisis of European science.* (D. Carr, Trans.) Chicago: Northwestern University Press.

HYCNER, R. (1985). Some guidelines for the phenomenological analysis of interview data. *Human Studies, 8,* 279-303.

KENDELL, R. (1984). Emotional and physical factors in the genesis of puerperal mental disorders. *Journal of Psychosomatic Research, 29,* 3-11.

MERLEAU-PONTY, M. (1956). What is phenomenology? *Cross Currents, 6,* 69-70.

OILER, C. (1986). Phenomenology: The method. In P. Munhall & C. Oiler (Eds.), *Nursing research: A qualitative perspective* (pp. 69-84). Norwalk, CT: Appleton-Century-Crofts.

SAKS, B., FRANK, J., LOWE, T., BERMAN, W., NAFTOLIN, F., PHIL, D., & COHEN, D. (1985). Depressed mood during pregnancy and puerperium: Clinical recogni-

tion and implications for clinical practice. *American Journal of Psychiatry, 142,* 728-731.

SPIEGELBERG, H. (1975). *Doing phenomenology: Essays on and in phenomenology.* The Hague: Martinus Nijhoff.

Spitzer, R., Endicott, J., & Robins, E. (1978). Research diagnostic criteria: Rationale and reliability. *Archives of General Psychiatry, 36,* 773-782.

SWANSON-KAUFFMAN, K., & SCHONWALD, E. (1988) Phenomenology. In B. Sarter (Ed.), *Paths to knowledge: Innovative research methods* (pp. 97-105). New York: National League for Nursing.

TILDEN, V., NELSON, C., & MAY, B. (1990). Use of qualitative methods to enhance content validity. *Nursing Research, 39,* 172-175.

WHIFFEN, V., & GOTLIB, I. (1989). Infants of postpartum depressed mothers: Temperament and cognitive status. *Journal of Abnormal Psychology, 98,* 274-279.

INTRODUCTION TO THE CRITIQUE

This research report "The Lived Experience of Postpartum Depression: A Phenomenological Study" by Beck (1992) is critically examined for its rigor in qualitative method, its contribution to nursing, and its utility in practice. The criteria identified in the box on p. 484-485 are used to guide the evaluation.

Statement of the Phenomenon of Interest

Beck (1992) clearly states that she is interested in studying postpartum depression. She describes the differences and similarities between the related concepts of maternity blues and postpartum psychosis. Beck states that it is important to study postpartum depression using a phenomenological methodology because nurses need a deeper understanding of the "world of women who experience postpartum depression" (p. 166). She further states that this understanding will offer insights not presently available.

In addition to understanding the world of women who experience postpartum depression, Beck (1992) suggests that the findings of her research can enhance the content validity of the quantitative scales that have been used to study depression.

The philosophical underpinnings of this research are stated. Beck (1992) refers to the work of Spiegelberg, Husserl, and Merleau-Ponty as guiding the inquiry.

These statements are important because they provide the reader with an understanding of the basic premises from which the research is derived.

Purpose

The purpose of the study is "to describe postpartum depression as it is experienced in everyday life and to answer the research question: What is the essential structure of the lived experience of postpartum depression?" (Beck, 1992, p. 166). The essential structure of the lived experience is the essence or the meaning of a phenomenon to those who live it. When searching for the essential structure, the phenomenologist is seeking the meaning units or critical themes that when related to each other create a pure description of the phenomenon under study.

The significance of the work as stated by Beck (1992) is that the data found "were used not only to describe the essential structure of postpartum depression but also to assess the content validity of some of these [depression] measurement scales" (p. 167). On the basis of these statements the significance of the study can be judged.

Phenomenological description of postpartum depression will offer insight into the lived experience of postpartum depression by the women who experience it. It also will be useful in providing insight into what the significant themes are. The identification of major themes provides an opportunity to compare them with developed instruments. This will allow researchers working in the area of postpartum depression to determine whether the instruments as developed represent the reality of what women who have postpartum depression experience or whether the instruments represent what developers of the instruments believe women experience.

Method

Beck (1992) used a phenomenological research methodology to study postpartum depression. The work of Colaizzi guided her inquiry. Because the purpose of the study is to describe the essential structure of postpartum depression, phenomenological methodology as identified by Colaizzi is an appropriate choice. Beck is interested in the lived experience of postpartum depression and Colaizzi's method will provide the direction for data analysis.

Beck follows the approach described by Colaizzi. She does not, however, report the exhaustive description. Reporting of the exhaustive description enriches the research report. In addition to providing the reader with an intimate view of the participants' lived experience, it demonstrates the relationships of the themes to each other.

Sampling

When the phenomenologist seeks participants to inform the inquiry, it is most important to be sure that those who are included have experienced the phenomenon. The term used to describe a sample of individuals who have particular knowledge of a phenomenon and have been selected for the purpose of sharing their knowledge is a *purposive sample.*

Beck (1992) used seven mothers who had experienced postpartum depression as informants. They were members of a postpartum depression support group. Six of the seven participants had been under psychiatric care for diagnosed postpartum depression. No information is provided to demonstrate that the seventh participant was suffering from postpartum depression. Because Beck states early in the report that it is important to distinguish among postpartum depression, maternity blues, and postpartum psychosis, the fact that one informant does not have a confirmed diagnosis of postpartum depression could raise the question "Was the seventh informant appropriate for the study of postpartum depression?"

Data Collection

Protection of human subjects was appropriately described. The procedure used to collect data is made clear in the report. The data were collected by means of private interviews using one guide question focused on the experience of postpartum depression. Data were collected until saturation occurred. *Saturation* is a term used to describe the point in data collection when no new themes are described and the ones that have been described previously become repetitive.

Data Analysis

Data were analyzed by using six procedural steps described by Colaizzi. **Credibility** was achieved by returning to three of the seven mothers who participated in the study and sharing the exhaustive description to see whether the participants agreed with Beck's (1992) description of their experience. Beck does not explain why she used only three of the mothers. Validation of the exhaustive description by all seven mothers would have strengthened her findings.

In the discussion section of the report, Beck (1992) states that she incorporated self-hatred and hypochondriasis at the request of one of the mothers "to more fully reflect her [mother's] experience" (p. 170). Colaizzi specifically includes this as one of his procedural steps. This activity further adds to the credibility of the findings.

Auditability refers "to the ability of another researcher to follow the thinking, decisions and methods used by the original researcher" (Yonge & Stewin, 1988, p. 64). Tables 1 and 2 are offered as examples of Beck's (1992) thinking process regarding themes. Beck also states she used a colleague experienced in phenomenological analysis to gain "intersubjective agreement" (p. 167) on interpretation of data.

Fittingness of the research refers to how well the findings fit outside the study situation. To demonstrate the fittingness of the findings, Beck (1992) reports that she sought out members of another postpartum depression support group who had experienced the phenomenon and were able to describe their experience. The reader is led to interpret from Beck's statement that the mothers in the second support group had similar experiences. However, this is not explicitly stated.

From Beck's (1992) report, one is able to determine that the data analysis strategy was compatible with the study and that she maintained rigor in the analysis.

Findings

The findings of Beck's (1992) research are presented in the context of the group that she studied: mothers who had experienced postpartum depression. The data are presented using both the informants' words and Beck's interpretation. Tables are provided to demonstrate how Beck arrived at her interpretations. When reading the report, the reader is able to get a sense of what mothers experiencing postpartum believe that the experience is. Beck also presents the current state of research related to instrumentation focusing on depression in general and postpartum depression specifically. The findings of this study are related to what is known already.

Conclusions, Implications, and Recommendations

The conclusions of this study are focused on explaining the limitations of quantitative instruments currently available to measure depression. The implications and recommendations are consistent with these conclusions. Beck (1992) stated, however, early in the research report that her intent was to describe postpartum depression and also to "assess the content validity of some of these [depression] scales" (p. 167). Her conclusions, implications, and recommendations are related only to the latter intent. Nurses choosing to use the data from this study are limited in the application of the findings because Beck provides only an explanation of the findings as they relate to instrument utilization.

The significance of the study to nursing is addressed from the perspective of the current state of depression instrumentation. Beck (1992) states, "Nurse researchers need to seriously consider whether to use a generalized depression scale in future studies on postpartum depression" (p. 170). However, nurse researchers interested in applying the findings to the practice of caring for women experiencing postpartum depression are left without a clear insight as to how the data are useful to their practice because there is no concluding statement summarizing the essence of the findings.

REFERENCES

Beck, C.T. (1992). The lived experience of postpartum depression: A phenomenological study. *Nursing Research, 41*(3), 166-170.

Hutchinson, S. (1986). Chemically dependent nurses: The trajectory toward self-annihilation. *Nursing Research, 35*, 196-201.

Miller, B., Haber, J., & Byrne, M. (1992). The experience of caring in the acute care setting: Patients' and nurses' perspectives. In Gaut, D., (Ed.), *The presence of caring in nursing* (pp. 137-156). New York: National League for Nursing.

Yonge, O., & Stewin, L. (1988). Reliability and validity: Misnomers for qualitative research. *The Canadian Journal of Nursing Research, 20* (2), 61-67.

Glossary

abstract　A brief, comprehensive summary of a study.

after-only design　An experimental design with two randomly assigned groups—a treatment group and a control group. This design differs from the true experiment in that both groups are measured only after the experimental treatment.

after-only nonequivalent control group design　A quasiexperimental design similar to the after-only experimental design, but subjects are not randomly assigned to the treatment or control groups.

alternate form reliability　Two or more alternate forms of a measure are administered to the same subjects at different times. The scores of the two tests determine the degree of relationship between the measures.

analysis of covariance (ANCOVA)　A statistic that measures differences among group means and uses a statistical technique to equate the groups under study in relation to an important variable.

analysis of variance (ANOVA)　A statistic that tests whether group means differ from each other, rather than testing each pair of means separately, ANOVA considers the variation among all groups.

animal rights　Guidelines used to protect the rights of animals in the conduct of research.

anonymity　A research participant's protection in a study so that no one, not even the researcher, can link the subject with the information given.

antecedent variable　A variable that affects the dependent variable but occurs before the introduction of the independent variable.

applied research　Tests the practical limits of descriptive theories but does not examine the efficacy of actions taken by practitioners.

assent　An aspect of informed consent that pertains to protecting the rights of children as research subjects.

assumption　A basic principle assumed to be true without the need for scientific proof.

auditability　The researcher's development of the research process in a qualitative study that allows a researcher or reader to follow the thinking or conclusions of the researcher.

axial coding　A data analysis strategy used with the grounded theory method. It requires intense coding around a single theme.

basic research　Theoretical or pure research that generates, tests, and expands theories that explain or predict a phenomenon.

beneficence　An obligation to do no harm and to maximize possible benefits.

benefit　Potential positive outcomes of participation in a research study.

bias　A distortion in the data analysis results.

bracketing　A process during which the researcher identifies personal biases about the phenomenon of interest to clarify how personal experience and beliefs may color what is heard and reported.

case study method   The study of a selected contemporary phenomenon over time to provide an in-depth description of essential dimensions and processes of the phenomenon.

chance error   Attributable to fluctuations in subject characteristics that occur at a specific point in time and are often beyond the awareness and control of the examiner.

chi-square (X^2)   A nonparametric statistic that is used to determine whether the frequency found in each category is different from the frequency that would be expected by chance.

CINAHL or the Cumulative Index to Nursing & Allied Health Literature   A print or computerized data base; computerized CINAHL is available on CD-ROM and OnLine.

close-ended item   Question that the respondent may answer with only one of a fixed number of choices.

cluster sampling   A probability sampling strategy that involves a successive random sampling of units. The units sampled progress from large to small.

computer data bases   Print data bases that are put on software programs that can be accessed OnLine or on CD-ROM via the computer.

concealment   Refers to whether the subjects know that they are being observed.

concept   An image or symbolic representation of an abstract idea.

conceptual definition   General meaning of a concept.

conceptual literature   Published and unpublished non–data-based material, such as reports of theories, concepts, synthesis of research on concepts, or professional issues, some of which underlie reported research, as well as other non-research material.

concurrent validity   The degree of correlation of two measures of the same concept that are administered at the same time.

confidentiality   Assurance that a research participant's identity cannot be linked to the information that was provided to the researcher.

consistency   Data are collected from each subject in the study in exactly the same way or as close to the same way as possible.

constancy   Methods and procedures of data collection are the same for all subjects.

constant comparative method   A process of continuously comparing data as they are acquired during research with the grounded theory method.

construct   An abstraction that is adapted for a scientific purpose.

construct replication   The use of original methods, such as sampling techniques, instruments, or research design, to study a problem that has been investigated previously.

construct validity   The extent to which an instrument is said to measure a theoretical construct or trait.

consumer   One who actively uses and applies research findings in nursing practice.

content analysis   A technique for the objective, systematic, and quantitative description of communications and documentary evidence.

content validity   The degree to which the content of the measure represents the universe of content, or the domain of a given behavior.

control   Measures used to hold uniform or constant the conditions under which an investigation occurs.

control group   The group in an experimental investigation that does not receive an intervention or treatment; the comparison group.

convenience sampling   A nonprobability sampling strategy that uses the most readily accessible persons or objects as subjects in a study.

convergent validity   A strategy for assessing construct validity in which two or more tools that theoretically measure the same construct are administered to subjects. If the measures are positively correlated, convergent validity is said to be supported.

correlation   The degree of association between two variables.

correlational study   A type of nonexperimental research design that examines the relationship between two or more variables.

credibility   Steps in qualitative research to ensure accuracy, validity, or soundness of data.

criterion-related validity   Indicates the degree of relationship between performance on the measure and actual behavior either in the present (concurrent) or in the future (predictive).

critical reading   An active interpretation and objective assessment of an article during which the reader is looking for key concepts, ideas, and justifications.

critical thinking   The rational examination of ideas, inferences, principles, and conclusions.

critique   The process of objectively and critically evaluating a research report's content for scientific merit and application to practice, theory, or education.

critiquing criteria   The criteria used for objectively and critically evaluating a research article.

Cronbach alpha   Test of internal consistency that simultaneously compares each item in a scale to all others.

cross-sectional study   A nonexperimental research design that looks at data at one point in time, that is, in the immediate present.

data   Information systematically collected in the course of a study; the plural of datum.

data base   A compilation of information about a topic organized in a systematic way.

data-based literature   Reports of completed research.

data saturation   A point when data collection can cease. It occurs when the information being shared with the researcher becomes repetitive. Ideas conveyed by the participant have been shared before by other participants; inclusion of additional participants does not result in new ideas.

deductive reasoning   A logical thought process in which hypotheses are derived from theory; reasoning moves from the general to the particular.

degrees of freedom   The number of quantities that are unknown minus the number of independent equations linking these unknowns; a function of the number in the sample.

delimitation   Those characteristics that restrict the population to a homogeneous group of subjects.

Delphi technique   The technique of gaining expert opinion on a subject. It uses rounds or multiple stages of data collection with each round using data from the previous round.

dependent variable   In experimental studies the presumed effect of the independent or experimental variable on the outcome.

descriptive/exploratory survey research   A type of nonexperimental research design that collects descriptions of existing phenomena for the purpose of using the data to justify or assess current conditions or to make plans for improvement of conditions.

descriptive statistics   Statistical methods used to describe and summarize sample data.

developmental study   A type of nonexperimental research design that is concerned not only with the existing status and interrelationship of phenomena but also with changes that take place as a function of time.

direct observation   A method for measuring psychological and physiological behaviors for purposes of evaluating change and facilitating recovery.

directional hypothesis   Hypothesis that specifies the expected direction of the relationship between the independent and dependent variables.

divergent validity   A strategy for assessing construct validity in which two or more tools that theoretically measure the opposite of the construct are administered to subjects. If the measures are negatively correlated, divergent validity is said to be supported.

domains   Symbolic categories that include the smaller categories of an ethnographic study.

downlink   A receiver for programs beamed from other agencies that allows a person to participate in telecommunications conferences.

element   The most basic unit about which information is collected.

eligibility criteria   Those characteristics that restrict the population to a homogeneous group of subjects.

emic view   The natives' or insiders' view of their world.

empirical   The obtaining of evidence or objective data.

empirical literature   A synonym for data-based literature; *see* **data-based literature.**

equivalence   Consistency or agreement among observers using the same measurement tool or agreement among alternate forms of a tool.

error variance   The extent to which the variance in test scores is attributable to error rather than a true measure of the behaviors.

ethics   The theory or discipline dealing with principles of moral values and moral conduct.

ethnographic method   A method that scientifically describes cultural groups. The goal of the ethnographer is to understand the natives' view of their world.

ethnography   A qualitative research approach designed to produce cultural theory.

etic view   An outsider's view of another's world.

evaluation research   The use of scientific research methods and procedures to evaluate a program, treatment, practice, or policy outcomes; analytical means are used to document the worth of an activity.

evaluative research   The use of scientific research methods and procedures for the purpose of making an evaluation.

ex post facto study   A type of nonexperimental research design that examines the relationships among the variables after the variations have occurred.

experiment   A scientific investigation in which observations are made and data are collected by means of the characteristics of control, randomization, and manipulation.

experimental design   A research design that has the following properties: randomization, control, and manipulation.

experimental group   The group in an experimental investigation that receives an intervention or treatment.

external criticism   A process used to judge the authenticity of historical data.

external validity   The degree to which findings of a study can be generalized to other populations or environments.

extraneous variable   Variable that interferes with the operations of the phenomena being studied.

findings   Statistical results of a study.

Fisher's exact probability test   A test used to compare frequencies when samples are small and expected frequencies are less than six in each cell.

fittingness   Answers the questions: Are the findings applicable outside the study situation? Are the results meaningful to the individuals not involved in the research?

frequency distribution   Descriptive statistical method for summarizing the occurrences of events under study.

generalizability (generalize)   The inferences that the data are representative of similar phenomena in a population beyond the studied sample.

grounded theory   Theory that is constructed inductively from a base of observations of the world as it is lived by a selected group of people.

grounded theory method   An inductive approach that uses a systematic set of procedures to arrive at theory about basic social processes.

historical research method   The systematic compilation of data resulting from evaluation and interpretation of facts regarding people, events, and occurrences of the past.

history   The internal validity threat that refers to events outside of the experimental setting that may affect the dependent variable.

homogeneity   Similarity of conditions.

hypothesis   A prediction about the relationship between two or more variables.

hypothesis-testing validity   A strategy for assessing construct validity in which the theory or concept underlying a measurement instrument's design is used to develop hypotheses that are tested. Inferences are made based on the findings about whether the rationale underlying the instruments' construction is adequate to explain the findings.

independent variable   The antecedent or the variable that has the presumed effect on the dependent variable.

inductive reasoning   A logical thought process in which generalizations are developed from specific observations; reasoning moves from the particular to the general.

inferential statistics   Procedures that combine mathematical processes and logic to test hypotheses about a population with the help of sample data.

informed consent   An ethical principle that requires a researcher to obtain the voluntary participation of subjects after informing them of potential benefits and risks.

institutional review board   A board established in agencies to review biomedical and behavioral research involving human subjects within the agency or in programs sponsored by the agency.

instrumentation   Changes in the measurement of the variables that may account for changes in the obtained measurement.

internal consistency   The extent to which items within a scale reflect or measure the same concept.

internal criticism   A process of judging the reliability or consistency of information within an historical document.

internal validity   The degree to which it can be inferred that the experimental treatment, rather than an uncontrolled condition, resulted in the observed effects.

interrater reliability   The consistency of observations between two or more observers; often expressed as a percentage of agreement between raters or observers or a coefficient of agreement that takes into account the element of chance. This usually is used with the direct observation method.

interrelationship studies   The classification of a nonexperimental research design that attempts to trace relationships among variables. The four types are *correlational, ex post facto, prediction,* and *developmental.*

interval   The level of measurement that provides different levels or gradations in response. The differences or intervals between responses are assumed to be approximately equal.

interval measurement level   Level used to show rankings of events or objects on a scale with equal intervals between numbers but with an arbitrary zero (e.g., centigrade temperature).

intervening variable   A variable that occurs during an experimental or quasiexperimental study that affects the dependent variable.

intervention   Deals with whether or not the observer provokes actions from those who are being observed.

interviews   A method of data collection in which a data collector questions a subject verbally. Interviews may be face-to-face or performed over the telephone, and they may consist of open-ended or close-ended questions.

item-total correlation   The relationship between each of the items on a scale and the total scale.

justice   Human subjects should be treated fairly.

key informants Individuals who have special knowledge, status, or communication skills and who are willing to teach the ethnographer about the phenomenon.

Kuder-Richardson coefficient The estimate of homogeneity utilized for instruments that use a dichotomous response pattern.

kurtosis The relative peakness or flatness of a distribution.

level of significance (alpha level) The risk of making a type I error, set by the researcher before the study begins.

levels of measurement Categorization of the precision with which an event can be measured (nominal, ordinal, interval, and ratio).

life context The matrix of human-human-environment relationships emerging over the course of one's life.

Likert scales Lists of statements on which respondents indicate whether they "strongly agree," "agree," "disagree," or "strongly disagree."

limitation Weakness of a study.

lived experience In phenomenological research a term used to refer to the focus on living through events and circumstances (prelingual) rather than thinking about these events and circumstances (conceptualized experience).

longitudinal study A nonexperimental research design in which a researcher collects data from the same group at different points in time.

manipulation The provision of some experimental treatment, in one or varying degrees, to some of the subjects in the study.

matching A special sampling strategy used to construct an equivalent comparison sample group by filling it with subjects who are similar to each subject in another sample group in relation to preestablished variables, such as age and gender.

maturation Developmental, biological, or psychological processes that operate within an individual as a function of time and are external to the events of the investigation.

mean A measure of central tendency; the arithmetic average of all scores.

measure of central tendency Descriptive statistical procedure that describes the average member of a sample (mean, median, and mode).

measure of variability Descriptive statistical procedure that describes how much dispersion there is in sample data.

measurement The assignment of numbers to objects or events according to rules.

median A measure of central tendency; the middle score.

medline The print or computerized data base of standard **med**ical literature analysis and retrieval system **On Line**; it is also available on CD-ROM.

metaanalysis A research method that takes the results of multiple studies in a specific area and synthesizes the findings to make conclusions regarding the area of focus.

methodological research The controlled investigation and measurement of the means of gathering and analyzing data.

modal percentage A measure of variability; percent of cases in the mode.

modality The number of peaks in a frequency distribution.

mode A measure of central tendency; most frequent score or result.

mortality The loss of subjects from time 1 data collection to time 2 data collection.

multiple analysis of variance (MANOVA) A test used to determine differences in group means; used when there is more than one dependent variable.

multiple regression Measure of the relationship between one interval level dependent variable and several independent variables. Canonical correlation is used when there is more than one dependent variable.

multistage sampling (cluster sampling) Involves a successive random sampling or units (clusters) that programs from large to small and meets sample eligibility criteria.

network sampling (snowballing) A strategy used for locating samples difficult to locate. It uses social networks and the fact that friends tend to have characteristics in common; subjects who meet the eligibility criteria are asked for assistance in getting in touch with others who meet the same criteria.

nominal The level of measurement that simply assigns data into categories that are mutually exclusive.

nominal measurement level Level used to classify objects or events into categories without any relative ranking (e.g., gender, hair color).

nondirectional hypothesis One that indicates the existence of a relationship between the variables but does not specify the anticipated direction of the relationship.

nonequivalent control group design A quasiexperimental design that is similar to the true experiment, but subjects are not randomly assigned to the treatment or control groups.

nonexperimental research Research in which an investigator observes a phenomenon without manipulating the independent variable(s).

nonparametric statistics Statistics that are usually utilized when variables are measured at the nominal or ordinal level because they do not estimate population parameters and involve less restrictive assumptions about the underlying distribution.

nonprobability sampling A procedure in which elements are chosen by nonrandom methods.

normal curve A curve that is symmetrical about the mean and unimodal.

null hypothesis A statement that there is no relationship between the variables and that any relationship observed is a function of chance or fluctuations in sampling.

objective Data that are not influenced by anyone who collects the information.

objectivity The use of facts without distortion by personal feelings or bias.

open-ended item Question that the respondent may answer in his or her own words.

operational definition The measurements used to observe or measure a variable; delineates the procedures or operations required to measure a concept.

operationalization   The process of translating concepts into observable, measurable phenomena.

ordinal   The level of measurement that systematically categorizes data in an ordered or ranked manner. Ordinal measures do not permit a high level of differentiation among subjects.

ordinal measurement level   Level used to show rankings of events or objects; numbers are not equidistant, and zero is arbitrary (class ranking).

parallel form (reliability)   *See* **alternate form (reliability).**

parameter   A characteristic of a population.

parametric statistics   Inferential statistics that involve the estimation of at least one parameter, require measurement at the interval level or above, and involve assumptions about the variables being studied. These assumptions usually include the fact that the variable is normally distributed.

path analysis   A statistical technique in which the researcher hypothesizes how variables are related and in what order and then tests how strong those relationships or paths are.

Pearson correlation coefficient or Pearson *r*   A statistic that is calculated to reflect the degree of relationship between two interval level variables.

percentile   A measure of rank; percentage of cases a given score exceeds.

phenomenological method   A process of learning and constructing the meaning of human experience through intensive dialogue with persons who are living the experience.

phenomenological research   Based on the investigation of the description of experience as it is lived.

phenomenology   A qualitative research approach that aims to describe experience as it is lived through, before it is conceptualized.

philosophical research   Based on the investigation of the truths and principles of existence, knowledge, and conduct.

physiological measurement   The use of specialized equipment to determine physical and biological status of subjects.

population   A well-defined set that has certain specified properties.

population validity   Generalization of results to other populations.

prediction study   A type of nonexperimental research design that attempts to make a forecast or prediction derived from particular phenomena.

predictive validity   The degree of correlation between the measure of the concept and some future measure of the same concept.

primary source   Scholarly literature that is written by a person(s) who developed the theory or conducted the research. Primary sources include eyewitness accounts of historic events, provided by original documents, films, letters, diaries, records, artifacts, periodicals, or tapes.

print data bases   Indexes, card catalogues, and abstract reviews. *Print indexes* are used to find journal sources (periodicals) of data-based and conceptual articles on a variety of topics, as well as publications of professional organizations and various governmental agencies.

probability   The probability of an event is the event's long-run relative frequency in repeated trials under similar conditions.

probability sampling   A procedure that uses some form of random selection when the sample units are chosen.

problem statement   An interrogative sentence or statement about the relationship between two or more variables.

process consent   In qualitative research the ongoing negotiation with subjects for their participation in a study.

product testing   Testing of medical devices.

program   A list of instructions in machine-readable language written so that a computer's hardware can carry out an operation; software.

propositions   The linkage of concepts that lays a foundation for the development of methods that test relationships.

prospective study   Nonexperimental study that begins with an exploration of assumed causes and then moves forward in time to the presumed effect.

psychometrics   The theory and development of measurement instruments.

purposive sampling   A nonprobability sampling strategy in which the researcher selects subjects who are considered to be typical of the population.

qualitative measurement   The items or observed behaviors are assigned to mutually exclusive categories that are representative of the kinds of behavior exhibited by the subjects.

qualitative research   The study of broadly stated questions about human experiences. It is conducted in natural settings and uses descriptive data.

quantitative measurement   The assignment of items or behaviors to categories that represent the amount of a possessed characteristic.

quasiexperimental design   A study design in which random assignment is not used but the independent variable is manipulated and certain mechanisms of control are used.

questionnaires   Paper and pencil instruments designed to gather data from individuals.

quota sampling   A nonprobability sampling strategy that identifies the strata of the population and proportionately represents the strata in the sample.

random access memory (RAM)   A computer's memory that the user can read or change.

random selection   A selection process in which each element of the population has an equal and independent chance of being included in the sample.

randomization   A sampling selection procedure in which each person or element in a population has an equal chance of being selected to either the experimental group or the control group.

range   A measure of variability; difference between the highest and lowest scores in a set of sample data.

ratio   The highest level of measurement that possesses the characteristics of categorizing, ordering, and ranking and also has an absolute or natural zero that has empirical meaning.

ratio measurement level   Level that ranks the order of events or objects and that has equal intervals and an absolute zero (e.g., height, weight).

reactivity   The distortion created when those who are being observed change their behavior because they know that they are being observed.

recommendation   Application of a study to practice, theory, and future research.

records or available data   Information that is collected from existing materials, such as hospital records, historical documents, or videotapes.

refereed journal or **peer-reviewed journal**   A scholarly journal that has a panel of external and internal reviewers or editors; the panel reviews submitted manuscripts for possible publication. The review panels use the same set of scholarly criteria to judge if the manuscripts are worthy of publication.

reliability   The consistency or constancy of a measuring instrument.

replication   The repetition of a study that uses different samples and is conducted in different settings.

representative sample   A sample whose key characteristics closely approximate those of the population.

research   The systematic, logical, and empirical inquiry into the possible relationships among particular phenomena to produce verifiable knowledge.

research base   The accumulated knowledge gained from several studies that investigate a similar problem.

research hypothesis   A statement about the expected relationship between the variables; also known as a *scientific hypothesis.*

research literature   A synonym for data-based literature.

research problem   Presents the question that is to be asked in a research study.

research utilization   A systematic method of implementing sound research-based innovations in clinical practice, evaluating the outcome, and sharing the knowledge through the process of research dissemination.

respect for persons   People have the right to self-determination and to treatment as autonomous agents; that is, they have the freedom to participate or not participate in research.

retrospective data   Data that have been manifested, such as scores on a standard examination.

retrospective study   A nonexperimental research design that begins with the phenomenon of interest (dependent variable) in the present and examines its relationship to another variable (independent variable) in the past.

review of the literature   An extensive, systematic, and critical review of the most important published scholarly literature on a particular topic. In most cases it is not considered exhaustive.

risk   Potential negative outcome(s) of participation in a research study.

risk-benefit ratio   The extent to which the benefits of the study are maximized and the risks are minimized such that the subjects are protected from harm during the study.

sample   A subset of sampling units from a population.

sampling   A process in which representative units of a population are selected for study in a research investigation.

sampling error   The tendency for statistics to fluctuate from one sample to another.

sampling frame   A list of all the units of the population.

sampling interval   The standard distance between the elements chosen for the sample.

sampling unit   The element or set of elements used for selecting the sample.

saturation   *See* **data saturation**

scale   A self-report inventory that provides a set of response symbols for each item. A rating or score is assigned to each response.

scholarly literature   Refers to published and unpublished data-based and conceptual literature materials found in print and nonprint forms.

scientific approach   A logical, orderly, and objective means of generating and testing ideas.

scientific hypothesis   The researcher's expectation about the outcome of a study; also known as the *research hypothesis.*

scientific literature   A synonym for data-based literature; *see* **data-based literature.**

scientific merit   The degree of validity of a study or group of studies.

scientific observation   Collecting data about the environment and subjects. Data collection has specific objectives to guide it, is systematically planned and recorded, is checked and controlled, and is related to scientific concepts and theories.

secondary source   Scholarly material written by a person(s) *other than* the individual who developed the theory or conducted the research. Most are usually published. Often a secondary source represents a response to or a summary and critique of a theorist's or researcher's work. Examples are documents, films, letters, diaries, records, artifacts, periodicals, or tapes that provide a view of the phenomenon from another's perspective.

selection bias   The internal validity threat that arises when pretreatment differences between the experimental group and the control group are present.

semiquartile range   A measure of variability; range of the middle 50% of the scores.

simple random sampling   A probability sampling strategy in which the population is defined, a sampling frame is listed, and a subset from which the sample will be chosen is selected; members randomly selected.

skew   Measure of the asymmetry of a set of scores.

snowballing (network sampling)   A strategy used for locating samples difficult to locate. It uses social network and the fact that friends tend to have characteristics in common; subjects who meet the eligibility criteria are asked for assistance in getting in touch with others who meet the same criteria.

social desirability   The occasion when a subject responds in a manner that he or she believes will please the researcher rather than in an honest manner.

Solomon four-group design   An experimental design with four randomly assigned groups—the pretest-posttest intervention group, the pretest-posttest control group, a treatment or intervention group with only posttest measurement, and a control group with only posttest measurement.

split-half reliability   An index of the comparison between the scores on one half of a test with those on the other half to determine the consistency in response to items that reflect specific content.

stability   An instrument's ability to produce the same results with repeated testing.

standard deviation   A measure of variability; measure of average deviation of scores from the mean.

standard error of the mean   The standard deviation of a theoretical distribution of sample means. It indicates the average error in the estimation of the population mean.

statistical hypothesis   States that there is no relationship between the independent and dependent variables. The statistical hypothesis also is known as the *null hypothesis*.

statistical reliability   An index of the interval consistency of responses to all items of a single form of a measure that is administered at one time.

stratified random sampling   A probability sampling strategy in which the population is divided into strata or subgroups. An appropriate number of elements from each subgroup are randomly selected based on their proportion in the population.

symbolic interaction   A theoretical perspective that holds that the relationship between self and society is an ongoing process of symbolic communication whereby individuals create a social reality.

systematic   Data collection carried out in the same manner with all subjects.

systematic error   Attributable to lasting characteristics of the subject that do not tend to fluctuate from one time to another.

systematic sampling   A probability sampling strategy that involves the selection of subjects randomly drawn from a population list at fixed intervals.

***t* statistic**   Commonly used in nursing research; it tests whether two group means are more different than would be expected by chance. Groups may be related or independent.

test   A self-report inventory that provides for one response to each item that the examiner assigns a rating or score. Inferences are made from the total score about the degree to which a subject possesses whatever trait, emotion, attitude, or behavior the test is supposed to measure.

testability   Variables of a proposed study that lend themselves to observation, measurement, and analysis.

testing   The effects of taking a pretest on the scores of a posttest.

test-retest reliability   Administration of the same instrument twice to the same subjects under the same conditions within a prescribed time interval, with a comparison of the paired scores to determine the stability of the measure.

theoretical framework   Theoretical rationale for the development of hypotheses.

theoretical literature   A synonym for conceptual literature; *see* **conceptual literature.**

theoretical sampling   Used to select experiences that will help the researcher test ideas and gather complete information about developing concepts when using the grounded theory method.

theory   Set of interrelated concepts, definitions, and propositions that present a systematic view of phenomena for the purpose of explaining and making predictions about those phenomena.

time series design   A quasiexperimental design used to determine trends before and after an experimental treatment. Measurements are taken several times before the introduction of the experimental treatment, the treatment is introduced, and measurements are taken again at specified times afterward.

time-sharing   Several users working on one mainframe via terminals at the same time.

true experiment   Also known as the *Pretest-posttest control group design*. In this design, subjects are randomly assigned to an experimental or control group, pretest measurements are performed, an intervention or treatment occurs in the experimental group, and posttest measurements are performed.

type I error   The rejection of a null hypothesis that is actually true.

type II error   The acceptance of a null hypothesis that is actually false.

uplink   The ability to broadcast conferences so that they can be attended from a distance.

validation sample   The sample that provides the initial data for determining the reliability and validity of a measurement tool.

validity   Determination of whether a measurement instrument actually measures what it is purported to measure.

variable   A defined concept.

Z score   Used to compare measurements in standard units; examines the relative distance of the scores from the mean.

Appendix A

The Abdomen, Thigh, and Arm as Sites for Subcutaneous Sodium Heparin Injections

Pamela S. Stewart Fahs and Marguerite R. Kinney

The purpose of this study was to evaluate three subcutaneous injection sites for low-dose heparin therapy (5,000 units). One hundred and one subjects were randomly placed in one of three groups. Group A received injections in the abdomen, Group B, in the thigh, and Group C in the arm. Each subject received three injections at the one site. Activated partial thromboplastin time (APTT) was measured prior to initiation of heparin and again four hours after the first injection. Bruising was measured at 48, 60, and 72 hours postinjection. There were no statistically significant differences among groups for either changes in APTT or bruising at 60 and 72 hours postinjection. Thus the clinical practice of utilizing the abdomen as the only or preferred site for subcutaneous heparin injections was not supported.

The effectiveness of low-dose heparin therapy (5,000 international units every 8 to 12 hours) has been well documented in the literature as standard medical therapy for hospitalized patients at risk for developing thrombophlebitis. Nurse authors frequently recommend the abdomen as the preferred injection site although the basis for this recommendation is unclear (Caprini, Zoellner, & Weisman, 1977; Chamberlain, 1980; Lundin, 1978). Use of the abdominal site for subcutaneous heparin injections may frighten the patient (Chamberlain, 1980) and inconvenience the nurse. Therefore, this study was undertaken to determine whether alternate sites were effective in accomplishing the goals of low-dose heparin therapy and to identify any differences in bruising at the injection site.

Literature Review

Brenner, Wood, and George (1981) studied two injection techniques to compare angle of injection, aspiration, and massage of tissue. Thirty-three white subjects received two injections into the abdomen. There was no statistically significant difference in bruising between the two techniques.

The effect of three techniques for administering subcutaneous low-dose heparin on the formation of bruises at the site of injection was investigated by Van-Bree, Hollerbach, and Brooks (1984). Forty-three white subjects received three subcutaneous injections into the abdomen. While no differences in bruising were found among the three techniques, women older than 60 years of age were noted to have a greater number of bruises and larger bruises than other subgroups of subjects.

Wooldridge and Jackson (1988) compared two techniques for subcutaneous heparin injections. Order of treatment was randomly assigned for 50 white subjects who served as their own control.

Reprinted from *Nursing Research*, 1991, Vol 40, No. 4, pp. 204-207. Copyright 1991. *American Journal of Nursing* Company.

While no difference in number of bruises was found, smaller bruises and fewer and smaller areas of induration were found in the technique employing a larger (3 milliliter) syringe, 0.2 milliliter air bubble, change of needle prior to injection, and sterile dry sponge for applying pressure after the injection.

The effect of needle size on bruising and pain of heparin injection was studied by Coley, Butler, Beck, and Mullane (1987). One technique was employed to administer heparin in the abdomen of 73 white subjects. No significant difference was found in bruising. Twenty-four hours after injection, a 28 gauge ½ inch needle, as opposed to a 25 gauge ⅝ inch needle, produced a significant difference in the number of subjects reporting pain and severity of pain with injection.

Only one study was found in which concentration of heparin and volume of injectate were reported (Mitchell & Pauszek 1987). A constant dose of heparin was administered to 49 subjects, with 24 subjects receiving 0.5 milliliters (10,000 units: 1 milliliter concentration) and 25 subjects receiving 0.25 milliliters (20,000 units: 1 milliliter concentration). Fewer and smaller bruises (measured by diameter only) were found in the group receiving the more concentrated dose with the smaller volume.

The relationship between techniques for administering low-dose heparin and the formation of bruises or hematomas has been addressed in two review articles (Hanson, 1987; Schumann, Bruya, & Henke, 1988). Both Hanson (1987) and Schumann, Bruya, and Henke (1988) conclude that, although numerous techniques are employed to administer subcutaneous heparin injections, few are based on scientific evidence. Kirch-hoff (1982) noted that it is important for nursing to reverse the direction in which practice flows. Currently, many nursing interventions are described in the literature without empirical evidence to support the practices. The use of sites other than the abdomen for subcutaneous heparin injections has not been empirically evaluated. Therefore, the nursing practice of using the abdomen as the only acceptable injection site for low-dose heparin therapy seems to be based on tradition rather than systematic inquiry.

Hypotheses

I. There is no difference in effectiveness of low-dose heparin therapy, as measured by activated partial thromboplastin time (APTT), when administered in three different subcutaneous sites.

II. There is no difference in the occurrence of bruise at injection site with low-dose heparin therapy when administered in three different subcutaneous sites.

III. There is no difference in size of bruises resulting from low-dose heparin therapy when administered in three different subcutaneous sites.

Method

Subjects: Data were collected on 105 subjects. Four subjects were dropped from the study. One had a bruise overlapping more than one injection site, another received intravenous heparin prior to measurement of subcutaneous injection site bruises, and two were nonwhite. Nonwhites were removed because there were so few and there was no interrater reliability for bruise measurements on dark skinned subjects. The final sample included 101 subjects classified as general medical/surgical patients. Final group sizes were Abdomen (A) = 33, Thigh (B) = 33, and Arm (C) = 35.

Sixty-two female and 39 male subjects received sodium heparin 5,000 units every 8 or 12 hours as prescribed. These subjects ranged in age from 20 to 94 years with a mean age of 65 years. Subjects' primary diagnoses were grouped into categories. Those with a diagnosis of cancer were grouped regardless of system affected. The number of subjects per category was: Cancer, 16; Neurological, 14; Respiratory, 14; Cardiovascular, 15; Gastrointestinal, 13; Muscoskeletal, 17. The other category included Gentiourinary, Endocrine, and Skin systems, with a total of 12 subjects.

Measures: Blood for calculation of APTT was collected by the laboratory personnel prior to initiation of heparin therapy. The APTT is a coagulation test that is used often as an indirect measure of effectiveness of low-dose heparin. The intrinsic portion of the coagulation system is assessed with the APTT (Hubner, 1986). The values of APTT considered to be within normal range at the data collection facility were 22-34 seconds. Phlebotomists collected all APTT samples. The procedure consisted of drawing 5 milliliters of blood, which was discarded if not used for other tests. Blood for the APTT was drawn via a vacutainer setup into a blue top tube containing .05 milliliters of 3.8% sodium citrate. The test was run on an automated precalibrated instrument. All samples in the batch were preceded by a control tube to assure the accuracy of the range established by the laboratory. A lyophilized preparation was used to determine whether reagents utilized were viable in validating patient val-

ues for each batch of samples. Activated Cephaloplastin was the reagent used in the APTTs for this study. Blood for two APTTs was drawn. The first sample was obtained prior to the beginning of heparin therapy and the second was drawn four hours after the first injection of subcutaneous heparin.

The injection sites were examined for bruising by the principal investigator or a research assistant 72 hours after the first injection, 60 hours after the second injection, and 48 hours after the third injection. The timing of assessment of bruising was consistent with the recommendations of VanBree et al. (1984). In the present study, a bruise was defined as a discolored, purpuric lesion. A bruise will change color and fade over a period of time, however, it does not blanch with pressure. The bruises measured in this study were soft tissue injuries resulting from the trauma of subcutaneous injections of heparin. A total of 105 injection sites were used to calculate interrater reliability over a period of 4 months. Ratings were done by the principal investigator and three research assistants. The Pearson correlation coefficients ranged from $r = 0.94$ to 0.99.

Bruises were measured by two methods. The first method was a measurement of the widest diameter directly on the skin. The second method was a trace of the outline of the bruise onto a piece of polyethylene wrap with a fine ballpoint pen. The outline was then traced onto a graph with the use of carbon paper. This outline was later used to calculate surface area by encircling the bruise with a compass, taking the radius, and calculating the area ($A = r^2$). Bruise surface area was reported in units of millimeters squared (mm^2). If no bruise was present, this finding was noted. The Pearson correlation coefficients computed between the two methods were $r = 0.86$ to 0.91. Calculations based on surface area presented a more accurate picture of bruise size, because surface area reflected the irregularly shaped bruise and thus was a more specific measurement. Surface area measurements were used in data analysis.

Procedure: To maintain standardization of the procedure, a videotape and a live presentation with a written script were reviewed with all nurses on all shifts. Training sessions were held for nurses new to the units as needed. Subjects were approached prior to initiation of prescribed heparin therapy. Informed consent was obtained as specified by the Institutional Review Board. Potential subjects were excluded if they had less than 25 millimeters of adiopose tissue at the injection site as measured by calipers. Based on normal limits at the data collection facility, anyone who had a pretreatment APTT greater than 34 seconds also was excluded from the study.

Nurses at the data collection facility administered all injections employing a technique congruent with the procedure manual at the facility. The skin was prepared by swabbing with an alcohol sponge. A roll of tissue was gently grasped between thumb and forefinger and heparin was injected at a 90 degree angle with a 25 gauge needle ⅝ inch long attached to the tuberculin syringe. Medication was injected without aspiration and the needle was withdrawn at the same angle as insertion. Gentle pressure with an alcohol sponge was applied to the site for less than 10 seconds, with no rubbing of site postinjection. Sodium heparin, 10,000 units: 1 milliliter solu-

tion was used to deliver the prescribed 5,000 units of heparin subcutaneously. The volume of heparin injectate delivered was 0.5 milliliters.

Three sites were used for subcutaneous injections of heparin. Subjects were assigned randomly to groups by use of a previously generated list of random numbers. Each subject received three injections in the specified site. Injection sites were selected using criteria from Sorensen and Luckmann (1986) Group A (Abdomen) injections were given into the adipose tissue of the lower abdomen or above the iliac crest; no injections were given within a two-inch diameter of the umbilicus due to the increased vascularity of this area. Group B (Thigh) injections were given into the adipose tissue above the vastus lateralis muscle or lateral thigh; no injections were given on the anterior thigh to avoid the possibility of accidental intramuscular injection. Group C (Arm) injections were given into the posterior adipose pad, one hand breadth above the elbow and below the axilla line, avoiding the area lateral to the deltoid muscle. A record was kept of all injection sites.

Results

Because cell sizes were not equal, the General Linear Model of ANOVA was used to analyze data. ANOVAS were calculated for each injection using the site as the value and injection as class.

APTT: All 101 subjects had pretreatment APTT measures of less than 34 seconds. The mean APTT level pretreatment was 24.65 seconds with a standard deviation of 3.18 seconds. The mean APTT level recorded four hours after the first injection was 25.71 seconds with a standard deviation of 3.61 seconds. There was a slight but statistically significant rise in APTT between pre- and postinjection measures at $p < 0.0001$. ANOVAS failed to show any statistically significant difference in rise of APTTs among the three sites of abdomen, thigh, and arm for Injections 1, 2, and 3. Hypothesis I was accepted.

Bruising: Subjects received a total of 299 injections. Data were missing on the bruising produced by the third injection for four subjects due to early discharge. Data from these subjects were included in the analysis for Injections 1 and 2 but treated as missing for Injection 3.

Of the 299 sites, 269 were bruised (89.97%) and 30 sites were not bruised (10.03%). There were no statistically significant differences among bruise occurrence of abdomen, thigh, and arm sites for any of the three injections. Table 1 shows the bruise occurrence by site and injection. Hypothesis II was accepted.

Size of bruise: Although the mean bruise sizes for the abdomen were smaller than the mean bruise sizes either for the thigh or the arm, the differences were not statistically significant, for Injections 1 and 2. Differences, however, were statistically significant ($p = 0.028$) for Injection 3. A post hoc analysis, The Duncan's Multiple Range test, was calculated for all three sites within each injection. Injections 1 and 2 showed no

statistically significant difference among mean surface area of bruises. The Duncan's Multiple Range test did show a significant difference in mean bruise surface area between the sites of abdomen and arm. Because Injection 3 bruises were measured 48 hours after injection and Injections 1 and 2 bruises were measured at 72 and 60 hours postinjection respectively, the question as to whether 48 hours was too soon to measure injection site bruise may be raised. Although the 48-hour time frame for measuring bruise size previously has been used in research (VanBree et al., 1984), Table 2 indicates that the abdominal bruises had not fully developed in size at 48 hours.

A repeated measure ANOVA was calculated to identify differences in bruise surface area of injection sites measured at 72, 60, and 48 hours, regardless of injection site. Again a statistically significant difference was noted for bruises at the three sites measured at 48-hours postinjection time frame. Table 3 provides the repeated measure ANOVA results. Hypothesis III was supported for bruise size measured at 60 and 72 hours.

Discussion

The rise in APTT between pre- and postinjection 1 was expected given the information on effectiveness of low-

Table 1   Bruise Count by Site for Each Injection

Bruise Present	Injection 1 ($N = 101$)			Injection 2 ($N = 101$)			Injection 3 ($N = 97$)		
	Abd	Thigh	Arm	Abd	Thigh	Arm	Abd	Thigh	Arm
No	05	03	04	05	02	01	05	03	02
Yes	28	30	31	28	31	34	27	28	32
TOTALS	33	31	35	33	33	35	32	31	34

dose heparin (Gallus et al., 1973). The acceptance of Hypothesis I indicates that the effectiveness of low-dose heparin therapy as measured by APTT is maintained whether the injection is administered in the abdomen, thigh, or arm.

There were no significant differences for occurrence of bruising among sites for any of the three injections. Eighty-nine percent (89%) of all 299 injection sites in this study did bruise. VanBree et al. (1984) reported a 55% bruising rate using a 10,000 units: 1 milliliter concentration, 0.5 ml volume, while Wooldridge and Jackson (1988) reported an 88% bruising rate using a 5,000 units: 1 milliliter concentration, 1.0 ml volume. In both of these studies, investigators administered all injections. One obvious difference in these studies was the concentration of dose and thus volume used to deliver the heparin. The present study used a 10,000: 1 milliliter concentration, 0.5 milliliters volume. Percentage of bruises produced, however, was similar to that reported by Wooldridge and Jackson (1988). The explanation may be

Table 2 Mean Surface Area (mm^2) and Standard Deviation by Injection and Site at Hour of Measurement Postinjection

	Injection 1 72 hours ($n = 101$)		Injection 2 60 hours ($n = 101$)		Injection 3 48 hours ($n = 97$)	
	M	*SD*	*M*	*SD*	*M*	*SD*
Abdomen	85.71	(295.57)	88.42	(368.94)	19.17	(44.94)
Thigh	95.15	(286.71)	200.20	(616.94)	118.69	(263.70)
Arm	219.39	(498.59)	151.69	(383.87)	176.07	(299.56)

Table 3 Repeated Measure ANOVA

Variable	ss	df	MS	F-Ratio	F-Value
SURFACE AREA (72 HOURS)					
Between subjects	386656.5	02	193382.3	1.37	.26
Within subjects	13870580.9	98	141536.5		
SURFACE AREA (60 HOURS)					
Between subjects	207055.5	02	103527.7	.47	.63
Within subjects	21532142.8	98	219715.7		
SURFACE AREA (48 HOURS)					
Between subjects	404498.0	02	202249.0	3.69	.03*
Within subjects	5038643.5	95	141536.5		

*$p > .05$

that staff nurses administered the injections in this study while the injections in the Wooldridge and Jackson study were given by the investigator.

In this study, staff nurses were used to give all injections not only because it was more cost-effective, but also because of the amount of variance in injection technique that occurs in practice. Because the hypotheses for this study proposed that there would be no difference among sites in bruise production and size of bruise as well as effectiveness of therapy, it was believed that using the standardized procedure administered by staff nurses in the clinical setting offered protection against artificially accepting the null hypotheses.

Forty-eight hours may be too soon to assess the full impact of bruise size produced by subcutaneous heparin injections. In future studies, examinations of bruise formation from subcutaneous heparin injections should use the 60- to 72-hour interval for measuring bruise size. Bruise size calculations that include surface area rather than diameter present a more accurate picture of the bruise: There are computer software packages available that will scan the surface area of a tracing to give a very precise measure. The cost of these programs was prohibitive for this study, but should be considered to increase accuracy of measurement.

In addition, the large standard deviation noted in Table 2 indicates a great deal of variability in bruise size. This occurred regardless of injection site and most likely was related to individual differences in bruisability. Future research should use a design that allows each subject to serve as their own control, thereby eliminating this source of variability. The use of only white patients in this study and in previous studies indicates a need for research in nonwhite subjects.

Further research is needed not only on patients' perceptions of bruises, but also on any discomfort they experience, whether physiologic or psychologic. The possible fear patients may have of injections in the abdomen, compared to the extremities, and the convenience to patients and nurses of using alternative sites should be studied. As with any clinical practice, patients' responses to subcutaneous heparin injections should be monitored regardless of the site of injection.

The alternate sites of arm and thigh, in addition to the abdomen, can be used safely for subcutaneous heparin injections. All three sites maintained effectiveness of the medication as measured by APTT. All three sites produced bruises, but when measured at 60 and 72 hours after injection, they were not statistically different.

REFERENCES

BRENNER, Z. R., WOOD, K. M., & GEORGE, D. (1981). Effects of alternative techniques of low-heparin administration on hematoma formation. *Heart & Lung 10*, 657-660.

CAPRINI, J. A., ZOELLNER, J. L., & WEISMAN, M. (1977). Heparin therapy-part II. *Cardio-Vascular Nursing, 13*(4), 17-20.

CHAMBERLAIN, S. L. (1980). Low dose heparin therapy. *American Journal of Nursing, 80*, 1115-1117.

COLEY, R. M., BUTLER, C. D., BECK, B. I., & MULLANE, J. P. (1987). Effect of needle size on pain and hematoma formation with subcutaneous injection of heparin sodium. *Clinical Pharmacy, 6*, 725-727.

GALLUS, A. S., HIRSH, J., TUTTLE, R. J., TREBILCOCK, R., O'BRIEN, S. E., CARROL, J. J.,

MINDEN, J. H., & HUDECKI, S.M. (1973). Small subcutaneous doses of heparin in prevention of venous thrombosis. *New England Journal of Medicine, 288,* 545-551.

HANSON, M. J. S. (1987). Hematoma associated with subcutaneous heparin administration. *Focus on Critical Care, 14*(6), 62-65.

HUBNER, C. (1986). Altered clotting. In V. K. Carrieri, A. M. Lindsey, & C. M. West (Eds.), *Pathophysiological phenomena in nursing* (pp. 367-389). Philadelphia: Saunders.

KIRCHHOFF, K. T. (1982). A diffusion survey of coronary precautions. *Nursing Research, 31,* 196-201.

LUNDIN, D. V. (1978). You can inject heparin subcutaneously. *RN, 41*(12), 51-54.

MITCHELL, G. S., & PAUSZEK, M. E. (1987). Effect of injectate volume on local hematoma formation during low-dose heparin therapy. *Critical Care Medicine, 15*(1), 87-88.

SCHUMANN, L. L., BRUYA, M.A., & HENKE, L. (1988). Administrative techniques for low-dose sodium heparin. *Dimensions of Critical Care Nursing, 3*(6), 333-339.

SORENSEN, K. C., & LUCKMANN, J. (1986). Administering parenteral medication. In *Basic Nursing* (2nd ed.) (pp. 1069-1098). Philadelphia: Saunders.

VANBREE, N. S., HOLLERBACH, A. D., & BROOKS, G. P. (1984). Clinical evaluation of three techniques for administering low-dose heparin. *Nursing Research, 33,* 15-19.

WOOLDRIDGE, J. B., & JACKSON, J. G.(1988). Evaluation of bruises and areas of induration after two techniques of subcutaneous heparin injection. *Heart & Lung, 17,* 476-482.

Accepted for publication January 5, 1991.

Research for this paper was supported by an Academic Research Enhancement Award from the National Center for Nursing Research, National Institutes of Health #1R15 NRO1880-01.

The authors acknowledge the assistance of Staci Covey, MSN, Kathy Bowen, MSN, and Terina Oman, MSN, Serdar Atav, PhD, Narayan Deshmukh, MD, Marguerite Kinney, RN, DNSc, and the nursing staff, laboratory personnel, administration, and physicians at Robert Packer Hospital, Gruthrie Medical Center, Sayre, PA. In addition we acknowledge Frances R. Brown, RN, PhD, Margaret Bruya, RN, DNSc, Karin T. Kirchhoff, RN, PhD, FAAN, Rick Madison, RN, MSN, CCRN, and Lorna L. Schumann, RN, PhD, CCRN, for their services as external reviewers.

Pamela Stewart Fahs, RN, MSN, is a DSN candidate at Decker School of Nursing, State University of New York, Binghampton, NY, and a lecturer at the University of Alabama at Birmingham.

Marguerite Kinney, RN, DNSc, FAAN, is a professor of nursing at the University of Alabama at Birmingham.

Appendix B

Coping and Adaptation in Children with Diabetes

Margaret Grey, Mary Emily Cameron, and Frances W. Thurber

The purpose of this study was to investigate the influence of age, coping behavior, and self-care on psychological, social, and physiologic adaptation in preadolescents and adolescents with diabetes. Children (N = 103) with insulin-dependent diabetes mellitus (IDDM) between 8 and 18 years of age and their parents participated in the study. Findings indicated that preadolescent children were significantly less depressed, less anxious, coped in more positive ways, had fewer adjustment problems, and were in better metabolic control than their adolescent counterparts. Age and secondary sexual development were related to psychosocial adaptation and metabolic control of the diabetes. Further, those who coped by avoiding their problems and who were more depressed were the most likely to have problems in both adjustment and metabolic control with 56% of the variance in metabolic control explained by the variables studied. These findings indicate that preadolescents and adolescents cope differently with a chronic illness, and that interventions should be designed to identify and help those with inappropriate coping styles.

How individuals cope with a long-term illness may be responsible for great variations in disease course and treatment responsiveness (Lazarus & Folkman, 1984; Moos, 1982). Coping skills develop and change as children mature (Garmezy & Rutter, 1983); thus, preadolescent children would be expected to respond differently to their illness than adolescents, and adolescents differently than adults. Preadolescent children tend to manage the self-care regimen of diabetes well, but rebellious feelings in adolescents may lead to neglect of self-monitoring, dietary recommendations, and insulin injections (Travis, Brouhard, & Schreiner, 1987). Thus, adolescents are at high risk for hospitalization and other problems. It is important to determine the factors associated with adaptation to illness in preadolescents and adolescents, because current approaches to the care of these children assume that the factors predicting adaptation are similar. If age and development influence adaptation to chronic illness, care should be varied appropriate to the age and developmental status of the individual.

The purpose of this study was to describe the adaptation of preadolescents and adolescents with insulin dependent diabetes mellitus (IDDM). It was proposed that adaptation would be influenced by age, coping behaviors, and self-care behaviors.

Review of the Literature

Adaptation is the degree to which an individual adjusts psychologically, socially, and physiologically to a long-term illness; it may include psychological and social functioning as well as alterations in health status (Pollock, 1986). Preadolescents and adolescents with diabetes may be at risk for problems with adapta-

Reprinted from *Nursing Research*, May/June 1991 Vol. 40, No. 3, pp. 144-149. Copyright *American Journal of Nursing* Company.

tion. Low self-esteem, social dependency, and poor ego development have been found to be more prevalent among children and adolescents with diabetes than among their healthy peers (Brown, 1985; Hauser et al., 1979; Sullivan, 1978). Further, both preadolescents and adolescents in poor metabolic control have been found to have more psychopathology (Swift, Seidman, & Stein, 1967), more dependency conflicts (Karlsson, Holmes, & Lang, 1988), and an increased likelihood of psychological disturbance (Burns, Green, & Chase, 1986) than either those in good control or a comparison group without diabetes. Preadolescents and adolescents who are in poorer metabolic control have significantly more anxiety and depression than either well-controlled patients or a non-diabetic control group (Olatawura, 1972; Sullivan, 1978). Kovacs and colleagues (1985) found that all newly diagnosed children with IDDM exhibited symptoms ranging from mild sadness, anxiety, a feeling of friendlessness, and social withdrawal to adjustment reactions with anxiety, depression, or mixed symptoms, and major depressive disorders.

Adaptation is a complex process involving internal and external factors (Pollock, 1984; Roy, 1976), such as the coping and self-care behaviors employed, that may influence psychological, social, and physiologic adaptation. Coping has been defined as "constantly changing cognitive and behavioral efforts to manage specific external and/or internal demands that are appraised as taxing or exceeding the resources of the person" (Johnson & Rosenbloom, 1982, p. 359). Diabetes creates increased self-care demands, and children with diabetes are expected to assume in-creasing responsibility for management of their disease (Travis, Brouhard, & Schreiner, 1987). Self-care of the diabetes may be a behavioral coping strategy. Appropriate skill in managing the necessary self-care regimen has been found to be associated with higher self-concept and better metabolic control (Saucier, 1984).

The child's ability to cope with a chronic illness may be affected by the way the family copes with the illness. McCubbin, McCubbin, Nevin, and Cauble (1979) reviewed the literature on family coping and found that family coping behaviors influence the child's developing coping skills. The extent of this influence, however, is not consistent across studies. Several researchers (Baker, Barcai, Kaye, & Hague, 1969; Burns, Green, & Chase, 1986; Grey, Tamborlane, & Genel, 1980) have concluded that the family has a profound effect on adaptation to diabetes. On the other hand, Hanson, Henggeler, Harris, Burghen, and Moore (1989) found that influence of the family was mediated by the duration of diabetes such that when duration was controlled, the influence of the family on metabolic control was substantially decreased.

While the presence of a chronic illness may not be sufficient to produce maladjustment, it may produce an at-risk state which increases vulnerability to the stressors of daily life (Green, 1968). Thus, the occurrence of stressful events may influence adaptation. Coddington (1972) demonstrated that there is a consistent increase in the number of stressful life events experienced as children increase in age. In patients with diabetes, stress scores have been shown to be positively correlated with blood glucose (Carter, Gonder-Frederick, Cox, Clarke, & Scott,

1985), triglyceride concentrations, Hemoglobin A1, and cholesterol (Chase & Jackson, 1981; Jacobson, Rand, & Hauser, 1983).

Little is known about the relative importance of these factors in preadolescents and adolescents with diabetes. Hanson (1983) studied 39 adolescents at a summer camp and found that perceived stressors and perceived ability to cope accounted for 11% of the variance in blood sugar above that accounted for by dietary intake, exercise levels, and insulin administration ($R^2 = .36$). In a study of stress, coping, and metabolic control in 32 adolescents, those teens in poor control were found to differ from their better controlled peers in that they used more wishful thinking, avoidance, and non-compliance with the diabetic regimen as ways of coping (Delameter, Kurtz, Bubb, White, & Santiago, 1987). Thus, coping and self-care behaviors may be associated with adaptation.

Age and developmental status may also affect the adaptation process. Stressful experiences (Coddington, 1972) and depression (Kovacs, 1985) are more prevalent in adolescents than in younger children. Further, adolescents have more problems with metabolic control and in psychological and social adaptation than do younger patients (Travis, Brouhard, & Schreiner, 1987). One potential reason for the increase in problems with metabolic control in adolescents is the hormonal storm of puberty. With the onset of puberty, increases in testosterone, estradiol, and androgen result in the development of secondary sex characteristics. These developmental changes follow the sequential pattern as described by Tanner (1962). The period of major hormonal change is in Tanner Stages 2 through 4. If the deterioration

in metabolic control and adaptation experienced by adolescents is a result of hormonal influence and not psychosocial development, preadolescence (Tanner 1) and maturity (Tanner 5) would be less likely to be associated with problems in control and adaptation. Burns and colleagues (1986) compared three small groups of children and adolescents with diabetes divided by age and found that parental and family factors had less importance in predicting hemoglobin A_1 in adolescents than in younger children, but they did not examine the influence of hormonal development. These authors also did not account for the length of time since diagnosis, which may also affect adaptation, since insulin reserves decrease with time (Travis, Brouhard, & Schreiner, 1987).

In summary, the literature supports the notion that multiple factors influence adaptation to a chronic illness such as diabetes during childhood and adolescence. The relative impact of these factors, however, cannot be determined by existing studies. Thus, the present study examined: the comparison of preadolescents and adolescents in adaptational factors by stage of sexual maturation; correlations of coping behaviors with adaptation; and, the relative influence of these factors on adaptation.

Method

Subjects: The sample was composed of 103 English-speaking patients between the ages of 8 and 18 from three diabetes treatment centers who assented and whose parents consented to their participation in the study and who met the following criteria: (a) had no other health problem than the IDDM; (b) in school grade appropriate to age within one year; and (c) managed with home blood glucose monitoring. Both metabolic and psychosocial data were collected during a routine clinic visit.

The children had a mean age of 12.9 (± 3.0) years and 52% were female; 62% of the sample was white, 10% black, and 28% Hispanic or Asian. Their families' socioeconomic status ranged from low to high, with the majority in the middle range ($20,000-$39,000).

Nearly all of the children were taking two injections of insulin per day, approximately evenly divided between Humulin[R] and pork/beef insulin. Clinical assessments of the level of metabolic control based on the history and physical examination ranged from poor to excellent, with the majority rated fair to good. Tanner stage of pubic hair development ranged from stage 1 to adult. Subjects had diabetes for an average of 5.3 years (range: 6 months to 16 years).

Instruments: All instruments were evaluated for reliability and results were consistent with previous reports. Social adaptation was determined with the Child and Adolescent Adjustment Profile (CAAP) and the Self-Perception Profile for Children (SPPC). The CAAP is a 20-item inventory which measures social role performance of children and adolescents in five areas (productivity, peer relations, dependency, hostility, and withdrawal) (Ellsworth & Ellsworth, 1981). Higher scores indicate poorer adaptation. Test-retest (.78-.89) and internal consistency (.78-.86) reliabilities are high for all subscales. The SPPC (Harter, 1985) is a 36-item scale consisting of six subscales tapping five specific domains of competence (scholastic competence, social acceptance, athletic competence, physical appearance, and behavioral conduct) and global self-

worth. Higher scores indicate higher perceived competence. The scale and its subscales have adequate internal consistency reliability (.71-.85).

Psychological adaptation was measured by the State-Trait Anxiety Inventory for Children (STAIC) and the Children's Depression Inventory (CDI). The STAIC is a self-report test for children between the ages of 8 and 19 which assesses state and trait anxiety (Speilberger, 1973). Each 20-item scale can yield a score from 20 to 60, with higher scores indicating higher anxiety. Internal consistency reliability ranges from .78-.85. The CDI (Kovacs, 1985) measures self-reported depressive symptoms in children and adolescents. It contains 27 multiple choice items that yield total scores from 0 to 54, with higher scores reflecting greater symptomatology. Kovacs established that the inventory has concurrent and discriminant validity, and the scale's internal consistency reliability is high at .71-.87. Physiologic adaptation was assessed by metabolic control as measured by glycosylated hemoglobin. Hemoglobin A_1 is routinely measured every three months as an overall assessment of metabolic control in all patients with diabetes mellitus (Daneman, Wolfson, Becker, & Drash, 1981; Travis, Brouhard, & Schreiner, 1987). Normal, nondiabetic individuals have less than 6.5% glycosylated hemoglobin (hgb A_1), whereas individuals with diabetes have higher levels. Those in good control can expect hgb A_1 levels to range from 8.5 to 12%, whereas those in poorer control will have levels over 12%. As is routine in the study settings, the test is performed by the microcolumn technique in the hospital laboratory on venous blood samples. Other factors which may influence metabolic control include the length of time since the diagnosis of diabetes and taking other medications (Travis, Brouhard, & Schreiner, 1987).

Coping, self-care, and recent stressors were measured with the Coping Orientation for Problem Experiences (A-COPE), the Coping Health Inventory for Parents (CHIP), the Self-Care Questionnaire (SCQ), and the Life Events Checklist (LEC), respectively. A-COPE is designed to identify behaviors children and adolescents find helpful in coping with problems or difficult situations (Patterson & McCubbin, 1983). The 54-item scale has 10 categories of coping behaviors, such as ventilating feelings and developing social support. Each behavior is rated as to how often it is used during a difficult time, with higher scores indicating more use of the behavior. The internal consistency for the scale is high at 0.90, and the scale reliabilities range from 0.67 to 0.78. The CHIP assesses parents' perceptions of their coping styles in response to having a chronically ill child or adolescent (McCubbin, McCubbin, Nevin, & Cauble, 1979). It is a 45-item self-report instrument with three factors (Family integration, maintaining social support, and understanding the health care situation through communication) replicable across samples. Cronbach's alpha has been acceptable at 0.75-0.87. The SCQ is a 15-item self-report inventory which measures self-care activities performed in managing diabetes (Saucier, 1984), such as insulin administration and blood glucose testing. Scores range from a low of 15 to a high of 60, and higher scores indicate higher compliance. Content validity was established by the author by having a panel of experts examine the scale. Coefficients of internal consistency have ranged from .63 to .85. The LEC

was developed by one of the authors (MG). Items from three child and adolescent life event scales (Coddington, 1972; Lewis, Seigel, & Lewis, 1984; Yamamoto, 1979) were evaluated for face and content validity by experts in pediatrics and stressful life events research. The 57 items which remained after this analysis were placed into a semi-structured interview format and pretested with healthy and chronically ill children and adolescents. Reliability of the scale as determined by Cronbach's alpha is .86. The two week test-retest correlation for the healthy sample was 0.84, whereas in the diabetic sample the correlation was 0.91. Six month test-retest reliability for the same events is $r = .63$ for the whole sample, and similar for children and adolescents. Concurrent validity assessments were made by comparing the responses to the items on the three instruments.

Demographic variables such as age, sex, and socioeconomic status were recorded, and sexual maturation was assessed with the Tanner stages. The five Tanner stages of sexual maturity are the standards for assessing and recording the development of secondary sexual maturation. These assessments are routinely made at each clinic visit, but if they were not available, self-reported Tanner staging was used. This method (Morris & Udry, 1980), in which the subject is shown pictures of the stages of adolescent development for pubic hair and the appropriate male or female genitalia and asked to report the correct stage of development for them, has been reported to have correlations of above .70 with physician ratings.

Analyses: Comparisons of preadolescents and adolescents in adaptation and coping were performed with analysis of variance. A model of hypothesized relationships was developed based on literature, and path analysis with the SPSS-PC statistical program was used to obtain the coefficient estimates of the predictors of adaptation. The t-test was used to test the significance of the estimated coefficient. Squared multiple correlations (R^2) indicate how well adaptation was predicted by the variables studied. If an interactive term was not significant, the term was dropped and analyses performed on the revised equation.

Results

Differences between preadolescent and adolescent children with IDDM are shown in Table 1, when the sample is divided by stage of secondary sexual development. Where subscales are not shown, no significant differences by stage of sexual development were found. Older adolescents, those in Tanner stage 5, reported significantly higher state anxiety and depression than younger children. Metabolic control worsened with increasing maturity. Younger children also reported significantly better peer relations than those in Tanner stage 2 through 4, and dependency was of concern for both the younger and the older subjects. Differences were found in self-perceived competence in behavior and school, with younger children, those in Tanner stage 1, scoring the highest. There were significant differences in the types of coping behaviors used. Ventilating feelings was more commonly used by children in Tanner stage 1, whereas avoidance behaviors (smoking, drinking, and staying away from home) and relaxation behaviors (daydreaming, listening to music, riding in a car) were used more often by those in Tanner stage 5. Parents of preadolescent children reported that family integration was more

Table 1   Differences in Adaptation and Coping by Stage of Sexual Maturation

Variable	Tanner 1 M(SD) (N = 34)	Tanner 2-4 M(SD) (N = 39)	Tanner 5 M(SD) (N = 25)	F-Value	p
State Anxiety	28.8(4.2)	30.8(4.4)	33.7(5.7)	6.10	.004
Depression	6.1(5.8)	6.2(5.6)	9.7(7.7)	5.71	.04
CAAP					
Peer relations	14.4(2.1)	13.4(2.7)	11.9(3.4)	5.95	.009
Dependency	9.4(2.2)	11.5(2.1)	10.8(2.5)	7.65	.001
SPPC					
School	19.6(4.4)	17.7(3.4)	15.9(4.2)	5.47	.006
Behavior	20.5(2.6)	18.6(3.5)	18.3(3.1)	4.15	.02
Hemoglobin A_1	9.8(2.9)	11.2(3.8)	13.9(4.4)	5.48	.007
A-COPE					
Avoid Problems	17.6(1.9)	18.0(2.6)	19.0(2.4)	3.96	.05
Vent. feeling	16.5(2.7)	13.4(3.4)	13.9(3.1)	8.11	.001
Relaxation	8.8(2.5)	9.8(2.4)	10.8(2.4)	4.64	.01
CHIP					
Fam. Integration	40.7(7.3)	41.3(7.6)	35.5(7.9)	3.75	.03
SCQ	40.0(6.5)	41.9(6.3)	43.1(5.9)	1.23	.29
LEC	8.1(6.4)	8.5(4.4)	7.7(3.9)	.15	.86

important and was used more often to cope than did the parents of pubescent and postpubescent children. No differences were found in the number of stressful events encountered in the most recent month or in self-care behaviors.

The relationships of specific coping behaviors measured on the A-COPE and adjustment, self-worth, and metabolic control were examined. Scores on the Self-Care Questionnaire and the parental coping scales were not associated with adjustment, self-worth, or metabolic control. Children who had higher scores on the CAAP and thus poorer adjustment were more likely to cope with behaviors of ventilating feelings (yelling, blaming others, and complaining; $r = .20$, $p < .05$) or avoiding problems by using substances as a way to escape ($r = .25$, $p < .01$). Higher self-perceived global self-worth was weakly associated with the use of humor ($r = .18$, $p < .05$), seeking spiritual support ($r = .16$, $p < .05$), and avoidance behaviors ($r = .18$, $p < .05$). Lower self-perceived competence was associated with the relaxation behaviors of daydreaming, listening to music, and riding in the car ($r = -.21$, $p < .01$). Poorer metabolic control as indicated by higher hgb A_1, was associated with several of the coping behaviors such as investing in close friends ($r = .25$, $p < .01$), avoidance behaviors ($r = .31$, $p < .01$), and daydreaming ($r = .23$, $p < .01$). Interestingly, better metabolic control was weakly associated with seeking professional support from a teacher, counselor, or health professional ($r = -.17$, $p < .05$) and with the use of humor by making light of the situation ($r = -.16$, $p < .05$). Correlations among the model variables and the demographic variables were computed using Pearson and point-biserial correlations (Table 2). To control for demographic variables, those having significant correlations with dependent variables were included in the analysis as dummy variables. Treatment center had the potential to be a confounding variable, and was also included in the analysis. The independent variables were examined for multicollinearity. Using Gordon's (1968) definition of multicollinearity of $r = .75$, age and Tanner stage were found to be highly intercorrelated ($r = .79$). Age alone was used in the remaining analyses because it is a continuous variable rather than ordinal as is Tanner stage.

The results of the path analyses are shown in Table 3. Coping is included as both predictor and dependent variable, as it was hypothesized to interact with age. The variance accounted for in hemoglobin A_1 was 56%, a substantial amount. Further, the model accounted for 28% of the variance in coping behaviors and 34% of the variance in adjustment. Family coping behaviors (CHIP), stressors, and self-perceived competence were removed because these paths were statistically significant.

The beta weights shown in Table 3 indicated: (a) Age has a significant association with adaptation and coping behaviors; (b) Age was associated with metabolic control through the mediation of coping behaviors as well as independently; (c) Both depression and anxiety were associated with coping behaviors and adaptation; and (d) Treatment center was significantly associated with metabolic control ($\beta = .64$, $p < .001$).

Discussion

Clearly, age and physical maturity have a significant impact on adaptation

Table 2   Variable Correlation Matrix N = 103

Variable	Age	Time	STAIC	CDI	LEC	SCQ	CHIP	COPE	CAAP	SPPC	M(SD)
Time since dx (Time)	.32										5.3(3.9)
State Anxiety (STAIC)	.40	.07									29.2(4.7)
Depression (CDI)	.15	−.10	.62								6.2(5.9)
Stressors (LEC)	−.01	.14	−.03	.14							8.2(5.2)
Self-Care (SCQ)	.06	−.17	−.11	−.07	.14						41.8(6.7)
Parent Coping (CHIP)	−.05	−.15	.14	−.25	−.29	.13					88.5(19.5)
Child Coping (COPE)	−.30	.06	.38	−.37	.19	.27	.20				171.0(25.9)
Adjustment (CAAP)	−.17	−.05	−.27	−.32	−.15	.12	.06	.10			67.4(14.1)
Self-Worth (SPPC)	−.15	.01	−.43	−.68	.11	.06	.07	.15	.38		19.8(3.4)
Hemoglobin A_1 (HgbA$_1$)	.43	.23	.34	.23	.12	.08	.04	.28	−.09	−.27	1.1(3.9)

Table 3   Standardized Regression Coefficients, t and R^2 Values for Coping and Adaptation

Endogenous Variable Predictor Variable	Beta (SE)	t-Value	p-Value
Coping[a]			
Age	.35 (.07)	2.36	.01
Anxiety	.39 (.10)	2.54	.01
Depression	.26 (.03)	1.68	.12
Adjustment[b]			
Age	.51 (.06)	2.67	.01
Self-Care	.41 (.03)	1.95	.06
Depression	.22 (.09)	1.25	.22
Diabetic control	.18 (.06)	1.14	.26
Age x self-care	.41 (.01)	1.95	.05
Diabetic Control[c]			
Treatment center	.64 (.19)	4.89	.001
Age	.41 (.17)	3.18	.002
Cope	.21 (.02)	1.74	.09
Depression	.24 (.08)	1.71	.09
Adjustment	.19 (.05)	1.40	.16
Age x cope	.41 (.03)	1.96	.05

[a]R^2 = .28; F = 2.43, p = .04; [b]R^2 = .34; F = 3.95, p = .0004; [c]R^2 = .56; F = 4.10, p = .01

to diabetes in childhood. Preadolescent and adolescent patients differ significantly in psychological, social, and physiologic adaptation. These data support some previous studies (Kovacs et al., 1985; Delameter et al., 1987) that anxiety and depression are common responses to diabetes and that both are more common in adolescent patients. As expected, metabolic control of the diabetes and psychosocial adjustment did worsen with increasing age, as noted by Travis and colleagues (1987). The lack of a comparison group precludes the conclusion that such problems in adaptation may be developmental rather than due to the illness. Such a conclusion awaits further study. The study does suggest, however, that approaches to management must be age-appropriate.

Little previous information was available on the coping behaviors of preadolescents and adolescents with diabetes. The findings of this study indicate that preadolescents and adolescents differ significantly in the manner in which they cope with the illness. Younger subjects in this study were more likely to cope by ventilating feelings through yelling, arguing, and the like, whereas older children were more likely to cope with avoidance behaviors of drinking, smoking, or staying away from home. These findings are supported by developmental theory, in that adolescents probably have more opportunity for avoidance behaviors than those who are younger. In addition, they further the understanding of diabetes management, because avoidance coping behaviors were significantly associated with poorer adaptation and metabolic control. These findings extend those of Delameter and colleagues (1987) who found in their small sample

of patients that wishful thinking and avoidance/help-seeking (avoiding being with people, getting away from it for a while) were more common ways of coping in those who were poorly controlled compared to those in good or fair control. These findings also support those of studies with adults (Felton & Revenson, 1984) that avoidant coping was associated with poorer health outcomes. It may be that those who are prone to avoidance as a method of coping are also more likely to be depressed, and that as these increase with age, the potential for difficulties in adaptation and metabolic control is exacerbated. An important extension of this study would be to follow children through the transition from preadolescence to adolescence to determine the process by which control deteriorates.

It was not expected that investing in close friends as a coping strategy would be associated with poorer metabolic control. Indeed, previous work in social support would suggest that supportive friends should be associated with better control (Burns, Green, & Chase, 1986). It is possible that this subscale of the A-COPE is a weak measure of social support, or that those children who invest in close friends use that investment as another avoidance mechanism. Thus, further work on the impact of both positive and negative social support is needed to determine the potential for influencing metabolic control in preadolescents and adolescents with diabetes.

Similarly, the finding that parental coping styles had no relationship to the children's coping or their adaptation is counterintuitive. Whether this finding is an artifact of measurement or valid for this population is not clear. It may be that since diabetes requires a large self-care commitment from the child, parental coping is less relevant than with other long-term illnesses in childhood. Alternatively, Hanson and colleagues (1989) found that the relationships between family variables and metabolic control were mediated by the duration of the illness, and the current study population had diabetes for a relatively long time.

The finding that neither self-care behaviors or intercurrent stressors were predictive of adaptation was also not expected. There are several plausible explanations for these results. First, in previous studies that examined these factors (Hanson, 1983; Jacobson, Rand, & Hauser, 1983; Saucier, 1984), either stressors or self-care were single independent variables. It may be that self-care behavior is simply another in the general coping pattern of the individual when faced with stressful situations, and thus, when both are studied, self-care is less important. This notion is supported by the work of Delameter and colleagues (1987). Second, although psychometric evaluation of both instruments demonstrated reasonable results, it may be that both suffer from problems with social desirability response sets.

The study has clear implications for practice with preadolescents and adolescents with diabetes. First, models of care, which address the developmental differences in response to the illness, must be developed and tested. Second, because those who cope by using avoidance behaviors are at greatest risk for both psychosocial and metabolic problems, children should be screened soon after diagnosis to describe their coping strategies, and preventive interventions

begun early, prior to the development of problems with adaptation.

REFERENCES

BAKER, L., BARCAI, A., KAYE, R., & HAGUE, N. (1969). Beta adrenergic blockage and juvenile diabetes: Acute studies and long-term therapeutic trial. *Journal of Pediatrics, 75,* 19-29.

BROWN, A. J. (1985). School-age children with diabetes: Knowledge and management of the disease, and adequacy of self-concept. *Maternal-Child Nursing Journal, 4*(1), 47-61.

BURNS, K. L., GREEN, P., & CHASE, H. P. (1986). Psychosocial correlates of glycemic control as a function of age in youth with insulin dependent diabetes mellitus. *Journal of Adolescent Health Care, 7,* 311-319.

CARTER, W. R., GONDER-FREDERICK, L. A., COX, D. J., CLARKE, W. L., & SCOTT, D. (1985). Effect of stress on blood glucose in IDDM. *Diabetes Care, 8,* 411-412.

CHASE, H. P., & JACKSON, G. G. (1981). Stress and sugar control in children with insulin dependent diabetes. *Journal of Pediatrics, 98,* 1011-1013.

CODDINGTON, R. D. (1972). The significance of life events as etiologic factors in the diseases of children. II. A study of a normal population. *Journal of Psychosomatic Research, 16,* 205-213.

DANEMAN, D., WOLFSON, D. H., BECKER, D. J., & DRASH, A. L. (1981). Factors affecting glycosylated hemoglobin values in children with insulin-dependent diabetes. *Journal of Pediatrics, 99,* 847-853.

DELAMETER, A. M., KURTZ, S. M., BUBB, J., WHITE, N. H., & SANTIAGO, J. V. (1987). Stress and coping in relation to metabolic control in adolescents with Type 1 diabetes. *Developmental and Behavioral Pediatrics, 8,* 136-140.

ELLSWORTH, R., & ELLSWORTH, S. (1981). *CAAP scale: The measurement of child and adolescent adjustment.* Palo Alto, CA: Consulting Psychologists Press.

FELTON, B., & REVENSON, T. (1984). Coping with chronic illness: A study of illness controlability and the influence of coping strategies on psychological adjustment. *Journal of Consulting and Clinical Psychology, 52,* 343-353.

GARMEZY, N. & RUTTER, M. (1983). *Stress, coping, and development in children.* New York: McGraw-Hill.

GORDON, R. A. (1968). Issues in multiple regression. *American Journal of Sociology, 73,* 592-616.

GREEN, M. (1968). The management of long-term non-life threatening illnesses. In M. Green & R. S. Haggerty (Eds.), *Ambulatory pediatrics* (pp. 443-451). Philadelphia: W. B. Saunders.

GREY, M., TAMBORLANE, W. V., & GENEL, M. (1980). Psychosocial adjustment of latency-aged diabetics: Determinants and relationship to control. *Pediatrics, 65,* 69-73.

HANSON, S. (1983). Perceived stress, coping ability, and diabetes control. *Diabetes, 32* (suppl. 1), 5A.

HANSON, C. L., HENGGELER, S. W., HARRIS, M. A., BURGHEN, G. A., & MOORE, M. (1989). Family system variables and the health status of adolescents with insulin-dependent diabetes mellitus. *Health Psychology, 8,* 239-253.

HARTER, S. (1985). *Manual for the self-perception profile for children.* Denver: University of Denver.

HAUSER, S. T., POLLETS, D., TURNER, B., JACOBSON, A., POWERS, S., & NOAM, G. (1979). Ego development and self-esteem in diabetic adolescents. *Diabetes Care, 2,* 465-471.

JACOBSON, A. M., RAND, L., & HAUSER, S. T. (1983). Psychosocial stress and metabolic control in diabetes. *Diabetes, 32* (Suppl. 1), 5A.

JOHNSON, S. B., & ROSENBLOOM, A. L. (1982). Behavioral aspects of diabetes mellitus in childhood and adolescence. *Psychiatric Clinics of North America, 5,* 357-369.

KARLSSON, J. A., HOLMES, C.S., & LANG, R. (1988). Psychosocial aspects of disease duration and control in young adults with type I diabetes. *Journal of Clinical Epidemiology, 41,* 435-440.

KOVACS, M. (1985). The children's depression inventory (CDI). *Psychopharmacology Bulletin, 21,* 995-998.

KOVACS, M., FEINBERG, T. L., PAULAUSKAS, S., FINKELSTEIN, R., POLLACK, M., & CROUSE-NOVAK, M. (1985). Initial coping responses and psychosocial characteristics of children with insulin-dependent diabetes mellitus. *Journal of Pediatrics, 106,* 827-834.

LAZARUS, R. S., & FOLKMAN, S. (1984). Coping and adaptation. In W. D. Gentry (Ed.), *The handbook of behavioral medicine* (pp. 282-325). New York: Guilford.

LEWIS, C. E., SIEGEL, J. M., & LEWIS, M. A. (1984). Feeling bad: Exploring sources of distress among pre-adolescent children, *American Journal of Public Health, 74,* 117-122.

McCUBBIN, H., McCUBBIN, M., NEVIN, R., & CAUBLE, A. E. (1979). Coping health inventory for parents (CHIP). In H. McCubbin & A. Thompson (Eds.), *Family assessment for research and practice* (pp. 171-192). Madison, WI: University of Wisconsin.

MOOS, R. (1982). Coping with acute health crisis. In T. Millon, C. Green, & R. Meager (Eds.), *Handbook of clinical health psychology* (pp. 129-151). New York: Plenum.

MORRIS, N. M. & UDRY, J. R. (1980). Validation of a self-administered instrument to assess stage of adolescent development, *Journal of Youth and Adolescence, 9,* 271-280.

OLATAWURA, M. O. (1972). The psychiatric complications of diabetes mellitus in children. *African Journal of Medical Science, 3,* 231-240.

PATTERSON, J., & McCUBBIN, H. (1983). *Coping orientation for problem experiences (Research instrument).* Madison, WI: University of Wisconsin.

POLLOCK, S.E. (1984). The stress response. *Critical Care Quarterly, 6,* 1-14.

POLLOCK, S. E. (1986). Human responses to

chronic illness: Physiologic and psychological adaptation. *Nursing Research, 35,* 90-95.

Roy, C. (1976). *Introduction to nursing: An adaptation model.* Englewood Cliffs, NJ: Prentice Hall.

Saucier, C. P. (1984). Self-concept and self-care management in school-age children with diabetes. *Pediatric Nursing, 10,* 135-138.

Speilberger, C. D. (1973). *Manual for the state-trait anxiety inventory for children.* Palo Alto, CA: Consulting Psychologists Press.

Sullivan, B. J. (1978). Self-esteem and depression in adolescent diabetic girls. *Diabetes Care, 1,* 18-22.

Swift, C. R., Seidman, F. L., & Stein, H. (1967). Adjustment problems in juvenile diabetes. *Psychosomatic Medicine, 29,* 555-571.

Tanner, J. M. (1962). *Growth at adolescence* (2nd ed.). Oxford, UK: Blackwell Scientific.

Travis, L. B., Brouhard, B. H., & Schreiner, B. J. (1987). *Diabetes mellitus in children and adolescents.* Philadelphia: W. B. Saunders.

Yamamoto, K. (1979). Children's ratings of the stressfulness of experiences. *Developmental Psychology, 15,* 581-582.

Accepted for publication December 10, 1990.

This study was partially supported by a grant from the University Research Foundation, University of Pennsylvania. It was presented in part at the Annual Meetings of the National Association of Pediatric Nurse Associates and Practitioners, San Francisco and the American Diabetes Association.

The authors acknowledge John Nicholson, MD, Lester Baker, MD, Kathryn Murphy, PhD, RN, Iraj Resvani, MD, and Terri Lipman, MSN, RN who facilitated access to the children.

Margaret Grey, DrPH, FAAN, is assistant professor, University of Pennsylvania, School of Nursing, Philadelphia, PA.

Mary Emily Cameron, MS, RN, is a doctoral candidate, University of Pennsylvania, School of Nursing, Philadelphia, PA.

Frances W. Thurber, PhD, RN, is assistant professor, University of Pennsylvania, School of Nursing, Philadelphia, PA.

Appendix C

Types and Meanings of Caring Behaviors Among Elderly Nursing Home Residents

Cynthia Poznanski Hutchison and
Sr. Rose Therese Bahr

This grounded theory study explored and described the types and meanings of caring behaviors engaged in by elderly nursing home residents. Data were derived from observation of participants and in-depth interviews with residents in one nursing home during a three-month period. One of two substantive theories—a categorical model of the various types of caring behaviors residents engaged in—is discussed. Engagement in caring behaviors was found to be a universally important means for residents to maintain their esteem, self-identity and continuation of personhood. The properties of caring which emerged included protecting, supporting, confirming and transcending.

Research in gerontology has accentuated the elderly's needs and demands on society rather than their social contributions outside the labor market (Kahn, 1983). Aged persons, especially nursing home residents, often are looked upon by younger individuals as a burden to society because they consume national resources but no longer contribute productively in the workplace (Kahn, 1983).

Besides the societal perception that nursing home residents (hereafter referred to as residents) have few or no skills to contribute to society, research has demonstrated that institutionalization has negative effects on the well-being of many residents. These include (but are not limited to): dependency reinforced by staff (Barton, Baltes, & Orzech, 1980; Lester & Baltes, 1978), helping behaviors among residents discouraged by staff (Noelker & Poulshock, 1984), increases in negative self-perceptions as length of stay increases (Koger, 1980) and loss of identity as length of stay increases (Kahana & Coe, 1979).

"Rolelessness" has been postulated by Rosow (1967) to be responsible for much of the deterioration, such as apa-

Cynthia Poznanski Hutchison, R.N., D.N.Sc., *Kappa* is a full-time mother and part-time consultant in Silver Spring, Maryland.
Sr. Rose Therese Bahr, R.N., Ph.D., *Kappa*, is Professor, Catholic University of America School of Nursing. Dr. Hutchison thanks her dissertation committee: Sr. Rose Therese Bahr, R.N., Ph.D., chair; Vickie Lambert, R.N., Ph.D.; Jean Toth, R.N., D.N.Sc.; and Christopher Hayes, Ph.D. Correspondence to 12820 Holdridge Road, Silver Spring, MD 20906.

Accepted for publication October 7, 1990

Reprinted from *Image: Journal of Nursing Scholarship,* Summer, 1991, Vol. 23, No. 2, pp. 85-88. Copyright *Sigma Theta Tau International,* Inc.

thy, withdrawal, isolation, loss of motivation, disorientation, depression and regression experienced by the elderly. Barns, Sack, and Shore (1973) described a "spiral of senility" which occurs in residents when others have few or no positive expectations of them.

In contrast, other studies indicate that a moderate (but unstated) percentage of residents seek opportunities to reach out to others and give of themselves in a productive way relative to their capabilities, in spite of the number and severity of losses they have had (Bininger & Kiesel, 1978; Laufer & Laufer, 1982; National Citizens Coalition for Nursing Home Reform [NCCNHR] 1981, 1985; Shore, 1972; Springer & Saylor, 1984). These types of behaviors, identified in this study as caring behaviors, are socially significant and are considered crucial to human development, human relatedness, self-actualization, health and survival across world cultures (Leininger, 1984).

Throughout the review of literature, no studies or reports were found that comprehensively focused on ways residents are socially productive through caring acts, or what it means personally to a resident to engage in caring kinds of behaviors. The purpose of this study was to explore and describe the specific types of caring behaviors engaged in by residents and the personal meaning of their involvement in these acts.

METHOD

The grounded theory method (Glaser & Strauss, 1967) was used to collect and analyze data in this exploratory and descriptive study. Data were gathered through interviews and observations in a nursing home. The purpose was to enter the world of the residents and to understand their view of caring. The grounded theory method of constant comparative analysis was used to identify patterns, develop categories and descriptions, and to create theoretical links with the goal of developing substantive theory on caring among residents. This method emphasizes concurrent data collection; coding; analysis; and allows for constant examination of conceptual interactions and linkages, and the conditions under which they occur.

Sample and Subjects

A 117-bed, non-profit, religiously-affiliated, long-term health care facility for the elderly in Washington, D.C. was the site for the study. It included a 17-bed independent living unit. Only elderly persons who are financially needy can be admitted. Nursing home residents who met the following criteria were included in the sample:

1. Age of 62 years or older.
2. Cognitively intact.
3. No severe hearing or speech impairment.
4. An expectation to live in the nursing home indefinitely.
5. A length of stay of at least two months.

No limitations were placed on the selection of the sample in regards to sex, marital status, ethnic background, race, religious affiliation, functional abilities or visual impairments. Theoretical sampling guided the researcher to study residents with a variety of demographic characteristics.

The guided interview included: the definition of caring and uncaring; types of caring behaviors residents stated they engaged in; reasons for performing them; relative personal importance of engaging in caring acts; perceptions of nursing home staff attitudes regarding residents' engaging in caring; perception of changes in their caring behaviors over time; the role of reciprocation, and other related questions. A pilot study at another non-religious nursing home, where nine residents were interviewed and many others observed, supported the topic, the methodology, and the questions on the interview guide. Because the grounded theory method instructs the researcher to continue data collection until saturation of data occurs, no predetermined number of resident interviews or observations were planned. Categories became saturated after the 20th subject was interviewed and after hundreds of informal and/or participatory observations.

Data Collection

Each formal interview was tape-recorded and transcribed verbatim. Verbal consent of participation was also recorded. The interviews became part of the observational notes along with any other significant observational data from the interviews which were non-verbal, such as facial expressions or actions. Other observational notes were written based on the numerous observations of most of the residents who lived at the nursing home but were not formally interviewed, or observations of interviewed residents at times other than the interview.

Theoretical notes also were written. They reflected the investigator's attempt to derive meaning from the observational notes which could bear on the conceptual aspects of the study. Methodological notes were written to critique the interview, observational methods and to make future modifications. Data collection took place over three months.

FINDINGS

Two substantive grounded theories emerged from the study. The first was a categorical model, (a typology or taxonomy) which lays out the various types of caring behaviors found among residents. The second theory is a process-oriented interactive model of the meaning of caring behaviors as expressed by the residents. The process model builds onto the categorical model by giving meaning to the numerous types of caring behaviors found among the residents. Only the categorical model is discussed here.

Properties of Caring

Four major properties of caring emerged. They were protecting, supporting, confirming and transcending.

Protecting

The definition of protecting as a caring behavior emerged from the data as a means of preserving the safety of or shielding another from injury through verbalizing concern, orienting, surveillance, eliciting help from others or providing physical support. The majority of these behaviors (reported or observed) were directed toward fellow residents. Others were directed toward visitors, staff or the investigator. For example, the protective behavior described as **orienting** included directing persons on

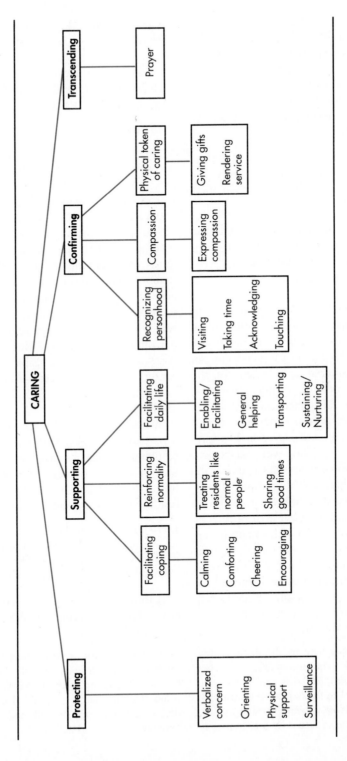

Fig. C-1   Categorical model of types of caring behaviors among nursing home residents.

how to find a specific place in the nursing home, as well as residents' own lay version of reality orientation for fellow residents who were confused and needed to be oriented to person, place, time or situation. Another protective behavior was termed **surveillance.** As described by one resident:

If someone refuses my help for walking, when they say 'No, thank you,' then I'm right in the back watching what she's doing so she doesn't fall.

This resident then said she would call for help if the resident she was concerned about "gets in trouble."

Supporting

Many ways were found that demonstrated caring behaviors through some type of support to another in need. The act of supporting as a caring concept can also be considered an element of the other properties of caring. However, three groups of conceptual categories emerged specifically as supportive acts of caring, each representing several specific caring behaviors. They were facilitating coping, reinforcing normality and facilitating daily life. The definition of supporting emerged as follows: to assist an individual in meeting her or his needs by reinforcing a 'normal' self-image in another; facilitating another's coping; facilitating another's daily life tasks through physical, emotional, mental, or other means. An example of *comforting* as a supportive way to facilitate coping was given by Mrs. B.:

There's a woman here by the name of Ida. She walks and walks and walks. . . . Then she'll start crying and I'll say 'What's the matter, Ida?'. 'I'm looking for my husband.' I say 'Listen Honey, your husband, he's in heaven. He went to heaven a long time ago.'

She said 'He did? Nobody told me.' I said 'Well, don't you cry. He's in heaven.'

Mrs. B. then said that she would stay with Ida and talk with her and hold her hand until she felt better.

Confirming

One of the most common and observable ways residents showed caring was through behaviors that expressed a way of confirming another as a respected and cared about fellow being. The definition of confirming as a caring act emerged from the data as: a way to validate the personhood of another in a manner that demonstrates care, respect, empathy or compassion, or through such actions as gift-giving, sharing or rendering service. Recognizing another's personhood, communicating love or compassion as well as visible tokens of caring were the conceptual categories that emerged as types of confirming caring behaviors.

A common example was visiting fellow residents, especially those who were confined to their rooms. For example, a woman severely debilitated with arthritis told the investigator how another resident's visits signified caring to her:

Every now and then she'll come around and see me and she'll bring me a sandwich or something, something good. She tells me, 'I went to the shop and thought of you.'

Another resident gave an example of how taking time represented a confirming caring act:

Down the corridor, a little colored woman, she likes to talk and talk and talk. People ask me how I put up with it. They say they couldn't stand that. . . . I said 'I know, but she wants somebody to talk to.' It won't hurt me. I'm a good listener.

Another example of confirming was rendering service. Several residents made religious articles for African missions or helped prepare meals in the home's kitchen.

Like the majority of caring behaviors found among the resident group, confirming behaviors usually did not require physical skills, strength or stamina. There were, however, caring acts such as some of the service activities (physical tokens of caring) which were largely physical. These included food preparation, folding laundry, sweeping the sidewalk, transporting a fellow resident in a wheelchair and running errands for fellow residents within the nursing home.

Transcending

Transcending caring was reflected in the almost universal response that residents prayed for others. Prayer was conceptualized as a transcending property of caring because it exceeded the limits of human caring interventions by seeking divine intervention for the benefit of others. The definition of the transcending property of caring emerged as the seeking of divine intervention for the benefit of others who are perceived as having needs that the person seeking intervention cannot supply due to his or her human limitations or human nature.

Like other forms of caring, prayer was made in various ways that were observable (religious services at the nursing home, grace before meals), reportable, as well as more personal, private and undefinable ways. Residents prayed for themselves, fellow residents, staff, family, friends, various groups and causes outside the nursing home and throughout the world.

Prayers were offered not only for people whom residents loved or were fond of, but also for those who were perceived as "mean," "uncaring," "insensitive" or "ignorant." As stated by one resident:

I pray daily for others, even those who are unkind to me so they could be more understanding and accepting. Jesus taught us to love those that hurt us and to pray for all.

Prayer was a universal way of caring among the residents except for one man who stated that he was agnostic. His lack of conviction in God, however, did not make him different from other residents in relation to engagement in caring behaviors.

DISCUSSION AND RECOMMENDATIONS

Caring emerged as a major way in which residents maintained their personal identity, sense of value and continuation of personhood. Based on the importance that residents in this study placed on self-engagement in caring acts, being able to act on one's caring feelings and desires can be seen as a quality of life issue for residents. That the study took place within a nursing home practicing the Judeo-Christian tradition is a limitation.

The categorical model has served to validate properties of caring previously discovered by other investigators (Aamodt, 1981; Gardner & Wheeler, 1981; Leininger, 1981, 1985; Rempusheski, 1985; Rempusheski & Phillips, 1985; Wenger, 1985). The similarities between the caring concepts in this study and previous studies support the refinement of the definition and description of caring as well as its universality among various groups and culture.

Although the categorical model requires further validation in the nursing home setting, it can be used by personnel and policy makers in several ways. It is an example of the numerous ways residents, despite disabilities, can continue to engage in meaningful social acts. Such a model points out capabilities that most residents have in the area of caring abilities. Admission and on-going assessments of residents could include an evaluation of how residents could or do function in a socially productive manner, in addition to the typical focus on problems, pathology and losses. By becoming more aware that interested residents can help themselves and benefit others through their caring, staff might be more likely to view them as both givers and receivers of care, which is a more accurate and socially equal position.

The findings also build on the extant theory of human needs as discussed by Maslow (1970). Caring, as an element of the higher level needs of love and belonging, self-esteem and self-actualization, was found to fit within Maslow's theoretical framework. Residents' statements about how important caring was to them supported Maslow's theory that higher level needs may become independent of their powerful prerequisites, physiological and safety needs. In this case, being caring toward others was important enough to residents that it kept them from focusing only on their pain, losses, and functional disabilities.

The total person needs to be understood when nurses and others work with residents. This study brought out the importance of the physical, mental, social and spiritual self as they relate to caring behaviors. Caring was demonstrated to be an important factor in the lives of the residents who were part of this study. How residents engaged in caring affected their personal identity. The results lead to speculation about the degree non-engagement in caring may be associated with the deterioration or "spirial of senility" often associated with people who reside in nursing homes (Barns, et al., 1972).

The study also has significance to nursing in general. Leininger (1981) said caring is the essence of nursing and Diers (1986) stated ". . . above all, nursing is caring" (p. 27). Although nursing research has focused on the concept of care recently, nursing as a discipline has yet to define what caring in nursing is to society. This study offers a beginning explanation of the meaning of the concept of care as related to a specific client group that engages in caring behaviors. But the questions remain. How is the care of a professional nurse different from 'generic care' that is engaged in by a lay person? What are the unifying properties of caring between nursing and other groups? The current findings as well as others are a source to compare lay care to nursing care, and it can be used as a base upon which to develop further studies to defining the concepts of care/caring.

FURTHER RESEARCH

The models proposed in this study require further validation and expansion in various nursing home settings. In addition, other specific questions are raised for future studies:

1. In what ways and to what extent does a nursing home milieu (philosophy, religious versus non-religious affiliation, quality and number of staff, privacy factors) affect caring behaviors among residents?

2. What variables can nursing home administrators influence to foster a caring environment?

3. How is depression related to engagement or lack of engagement in caring behaviors in residents?

4. Are self-esteem/self-concept levels higher in residents who perceive themselves as caring individuals?

5. What is the relationship between the caring behaviors residents engage in and the extent to care they perceive they receive from others?

6. How do mentally impaired residents express caring and what role does caring play in their lives?

REFERENCES

Aamodt, A.M. (1981). Neighboring: Discovering support systems among Norwegian-American women. In D. Messerschmidt (Ed.). *Anthropologists at home in North America: Methods and issues in the study of one's own society* (pp. 133-152). New York: Cambridge University.

Barns, E., Sack, A., & Shore, H. (1973). Guidelines to treatment approaches: Modalities and methods for use with the aged. *The Gerontologist,* Winter, 513-527.

Barton, E.M., Baltes, M.M., & Orzech, M.J. (1980). Etiology of dependence in older nursing home residents during morning care: The role of staff behavior. *Journal of Personality and Social Psychology, 38,* 423-431.

Bininger, C. & Kiesel, M. (1978). Assessment of perceived role losses in the gerian. *Journal of Gerontological Nursing, 4, 5,* 24-27.

Diers, D. (1986). To profess—To be a professional. *Journal of Nursing Administration, 16,* 25-30.

Gardner, K. & Wheeler, E.C. (1981). Nurses' perception of the meaning of support in nursing. *Issues in Mental Health Nursing, 3,* 13-28.

Glaser, B.G. (1978). *Theoretical sensitivity,* Mill Valley, CA: The Sociology Press.

Glaser, B.G., & Strauss A. (1967). *The discovery of grounded theory.* Chicago: Aldine.

Kahana, E. & Coe, R. (1969). Self and staff conceptions of institutionalized aged. *Gerontologist, 9,* 264-267.

Kahn R. (1983). Productive behaviors: Assessment, determinants, and effects. *Journal of the American Geriatrics Society, 31,* 11, 750-757.

Koger, L.J. (1980). Nursing home life satisfaction and activity participation. *Research on Aging, 2,* 61-72.

Laufer, E.A. & Laufer, W.S. (1982). From geriatric resident to language profesor: A new program using the talents of the elderly in a skilled nursing facility. *The Gerontologist, 22,* 548-550.

Leininger, M. (1981). The phenomena of caring: Importance, research questions, and theoretical considerations. In M. Leininger (Ed.), *Caring: An essential human need, Proceedings of Three National Caring Conferences* (pp. 5-20). Thorofare, N.J.: Charles B. Slack, Inc.

Leininger, M. (1984). *Care: The essence of nursing and health.* Thorofare, N.J.: Charles B. Slack, Inc.

Leininger, M., Editor (1985). *Qualitative research methods in nursing,* New York: Grune & Stratton.

Lester, P.B. & Baltes, M.M. (1978). Functional interdependence of the social behavior of the institutionalized aged. *Journal of Gerontological Nursing, 4,* 23-26.

Maslow, A. (1970). *Motivation and personality* (2nd Ed.). New York: Harper & Row.

National Citizens' Coalition for Nursing Home Reform (1981). *Nursing home projects for Area Agencies on Aging.* Washington, DC: NCCNHR.

National Citizens' Coalition for Nursing Home Reform (1985). *A consumer perspective on quality care: The residents' point of view.* Washington, DC: NCCNHR.

Noelker, L.S. & Poulshock, S.W. (1984). Intimacy: Factors affecting its development among members of a home for the aged.

International Journal of Aging and Development, 19, 177-190.

Peck, R. (1968). Psychological developments in the second half of life. In B.I. Neugarten (ed.). *Middle age and aging: a reader in social psychology.* 88-92 Chicago: University of Chicago Press.

Rempusheski, V. (1985). *Exploration and description of caring for self and others with second generation Polish American elders.* Unpublished doctoral dissertation, University of Arizona, Tucson.

Rempusheski, V. & Phillips, L. (1985). Care: A description by caregivers of home-based elders. Presented at the National Symposium of Nursing Research, San Francisco, CA, November 14, 1985.

Rosow, I. (1967). *Socialization to old age.* Berkeley: University of California Press.

Shore, H. (1972). *Adventures in group living.* Dallas, Golden Acres: The Dallas Home for the Jewish Aged.

Springer, F. & Saylor, H. (1984). People need to give as well as to receive. *American Health Care Association Journal, 10,* 8-11.

Wenger, A.F.Z. (1985). Learning to do a mini-ethnonursing research study: A doctoral student's experience. In M.M. Leininger (Ed.), *Qualitative research methods in nursing.* Pp. 283-316. New York: Grune & Stratton.

Index